Psychosocial Nursing

THIRD EDITION

Psychosocial Nursing

THEORY AND PRACTICE IN HOSPITAL AND COMMUNITY MENTAL HEALTH

Frances Monet Carter, R.N., Ed.D.

Professor, School of Nursing / University of San Francisco

MACMILLAN PUBLISHING CO., INC.

New York

Collier Macmillan Publishers

London

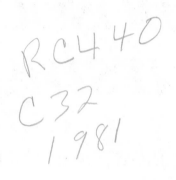

Macmillan Publishing Co., Inc.
866 Third Avenue, New York, New York 10022

Collier Macmillan Canada, Ltd.

Library of Congress Cataloging in Publication Data

Carter, Frances Monet.
  Psychosocial nursing.

  Includes bibliographies and index.
  1. Psychiatric nursing. I. Title. [DNLM:
1. Community mental health services. 2. Psychiatric nursing. WY160 C323p]
RC440.C32   1981   610.73′68   80–15311
ISBN 0–02–319660–2

Printing: 1 2 3 4 5 6 7 8   Year: 1 2 3 4 5 6 7 8

In loving memory of
my brother James

Preface

The focus of this book is upon psychosocial concepts of behavior as they apply to the nursing care of patients. This book concentrates on some of the major problems seen in nursing practice. Written from an eclectic theoretical base, it contains psychoanalytic and psychosocial theories, emphasizing intrapsychic, developmental, and sociocultural points of view. It contains values of Western humanism—that the helping professions do what they can to prevent human pain and suffering and that, when people come to, or are brought by others, to the helping professions when they can no longer manage on their own the professions are committed to helping them.

This edition retains the original organization. New chapters on psychotherapy, group psychotherapy, and somatic approaches to treatment make explicit major therapeutic modalities for psychiatric patients. A chapter on psychogeriatrics has been added. Original chapters and bibliographies have been updated. Some of the new topics added to this edition are: catastrophic stress, anticipatory grief, hospice, urban transients, alternatives to hospitalization, psychodrama, and the Problem-Oriented Medical Record. Deinstitutionalization and its consequences, as well as other topics, have been expanded upon. The appendix contains new material.

This book has been written for nursing students and is designed to provide some of the basic psychosocial concepts necessary for the practice of psychiatric nursing.

Acknowledgments

The understanding and significance of development throughout the life span, of personality structure, defense mechanisms, dynamics, and symptoms have better equipped us to aid in the relief of pain and suffering of persons experiencing stress and mental disorder. Without these understandings, the therapeutic approaches in this book could not have been written.

I wish to express appreciation to my patients, students, teachers, and mentors for their assistance in helping me to better understand the human condition.

I am also indebted to Annie Laurie Crawford, Esther A. Garrison, and Marion E. Kalkman and others not mentioned here for sharing with me their insights into history.

Appreciation is hereby expressed to the staff of the Macmillan Publishing Co., Inc. for their thoughtful, responsive expertise.

Thanks are also due to Glenna M. Richards, Sharron Godbois, and Gloria Stracke for their help in typing the manuscript. To those authors whose works are quoted in this book, I am especially thankful.

Frances Monet Carter

Contents

List of Tables

List of Figures

1

Human Development and Crisis Points

LEARNING OBJECTIVES / Persons studying this chapter should be able to:

1. Describe Freud's topographical, structural, and psychosexual theories.
2. Describe the life cycle point of view of growth and development of the person in each phase of life (i.e., infancy and early childhood, middle childhood, adolescence, early adulthood, middle age, and older age), according to Havighurst, Erikson, Piaget, and Kohlberg.
3. Describe crisis theory in terms of developmental crises (expected) and unexpected crises.
   - Name four characteristics of a crisis.
   - Name four phases of a crisis.
   - Describe the role of the nurse.
4. Relate theories of growth and development to one's own life and health.
5. In nursing practice, assess growth and development of persons according to developmental milestones.
6. Describe the following concepts as they relate to the older person; outline nursing implications:
   - Life review
   - Retirement
   - Housing
   - Relocation and separation anxiety
   - Loss of spouse
   - Explanation
   - Desolation
   - Poverty
   - Independence-dependence
   - Social isolation
       Institutionalization
           Nursing homes
   - Constriction
   - Loneliness
   - Death

Most developmental theorists in Western society recognize a set of stages called infancy, preschool, childhood, adolescence, adulthood, middle age, and older age. In the developmental life cycle point of view, transition points or tasks are experienced by the individual for each stage and are expected to be accomplished by everyone; if they are not achieved, problems emerge for the individual for subsequent stages. The nurse's role in the prevention of mental dis-

order, in the maintenance of positive mental health, and in the restoration of health requires knowledge of the developmental life cycle point of view. Considering aspects of human development and some of the crisis points of the life cycle may stimulate the reader to perceive the role of the nurse in prevention of mental disorder and to be better able to assist individuals in stress. Not only can the developmental life cycle point of view assist in development of knowledge, understanding, and skills of the clinician, it can also, in a humanistic sense, aid in self-understanding.

Physiological development and psychosocial development do not necessarily coincide. Although physiological aspects of human development are not emphasized in this chapter, their importance is not to be minimized. Growth and development has been an essential component of psychiatric nursing since the publication of the first curriculum guide. (National League of Nursing Education, 1917). The importance of all aspects of growth and development for nursing practice cánnot be overestimated.

Although much human relations study is currently directed toward the "here and now," what we are today has its roots in our past. Certain characteristics of adulthood can be traced to babyhood. For instance, when an adult gets very thirsty, he may drink with the noises and passion he evidenced when he was a baby. With the collection of many similar observations, the study of human behavior asserts that _the early behavioral patterns are never destroyed; they are modified._

A theoretical frame of reference helps to organize observations about manifestations of behavior, treatment of people who have problems, and the etiology of the disorder. Theory is a mixture of facts and interpretations. It helps to explain what has been observed before and to anticipate what may occur next. It also helps us to communicate about what we observe and do. Most major theories used in working with people who have psychiatric problems relate to the intrapsychic, motivational point of view; the developmental, sociocultural; learning theory; and the physiological. Most theorists agree that there are biopsychosocial aspects of every human problem and that these play a part in all normal and psychopathological processes of human behavior. New theory may be generated by those who work with people and therefore contribute to a better understanding of the human condition.

This chapter emphasizes selected theories of developmental phases and crises that are pertinent to nursing, with more attention given to later periods of the life cycle. Since Freudian theory is the basis of developmental theory, some aspects are presented here.

Topographical Theory

Freud's topographical theory refers to the concepts: _conscious, unconscious,_ and _preconscious. Unconscious_ refers to anything about the person of which the individual is unaware. _Conscious_ refers to awareness of self in relation to the outside world. _Preconscious_ refers to that part of the self that is not consciously aware but that can easily be brought to consciousness. One of the major maxims of psychoanalytic treatment is that unconscious aspects of the mind can become a reality.

Structural Theory of the Mind: Id, Ego, and Superego

Later, in the development of psychoanalytic theory, Freud postulated the structural theory of the psychology of the individual: the _id, ego,_ and _superego._ In psychoanalytic theory, the id refers to the energy of the primary instincts, the biological urges, drives,[1] or needs, for example, sex, aggression, hunger, and self-preservation. Corresponding to the unconscious, instinctive desires, and strivings of the person, it is identical with the unconscious (Potter, 1962).

The ego is defined in terms of the control of functions and processes: thinking, perception, motor activity, understanding, communication, and defenses. The ego is the rational aspect of the pesonality; it helps to maintain biopsychosocial balance. It develops as the child explores his environment, grasps a part of himself, and perceives that it is his body, different from his surroundings. It marks the combination of the eye perceiving an object, the arm reaching for it, the hand grasping it and bringing it back to the mouth. There are observation, perception, execution, and reception of an object. The entire process requires the breaking down of the simply pleasurable

[1] A drive refers to the urge to act.

rhythmical movements for the accomplishment of something in which several things are combined.

The ego helps the individual delay gratifications. It functions to preserve the sense of reality, to feel the actions of the world, to mediate between the id and the superego, and to keep a person on an even keel (Menninger, 1963). It thereby aids in adaptation, adjustment, and survival.

The ego refers to the psychological functions that relate to the environment. It is a mediator between the self and the outer world; it refers to memory, movement, perception of the self, and knowledge of the self as distinguishable from the outer world. The ego is thought to be developed after one year of life and continues development throughout the life cycle. It affords the person a sense of individuality, autonomy, and identity. It becomes the organized experience of the self and enables us to do rational planning, for example. It is thought that one of the main dynamic processes of a compulsion neurosis is a development of the ego ahead of the drives.

The superego, developed later in childhood, derives from and centers around the moral demands of—particularly prohibitions—parents and their aspirations and ideals as well as those of society. An unconscious force that blocks unacceptable drives, it is concerned with the "do's" and "don't's" given to the child from parents and his culture. The superego represents the internalization of all the restrictions in which the ego is constrained, for example, parents, teachers, and others. It represents the ego ideal; therefore, it represents both a *force* and *image* and acts as a control to keep the id balanced. Ethical values are internalized and the superego provides us with feelings of guilt. The ego and the superego are the two structures for the distribution of love and hate. In the hostile part of the superego, object hate is turned against the self into self-hate. The beloved aspect of the superego is transformed into self-love (narcissism) and becomes pride and security in relation to society as well as one's conscience (Schafer, 1960).

Freud (1923) stated that the "ego is first and foremost a bodily ego; it is not merely a surface entity, but is itself the projection of a surface."[2] A footnote, described as authorized by Freud, adds that the "ego is ultimately derived from bodily sensations, chiefly from those springing from the surface of the body. It may thus be regarded as a mental projection of the surface of the body, besides, as we have seen above, representing the superficies of the mental apparatus."[3] Freud's description of the ego encompasses the concept of body image as presented in this book.

Body Image

As the child differentiates his own body from his environment, his body image[4] is formed; *tactile, optic, auditory,* and *kinesthetic* impressions aid in its development. One of the earliest controls is that of the image of the body—the libidinal pleasures of sucking, for example. Other special senses—olfactory, gustatory, visceral, and body sensation—also contribute to the development of body image. Gorman (1969) states that all the sensory functions and the development of the ego work together dynamically from birth to form the body image.

Erotogenic Zones

In addition to the concepts of the topographical and structural theory, other aspects of Freudian theory are important in psychiatry today, for example, the development of the *libido*[5] or psychosexual development.

The *erotogenic zone* hypothesis of *oral, anal,* and *phallic* stages of development is a Freudian contribution to the understanding of the

[2] Freud, Sigmund: "The Ego and the Id," *Standard Edition of the Complete Psychological Works of Freud.* Vol. XIX. London: The Hogarth Press, 1961, p. 26.
[3] Freud, ibid., p. 26.
[4] The concept of one's body, based on conscious and unconscious aspects of experience.
[5] Libido refers to the total energy available to Eros, the love instinct. Freud postulated that the libido seeks expression and that it is gratified through the erotogenic zones.

mental life of the individual. This hypothesis states that sexual life begins at birth. It is important to understand that the social life of each individual also begins at birth. The *pleasure principle* refers to the condition in which what feels good is that which at the moment feels good. Freud's theory also includes the concept of the *reality principle,* the consideration that all intrapsychic and outer developments coalesce and create a possibility of a more permanent feeling of well-being. These two principles are basic and regulative to the human psyche. In Freud's theory, mental processes are the result of an interaction of forces that are originally instinctual and the mental representatives of the instincts have a charge.

In the first year or year and one half of life, the baby's libido is centered in the oral zone, the first psychosexual state of development, the *oral stage.* Need gratification is achieved primarily through the mouth by sucking, eating, chewing, and so forth. The *anal stage* begins in the second year of life and continues for about one year until about the age of three. Need gratification in this stage occurs around bowel training. Love and approval are centered on bowel control, as voluntary control of the sphincter becomes possible. The third stage, the *phallic-oedipal stage,* begins around the third year and ends about the sixth. It is during this stage that the Oedipus complex emerges.

The story of Oedipus from which the complex derives is one in which the abandoned son slays his father and unknowingly marries his mother, Jocasta. They had four children and lived peacefully for many years. Then a scourge came upon the land and finally the true story emerged. Jocasta then hung herself and Oedipus, grieved by her death, tore the gold clasp from her robe and pierced his eyes. Thus blinded, he wandered throughout Greece and gave himself to the underworld (Schwab, 1946). The story of Oedipus was written by Sophocles as *Oedipus Rex.*

During the oedipal state, the boy has intensive feelings for his mother, but as he grows older, he is more aware of the father and the intensive, positive feelings for mother are interfered with by the father. The boy develops a feeling of hate for the father and wishes to have the mother all for himself. The *castration complex* emerges

in that the son wishes to cut off his father's penis and, in turn, feels that the father would like to do the same to him. The child solves the conflict by *identification* with the father, giving up the mother, and seeking love objects elsewhere. The song "I Want a Girl Just Like the Girl That Married Dear Old Dad" exemplifies some of the feelings of this stage.

Trouble develops if the child does not make the identification with the father. In fact, then the child is fixated at this stage and is unable to take up the traditional masculine role in society. Instead, he at the age of 40 or 50 may still be single, very attentive to his mother, and unable to be interested in other women. Hostility may arise in which men cannot get along with their superiors due to an unresolved oedipal complex.

With the girl child, the oedipus complex is more complicated. In the first place, she is close to the mother but in the phase of sexual curiosity learns that she does not have a penis. So she begins to feel that her mother left something off at her birth and develops ambivalent feelings toward her of love and hate. This is the so-called experience of penis envy. Therefore, she turns toward the father for attention and her greatest wish is to be her father's favorite. Gradually, however, she identifies with the mother and enters into a very close relationship with her. The father is given up and the girl seeks love objects elsewhere. Thus, the girl's resolution of the oedipal complex is more difficult: She begins with the mother, moves to the father, and returns to the mother in her normal resolution. Like the boy, the girl child may not resolve the oedipal complex. If she remains identified with the father, she may become masculine and an overt homosexual, or there may simply be a lifelong attachment to the father in which the girl feels that no man can ever fill his shoes. The oedipal stage helps teach tenderness, self-sacrifice, consideration for others, and a tolerance for frustration.

The *latency* stage occurs between five or six years and the age of eleven or thirteen. This is the state of quiet and relative inactivity of the sexual drive. Infantile sexual activity subsides and major direction of drive is focused or directed into socially approved activities, especially learning. The ego is further developed and ideals become formed. In this stage, need for belonging to a group is very strong and brings gratification to the developing and differentiating individual.

The *genital phase* of development begins with adolescence when the individual is about thirteen. The person is now physiologically capable of orgasm and this is the final phase of psychosexual development. The maturity of this phase is possible only after successful resolution of the conflicts of adolescence and the earlier phases. Usually, the emerging adolescent has a good friend of the same age with whom he becomes very close. Group relationships again play a significant role in the developing maturity of the individual, and life's values are formed.

This theory has been shown to be helpful in the understanding of some of the early influences of the parent–child relationship. It is generally accepted by dynamic psychiatry in our culture.

Psychoanalytic concepts help us to better understand (1) anxiety and the mechanisms of defense, (2) the role of the first five years of life, (3) that conflicts of early childhood may result in difficulty, (4) the role of repression in unconscious life, (5) that mental disorder and normality are different in degree only, and (6) how to differentiate the normal from the abnormal. They also give us a research tool for the study of human behavior.

Cognitive–Development Theory

Jean Piaget has spent most of his life studying, recording, and writing about how children learn to comprehend the world. He postulated stages by which children learn to comprehend and deal with the world around them. As they attempt to deal with the world, they take in or *assimilate* what they have encountered and use it. Also, they *accommodate* their own efforts to the resistances that they encounter. Piaget views intelligence as development that occurs when the child attempts to assimilate new situations and experiences disequilibrium. In response to the disequilibrium, new structures are created, and a new equilibrium reached.

In cognitive–developmental theory, thought is considered as a central element in all phases of growth; cognition and development are parallel. Development emerges from initiative and action in addition to experience and biophysical readiness. Fundamental to cognitive theory is the assumption that a person's behavior is based upon an act of knowing or thinking (Rohwer et al., 1974). According to Piaget (1970), as the child develops, the passage is ordered and constant from one stage to the next and results in new structures, but the age at which a stage occurs cannot be fixed. Piaget describes four stages of cognitive structure based upon the concepts of equilibrium–disequilibrium as in Table 1.

In the first stage, the *sensorimotor* period, the infant graps, pulls, pushes, looks, and uses these actions to retrieve objects. If an object is hidden from view, the infant no longer looks for it. In this stage, cognition and behavior are not clearly differentiated. Objects are at first transitory (i.e., it is thought about only if the infant is in sensory contact with it). Later, object permanence is achieved (i.e., the child forms a mental picture of an object without immediate sensory contact with it). Practical intelligence assists in dealing with the environment in this stage.

In the second stage, the *preoperational* period, the child learns that one thing can signify another. The past and future are put together and the child can imagine. The child's thinking centers on one aspect of a system.

In the third stage, the *concrete operations* period, the child develops thinking that enables adding and subtracting, for example, and the child can perceive relationships between things. Early in this phase, the child learns that, for example, the same amount of liquid poured into two glasses of different diameters *is* the same amount (conservation of amount), but thinking in this phase applies only to actual (concrete) situations.

In the fourth stage, *formal operations,* reasoning about abstract possibilities is developed (Piaget, 1973).

According to Piaget, the four stages occur when the child has new experiences and

Table 1. Piaget's Stages of Intellectual Development

I. *Sensorimotor* (from birth until age 2)
- A child learns to retrace his actions to find a toy
- Practical intelligence

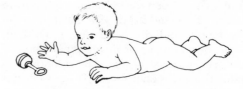

II. *Preoperational* (ages 2 to 7)
- Fact and fantasy and play and reality are not clearly separated
- Things are as they appear
- Animism
- Unconcerned about logic

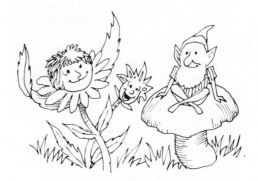

III. *Concrete operations* (ages 7 to 12)
- Orientation toward concrete objects
- Activity is toward organization and order
- Logic becomes based upon objects

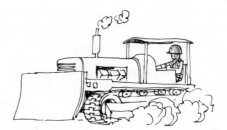

IV. *Formal operations* (ages 12 and up)
- Abstract thinking occurs
- Can consider the real vs. the possible
- Can make hypotheses

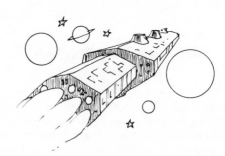

attempts to deal with the resultant disequilibrium. The new thought and new equilibrium is called *equilibration*.

Cognitive–developmental theory is important to nursing, because nursing care for patients at varying levels of intellectual development must be planned and carried out according to the person's ability to understand what is happening to him.

Moral Development

In recent times, moral and ethical issues have a renewed importance within the professions. Kohlberg (1964) describes six stages of moral judgment in three levels of development as in Table 2.

Level one, the *preconventional* level, is

Table 2. Kohlberg's Levels and Stages of Moral Growth.

I. *Preconventional* — (dominant between ages of 4–10)
  ● Responds to labels of good and bad

Stage 1: Punishment and obedience

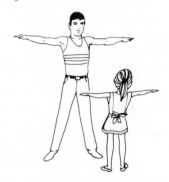

Stage 2: Instrumental relativist —
do that which satisfies self
and sometimes others

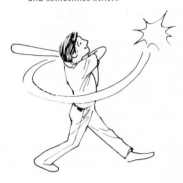

II. *Conventional* — (dominant in preadolescence)
  ● Conformity and loyalty to the family or group

Stage 3: Interpersonal concordance —
good behavior is that which
assists others

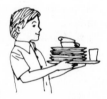

Stage 4: Law and order orientation —
approval is gained by being nice

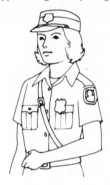

III. *Postconventional* — (early adolescence on)
  ● Universal moral values and principles

Stage 5: Social contract orientation

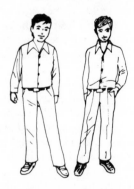

Stage 6: Universal ethical principle orientation

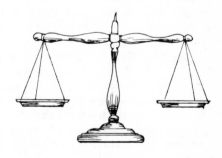

where the child responds to labels of good and bad and views them in terms of punishment and reward. This level has two stages: Stage one is punishment and obedience, and stage two is instrumental relativist (i.e., the right thing is that which gratifies one's own needs and sometimes the needs of others).

Level two, the *conventional* level, describes conformity to the family, or group. Two stages occur in this level, stage three is described as interpersonal concordance (i.e., conformity to avoid disapproval) and stage four, the law and order orientation (i.e., doing right and maintaining order for its own sake).

Level three, the *postconventional* level, is the autonomous level and the last two of the six stages occur here: stage five, the social contract orientation stage (i.e., doing the right thing according to individual rights and those agreed upon by the society), and stage six, the universal ethical principle orientation. In this, the last stage, the universal principles of justice and the respect for the dignity of human beings as individual persons are gained. Kohlberg's hierarchy of stages adapts Piaget's concept of equilibration.

As the professions now have a renewed interest in ethics, moral growth of the individual has assumed a new importance in nursing. Objectives of nursing curricula often involve stage six expectations in the beginning courses. According to Keniston (1971), most Americans do not reach this highest level of moral development. Thus, nursing students are, at the outset, expected to have higher ethical principles than most of their peers.

Life's Crises

Freud believed that the personality of the individual was formed in early childhood. Although great literature of the past had given us a picture of the inner person, it remained for Freud to construct psychological theory. Additional theorists have followed, but Freud's theories remain fundamental to an understanding of the mental life of individuals. Erikson (1963) has formulated a theory that purports that the personality continues to develop throughout the life arc. He identified eight ages that represent psychosocial developmental stages in the life cycle. Thus, a series of stage-specific crises may be anticipated by everyone; they are considered to be pancultural. In Erikson's (1968) theory, a crisis refers to developmental aspects of the individual, not a catastrophic threat.

Crisis Theory

Crisis theory is built upon recognition of developmental crises, crises at role-transition points, for example, birth of a child, leaving one's family for college, marriage, events that occur without warning. At these points, new relationships are formed and old relationships take on new aspects. Crisis theory identifies that all people have certain things to face: developmental ages, tasks, crises, and role-transition points. A crisis used in the *developmental sense* connotes a turning point, a crucial period of vulnerability and heightened potential that represents, therefore, not a catastrophic threat, but a point in development at which time a person may increase his potential or may become maladjusted (Erikson, 1968, p. 96).

In addition to the developmental crises and psychosocial transitions that occur to everyone and therefore may be anticipated, crises may occur to some individuals that are unexpected, for example, sudden infant death, loss of home, and the like.

An important contribution to social psychiatry is the now widespread crisis theory for which the base was laid by Freud (1957), particularly in the paper "Mourning and Melancholia," first published in 1917. Concerned with the effects of anxiety produced within the individual whose ego is in conflict with its id, he showed how acute the condition is in individuals suffering from a personal sense of loss. Lindemann (1944, 1952) and his associates, who observed and helped those bereaved by the Cocoanut Grove fire victims of 1944 in Boston, made observations that added to crisis theory.

The reaction of the person undergoing the crisis is the main point of focus for the helping person. Cultural background, experience, ego strength, and available resources are some factors involved in whether or not the crisis results in healthy resolution or whether a crisis is perceived by the individual. Crisis intervention offered by psychiatric residents to families who lost their homes in the 1970 Malibu Mountain fire in California was ignored in preference to dependency gratification from their emergency housing officials (Goldsmith, 1973).

The idea of achieving emotional growth by surmounting a crisis is a new one in theory but old in life's experiences. We all know people whose lives were radically changed toward self-realization and emotional growth by an emotion-laden event. On the other hand, psychiatric practice is filled with those who, instead, became disorganized. The following is a description of the effect of the horrors of war on a Polish refugee as the advances and retreats were made by the Russian armies, August 30, 1915, at Kuzmy, Poland, by an English nurse, a member of the Imperial Russian Red Cross.

The woman was suffering from the madness of despair. She looked at me with vacant wandering eyes which were never still. I tried to converse with her, but her voice was monotonous and she murmured rather than spoke. Her husband explained that she thought that she had committed a great sin which had bereft her of body and soul and, although living, she believed herself to be dead; she was constantly asking how she could go on living when her body and soul were dead.[6]

Since the profession of nursing originated, nurses and others have observed and helped people in crisis situations. Now a theory of crisis resolution has developed, useful to all those in the helping role.

What a Crisis Means to a Person

A crisis occurs when a person faces an insurmountable obstacle and the usual methods of coping and problem solving do not work (Caplan, 1961). Therefore, the person becomes upset and disorganized and seeks a solution. In the search for a solution, which is time limited (from four to six weeks), the person may move toward healthy adaptation or toward maladaptation. To move toward healthy adaptation, the person in crisis may need assistance at once.

[6] Farmborough, Florence: *Nurse at the Russian Front: A Diary 1914–18.* London: Constable, 1974, p. 139.

A crisis is composed of the following characteristics:

1. It is a threat or danger to life goals.
2. It creates mounting tension and/or anxiety and the affects of fear, guilt, or shame are felt subjectively.
3. It evokes or awakens unresolved problems in the past.
4. It is a turning point in which the person may achieve emotional growth or become further disorganized.

People often are made vulnerable by situations characterized by significant losses, for example, loss of a loved one, home, job, status, country, or body part. Caplan (1964) describes four phases of a crisis:

1. Tension arises as the usual coping mechanisms and problem-solving techniques are used.
2. Tension continues to rise as the usual coping mechanisms and problem-solving techniques fail and the person feels upset and perplexed.
3. Emergency problem-solving mechanisms are brought into play, the individual searches for assistance, and the person calls on all reserves of strength. As a result, the problem may be solved and equilibrium restored.
4. If the problem is not solved, tension and/or anxiety mounts and major disorganization of the personality occurs.

The process of helping someone in crisis follows the steps of problem solving: (1) assessing biopsychosocial needs, (2) making a plan to intervene, (3) intervening, and (4) helping the patient plan for the future. When trust is developed, by use of the interpersonal relationship, the patient is helped through the crisis. Catharsis may help the patient to accept help, confront the crisis, and accept reality (Cadden, 1964). The reality may be that in addition to the improvement of his emotional state, the patient may need a place to stay, some money to live on, and something to eat. Basic needs of people have to be met before much else can be done. Throughout the process, catharsis helps the person gain a new perspective about himself.

In Erikson's developmental life cycle model, each phase of life has a crisis introduction and a task to be accomplished. As the crisis is resolved and the task met, the individual is better equipped to move on to the next phase. It is important for the reader to distinguish between the stage-specific crises of Erikson (1963), which have to be met by everyone, and can therefore be *expected* (i.e., developmental) crises and those that are *unexpected.*

INFANCY AND EARLY CHILDHOOD

In infancy, the child at first seems to want mostly to rest. The embryonic life has been broken by birth, hunger, cold, and other discomforts, each of which acts as a stimulus. The infant reacts to remove the disturbing stimulus and to return to rest. At this time the general action is one of defense.

Two principal defense reactions occur: (1) destruction (devouring food is an example), and (2) flight (e.g., closing the eyes, turning the head). They comprise the aggression instinct; in adulthood, this may be referred to as hate. The opposite reaction that develops is love. The infant hears and seems to like certain sounds. By rhythmical repetition, he begins to find some actions desirable to which he formerly objected.

The human face and figure combine sound and motion; this combination is one of the most constant aspects of the infant's environment, providing certain satisfactions such as contact comfort, motion stimulation, and food. It is logical, therefore, that the infant's first love object is the mother or the mother substitute. The developing child needs the assistance of another person to whom he may become attached. Following, clinging, and feeling secure in the presence of this person and depending on him all are indications of attachment behavior. Crying in the absence of the person or at intimations of absence occurs readily and ceases when the person returns (Bowlby, 1969).

The concept of the love object is based upon the love of the child for the mother or mother substitute. It derives from Eros and represents the urge for union with ob-

jects in the world. Love objects originally serve primitive instinctual needs whereas object choice,[7] which comes later, carries with it additional emotional commitments. *Object constancy* refers to the ability of the child to integrate both "good" and "bad"[8] objects as well as self-images without splitting them up and introjecting them as "good" and "bad." It occurs as part of healthy maturity and refers to equilibrium balance. The ego itself establishes object relationships, assesses dangers to these relationships, and acts to protect them. The absence of or lack of adequate object relationships and the loss of love as well as the object loss itself in infancy may be life threatening and result in irreversible changes in areas of maturation (Kris, 1950).

Mahler (1952, 1961) thinks that childhood psychosis rests on early experiences where object relations appear so threatening that the child fixates or regresses at the autistic or symbiotic stage. More discussion of Mahler's theory will follow in Chap. 10.)

Love appears later than defense. This progressive tendency Freud called sex, or libido, the impulsive energy of man. It is during this phase of life that developmental aspects of anxiety occur. The smiling response shows the infant's awareness of another human being; it is the beginning of the differentiation of animate from inanimate objects. During the first year of life eighth-month anxiety also develops. Object constancy has developed with the mother or the mother substitute as the major object in his environment. It is here that the child is calm with the mother and uncomfortable with strangers. *Stranger anxiety* may reach its peak at twelve months.

Separation anxiety also develops in the infant phase and continues throughout life to old age. Separation anxiety refers to feelings of abandonment—being alone, unloved by, and alienated from others. It can occur in the normal individual as well as in the most regressed psychotic person. In later life, an extreme degree may result in formation of

---

[7] *Object choice* refers to objects, usually persons, upon whom psychic energy is centered.

[8] *Good* versus *bad* objects arise from superego evaluations, that is, to morality and conscience.

delusions. The infant may express separation anxiety by crying every time a person enters the house with his coat on. I have observed this phenomenon while visiting a home for children who were abandoned by their mothers. Crying when the mother leaves is another common sign of separation anxiety. The listlessness of babies in a foundling home described by Spitz (1945) and Ribble (1965) and the turning away from food may be other indications. Bowlby's (1952) study of a two-year-old in a hospital documented reactions to separation from family. His later work delineates his theory and surveys the literature (Bowlby, 1969, 1973).

The first feelings of wanting to be like others are developed during the first year. The erotogenic pleasures are mostly derived from this oral phase of development where the mouth is involved. Other areas of the body, the eyes, and the skin also give pleasure. The oral phase involves (1) passive receptivity (Erikson calls it the getting phase) and (2) incorporation (the child learns that his own activities can destroy, for example, biting). This phase is the period of origin of the concepts of the good and bad mother, the "good me" and the "bad me" derived from the concept of the good and bad mother.

Achievements of the first year of life relate to the pleasures of the erotogenic zones, development of the ego and body image, the differentiation between the id and the ego, and the formation of defense mechanisms.

DEFENSE MECHANISMS[9]

The defense mechanisms of the early life of the child can be divided into primary process and secondary process. Primary processes are the most rudimentary ways that infantile ego is defended or tension and anxiety handled. Dreams and psychoses also represent primary process thinking. Symbolization, displacement, condensation, and incorporation are examples of primary process defenses.

"*Symbolization* is an unconscious mental

process operating by association and based on similarity and abstract representation whereby one object or idea comes to stand for another through some part, quality, or aspect in which the two relate. The symbol carries in disguised form the emotional feelings vested in the initial object or idea."[10]

Incorporation is a defense mechanism in which the psychic representation of a person or parts of him are figuratively ingested. An example is the infantile fantasy that the mother's breast has been ingested and is part of one's self. *Displacement* is an unconscious defense mechanism, in which an emotion is transferred from its original object to a more acceptable substitute. *Condensation* is a psychological process in which two or more concepts are fused so that a single symbol represents the multiple parts (American Psychiatric Association, 1975).

Secondary process defenses occur when the ego is older and more able to tolerate tension and frustration; they enable the ego to deal with these. The following paragraph describes certain secondary process defenses.

Identification is a defense mechanism operating unconsciously by which an individual attempts to pattern himself after another. It is to be differentiated from imitation, which is a conscious process. *Projection* is a defense mechanism, operating unconsciously, whereby that which is emotionally unacceptable in the self is rejected and ascribed to others. *Repression* is unconscious forgetting. Many stored and forgotten events are repressed. Repression represents an internal flight of painful material and it is sometimes used to refer to all the defense mechanisms. It is sometimes confused with suppression. *Suppression* is a conscious process of crowding out undesirable material from consciousness, controlling it, and forcing it completely out of memory into the unconscious. *Denial* is a defense mechanism, operating unconsciously, in which conflict and anxiety are resolved by disavowing thoughts, feelings, wishes, needs, or other reality factors that are consciously intolerable.

[9] See "Glossary," Appendix B, for additional defenses.

[10] American Psychiatric Association: A *Psychiatric Glossary,* Washington, D.C.: American Psychiatric Association, 1975, p. 146, by permission.

DEVELOPMENTAL TASKS AND DEVELOPMENTAL STAGES

Developmental tasks, faced by everyone in the course of growth and maturation, are things that each person has to accomplish for himself. They are pancultural insofar as people around the world must come to terms with them in one form or another. Different practices in different societies affect the perceptions and resolutions of the tasks, but all must be faced.

Havighurst (1953) was one of the first to ascertain the tasks of life. He identified a series of developmental tasks for individuals to achieve in the life cycle. His principal aim was to provide a theoretical framework in opposition to the permissive theory of education that the individual develops best if left as free as possible. He emphasizes the importance and necessity of learning new roles as one progresses through the various stages of life. Each developmental task has its roots in biological, psychological, sociological, and cultural components of the necessities of human life. Development, therefore, is learning to live with yourself as you and your society change. This list of developmental tasks was worked out at the Institute of Human Development at the University of Chicago and is biopsychosocial. Other lists of developmental tasks are often either biological, psychological, or social. Havighurst's list combines some aspects of each. It is included here for reference when you are assessing maturity levels of patients (see Appendix A). The tasks are divided into six periods. Each period brings with it the new tasks and roles for that phase of life. For the first period, the tasks and roles for infancy and early childhood (ages birth through six) are as follows:[11]

1. Learning to walk.
2. Learning to take solid foods.
3. Learning to talk.
4. Learning to control the elimination of body wastes.

5. Learning sex differences and sexual modesty.
6. Achieving physiological stability.
7. Forming simple concepts of social and physical reality.
8. Learning to relate oneself emotionally to parents, siblings, and other people.
9. Learning to distinguish between right and wrong and developing a conscience.

Developmental stages of the person described by Erik H. Erikson build upon Freud's psychosexual theories. The eight ages represent a continuum from the beginning to the end of life and there is a stage-specific crisis for each phase (Erikson, 1963, Chapter 7). Each stage of life has a phasing out and a phasing in where psychic energy is used. Each person has to face these crises. Each phase has an aim and a crisis to overcome before movement on to the next phase. Healthy resolution of each crisis is essential for positive mental health and for the successful resolution of the succeeding phase of the eight ages; the following are three ages of infancy and early childhood described by Erikson: (1) basic trust, (2) autonomy, and (3) initiative.

Basic trust is developed where the infant knows that someone is there to meet his needs. The crisis is *mistrust.* Infants who have neglectful mothers or mother substitutes may not be able to resolve this phase. This stage of learning to trust others coincides with the oral phase of development described by Freud.

The following child was in crisis in the oral and basic trust phases of development, and the succeeding ones as well.

J. was born of parents who considered him an intruder in their lives and a threat to their aspirations. He was thus unwanted, and in addition to being unwanted, most likely felt it keenly. The mother had a postpartum depression for several months. Being breast-fed, J. was described by his mother as being loud, irritable, and demanding during the breast-feeding period. He said "Daddy" at the age of thirteen months but did not learn any more new words. At the age of two years, he, according to the mother, "stared right through" her. Shortly after he was four, his brother was born. In nursery school, J. was noted to be uninterested in other children and did not relate at all to other individuals.

---

[11] Havighurst, Robert J.: *Human Development and Education.* New York: Longmans Green and Co., 1953, pp. 16–19, by permission. New York: David McKay Company, Inc. (See Appendix A for the tasks from infancy through later maturity.)

He turned away from others and played with toys. The nursery-school teacher mentioned it to the parents, who contacted the pediatrician, who sent them to a psychologist, who, in turn, referred them to a psychiatrist.

In order for a child to grow and develop, the mother or mother substitute helps the child to meet this need and therefore a sense of trust is developed within the child and the child also develops trust within himself and an ego in touch and tune with reality. This child felt the negative feelings within the parents and this could have been the initiation of withdrawal. Withdrawal defends against anxiety but it leads to a stunting of the ego functions, and the result is lack of development of a clear body image, identity, and ability to perceive who he is and where he is in time and space. Withdrawal therefore affords the child avoidance of painful exposure of low self-esteem by diminishing interpersonal contacts.

This child was admitted to the inpatient unit unable to handle the structure of language due to his underdeveloped ego; he exhibited echolalia, pronominal reversal, tonelessness, limited verbalizations, and very little emotional expression of any kind except anger. His speech was impaired and this added to the withdrawal because others around him could not understand him. Bettelheim (1967) believes that the child's reluctance to talk and the avoidance of the correct use of "I" and "you" may be due to fear of communication of his thoughts. Szurek (1967) is of the opinion that the psychotic child feels the hatred of his parents, introjects this hatred, which then becomes self-hatred and a hatred for others, and may withdraw. When his needs are not being met, his defense is an attack to show others that he is powerful; therefore, he may strike out and hurt others.

Autonomy is the next phase and is characterized by the achievement of defiance and independence. The crises are *shame* and *doubt*. It coincides with the period of life in which the child is in the "no, no" stage. Children in this phase will say "no" to almost everything asked of them.

Initiative is characterized by the development of love and hate for the parent of the opposite sex. The crisis is *guilt*. This phase coincides with the Oedipal phases of development as described by Freud.

MIDDLE CHILDHOOD

The next stage marks the midpoint of Erikson's eight ages of the person; it is called industry. This phase corresponds with the *latency* period[12] described by Freud. Here the child is eager to learn and searches for reasons why things are as they are. The crisis is *fantasy*.

FANTASY

Fantasy is one way of handling tension and anxiety. The infant has difficulty differentiating between wish and reality. During infancy one learns to wait; it is thought that hallucinated images of the mother permit monetary delay and temporary satisfaction. The infant may indulge in thumb sucking, which satisfies him temporarily. Through experience one learns that real things have taste, odors, are hot or cold and these real things become more vivid than those of the imagination.

Later on, children may hit parents and berate them. Some parents need help to perceive that a child must relieve tension. There are dangers of overpermissiveness where a child is permitted to get into trouble and feels that the parent does not care for him. A confused superego may result. Some parents cannot tolerate expression of tension. The child may then retreat into fantasy. To him, to think his bad thoughts about his parents is often as bad to him as actually carrying out his thoughts. This is called *magical thinking* and is normal in certain amounts. Our culture demands some sharp distinctions between the real and the unreal, but there are cultures where magic, symbols, and fantasies play a larger part in life. When symbolic action is a belief, magic exists. We tend to keep fantasies of the good parent. In fairy tales, the fairy godmother is the fantasy of the good mother. Bettelheim's work (1976) on the benefits of fairy tales for the growth and development of

---

[12] Latency is the period between the phallic phase and the turbulence of puberty and adolescence.

the child emphasizes the power of polarities such as good and bad to aid the child to distinguish between the two. Fairy tales delineate the most complex of situations in simplified form and this unique art form is easily understood by children. Identification with characters in fairy tales and fantasizing about their situations and obstacles can assist in the emotional development of the child. According to Bettelheim, fairy tales convey to children that life is a struggle but if one meets the challenges, victory is possible.

The play of the preschool child who reacts to his environment as though people and situations were present when, in actuality, they are not, gives impressions of hallucinatory activity. The imaginary playmate to whom the child speaks and for whom he does things also has this quality. However, when asked, the child readily distinguishes his activity as play and as imaginary. For the second of Havighurst's six periods, the developmental tasks for the age group six to twelve are as follows:[13]

1. Learning physical skills necessary for ordinary games.
2. Building wholesome attitudes toward oneself as a growing organism.
3. Learning to get along with age mates.
4. Learning an appropriate masculine or feminine social role.
5. Developing fundamental skills in reading, writing, and calculating.
6. Developing concepts necessary for everyday living.
7. Developing conscience, morality, and a scale of values.
8. Achieving personal independence.
9. Developing attitudes toward social groups and institutions.

Excessive aggression in this phase may act as a defense against passivity or dependence (Engel, 1962).

Very often the first person to notice that something is wrong is the teacher in kindergarten and this heralds the many visits to multiple professionals to define the problem presented. It is difficult for diagnosticians to differentiate between mental retardation,

[13] Havighurst, ibid, pp. 28–40.

brain damage, and early psychosis. The following is an example of a child attempting to cope with his developmental tasks.

D., a six-year-old, started kindergarten last year and it was at this time that some of his behavior was noticed. He was noted to have some difficulty with motor coordination. Upon referral to the local speech and learning center for evaluation, the psychiatric evaluation was as follows: "Rapport was easily attained; his motor activity was average; his attitude was cooperative; his attention was variable; his response to failure bothered him moderately; his problem-solving methods were variable; his tasks need constant direction and praise; his verbal activity is average; he is easily distracted and his performance fluctuates with deterioration." He stated that his greatest worry was doing well in school. He was found to be superior in verbal conceptual ability but all performance scales were severely depressed. He was low in practical knowledge and social judgment and immediate auditory memory. His reponses were bizarre and only directly related to a question. In the human figure drawing, D. chose to draw a picture of a little girl indicating an anxious concern or conflict in relation to the child.

On a home visit by the nurse, an assessment was made of the family. It was found that the family lived about ten yards from the entrance to school, that D. was the older of two boys, and that the mother was about ready to deliver the third child. The father was found to have been in outpatient psychiatric treatment and, in addition, was working as a longshoreman and part-time janitor at two jobs for seven days per week. The family had done little traveling or exploration of the environment about them, for example, outings, vacations, and the like. The mother had also been working.

D., in this period of industry, had failed to gain patterns of industry and was not able to measure up to his peers in school and on the playground; a sense of inferiority was instilled. Since group play activities provide for gradual growth and pleasure in the companionship of others, the child who suffers in this interaction may respond in a way that deepens the existing reactions to frustrations at home. The expectation of identifying more strongly with the parent of the same sex along masculine or feminine lines is there. At this time, it is important that the child have close association with a parent of the same sex. It is also during this period that the child's training in the customs and attitude of society are progressively developed. The ego continues to develop in relation to growth and education and experience and inner control of aggression is attained.

In a consultation visit with the teacher, she described D. as presenting himself in a passive, nonsocializing manner. He was noted to sit in class without talking to other students, appeared to be a "loner" with the exception of a few friends. In class he appeared to be "in another world." She had to raise her voice before he would respond, and the response was with a very startled expression. D. had great difficulty in completing assignments and following directions. When confronted about his lack of performance, he stuttered, fidgeted, and gave no explanation. On the playground he was not well coordinated.

D. was found to have difficulty in relating to his family group. He was constantly daydreaming, a characteristic one finds primarily in the preschool child. It was also learned that the family did not give the children any tasks to do except to make their own beds on the weekend; therefore, no regular task performance had been given to either of the children to nurture the self-image within the family group.

D.'s Caucasian father was born and brought up in the midwest. His Philippino mother ran away from home to America. It was also observed in the home visit that neither child responded to either parent unless they spoke in an extremely loud voice. When D. was asked what he did with his father, he stared with a blank expression. He did say that his mother only screamed at him. The father stated that since D. was the oldest that he must do well and be a good example to the other children; he had therefore put a lot of responsibility on D. It seemed that the only escape for D. was his dream world. The parents, in their efforts to mold their children, had not thought about what D. was like as an individual and what he himself thought about and was concerned with. When the subject of the new baby came up, D. said that he was happy but had a strange grimace on his face and changed the subject. The only other time he smiled was when he made his five-year-old brother fight and scream.

As a result of a family conference with the psychiatric team, a decision was made that the family should be seen in outpatient treatment and some assistance provided to the family with regard to helping the father–son relationship.

Success in task attainment of the preceding development stages is considered necessary or desirable if the individual is successfully to meet later ones. There is variation between individuals in ways of attainment of specific developmental tasks. Different societies present unique patterns of developmental task attainment.

SEPARATION ANXIETY DISORDER: SCHOOL REFUSAL

Where school refusal is due to separation anxiety, the child has difficulty being apart from family or home on a variety of occasions, school being one of them. This condition has been referred to in the past as school phobia. A differentiating factor between school refusal due to separation anxiety and school phobia is that in school phobia the child is afraid of school even though accompanied by the parent. School refusal due to separation anxiety is not truancy and must be clearly differentiated from it. Children with this condition are usually of average or above-average intelligence; they respect authority and are from an achievement-oriented home environment. Truants usually come from home environments where there is little emphasis on achievement, where behavior is oriented against authority, and where there is general indifference to the school.

School refusal is most commonly seen upon entrance to school and usually revolves around separation from mother. The mother and child are excessively dependent upon each other, and the mother may unconsciously bind the child to remaining at home although she tells him he must go to school. Thus, the ego of the child struggles with the hostile wishes, especially the death wish, toward the mother and deals with it by an inability to leave the mother. The child verbally declares his avoidance of school and does all he can to remain in the security of the home. He will verbalize fear of school or somaticize with complaints of headache, nausea, fainting, or stomach pain.

In the treatment of these children, the whole family is involved. Usually parents have not aided or permitted the child to achieve autonomy comparable to that of his peers. After assessment of the particular family situation, and development of rapport with the child himself, nurses may be able to help the family or to make a referral.

The child may be able to relate directly why he is afraid.

Bulbulyan's (1967) work with school phobic children was part of her role in community mental health nursing. In communities where school nurses are employed, the school nurse may be this helpful figure. Treatment consists of returning the child to school as soon as possible. Accompanying the child to school or having him stay one day with the principal eases him back into the situation. Changing schools is not the answer. Going to the home at the time the child has to leave the house may give the emotional support to the mother and child that is required for the separation. Giving emotional support to the mother who must accept the separation will help her to adapt. Helping her to rebudget her time around other things when the child is absent may give equanimity to the family situation.

ADOLESCENCE

Trust thyself; every heart vibrates to that iron string.

Ralph Waldo Emerson

In adolescence, the crisis of *identity* manifests itself (Erikson's fifth age). The young person searches for a unity for himself, a place in the social order. He also seeks to make two major decisions in life: What will his occupation be and whom will he love? The crisis is *nonidentity* or *identity diffusion* (Erikson, 1963). Nursing and other professional students such as those in medicine may have partly solved their identity crises by deciding upon their professions early in life. Others may not be so fortunate. Whom to love and what to be now have to be decided upon rather early in life. The requirements of specialization in a technological society demand that the adolescent decide in high school what he will do in college in order to take the necessary courses so that he will be able to compete with others in college entrance.

Adolescence, one of the most painful periods of life, is heralded by the relatively short puberty period. The legend of Romeo and Juliet epitomizes the intense feelings of the adolescent about self, family, culture, lover, and spouse. In this period, stereotyped behavior may serve as a defense against identity diffusion. There is doubt of self and of the future, there are strong emotions of shame about changes in one's body, guilt is prevalent, and feelings of inferiority are great. The formation of friendship groups or cliques aids in the establishment of identity. A negative identity may result in an adolescent's being a temporary thief or a member of a gang destructive in other ways.

There is a strong need to form an identity that is free of parental influence. New coping mechanisms are called for in the turmoil of relinquishing the latency period for heterosexuality.

Mass society makes its contribution to the identity crisis where most urbanized American schools are very large and daily contacts are with large numbers of people on a superficial basis. Young people are now handling aggressive impulses by the use of drugs, which help to counteract feelings of anger and frustration with parents and school.

For the third of Havighurst's six periods, the developmental tasks of the age group (twelve to eighteen) are as follows:[14]

1. Achieving new and more mature relations with age mates of both sexes.
2. Achieving a masculine or feminine social role.
3. Accepting one's physique and using the body effectively.
4. Achieving emotional independence of parents and other adults.
5. Achieving assurance of economic independence.
6. Selecting and preparing for an occupation.
7. Preparing for marriage and family life.
8. Developing intellectual skills and concepts necessary for civic competence.
9. Desiring and achieving socially responsible behavior.
10. Acquiring a set of values and an ethical system as a guide to behavior.

The following are two examples of patients who did not achieve some of these developmental tasks. One example, given

[14] Havighurst, ibid, pp. 111–47.

as follows, shows a patient struggling with developmental tasks.

A patient, S., age eighteen, was hospitalized for depression. His girl friend had been killed in an automobile accident four months previously. He is suicidal and unable to carry on the activities of daily living. The history revealed a conflict within the family related to religion. The parents had refused their consent for marriage because the girl friend was not Catholic. Part of the treatment plan was to help him achieve his developmental task of emotional independence of his parents so that he could make his own decisions about his life in the future.

The problems of the following patient are connected with the later effects of unfinished developmental tasks of this period of life.

A patient, M. G., now forty-five years old, was admited to the psychiatric hospital in a manic state. In reviewing her life history, her problem was thought to be derived from an identity crisis in adolescence at which time she was institutionalized in a state mental hospital. Although adored by her father and a brilliant student in a private university, she had met few of the developmental tasks of adolescence. During adolescence, she had few friends other than her father; she was interested in one young man who, instead of asking her to go out with him, dated one of her sisters. Therefore, her new feminine role for this phase of development did not emerge. She also thought she was ugly and compensated by humorously referring to people whom she met by whatever name they brought to her mind. She was still very emotionally dependent upon her father and had made no plans for a life goal or purpose so that she could become emotionally and economically independent of her parents.

During her twenty years of hospitalization, marriage and preparation for family life were denied her by hospitalization and her emotional state; intellectual skills were delayed and socially responsible behavior was affected by the stigma of hospitalization. She did, however, have a very strong set of values and ethics exemplified in her desire to help those less fortunate than herself, for example, always taking the part of the underdog, assisting in the care of older people who were institutionalized, and playing the piano for special events.

Since the tasks of the adolescent period were unmet, and therefore not incorporated in M. G.'s daily living, she was unable to cope successfully with early adulthood and middle age. Now economically secure through a trust fund established through her deceased father's estate, her plan of therapy included helping her to work through some of the unmet developmental tasks of adolescence and to meet some of the tasks of middle age. She was, for example, encouraged to keep in touch with her nieces so that she would have definite contact with the upcoming generation. Talking about the physiological changes of the climacterium was part of the plan to help her accept and adjust to them. She was also encouraged to renew contacts with some people whom she knew during her adolescent years in an effort to work through some of the problems of that period.

Adolescence is a vulnerable phase for mental disorder. During 1975, 25,252 persons under the age of eighteen were admitted to the inpatient services of state and county mental hospitals (U.S. Department of Health, Education, and Welfare, 1977). For both sexes combined, under eighteen years of age, the total number of additions to state and county mental hospitals decreased during the period 1969–1975 (U.S. Department of Health, Education, and Welfare, 1978). On the other hand, in 1975, for all mental-health inpatient and outpatient services combined, there were 655,036 admissions under eighteen years of age, representing almost a 50 percent increase over the 433,372 admission in 1971 (see Table 3).

The central problem of adolescence is definition of the self, for this is the period of life in which one learns who he is and identifies how he feels. It is the time that he differentiates himself from his family and detaches himself from his family. By becoming an individual in his own right, he is able to experience intense interpersonal relationships with others. He is often consumed with the intensity of his feelings toward others. It is the process through which the self is defined through experience and through clarification of experience. Maturity seldom arrives to those with minimal life experiences. Friedenberg (1959) pointed out that the basic unit of a continuing community is a stable self to respect. It is through this phase of life that the stable self emerges.

All of life's experiences are meaningful in the development of the individual. Reso-

Table 3. Number of Admissions and Percent Change in Number to Selected Mental Health Services* of Individuals under 18 Years of Age, U.S.A., 1971 to 1975.†

Type of Service	Number of Admissions		Percent Change
	1971	1975	1971–1975
All Services	443,372	655,036	47.7
State and County Inpatient	26,352	25,252	−4.2
General Hospital Inpatient	44,135	42,690	−3.3
Private Psychiatric Hospital	6,420	15,426	140.3
Community Mental Health Centers (all services)	113,082	213,607	88.9
Outpatient Psychiatric Services	253,383	358,061	41.3

* Includes inpatient services of state, county, and general hospitals, private psychiatric hospitals, all services of community mental health centers and outpatient psychiatric services. Excluded are Veterans' Administration services and those of residential treatment centers for emotionally disturbed children.

† Source: U.S. Department of Health, Education, and Welfare: *Memorandum #37*. Bethesda, Md.: National Institute of Mental Health, 1978.

lution of one crisis prepares one for the next phase, a process that continues until death.

EARLY ADULTHOOD

Intimacy is the next stage and occurs in early adulthood (Erikson's sixth age, 1963). It portrays the need for closeness and sharing and defines the stage of heterosexuality. The crisis is *isolation.* In the culture of the United States, intimacy is often never achieved. As adolescence is being phased out, intimacy is being phased in. Psychic energy is used in both phasing out and phasing in. In all these stages, overlapping may occur. There is no clear line of demarcation. In adolescence, attachment to other boys and girls is likely to be one that fosters relationships that help define identity. In young adulthood, as a contrast, attachments involve real sharing. Our culture perhaps places little emphasis upon this state; yet, earlier phases receive much attention. Thus, many young people never adequately solve the problem of development of intimacy.

They many attain all other aspects but fail in intimacy and therefore be painfully isolated from others. This may account in part for the alienation felt in our society and for the popularity of encounter groups where individuals take off their clothes in efforts to be close to others. If the crisis

of this stage, *isolation,* is not conquered, subsequent stages of life involve painful loneliness.

As a nurse you will have occasion for much physical contact with patients. What are *your* feelings about the intimacies associated with nursing? People confide in you, they bring their life's sorrows to your attention. In nursing, you perceive the inside of people, the intrapsychic functions. You also assist others with their body functions. In ordinary life you probably do not see the various parts of the body as you do in nursing. It will have an impact on you. Identify your own feelings about some of these experiences and discuss them with a friend. In nursing, you cannot avoid intimate contacts.

The young adult who is sure of his own identity can share satisfying intimate relations with others. The loneliness of subsequent stages of life may be due to the fact that the isolation crisis was never resolved.

For the fourth of Havighurst's six periods, the developmental tasks of this phase of life (ages eighteen to thirty-five) include:[15]

1. Selecting a mate.
2. Learning to live with a marriage partner.
3. Starting a family.

[15] Havighurst, ibid, pp. 259–66.

4. Rearing children.
5. Managing a home.
6. Getting started in an occupation.
7. Taking on civic responsibility.
8. Finding a congenial social group.

The following patient had a mental break at the age of twenty-eight after a marriage of nine years had ended in divorce.

G.M. had one abortion and one child now five years old. According to the parents, she developed normally. Although she had coped for nine years of marriage, G.M. now states they were divorced because, "He used to hit me and I couldn't stand the blood any more." Against the wishes of her Catholic parents, she had married in the Russian Orthodox church. G.M. met the tasks of her age group as follows: married, started a family, was rearing a family, and was now managing a home with the help of a babysitter while she worked as a secretary. However, she did not come to terms with her *ethical values* and had not identified with a *social group*. To compensate, she began joining several churches. Needing help with the work at home, she took in her teenage brother, and two other teenage boys, began smoking marijuana, and told her daughter that she had been to heaven. One day she threw her suitcase out the window and threatened to jump, at which time the parents brought her to the hospital.

On admission she expressed feelings of guilt about disappointing her parents, the abortion, her divorce, and going against her religion.

University life for many young people is on a mass basis. Students may arrive on campus with hopeful expectations that they will be able to choose a variety of desired courses only to find a highly structured course requirement that gives little leeway to them as individuals. A student may also find himself in class with twelve hundred other students who are in the same mass life at mealtime, at the library, and in their living quarters. In the search for meaning, the university environment itself contributes to psychological numbness (Keniston, 1967). Students may be so unknown to faculty and administration that just being called by name is significant. During my student days, arrival on campus was designated "Berkeley shock," and very little time was spent there except for classes and concerts. "Sitting in" at that time meant something entirely different from what it means now. To overcome the *ennui* of required courses in the constricted curriculum, "sitting in" meant attending other more interesting classes out of my major taught by prominent and internationally known professors on campus.

Rebellion against some of these aspects of university life was widespread in this country in the sixties, following the example of the civil-rights movement in the southern United States. Mass protests against rent, national policies, police power, and the rights of institutions in planning for the use of its property documented these times.

As America becomes more and more urbanized, ways for young people to meet and select mates become increasingly difficult. Lonely hearts clubs and computer dating are indicators. It must be stated here that selection of a mate is not limited to early adulthood in any sense. The high divorce rate and the earlier death of men results in many people throughout the life arc selecting a mate. Nurses themselves are in this category and should be particularly aware of developing all aspects of themselves so that they are interested in and can discuss something more than their profession. The curriculum of most nursing schools and other preprofessional and professional students leaves little time for pursuit of other interests. The amount of required reading alone is enormous and the push for grades for eligibility for graduate school adds stresses. Keniston (1967) calls this compulsive professionalism.

A balance of work, study, and play is necessary for positive mental health and should be achieved even if one has to take less than a full semester's load in college.

Taking up a new interest after high school and college or joining a club provides fun and an opportunity for meeting others.

In this phase of development, marriage brings a new set of adjustments and, as nurses, people confide in you. Cathartic listening can often aid the person with marital problems who, having a sympathetic ear, can then do his own problem solving quite effectively. For more severe problems, referral to a marriage counselor may be required. Nurses also aid in family planning. The nurse may assist the family or help them to get the aid that they need. In turn, the nurse needs someone to whom to turn to discuss problems encountered in professional practice. The constant work with the crises and problems of individuals and families elicits needs in all professionals for checking perceptions with colleagues and/or consultants. Nursing students turn to their instructors and to their peers for this help.

In the rearing of children there are many facets that involve nursing. Helping mothers and children to be healthy is a traditional part of nursing all over the world. Helping parents to perceive the importance to children of love may set a firm foundation for the healthy emotional growth of the child. The needs of parents, especially young mothers, to have time to themselves for rest and relaxation cannot be overemphasized. The suburban housewife unable to find a babysitter may suffer stresses similar to those of the ghetto mother who lives in a crowded area and is constantly bombarded by stimulation from others.

Managing a home, making a budget, and organizing the home to meet the needs of the various family members have to be learned. Cooking and managing a food budget are important items of homemaking. The knowledge that nurses have of normal nutrition can be used to assist families to develop normally.

The nurse may also be able to help the busy mother with many children find time to be alone with each child frequently. Some mothers are able to take yearly trips with each child. Others can use time for errands and outings to take a child along so he has some time all to himself to be with his mother. The husband and wife also need time alone together. The importance of space assignment to children is also vital— a room or some part of a chest of drawers, even a box where a little boy can keep his bugs or rocks where no one else has entry, fulfills a basic need. Attention to this space for personal property aids the child to develop a sense of who he is and what he wants to be.

In some cultures, it is expected that women contribute to the economy of the country as well as to its progeny. In the Soviet Union, for example, women are given pregnancy leave and return to work within the year after the birth of a child. A well-developed and carefully run system of nursery schools enables mothers to do this. In our own country, nursery schools and child-care centers are likely to be for the poor or the very rich or run on a cooperative basis by parents. Few provide weekend and overnight care, which means that the working mother has additional hardships to deal with if she works. Suitable babysitters are both hard to find and expensive. The nuclear family has no old aunt, cousin, or grandparents to turn to for help. Some help is provided to families with handicapped children in certain communities. Respite from the continuous task of caring for retarded children is needed on a widespread basis. The working husband and wife who return to suburbia after a long day's work and often an even more stressful period of commuting may have few reserves for civic responsibility.

Some young people in this decade who have grown up in the affluence of a home environment where parents work to provide more material things for themselves and for their families are becoming disenchanted with the whole idea and are establishing a life more meaningful to themselves in communes and in rural life styles.

New dimensions of the life cycle of adult men have been investigated by Levinson and colleagues (1978). Their study of forty men with varying backgrounds describes the life cycle and its seasons, and focuses on the individual and his development over the adult years. Transitions to each phase are described and midlife individuation is emphasized. In Levinson's study of the adulthood of men, three developmental periods occur, each with its own transition: (1) *early adulthood* from the ages of seventeen to twenty-two where the tasks are to end preadulthood and begin early adulthood. A variety of separations occur here and the young man makes choices for adult living. From ages twenty-two to twenty-eight, he needs to explore options for adult living and create a stable life structure. Some men have a smooth age thirty transition but most men in Levinson's study had an age thirty crisis. Levinson refers to these fifteen years as the novice phase of early adulthood; following this phase is the set-tling down period from ages thrity-three to forty. Thereafter, the next developmental period begins with a midlife transition, (2) *middle adulthood,* the era in which he makes a place for himself in society and works at "making it" to the top rung of the ladder. Ages forty to forty-five bring a new set of developmental tasks where reassessment of life takes place. For the majority, this is a phase where struggles occur. Choices that have been made have been done at the cost of others and those choices are now ques-tioned. Therefore, the period of forty-five to fifty years requires a new life structure. Some men are on the decline while, for others, it is the most creative phase. Levin-son's study does not go beyond the late for-ties. However, he does describe the subse-quent periods. From ages fifty to fifty-five, the age fifty transition affords a time to mod-ify life and to work more on the tasks of midlife transition. From ages fifty-five to sixty, a second middle adult life structure is built. For those who have inner resources, the fifties can bring self-fulfillment. From ages sixty to sixty-five, middle adulthood is ended and a basis set for the third period, (3) *late adulthood.* With each transition, a new season occurs. Four polarities of midlife transition occur and have to be dealt with by each person: (1) young/old, (2) destruc-tion/creation, (3) masculine/feminine, and (4) attachment/separateness. Levinson's study offers specific insights into how adult men change and adds to our knowledge of the human life cycle.

MIDDLE AGE

Generativity is the stage in which one be-gins to look at what he has done and assesses it as worthwhile or as deficient (Erikson's seventh age, 1963). If one feels his life is good and rewarding, he surmounts the crisis of *stagnation* or *self-absorption.* Generativity occurs in middle age and is related to pro-ductivity and creativity. It is during this pe-riod that individuals review what they have accomplished and what has yet to be done. It is a time where a life review occurs, and the individual realizes that, with the ap-proach of the half-century mark, there is

not much of life left to achieve all the hopes and desires of youth. One of the primary concerns of generativity is the guidance of the succeeding generations. The drive of generativity thus seems to be related to pass-ing on one's influences to children, as in a family; to the next generation, as in teach-ing; to society, as in the Marxian sense; or to all succeeding generations, as Botticelli, Michelangelo, and da Vinci.

The *empty nest* phase occurs when the youngest child is in high school and the parents face their remaining years alone (Spence, 1969). It is the time when children leave the home for their own lives and par-ents face each other as a couple again. Moth-ers and fathers who have devoted them-selves to their children to the exclusion of other interests may have a particularly diffi-cult time in this phase. Adaptations relating to the *empty nest* represent only one aspect of those required for this stage.

For the fifth of Havighurst's six periods, the developmental tasks (ages thirty-five to sixty) are:[16]

1. Achieving adult civic and social responsi-bility.
2. Establishing and maintaining an eco-nomic standard of living.
3. Assisting teen-age children to become re-sponsible and happy adults.
4. Developing adult leisure-time activities.
5. Relating oneself to one's spouse as a per-son.
6. Accepting and adjusting to the physio-logical changes of middle age.
7. Adjusting to aging parents.

The empty-nest phase of life and genera-tivity seem to be part of the same period and relate to similar problems and growth points. However, the empty-nest phase can only relate to individuals with children, whereas generativity relates to all individu-als.

The middle years bring with them all the growth from the earlier phases of the life cycle; unresolved conflicts are also brought into this phase.

Middle age brings many physiological changes within the body. Vision changes

[16] Havighurst, ibid, pp. 269–74.

and eyeglasses have to be worn. Hearing changes are evidenced and metabolism slows down. Jokes are made about gray hair, wigs and toupees are considered, and dyes are used experimentally. In an attempt to keep up with the intensity and pace of earlier years, people of this age group often die on the tennis courts or during the furious early-morning bicycle ride. In our youth-oriented culture nursing students who are themselves young and physically active need to thoroughly understand that physical overexertion can kill a middle-aged and older person, especially when it is engaged in on an irregular basis. Pursuit of earlier intense interests with moderation and with less competitive spirit should, however, be encouraged here. The space program and the current popularity of jogging have resulted in renewed attention being given to physical fitness.

In middle age, one begins to feel there is not much time left to accomplish all the things that one wishes to experience and new priorities are set in terms of time. It is a period of life when women who have heretofore been otherwise occupied often blossom into new careers and develop their creative abilities. A new sense of fulfillment is therefore possible.

Climacterium

In women, the climacteric appears usually in the mid or late forties. Ovulation ceases and menstrual cycles may be irregular for one or two years; periods of heavy bleeding alternating with amenorrhea may occur. Hot flashes, associated with chilly sensations, perspiration, insomnia, muscle cramps, and manifestations of anxiety may appear. Cyclic therapy with progestin regulates the cycle as the decline in ovarian function progresses to the state of amenorrhea (Goodman and Gilman, 1970, p. 1546). Estrogen replacement therapy is prescribed by some physicians. However, recent studies on the use of estrogen affirms that menopausal and postmenopausal women who take estrogen increase their risk of having endometrial cancer (U.S. Department of Health, Education, and Welfare, 1979). Others prescribe small doses of phenobarbital and reassurance.

In men, although there is no consensus about the occurrence of the climacterium, the andropause has been fully described by Szalita (1966), who says that it is an inevitable phenomenon for every man who reaches advanced age. The gonads gradually decline in function, and there are disturbances in the endocrine balance, various emotional reactions, and a decline in sexual activity. The andropause is thought to occur later in men than the menopause in women.

For men and women, there is a decline in physical capacity, depressive moods are prevalent, and both depression and alcoholism are common in this age group.

Sexual activity may be increased with new partners or it may decrease. For some people the anxiety of proving themselves may lead to other impulsive bahavior, e.g., exhibitionism.

Because women live longer than men and the sexual peak for women (ages thirty to forty) is later than men (ages eighteen to twenty-five), Stevenson (1977) suggests it might be more reasonable for thirty-year-old women to marry eighteen-year-old men.

Preparation for Growing Older

Each phase of the life cycle has a period of phasing in and phasing out. The attitudes of middle-aged persons toward growing older were studied by Neugarten and Garron (1959). In their sample, fear of aging meant fear of dependency involving loss of income and loss of health. Their data were analyzed for positive, negative, and neutral attitudes toward aging. Twelve percent of women and men in their study considered their health to be worse than that of others of the same age. These individuals also held negative attitudes toward the future. An interesting finding of the study was that the *fear of death was never alluded to,* nor was social isolation. Middle-aged people usually have to face death and the reminder of their own age and death through meeting the developmental task of adjusting to aging parents. Although Medicare now assists with their care, older people also need the care and concern of their children. Role reversal may therefore occur and offer opportunities for interpersonal growth and for regression as well. In this role reversal, the parent becomes dependent on the child, and the child relinquishes his longing to return to childhood (Sheps, 1959). The parent ceases to be seen as the all-powerful person and is, instead, perceived as a human being. Before the advent of Medicare, the financial strain of helping children through college and of assisting aging parents simultaneously was often a much more difficult problem.

The empty-nest phase probably affects women more than it does men, but it involves both. Consideration of life without the children requires adaptation to new identities. Divorce is common at this point when readjustment to old roles often does not work out and new identities emerge.

OLDER AGE

Ego Integrity

Older age, the last phase of the life cycle, culminates all phases. *Ego integrity,* Erikson's (1963) eighth and last age of the person is the one in which life is accepted as one's own, dignity and meaning of one's life style is defended, and a new perspective of parents is achieved. The crisis is *disgust or despair.* Fear of death, despair, depression, and suicide are all related to disgust. Ego integrity implies a state of mind in which the person is involved in "followership" in addition to the acceptance of leadership. Preparation for this phase of life begins with childhood; successful achievement of previous crises readies one for this period.

It is often possible for a person to overcome earlier handicaps in his development and rather late in life achieve feelings of identity, intimacy, and integrity. Individuals with children and grandchildren may be better able to understand and work out their earlier conflicts as they interact with the two generations. Helping others to work out conflicts may also give insights into one's own. It is no longer thought that persons in the older years cannot undergo behavioral changes but recent behavior is probably more amenable to change than behavior that has occurred many years previously. It is now held that new crises may call for new types of ego defenses in the older age

group. The adage that persons in the older group will meet their problems with the same defenses that served them in their earlier years no longer holds. A new field of psychogeriatrics has therefore emerged. The nursing care of people in the older age group calls on all the known psychiatric skills.

For the sixth and last period of life as described by Havighurst, the developmental tasks (ages sixty to death) are:[17]

1. Adjusting to decreasing physical strength and health.
2. Adjusting to retirement and reduced income.
3. Adjusting to death of spouse.
4. Establishing an explicit affiliation with one's own age group.
5. Meeting social and civic obligations.
6. Establishing satisfactory physical living arrangements.

Older people now are mostly work oriented. They have lived through the Depression, where just having a job was sometimes a lifesaver. They have seen two World Wars, the Spanish-American War, the Korean conflict, and the war in Vietnam. If they are from other countries, they are likely to have come to America in order to make better lives for themselves. Often a person's sense of identity is associated with his job and an organizational structure.

Discrimination in employment because of older age is *ageism* (Butler, 1975). Factors contributing to ageism are: bias in hiring, bias in acceptance into educational programs for retraining, ceilings on earnings or the threat of loss of Social Security, and unemployment rates of younger persons. *Institutional ageism,* where psychiatric services are not offered to older persons occurs often. Knowledge of the needs and problems of older persons should receive more emphasis in the curricula of professionals and health service planners.

The Life Review

The point at which one arrives at the acceptance of his life is reflected dramatically in the later years. The reflection on the high

[17] Havighurst, ibid., pp. 277–281.

and the low points of life—achievements as well as disappointments—occurs in this phase. The life review helps the older person perceive how his life has been spent and to see his own parents and himself as part of the flow of humanity. What one has done and cannot do and a review of these activities aid in the resolution of this phase. Depression is a form of disgust. It is not always manifestly expressed. An overconcern with body symptoms or psychological invalidism may indicate an underlying depression. A constant preoccupation with the state of affairs of being old and lonely indicates depression in the older person. Remarks such as "I am just in the way" and "Why does someone like you want to visit the likes of me?" are common.

In aging there is a renewed ability to free-associate (Bernfeld, 1951) and a reliving of earlier experiences while putting one's life in perspective. Butler (1968) and others refer to this process as the life review, which is part of the preparation for death. One older person at the age of seventy confided in me that she dreamed of her classmates in the second grade and woke up wondering where they all were. It is not uncommon for older people to give their life review from birth until the present within a few minutes whether it is at the bedside at the time of crisis or at other times when there is someone to listen.

The life review is a phenomenon of old age that, in the past, was thought to be due to the loss of recent memory and clearly one of the cardinal signs of senility. It is now clearly established to be a universal mental process of aging. The life review is not relegated solely to the years of later maturity but can come at times of stress and threat, such as impending death, during the earlier years. A salient point made by Butler (1968) is that retirement, along with removing the defenses of work, may provide the necessary time for the life review. Relationships with others are remembered and dreamed about. Yearnings to see former classmates and acquaintances and to know what they have done with their lives, whether they are alive or dead, become a preoccupation. Conflicts with others, especially with family members, are recalled and sometimes a new and more mature perspec-

tive is attained through this introspective process.

The life review is aided by the renewed ability to free-associate and to remember in detail the myriad of earlier events and experiences. The life review may result in a negative view of what one has accomplished, accompanied by anguish and depression. On the other hand, it may result in settling long-standing family feuds, resolving conflicts with old enemies, philosophizing about life and personal growth. Nurses should be aware of the value of life-review therapy at various phases of life, but especially for the older person, and incorporate it in their practice. Reviewing life events is the therapy. A nursing student held a reminiscence group with older women (ages seventy-five to eighty) in a small, private, convalescent hospital. The goals of this group centered around catharsis and socialization. In one session, the nursing student structured the group along the theme of contrasting adolescence today with their experiences. Mrs. Jones said that young people of today are always in a hurry to go somewhere and that she could not tell the boys from the girls. She said that when she was young, she and her brothers and sisters (thirteen in all) were too tired to go anywhere because they worked all day on the farm. She recalled:

"When I was a girl, one Easter my mother made me a yellow gingham dress. It was so lovely, down to my ankles, all ruffles and lace. Not like today, we made our own clothes in those days and we had plenty of fresh food; we churned milk for butter, made our own bread, and cooked on a wood-burning stove."

All the group members smiled at the mention of the dress and recalled the colors and styles of their own Easter dresses when they were adolescents.

My grandfather reviewed life events by telling stories and jokes about his life; sometimes he told them to his horses! Gramp and Grandmother married at age eighteen and sixteen respectively and in older age often reviewed their lives together, although they did not always agree on the details. A rich and colorful tapestry of life emerged for anyone who would listen. They grew up in rural western Kentucky where storytelling was an art; it reflected the social activities of the times: shivarees, musicales, play parties, church socials, deaths, and baptisms. Stories about clearing land, building log houses, travel by horse and buggy and steam trains, wheat threshings, droughts, floods, blizzards, family experiences during the Civil War, cyclones, and hunting were truly hair-raising. Home births of siblings, and sibling relationships were gone over in detail. Remembrances of classmates and earlier loves were related gleefully as though they had happened just yesterday. Illnesses were fearsome experiences: Diphtheria, croup, flux (dysentery), typhoid fever, scarlet fever, and tuberculosis claimed many children and adults. Recently, when I had lunch with an uncle in the local nursing home, we started talking about wheat threshing. Smiles lit up on old faces around the room; one could almost smell the fresh straw, and taste the peach cobblers, ham, and freshly made bread, all available at wheat-threshing time as these older persons reminisced.

Various ways are used to achieve the life review. Making a scrapbook of oneself is another approach. A study of one's geneology may be accomplished as a legacy for living family members. Perceiving the progression of life from one phase to the next can result in a different feeling about one's identity, intimacy, autonomy, and all the other phases through which one has developed. Sharing life's experiences with another interested human being leaves one with the feeling of not being all alone and also of having an effect on that person. The relating of conscious past experiences helps one to see his life as it is and to accept it for its worth. It is important for the younger generation to remember this process and lend a patient ear to the reminiscing person. It lessens the alienation that an older person feels when there is no one else around who understands what times were like during the parts of his life when he was more ego-involved.

Taking photographs of older people aids them to perceive their changed self-image in comparison with younger years. A videotape made of a home visit by the writer to an older person living in a downtown hotel records the facets of his life review, beginning with his birth in a sod house.[18]

RETIREMENT

Once a person loses his position by retirement, he no longer has a place in a meaningful organizational structure and therefore must make adaptions and adjustments to a new role. Retirement age in this country is generally set for sixty-five, although required retirement at sixty-five is now changing. Preparation for retirement should begin early in life, and those who in their earlier years develop their inner resources will be better equipped for this period.

The older population in this country is becoming more isolated as their knowledge and skills become obsolete. Their world and their values have become increasingly irrelevant in a highly technological society with rapidly changing customs. If we are to counteract the dehumanizing aspects of contemporary society, one pathway is through care and concern for the aging members.

People now live longer and therefore have an increasingly higher number of retirement years. Twenty more years of life are expected now than at the turn of the century. Many Americans are unprepared for retirement and have numerous difficulties during this period of life. We need to know more about retirement and its effect upon persons and upon the society in which they live.

Persons who have the ability to obtain a good education, who have developed diverse interests, and who are in a high socioeconomic status group are more likely to adapt successfully to retirement.

The attitude that each person has toward the later years of life influences the quality of life of those years. The importance of time in our technological society points the way toward the need for planning the time of the retirement years. Carp (1968) emphasizes the need for more study of these emerging phases of the life cycle. Allocation

[18] The play *Krapp's Last Tape* by Samuel Beckett is a good example of the life review: *Krapp's Last Tape and Other Dramatic Pieces*. New York: Grove Press, 1960. The epilogue by Arnold Toynbee in *Man's Concern with Death* provides a life review (London: Hodder and Stoughton, 1968).

of leisure time and taking on new careers are in order for the most effective use of the retirement time budget.

A variety of activities is necessary in any given community for effective use of leisure; different leisure activities can have the same significance for certain people (Havighurst, 1957). In this study, social class was determined to be an important factor in how people spent their leisure. Among the findings of the four social classes studied, for example, reading was favored equally by the two middle classes and the upper–lower. Since suitable leisure activity helps maintain life-style and level of integration, it especially needs attention in the middle and later years. Kreps (1968) raises the question of the dilemma of increased time in the older years when income is also reduced.

A target group of individuals who need special assistance in retirement planning are women who are social overachievers: ". . . they seem to have reached for statuses beyond their capabilities and, as a result, they tend to view themselves as failures (indicated by feelings of low self-esteem)."[19]

Preretirement education and counseling need to be done on a widespread basis. Nurses in occupational health practice have ready access to individuals at this time of life. The first longitudinal study of the effect of preretirement education was made at the University of Michigan's Division of Gerontology. Preretirement education reduced dissatisfaction with retirement and worry about health. It encouraged participants to engage in all kinds of activities but especially social activity with friends and family (U.S. Senate, 1969).

The retirement time budget should include renewal of social contacts with old friends, maintaining relationships with friends and family, and reaching out for new acquaintances. Travel is now possible for many older people and life-long wishes to visit foreign countries are being fulfilled. Plans for visits to the "old country" or to scenes of childhood and those of intervening years help to give a perspective on life and a renewed sense of self. Perception of

self in relation to these earlier contacts with friends, family, and place of birth aids in making the life review and surmounting the crisis of ego integrity. Contacts and renewal of contacts with younger family members can also aid the younger ones to come to terms with their developmental tasks and thereby further enhance the sense of self.

There is some evidence that the alternative generations get along better together than the contiguous ones; therefore, ways must be found for the older and the younger generations to get together. Much mutual education can be accomplished by this interaction (Evans, 1969). Friendly visiting programs are also helpful. The Foster Grandparents plan puts the two generations into contact with each other and, in addition, gives older people an opportunity to do community service. Foster Grandparents may work in hospital pediatric units, helping with the sick children. Others work in juvenile centers and mental hospitals giving love and help to rejected children and those without significant others. Numerous volunteer programs are available for making one's contribution to society. The American Cancer Society, the Heart Association, and various next-to-new shops raising money for specific causes all have work for older people, just to name a few. More older people will now continue to work as efforts have been made against forced retirement. As physical fitness is now highlighted in the U.S.A., the retirees may spend leisure time jogging, swimming, or on the tennis court.

Additional programs have been developed to provide continued usefulness. Large companies and other institutions such as universities use retired individuals for consultation, lecturing, and so forth. Retired vice-presidents and presidents clubs exist in some areas. For example, the Fromm Institute of the University of San Francisco provides classes for older people taught by retired professors. Tuition, in this case, is minimal.

In the Soviet Union retirement age is sixty for men and fifty-five for women. Although they have an earlier retirement than we do, emphasis is put upon the retired person contributing to the economy of the country by helping in the nursery schools, museums, and other places. Returning to

[19] Spence, Donald L.: "Patterns of Retirement in San Francisco," in Carp, Frances M., ed: *The Retirement Process.* Washington, D.C.: Superintendent of Documents, 1968, p. 73.

their old job for a few weeks each year is encouraged. This keeps the retiree in touch with his occupation, relieves others for vacations, and provides additional income. In our society, however, we have an unemployment rate that poses a different problem for us. In Denmark and Sweden, careful provisions are made for older people in terms of free health care, living arrangements in their home communities, and availability of health care in the place where they live.

For the nurse, preventive work is the focus. Find out what retirement means to each individual. There are cultural differences. In the American rural South, some professional workers still attempt to get retired older people to learn a hobby, join a club, or get involved in civic work. In practice, it is part of the culture to do nothing when one retires. The older person stays at home and others are expected to come to him, to seek him out for comments on life and for his connection with the past. A pattern learned early in life, that an older person sits in his porch swing and lets others visit him and seek him out for advice, is difficult to change overnight. In urban areas the activity rooms of churches in some instances have become "front porch swings." They provide places where older people living in crowded cities in their own homes, apartment houses, and residential hotels can get together to visit, talk, have a hot lunch, and create something with their hands if they wish.

Helping the person who is retiring to talk about retirement, how his day will go when he no longer works, will help. In a time-oriented society, most people place high priority on this item. It is ironic that the retirement gift is often an elaborate and expensive watch! Wives who traditionally have done all the homework and who have had their days free to do as they please may find it particularly difficult to have a retired husband around the house all day with nothing to do. However, many constructive tasks can be done around the house. Redoing the cabinet space, refinishing furniture, and gardening are all useful and creative. Rearrangement of living space provides room for each person to do his thing and asserts his territorial rights. Sharing house-

hold tasks and cooking may help solve this problem of some older couples; this practice is best begun in earlier years. Since women are more likely to fit into the household tasks upon retirement, they do not have the difficulty that men do in making adaptations. As more women enter the labor force, retirement begins to pose a different problem for them. Now, we are beginning to see a new phenomenon, the mother in her eighties who sees her children retire.

HOUSING

The cities are becoming more and more uncomfortable for retired people who may be repeatedly robbed of their purses and wallets, whose mailboxes are burglarized on the day they receive their checks, and who may be knocked down and severely beaten if they do not have enough money to satisfy a thief. Even the elegant and expensive apartments with doormen and television observation of entering visitors are subject to terror. A person might be safe inside his tower, but the outside streets sometimes make it impossible for him to take a walk in his own neighborhood, shop, or go to church. Taxi service is expensive and not always as fast as the bus or subway.

Much housing for the elderly is financed by private means and is therefore designed for profit. Older people who are well off financially have a greater choice of housing. Two examples of housing planned for the affluent are: Rossmoor at Walnut Creek, California, and the Sequoias, San Francisco.

Many, however, do not have this choice, and therefore have to make other arrangements such as downtown hotels or public housing. A study by Wilner et al. (1968) of all the retirement housing in California concluded that this type of housing presents a solution for older persons who are alone and without families. The same study noted that the kind of retirement housing chosen was likely to reflect previous life arrangements. For example, those who owned their own homes were most likely to buy homes in their retirement years; those who had previously rented were likely to continue to rent. Therefore, it is clearly established that older people need diverse types of housing. Many government projects are designated for housing for the elderly but they are not keeping up with the need and there are long waiting lists for these places.

Conversion of affordable inner-city apartments to condominiums and high rents are now forcing some older persons to find other housing. Development of old, established neighborhoods into resorts, for example, Atlantic City, puts pressure on retirees in established neighborhoods to relocate. Mobile homes are popular in California, and although their communities may not be designed only for older persons, they may be described as "adults only" (for example, "Youngstown Adult Mobile Home Community—for the young in heart"). Diverse activities are planned within the mobile communities, and residents are encouraged to develop and pursue hobbies. A swimming pool is a "must" in California and golf, folk dancing, sewing, art work, and writing are encouraged. For those who own their homes, the rising cost of repairs and utilities make continued ownership difficult, even though tax breaks do help.

Decreased income as well as other factors in the years of later maturity may require a move from a large to a smaller house for those who are able to afford their own home. For others it may mean moving from a rented apartment to a downtown rented hotel room either with meals included or without meals in which the older person must then depend on local restaurants for all of his meals. For people who live in cold climates, the high cost of fuel and inclement weather pose additional hardships. The need for warm clothing and the navigation of icy areas can lead to serious problems for the older person. A change in life-style may mean moving to smaller quarters and therefore giving up old furniture to which one has become attached. One older person living in a high-rent area of the city attempted to keep all of her furniture in a small, expensive apartment and was desperately working long hours to maintain her former life-style. Her money was so tight she could not afford even Part B of Medicare. This is an example of an inability to adjust to decreased income and a change in life-style due to loss of spouse.

Older people of diverse ethnicity need to live in an area where they have contact with language, food, and other aspects of the daily life. The older Italian or Chinese person, for example, will surely wish to be in an area where he can speak his native tongue and where he feels a cultural affinity for those around him. Some older individuals are mobile enough to make the daily return by bus or on foot to Chinatown or the Italian area for sidewalk talks with peers about the price of food, what store closed, and which one opened, as well as other changes in the old neighborhood. Newspapers and other reading material in their maternal languages are readily available, and nodding and speaking acquaintances are maintained. Other older people, in relocated neighborhoods and less mobile, may withdraw.

RELOCATION AND SEPARATION ANXIETY

Urban redevelopment and renewal have hit the central areas of cities and the retirement hotels where many old people have found places for themselves close to bus stations, other public transportation, inexpensive restaurants, physicians, and movie theaters with reduced rates for the older person. Emotional ties made with landlords, visiting nurses, the local church, and storeowners may help maintain independence at a time when physical vigor is declining. Once the older person is relocated, he may not be able to reestablish these kinds of relationships, and his desolation and separation anxiety therefore may be further increased. Forced by urban development to move to new areas even more convenient to them poses a threat to the self-system. Some older persons are now organized in protests of bulldozing for redevelopment and of conversion of their apartments to condominiums.

For single older persons who comprise one half of all relocated older individuals, and who have been somewhat neglected by relocation programs, catastrophic results are likely to ensue (Niebanck, 1966). A study by Smith (1966) of the relocation of elderly persons living in an area planned for redevelopment reports the wide spectrum of problems faced by older people who live in the central areas of cities.

The break with old neighborhood ties and acquaintances and the routine of the day can result in separation anxiety. Older people from ghettos containing many different ethnic groups may feel the loss of contact with their particular group in their daily association with the others in the next-door apartment, at the neighborhood drugstore, or at the grocery. Inability to secure foods that are common to a particular cultural group further adds to the separation. It may be manifest in an inability to participate in the life of the new location and a further withdrawal from those around him. Mistrust of new neighbors and a constant verbalization of a longing for old friends may be evidence of separation anxiety. Inability to participate in senior centers in new neighborhoods where one does not find members of one's own ethnic group may also be evidenced.

Middle-class America creates some of its own problems; suburbia leaves the poor and the elderly in the cities. Retirement communities therefore become defensive reactions to noninvolvement in society. They have been built in large numbers over the country, often far away from medical care, public transportation, and hospitals. Health-care facilities are needed more and more by the older age group, many of whom may have a number of chronic diseases.

Nurses have a responsibility to acquaint themselves with the various types of housing available for older people and to help them decide to move and find new places if their present living quarters are not suitable.

LOSS OF SPOUSE

The sickness or death of a relative, or of a *significant other,* may precipitate a crisis. Anderson's study (1964) of six hundred well persons over sixty years of age and six hundred older people in the same age group with a diagnosis of mental disorder showed that the death of a relative was the *most stressful event.* Older persons are therefore in need of aid relating to problems associated with grief, mourning, and bereavement. Grief work may take longer to accomplish than in the earlier years. The following is an example of what occurred

with one older person upon the death of his wife.

Mr. A., a somewhat melancholic man who has been retired from law practice for several years, lost his wife of thirty-five years. Although she had been ill for several months, her death came to him as quite a blow. Since he was the second husband, there was a question as to whether he would be able to remain in the house since the children of the dead wife were to inherit part of the estate.

In his grief for his lost spouse, he felt that his pain was the worst that anybody ever had. He was also highly critical of the church where his wife had been a regular member. He felt that no one cared for him; no one came to see him, and he just did not know what to do. Nursing interventions that helped Mr. A. centered around the problem of loneliness. Going to visit with him, telephoning, listening, and encouraging him to speak of former times when his wife was alive built up a pool of *shared images* so that he could speak freely of times in which he had been happier.

Mobilizing the minister of his deceased wife's church to visit and telephone more often aided in emotional support that he also was receiving from his physician of many years. Although there were many contacts made by these caring people to Mr. A., it was his *feeling of loneliness* and of being abandoned that had to be worked through. All were in touch with each other by telephone and encouraged each other. He was encouraged to get someone to help him with the housework and cooking and subsequently found someone on his street to do this for him and thereby maintained his independence. With the passage of a year, his loneliness became less intense and he resumed his former pattern of life with daily walks, contacts with war veterans, playing his guitar, and singing.

Many older people, in times of emotional need and great emotional stress, may not know that they need help or understand just what a psychiatrist can do to help. They have grown up in an era when there were few psychiatrists and where psychiatrists were used only for those who had to be admitted to the "asylum." They may have the idea that no one really needs a psychiatrist for the problems of life. Community mental-health services and senior centers now make psychiatric care more accessible to older people whose needs may have formerly been unknown except to public-health nurses and general practitioners.

Older people who have long depended upon a spouse to attend a certain business aspects of life such as filling out forms, cashing checks, and keeping books may be rather overwhelmed with the prospect of assuming this responsibility upon the death of the mate. Papers for Medicare, for example, are quite complicated for old eyes to read and fill out properly. Mt. Sinai Hospital, at Baltimore, Maryland, has a Service Center to help older people with the multiagency problem, not just the medical care that they need. I have advised many older people to get their medical care at a clinic or a medical center where they only have to "open one door" and pay one fare for the trip. If an older person has may ailments, it is more convenient to visit physicians who have group practices with all offices of the specialists in one building.

Although older couples often speak of what each of them will do "if he (she) dies first" and have their funeral arrangements made and burial clothes in order, the full impact of losing a spouse only occurs upon return to the empty house.

POVERTY

In our affluent and progressive society we have many poor older people. In 1977, the official poverty level was $2,572 annual income; for two, it was $3,232. Due to federal assistance the number of older people below the poverty level decreased from one in three in 1967 to one in six in the mid-seventies (Aiken, 1978). Ethnicity and economic status are related, with Blacks, native Americans, Mexican-Americans, and Puerto Ricans making up the largest poor ethnic groups.

Of the total population of 208.8 million in the United States, 20.9 million are over sixty-five years of age (U.S. Bureau of the Census, 1973). Their number is expected to total 25 million by 1985, and be 27,-567,000 by 1990. By 1990 about one person in eight will be of retirement age whereas in 1960 only one person in eleven was this old (Bogue, 1969, p. 893). A new wholly federal program of supplemental security income was instituted January 1,

1974, which resulted in increased grants to the aged, blind, and disabled. In a money-oriented society, poor older persons are economically useless and thereby without the status of younger persons. Through Medicare and Medicaid professionals are now more aware of older people, who, previous to its adoption, went without proper care and therefore were often invisible in the urban medical community. We now know more about their needs and problems. More help is available from the federal government. For example, the Older Americans Act of 1965 (Public Law 89–73) was established "to provide assistance in the development of new or improved programs to help older persons through grants to the States for community planning and services and for training, through research, development or training project grants, and to establish within the Department of Health, Education and Welfare an operating agency to be designated as the Administration on Aging." Various conferences, task forces, and commissions were formed to carry out the intent of this act and the decade of the seventies targeted to improve adequacy of income for older people. The Older Americans Act Amendments of 1968 provided for service roles in retirement. The Office of Economic Opportunity provided aid to the older age group through various self-help projects. Benefits to the elderly are contained in the Comprehensive Older Americans Act Amendments of 1978 (PL 95–478). Title III consolidates services on nutrition, multipurpose senior centers, and social service. A required 50 percent of Title III funds must be spent on in-home services, transportation, information and referral, outreach, and legal services. Allocations are required for older persons living in rural areas and for state-wide long-term *ombudsman* programs. Nutrition programs must provide meals in congregate settings and establish outreach efforts. The amendments provide funds for various other types of services.

The conclusions and recommendations of the U.S. Senate's Special Committee on Aging (1969) warned against the acceptance of low income among older persons as an inevitable component of life. Suggestions made by this committee have now become viable programs and attention is being given to the needs of older people in our society in an attempt to provide them with a better life. The White House Conference on Aging (1971) met to arrive at a system of national policies to spearhead action on behalf of older people at national, state, and county levels.

One of your principal tasks as a nursing student is to learn the needs and problems of each older person under your care and help him meet them. As you make an effort to get to know the older individuals around you, they become visible to you, whereas before learning about them, you probably passed them up without scrutiny.

Proper nutrition becomes a problem for the older person who is poor, especially if he lives alone. It is not uncommon for older people to subsist on two meals a day or even one, eating dry foods as breakfast snacks in hotel rooms where cooking facilities are not permitted. Rising food costs leave little leeway for food planning at lower costs, and changes in taste, denture problems, and eating alone are not conducive to the best nutritional states. Because of the cost of eating out, older people living in hotels that close their dining rooms on holidays and weekends often go without meals during these periods. Decreased strength or infirmities and lack of transportation make grocery shopping impossible for some older people. The Housing and Community Development Amendments of 1978 provide for congregate housing services. These services must include congregate meals and may include housekeeping and other services necessary for maintenance of independent living.

Senior centers may offer a hot midday meal to members. For some, this may be the main meal that day. Cities have developed programs for the delivery of hot meals on a regular basis to those individuals who are homebound. Classes in nutrition and meal preparation are often part of senior-center programs.

The cost of medication may be a big item in the budget of an older person. Telephone shopping may prove valuable in the purchase of drugs and should be encouraged. Generic prescribing also helps in this cost since many drugs cost less when prescribed under their generic name instead of by brand name (Task Force on Prescription Drugs, 1968, p. 80).

Many older individuals without aid and sustenance are often ashamed to ask for assistance and should be encouraged to use resources that are set up for them. Wiltse (1963) found that the "hard-to-reach" client of later maturity for public assistance was the man on old-age assistance. The fierce independence of the entrepreneurial system may keep needy persons on starvation diets, without electricity and without running water or gas, right in the middle of our cities. Inflation and the astronomical cost of fuel have greatly added to the financial problems of the older person. Older people have been found frozen to death in cold areas because their heat had been turned off due to unpaid bills. Recently, ACTION, a nonprofit housing corporation in Marquette County, Michigan, supplied forty-five poor elderly families with ten cords of wood each, cut and delivered by youth, for their wood-burning stoves, their sole sources of heat (ACTION, 1978). Trusting others may be the first hurdle to getting aid. After gaining trust, pride may be the intervening force unless persuasive arguments portray their right to aid.

INDEPENDENCE–DEPENDENCE

Older people now are maintaining independent existences longer than ever before. Medicare and other federal assistance give a new independence to the elderly poor. Older people who previously were unable to receive medical care except through "charity" now can receive this by their Medicare cards. These enable them to receive cut rates at some downtown cafeterias and pay lower bus fares in major cities. The card itself is shown proudly by some older people in the same way that a younger person might display his club card. Formerly, poor older patients in county hospitals were not likely to complain about any procedure, whereas now they feel more free to speak up since their care is financed differently.

Falling symbolizes loss of independence and the beginning of infirmity. Falls, however slight, are discussed and reviewed many times by the victim. Bringing to mind loss of self, the possibility of a broken bone, hospitalization, and pictures of the incapacitated and bedridden older person, they are therefore a great threat to the ego and the sense of security. Outings such as visits to physicians and senior centers may be canceled due to fear of falling with its consequences.

Nurses, who have a definite role with the older person in helping him to prepare for dependence and helplessness, should be aware of available community resources. Listening to older people's fears and concerns about medical care, physicians, hospitals, convalescent centers, nursing homes, and other living arrangements help them to sort out the real from the unreal and to accept help when it is needed. Talking about infirmity and what to do if it comes is important, along with discussing some of the positive aspects of various living arrangements. If possible, the older person should be in contact with his own culture; with orthodox Jews, for example, the availability of appropriate food and religious services gives a connection with self and the past.

Loss of independence can be a crisis and should be thoroughly assessed by the nurse. Adaptation from independence to dependence and vice versa varies with levels of wellness, motivation, and life-style. In Clark and Anderson's study (1967) of older San Franciscans, two basic goals were found in aging persons, survival and self-esteem. The study emphasized the linking together of self-esteem with the cultural and personal value of independence–autonomy and self-reliance for the present generation of older Americans.

Maintaining independence is therefore necessary for self-esteem. If institutionalization is required for survival, the challenge then becomes one also for society to help older institutionalized persons to maintain their independence in the way most meaningful to them and the preservation of their self-esteem.

The studies of Lieberman (1968) show that older persons require a year or more of preparation before entering a nursing home if they are to survive the first six months of adaptation. The preventive work of the nurse is therefore clearly drawn.

SOCIAL ISOLATION

Institutionalization brings with it a loss of status and social roles; independence is given up, and the older person feels abandoned by family and other loved ones. The reality of the nuclear family's limitations in being able to care for its aging relatives is manifest, and the older persons' feelings of being "in the way" and "unwanted" are reinforced. Visits, flowers, letters, and other contacts and symbols help, but they do not overcome the reality of social isolation by institutionalization.

Institutionalization. Institutionalization refers to the provision of custodial facilities for those individuals who can no longer care for themselves.

For a contrast with present practices it must be remembered that up into the 1960s many confused older persons without finances and without caring families were sent in large numbers by the counties to state mental institutions. In my county the practice was to empty out the county psychiatric wards on Fridays. Twenty or more patients transported in police "black Mariahs" might arrive at the state hospital, in one group, the old, the young, and the middle-aged together. Once some of the older persons got three meals a day and their insulin regulated, etc., their confusion cleared up but rarely did they get back to their home community.

A geriatric ward in a large state mental hospital might house from one hundred to one hundred and fifty patients. During those years, patients over sixty-five comprised from one fourth to one third of the patient population in some institutions. Some units were open, clean, and homelike. Usually one unit was the showplace with antique furniture in the day room, waxed floors, plants in abundance, and patients who were physically and mentally able to help the nursing personnel keep the ward and clothes clean. These same patients were able to go out on the grounds of the institution, to the canteen, to church, and the like. Clothes were issued by the state or secured from the next-to-new shop on the hospital grounds. Each person had a shelf for clothes in the clothes room, which was kept locked.

Closed wards were another picture. Crowding was evident where the dormitories sleeping one hundred patients were locked during the day and all the patients were then sitting or lying in the small day room or in the hallway. Toilets and bathing facilities were kept locked and patients bathed during the evenings once per week as scheduled. On sunny days patients were locked in the inner courtyard and the din of voices was very loud. Women patients often carried their personal belongings such as combs, apples, and oranges in their brassieres. Meals were served in a common dining room and the schedule was staggered for different wards. The noise in the dining room was indescribable. On their way back to their wards from the dining room, some patients fed the rats that were waiting for them in the shrubbery.

A program for resocialization of the elderly psychotic patient in a large state mental hospital was developed in the 1960s by W. A. Oliver, M.D.,[20] and associates. In this program both men and women patients were transferred from back wards to a smaller homelike cottage unit and divided into groups for assignment to nursing personnel. All activities were performed in a group. Patients were assigned their own tables by group in the dining room. All meetings, activity groups, and occupational therapy groups were held together. Patients were encouraged to know their staff members as well as each other. This program was responsible for the deinstitutionalization of many otherwise forgotten people.

Only small proportions of older persons live in institutions—about five percent in the United States. The sad element of this process is that it is often irreversible: Institutions for the aged are seldom rehabilitative, and once the older person begins custodial care, he rarely returns to an independent state. The older individual in his own home who forgets to take his medication, whose special diet is not followed, who forgets to

turn off the gas, and who seems unable to handle his money may be thought by nurses and other helping persons to be better off in an institution. There are two schools of thought on this point: Some urge institutionalization, and others recommend it only as a last resort. What do we gain by having a well-fed older person in a communal dying house who loses his will to live? From a humanitarian point of view, even in the most cluttered and unsanitary hovel a person can maintain the identity and self-concept that are lost in an institution.

Older people who begin to lose their memory and ability to care for themselves are often aware of the drawbacks of institutionalization and sometimes delay getting needed medical care in fear of being "put away in a home." Once the older person leaves his home for a hospital, he feels he has less and less to say about his own destiny. Some older persons, aware of this process, may finally agree to enter a hospital but will then sign themselves out after two or three days. Others, persuaded by family members to leave their houses and live in custodial institutions, simply leave them and return to their former homes. One man, aged ninety, sent to a convalescent home in a nearby county, was visited by his older friend. This friend had to make the trip a day's journey, taking the bus and walking. On his arrival, he found his friend without his teeth, mumbling, and wanting to leave. The physician did not return the friend's call. So the friend rang up someone with a car and took the old patient home to his apartment. Another incident occurred at one convalescent home where a volunteer, touched by an old man's wish to return to his home, was apprehended pushing him rapidly down the street in his wheelchair.

NURSING HOMES. The question of institutionalization is a family crisis and various children hesitate to be the one to insist on it. Sometimes inheritance of property is a big issue and a deterrent to action because of fear of being disinherited. Approximately one million older people now live in nursing homes. The federal government began to pay for nursing-home care in the 1960s and nursing homes have rapidly become a lucrative business. Through Medicare and Medicaid two types of nursing homes re-

[20] Associate superintendent, Napa State Hospital, and later, senior psychiatrist, Napa State Hospital. It is noteworthy that Dr. Oliver, as he approached retirement age, asked for a demotion so he could work directly with older people. A highly professional psychiatrist, he was dedicated to the improvement of conditions in state hospitals.

ceive financial aid from the federal government: skilled nursing facilities and intermediate-care facilities. A skilled nursing facility administers nursing care under the supervision of a registered nurse. An intermediate-care facility provides more than board and care but less than a skilled nursing facility.

During the 1960s 30 percent of patients in state and county mental hospitals were over sixty-five years of age, whereas, now, 28 percent are sixty-five or over although the total number of patients has dropped markedly. Many older persons who formerly would have been in state and county mental hospitals are now in nursing homes. Nursing homes have a high mortality rate, as any local funeral parlor director can substantiate, and many patients die early in their stay in these places. The death rate following admission to an institution has been found by Lieberman (1961) to be two and one half times higher than in the waiting period.

The Medicare programs under Title XVIII and the programs for help to older people in institutions for mental disorders under Title XIX reinforce the efforts for local care in the older person's home community. Title XVIII discourages the use of state hospitals for long-term care; it facilitates the use of general hospitals, skilled nursing facilities, and services provided by home health agencies for the care of the mentally disordered older person. A limit is made upon the number of days that an older person can spend in a psychiatric hospital during his lifetime; however, no limit is made on the number of illnesses that one may be treated for in a general hospital. Each hospital must have a hospital utilization committee that reviews admissions; length of stay is noted as well as the care provided for each individual who remains over a long period of time. The legislation is aimed toward reducing the custodial elements of mental hospital care by requiring treatment plans and programs for each patient and the use of alternative facilities for hospitalization. It is directed toward securing a variety of sources of care within the home community and a reduction of mental hospital long-term care. For a state to qualify for medical assistance under Title XIX, certain standards must be met.

Medicare and Medicaid have given visibility to the problems of aging. Problems of development of preventive services and continuity of care are still with us. The issues of personnel shortage, and training of professionals in gerontology and geriatrics have not been solved. Problems of adequate nutrition, drug dependence, suicide, and adequate health-care delivery remain. Some populations at risk in older age are the poor, those without much education, some who are retired, bereaved, single, separated, divorced, socially isolated, the alcoholics, the physically ill, and those who have made suicidal attempts.

Many older people were formerly sent to state mental hospitals simply because the state paid for their care and the counties had not developed any alternative to state hospital care. A Geriatric Screening Program (Rypins and Clark, 1968) was established in 1963 in my own county to provide alternatives to state hospitalization. This practice was conceptualized by W. A. Oliver, M.D., formerly associate director of Napa State Hospital, Imola, California. In this program, a staff dedicated to helping older people find solutions to their problems saw the patients in their own homes. This practice was patterned after the Amsterdam plan originated by Professor A. Querido (1961). Sociopsychiatric nurses carried out precare and aftercare in the Amsterdam plan (Evans, 1968).

It is significant that the geriatric screening project, without being involved in the direct care, mobilized community services to come to the aid of the disturbed older people; 44 percent were able to be maintained in their own homes. Lieberman's study (1968) shows the deleterious effect of extensive change from residence in the community to an institution and transfer from one institution to another. He indicates that the crucial time for the person who needs institutional care is the waiting period before he is admitted. At least one other study indicates the hazards of relocation (Aldrich and Mendkoff, 1963). Nurses have an important job to do in this area: to help better prepare aging individuals and their families for accepting assistance. Older people in this country speak of the "poorhouse" and remember what happened to family and acquaintances before them; such images are not easily removed from their memory. If nurses have visited the nursing homes, they are in a better position to explain what life is like in these places.

A cross-cultural study by Kayser-Jones (1979) on the care of institutionalized older persons in Scotland and the USA found that Scottish individuals were more independent than their American counterparts due to the structure of the health care system and the institution. In Scotland, more emphasis was placed upon the older person making useful objects that they could give in exchange for services.

Nurses should see for themselves the conditions of a nursing home before referring any patient to it. Subsequent visits may be necessary to keep up with the changes. It is important to know if the home and administrator are licensed by the state and if the home is certified for financial assistance from the government.

In the selection of a nursing home, many factors should be taken into consideration: the nurse–patient ratio, staffing patterns, the quality of nursing care, the quality of the food, availability of linens, creative arts, beauty parlor, physical therapy, and the physician–patient ratio. Proximity to friends and relatives should be a major factor. Plants, table games, telephone, newspapers, clocks, calendars, and activities on major holidays are indicators of attempts to provide a humanistic environment. The number of patients out of bed is an additional indicator of caring. There is no substitute for a field visit to institutions to determine what they are like.

Institutionalization, although providing for the physiological needs of the aging, in many instances leaves much to be desired in the psychosocial realm. With institutionalization comes social impoverishment. The institutionalized older person may be cut off from his past and cared for by people who have little understanding of what life was like for him. There is likely to be little interpersonal behavior among peers when aged people are in institutions. Apathy therefore easily occurs, and regression is in full swing. With lack of a future perspective, depression is widespread. An imposed constriction of activities resulting in withdrawal from other activity leads any adult to preoccupation with himself. Institutional practices may reinforce regression or immature behavior to aid in the passive adaptation to institutionalization. The aged woman with her hair tied with a child's ribbon is one example and use of first names by nurses who are fifty or sixty years younger is another. Making all decisions for patients is one of the most lethal. A study by Langer and Rodin (1976) on the relationship between attitude and ability to make choices showed significant increases in alertness and activity for the group that made decisions for themselves, whereas the attitude of the group without control over choices decreased in alertness and activity. Older people in institutions are like displaced persons without hope of ever finding another place to live. The most critical period of adaptation and adjustment is in the first few months of institutionalization. Encouraging ventilation and offering control over choices cannot be overemphasized as part of nursing care of the older person in institutions.

ORIENTATION. Efforts by nurses to maintain orientation[21] can aid in healthy adaptation. The use of clearly visible calendars and clocks in rooms and lounges helps residents to maintain contact with time. Daily hometown newspapers help them to keep in touch with the events of their community.

Provision of recreational facilities aids the institutionalized person to better deal with his time and television helps those who enjoy it. Music can aid the older person in catharsis where earlier and happier times are evoked by hearing a familiar tune. All can now have their own radio or television, complete with earphones for individualized listening. At other times, watching universally liked programs such as the news in a communal lounge encourages socialization and is an area where current affairs can be discussed with others. If childhood table games are available, some older people will spend hours at these pursuits. Many institutions, newly built, are unknown to older people. Knowing their location and who owns and operates them helps the older resident to maintain orientation as to where he is.

Acknowledgement of birthdays aids in maintaining identity. Nurses should find out about the life of each person and acknowl-

---

[21] Orientation refers to awareness in three spheres— time, place, and person.

edge to him some of his earlier achievements; encourage him to air his feelings about who he is and where he is. Bridging the gap between him and other residents through introductions and telling each a bit about the other may help the new resident to find a new friend. Grouping people together in the dining room who have similar interests and who know others in common is also important. Keeping one's clothes and some belongings and arranging these as desired within one's own room aids in the maintenance of some autonomy, which is essential to mental health. Use of the telephone as a means of contact with the outside world, for both incoming and outgoing calls, is of central importance in the retention of sense of self. The institutionalized older person with decreasing emotional response needs to be encouraged to telephone others. Suggesting that he do so may be the impetus that he needs. Helping to get stationery and stamps and writing letters for those who are unable to do so themselves may result in their receiving much desired mail.

Increased preoccupation with body responses can be diminished by listening to patients, investigating and assessing complaints, but also discussing something else. If the older person can make decisions about himself and his needs, the institution should encourage him to do so. If he has hope for return to an independent life, he will probably be more motivated toward autonomy than the individual who has no hope for independence. You may sometimes have to listen to the recital of malfunctions of each organ of the body before being able to move on to other subjects.

Some homes for the aging regularly have open houses and other programs that interested persons can attend, thereby seeing for themselves what it is like to live there. Older people can be helped to make a plan for themselves if infirmity comes. Human beings can adapt to great stresses in a more effective way if they have some time and help to prepare for them. Use of the *reportorial* approach here is useful; i.e., the nurse can freely speak of what another person has done in preparation for the time when he can no longer manage things on his own. Older well-known national figures who are going through illness, hospitalization, and infirmity can form the basis for preparation for accepting help. If the nurse is familiar with the peer group of the older person, talking about what plans others have or have not made for their helplessness aids the individual to come to terms with his own plans. Asking the older person to think about his parents and other older relatives often is of assistance in aiding the individual to come to terms with his inability to do the things he once was able to do quite freely.

CONSTRICTION

Because of the mental and sensory changes caused by aging in the individual, his circle of movement is likely to become constricted in some manner. Thought, movement, and activities are necessarily changed by the process of aging. Individuals who have been resourceful in their earlier years are likely to be more able to draw upon these resources in older age than those who lack them. Those who are financially better off and those with good education are also more likely to be able to avoid mental constriction. Patterns of involvement in early life may continue in the older phase— for example, membership in clubs or organizations. These continuing memberships may widen the horizons of older people and aid them in the establishment of an explicit affiliation with their age group.

Illness and infirmity are two conditions that cause constriction. The aging process itself produces changes in the sensory, motor, and mental activities of the individual. Arthritis, which is very common in older people, limits activity. One older woman, Mrs. S., depressed because of her physical decline, prayed every day that "the good Lord take me." Many older persons may have as many as four or more chronic diseases. The adaptations that older people must make because of illness may add to a diminishing circle of activities.

Pets and Plants. In the lives of older people, pets and plants may assume great importance; they often become totems to older people. The nonhuman environment may become more important to the older person than ever before. The caged bird can be identified and sympathized with due to the fact that it also is a prisoner and unable to fly freely about the earth. Parrots can also be taught words to greet others who enter the home. Cats and dogs, although more expensive to care for, like to be caressed and cuddled, and they show steady affection.

Animals may become substitutes for affection for deceased spouses, especially if the animal was also a pet of the deceased. They demand care and make the person feel needed when they greet him on his return home. They also listen and give the older person the feeling of being understood. Plants are also alive and thrive under a careful green thumb. They grow, reproduce, and die. Mrs. A. spoke of removing leaves from the mother plant, planting the small leaves while the mother plant then died. She spoke of the mother plant doing work and not being needed any more, as if she were symbolically speaking of her own situation.

Cumming and Henry conclude that "disengagement is an inevitable process in which many of the relationships between a person and other members of society are severed and those remaining altered in quality."[22] Levine (1969) studied the relationship between the abandonment of life's central roles and disengagement. In this study, disengagement was defined as decreased interaction between the aging individual and others in his social system. Levine showed that older persons have severed many of their relationships with other people; their low morale was found to be connected with living alone, widowhood, and retirement.

On the other hand, Clark and Anderson's study (1967) did not find that acceptance of decreased social involvement in old age and willful disengagement from the social system was adaptive. Instead, it concluded that social engagement is more clearly related to psychological well-being and that without social contacts older persons become anxious and pessimistic.

[22] Cumming, Elaine, and Henry, W. E.: *Growing Old—The Process of Disengagement.* New York: Basic Books, Inc., 1961. p. 211.

EXPLANATION

When misfortune occurs and the older person cannot find an acceptable explanation for what has happened to him, he is in the crisis of explanation. The inability to explain the misfortune rather than the misfortune itself creates the crisis. This can happen to people who have not given any serious conscious thought to aging; they do not think of themselves as old.

The crisis of explanation was described by Kastenbaum (1964) as occurring when a person finds himself old and different from earlier years but cannot find any reason for it. It is the inability to explain the misfortune of old age. In this crisis the individual is faced with the very difficult task of explaining to himself and others that he is "not what he used to be" or is not, like the motto of one man's club in London, "the older the bolder."

The following is an example of an individual experiencing the crisis of explanation and the beginning of its resolution.

D.F. aged seventy, is dressed in tattered light blue faded denims with patches and an old studded denim jacket. He wears a rather long black wig and dyes his mustache black. He also wears several ornate rings and an old red beret. A certified public accountant all of his working years, and in good health since retirement, he has suddenly abdicated family, home, friends, church, familiar surroundings and activities and now spends much of his time as a street artist selling macrame. He frequents the local café where the young people hang out and stays out until the wee hours of the morning. A widower for several years, he now lives with his son, daughter-in-law, two granddaughters, and a grandson. He insists that they all call him by first name, sees very little of them, and when he does see them refuses the role of father and grandfather. On a series of home visits to assess the needs of the family, the nurse observed the tense family relationships, the exhausted appearance of Mr. F.; she gained rapport and guided him to speak for himself. Mr. F. had not accepted the fact of his advancing age. The nurse helped him, through a discussion of the ages of man and developmental tasks faced by all, to take a new look at himself and his family relationships. He subsequently renewed his generational role with his family and began to assist the grandson with his stamp and coin collection, slept better, and was more at peace with himself.

DESOLATION

The crisis of desolation, which may begin in middle age, continues until one's death. Desolation has been described by Townsend (1963) as being the underlying reason for loneliness in old age. He defined it in terms of deprivations by death, illness, or migration of the company of someone who is loved, e.g., a spouse or a child. Other dimensions may be added such as the requirement of the older person himself to change his ecological unit. For example, having to move from a condemned hotel or from an area that is being redeveloped or giving up a home for institutional living as in a nursing home. Desolation is expressed by many as: "I'm the only one left, all the others are dead." Or (speaking of a spouse), "I never thought she would die before me." One older person, Mr. M., who now lives in an area of the city formerly heavily populated by the Irish, said: "They are all dead now. Their children have moved away, and I have lost contact with them. There is no one to help me. There is no Irish mayor, and there is no one on the board of supervisors who is Irish. I don't know who to ask for help."

Relocation of older people from their familiar areas of the city can result in desolation since they can no longer visit old friends and familiar places.

Parents and siblings die, and desolation may be intensified if the individual himself has no progeny.

LONELINESS

. . . man can fulfill himself only if he remains in touch
with the fundamental facts of his existence, if he
can experience the exaltation of love and solidarity,
as well as the tragic fact of his aloneness and of the fragmentary character of existence.[23]

Loneliness has been described as a "state of mind in which hope that there may be

[23] Fromm, Erich: "Alienation Under Capitalism," in Josephson, Eric and Mary: *Man Alone: Alienation in Modern Society.* New York: Dell Publishing Co., 1963, p. 71.

interpersonal relationships in one's future life is out of realm of expectation or imagination" (Fromm-Reichman, 1959). To be lonely is to be without the feeling that someone cares. Loneliness can occur at any time throughout the life cycle, but it is intensified in adolescence, early adulthood, and old age. It can be felt by émigrés and has been referred to as "cultural shock" by anthropologists. Loneliness felt upon the death of a loved one or by the dying person himself can be very intense. In the era of the organization person, it can be felt when one loses one's place through retirement.

One older person, Mrs. P., expressed her loneliness thus: "You come and visit me any time. You know when I start talking, I am just like a record, I can't stop. You know, the telephone doesn't ring very often." She had just spent forty-five minutes explaining in detail her sister's stroke, subsequent hospitalization, and condition at this time, all staccato without stopping for a pause.

Loneliness is felt by everyone at some stage of life. Nurses can help older people lessen this feeling by being interested in them, caring about them, and sharing the thoughts of their generation with them. Some young people in our society have never really talked with an older person. Although the mass media now act to keep older people in touch with the times, contact with others in the younger age group may be tenuous or nonexistent. Visiting with older people, showing care and concern for them, can aid in overcoming loneliness (Evans, 1969). Since people in the older age group are populations at risk in terms of being vulnerable to mental disorder, attention to their psychosocial needs and care is primary prevention. The interpersonal relationship is a means by which loneliness can be conquered.

Senior centers are places in which older persons can meet, plan interesting activities, and maintain usefulness and worth. Group work with older persons further encourages interpersonal well-being. Senior centers provide a place where one is known, expected, and missed when absent. When one is lonely, helping someone else may help relieve the pangs of loneliness. The Foster Grandparents idea is in this direction as are the organized helping groups within senior centers where homebound persons telephone others who live alone, at a designated time every day, just to see how they are and if they need anything. Those who are healthier may organize monthly meetings and programs for the homebound themselves in which the Red Cross offers transportation to and from the centers.

Monthly birthday parties are given in the centers, and all who have a birthday in that month have a group party and cake. Each is therefore recognized and remembered. During holidays, when loneliness may become almost unbearable, members of senior centers may cook their dinner together or reserve a large banquet hall in downtown restaurants for this occasion.[24]

DEATH

Older people are most likely to be the age group where death is thought of rather frequently and openly and freely discussed. To die and not to die alone is a central issue of humankind and especially for the person of later maturity who lives alone and ponders about dying and the possibility of his death not being discovered for a long time. The beginning of grief and mourning for one's own death occurs in later maturity. Reading the obituaries becomes a daily habit, and interest in the details of funerals is manifest. One older widow, Mrs. L., went to the funeral parlor and to all the funerals in her parish for several years, even though many of the deceased were strangers to her.

Funerals are important ceremonies in our culture and serve as social events as well as farewells to the deceased. Comments are made on the "natural look" of the dead, cards are read, and floral arrangements counted to determine which family and friends "remembered." The coffin is scrutinized for quality and cost, and comments are made on whether the children thought

enough of the deceased to "put him away nice." Younger men are called upon to be pallbearers because the older ones are often too infirm to do the required lifting. Mourners view other mourners and wonder who will be next. Funerals bring to mind the need for preparation for one's own demise, and subsequent visits to the graveyard spur those remaining to write their own epitaphs.

To know that someone will mourn for them and to have an effect on younger people meet the need for *creative expansion* (Buhler, 1962)[25] in older people. Memorials may be established before death in the form of buildings and foundations, if the person is wealthy. For others, knowledge that one can live on in his progeny and in the memories of others may suffice. Most older people have mementoes of their past that they like to share with others. Helping them to decide to whom to leave their things is an important part of preparation for death.

Nurses can assist the elderly individual to arrange for a funeral suitable to his income and help him to talk about his own death. Every funeral director has an inexpensive funeral service if one demands it and refuses the four-car cortege and other expensive items. The return to the use of the plain pine coffin is refreshing. Some nurses may find the subject acutely uncomfortable and avoid it by keeping busy with other things. (This was a central finding of a study by Glaser [1966] of nurses in hospital settings.) Noting expressive symbols of religion in the immediate environment of the older person may help to raise the subject of whether the older person believes in an afterlife. In previous years it was commonly thought that the elderly immersed themselves in religion in preparation for death. While some may certainly do this, many, on the other hand, may feel that they have gone to church enough and now pray

[24] An excellent publication—Vickery, Florence B.: *Creative Programming for Older Adults: A Leadership Training Guide.* New York: A.C.S.W. Press, 1972— is a guide for professional and volunteer leaders of social-activity programs for older people. The author did some of the pioneer work during her twenty years with older people at the San Francisco Senior Center (1947–1967).

[25] Buhler described the tendency toward creative expansion first occurring in the child at about eight months. The child begins to realize his own potentialities and will choose a toy that he can do the most with—e.g., a rattle that he can swing best. Although Buhler describes old age as a contracting tendency, I think creative expansion continues as long as there is life.

at home. Many attend several churches or go to the churches of their friends. Clark's study (1967) of aging people in San Francisco supports this.

At the end of life, in this age group, the most that one can do is to help in the preparation for death, to provide as much comfort as possible, to stand by, and to be present when death comes. Would that the humanistic aspects of the hospice movement spread to nursing homes!

COMMUNICATION WITH OLDER PERSONS[26]

In communicating with older persons, conversations should deal with (1) something of the past, (2) something of the present, and (3) something of the future. Discussion of the past emphasizes times that the older person was perhaps more ego-oriented and involved.[27] Discussion of the present relates to how things are now, and discussion of the future relates to hope.

Older persons may not hear all you have to say; so speak slowly, use short sentences, enunciate clearly, and pause for response. Face-to-face communications will help those who have hearing problems. If they are in bed, position them to face you. All aspects of therapeutic communication apply in your relationships with older people (see Chap. 4).

There are various aids and devices available to help compensate for failing sight and hearing. For example, a flashing light on the telephone for the hard-of-hearing draws his attention to the instrument. Special earphones for television sets amplify sound for the viewer who watches with others. Amplifiers for telephone conversations help, as do lip-reading classes given by various adult-education programs. Hearing aids and eyeglasses assist many older people to maintain social contacts.

Telephone visits are often welcome and very much enjoyed if they are timed appropriately. A bedtime hour of 8:00 P.M. or even earlier is quite common for older persons. Letters and cards for special holidays and other events are symbols of love to older people who may receive very little mail.

Discussion of all the little things that happen in life aids in health maintenance. Having a confidant helps relieve loneliness.

The use of touch is essential; shaking hands as you come and go aids communication. Effective communication is also achieved through control of the complexity, timing, and amount of communication. A topic that requires serious consideration should be mentioned at the beginning of a contact so that all facets of it can be reviewed. If an older person brings something to you that you cannot handle, help him get assistance elsewhere. For the older individual, anticipating a visit, the visit itself, and thinking about the visit help overcome loneliness.

Blocks to communication with the older individual include your own attitudes and feelings. Persons in the therapeutic role are sometimes irritated that they must shout to be heard. There may be difficulty in acceptance of limited goals and the fact that very small things mean so much and count a lot in therapeutic care. There may be a feeling of futility that change is not possible. Stereotypes may block us in that we expect an older person to behave in a certain manner.

Table 4. Stereotypes of Older People

- Most are in their second childhood
- Most live in the past
- Most are hypercritical of youth
- Most are sick and helpless
- Most are confused and live in institutions
- Most are set in their ways and cannot change
- Most have no sexual desires

Our feelings about parent–child or grandparent–grandchild get in the way. This is called countertransference.[28] It may be difficult to accept the social, physical, psycholog-

[26] The reader is referred to Chapter 4 for concepts of therapeutic communication.

[27] In later years, the ego has less energy to involve in activities outside the self; there is a decreased investment in living in that gratifications tend to be more vicarious than direct (Rosen and Neugarten, 1960).

[28] Countertransference refers to the conscious or unconscious reaction of the nurse toward the patient, as if he were a significant other in the nurse's earlier life. It is a temporary identification with the patient.

ical, and economic dependency that one sees in aging. Attitudes of professionals toward older people have often been developed by contact with those whose symptoms have been labeled as being due to senility with the feeling that nothing can be done.

In working with older people, it is important to "fan the flame" that keeps the ego organized in order to help maintain the sense of self for as long as it exists.

Summary

This chapter emphasizes the psychosocial developmental tasks and stage-specific crises for the phases of the life cycle from infancy through old age, with special emphasis upon old age. Some major aspects of developmental theory are included. Crisis is presented in terms of the expected and the unexpected. As nursing is involved with the care of individuals from womb to tomb, knowledge of life's crises is required for quality nursing care. Some of the crisis points in each developmental phase are included here to aid the nursing student to recognize these crises so that help can be given to patients and families in the attainment of developmental tasks, in life's crises, and in early crisis resolution. Examples of patients with problems in the phase-specific periods exemplify the theory.

References

ACTION: "Action Housing's Woodcutting Project." *Aging,* Nos. 289–290, November–December, 1978, p. 42.

AIKEN, LEWIS: *Later Life.* Philadelphia: W. B. Saunders Company, 1978, p. 144.

ALDRICH, C. K., and MENDKOFF, E.: "Relocation of the Aged and Disabled: A Mortality Study," *Journal Geriatrics Society,* 11:3, March 1963.

American Psychiatric Association: *A Psychiatric Glossary.* Washington, D.C.: American Psychiatric Association, 1975.

ANDERSON, BARBARA GALLATIN: Death as a Subject of Cross-Cultural Inquiry. Paper presented at the First International Congress of Social Psychiatry, London, 1964.

BECKETT, SAMUEL: *Krapp's Last Tape and Other Dramatic Pieces.* New York: Grove Press, 1960.

BERNFELD, SIEGFRIED: Notes taken from case presentation, 1951.

BETTELHEIM, BRUNO: *The Empty Fortress.* New York: The Free Press, 1967, p. 427.

———: The Uses of Enchantment: *The Meaning and Importance of Fairy Tales.* New York: Alfred A. Knopf, 1976.

BOGUE, DONALD J.: *Principles of Demography.* New York: John Wiley & Sons, 1969.

BOWLBY, JOHN: A Two-Year-Old Goes to the Hospital. *The Psychoanalytic Study of the Child,* 7:82–94. New York: International Universities Press, 1952.

———: *Attachment and Loss. Vol. I.: Attachment.* New York: Basic Books, Inc., 1969.

———: *Attachment and Loss. Vol. II.: Separation; Anxiety and Anger.* New York: Basic Books, Inc., 1973.

BUHLER, CHARLOTTE: *Values in Psychotherapy.* New York: The Free Press of Glencoe, 1962.

BULBULYAN, AGAVNI: "One Aspect of Psychiatric Nurses' Participation in Community Mental Health Program: School Phobic Children," in *ANA Clinical Sessions.* New York: Appleton-Century-Crofts, 1967, pp. 164–71.

BUTLER, ROBERT N.: "The Life Review: An Interpretation of Reminiscence in the Aged," in Neugarten, Bernice L.: *Middle Age and Aging,* Chicago: University of Chicago Press, 1968, pp. 486–96.

———: "Old Age," in Arieti, Silvano, ed.: *American Handbook of Psychiatry,* Vol. I, New York: Basic Books Inc., 1974, pp. 646–61.

———: *Why Survive? Being Old in America.* New York: Harper & Row, Publishers, 1975.

——— and LEWIS, MYRNA, I.: *Aging and Mental Health: Positive Psychosocial Approaches,* 2nd ed. St. Louis: C. V. Mosby Company, 1977.

CADDEN, VIVIAN: "Crisis in the Family" in Caplan, Gerald: *Principles of Preventive Psychiatry.* New York: Basic Books, Inc., 1964, pp. 288–96.

CAPLAN, GERALD: *An Approach to Community Mental Health.* New York: Grune and Stratton, 1961, p. 18.

———: *Principles of Preventive Psychiatry.* New York: Basic Books, Inc., 1964, pp. 40–41.

CARP, FRANCES M. ed.: *The Retirement Process.* Washington, D.C.: Superintendent of Documents, 1968, pp. 1–26.

CLARK, MARGARET, and ANDERSON, BARBARA GALLATIN: *Culture and Aging.* Springfield, Ill.: Charles C. Thomas, 1967.

CUMMING, ELAINE, and HENRY, W. E.: *Growing Old—The Process of Disengagement.* New York: Basic Books, Inc., 1961.

————: "New Thoughts on the Theory of Disengagement," in Kastenbaum, Robert, *New Thoughts on Old Age.* New York: Springer Publishing Co., 1964.

EMERSON, RALPH WALDO: "Self Reliance," in Lindeman, Edward C.: *Basic Selections from Emerson.* New York: A Mentor Book, 1954, p. 54.

ENGEL, GEORGE L.: *Psychological Development in Health and Disease.* Philadelphia: W. B. Saunders Co., 1962, p. 134.

ERIKSON, ERIK H.: *Childhood and Society.* New York: W. W. Norton & Co. Inc., 1963, pp. 247–84.

————: *Identity: Youth and Crisis.* New York: W. W. Norton & Co., Inc., 1968, p. 96.

EVANS, F. M. C.: "Visiting Older People—A Learning Experience," *Nursing Outlook,* 17:3:20–23, 1969.

————: *The Role of the Nurse in Community Mental Health.* New York: Macmillan Publishing Co., Inc., 1968.

FARMBOROUGH, FLORENCE: *Nurse at the Russian Front: A Diary 1914–18.* London: Constable, 1974, p. 139.

FLAVELL, JOHN H.: *The Development Psychology of Jean Piaget.* New York: Van Nostrand Rheinhold Company, 1963.

FREUD, SIGMUND: "The Ego and the Id." *Standard Edition of the Complete Psychological Works of Freud,* Vol. XIX, London: The Hogarth Press, 1961.

————: "Mourning and Melancholia," *Standard Edition of the Complete Psychological Works of Freud,* Vol. XIV, London: The Hogarth Press, 1957, pp. 243–58.

FROMM, ERICH: "Alienation Under Capitalism," In Josephson, Eric and Mary: *Man Alone: Alienation in Modern Society.* New York: Dell Publishing Co., Inc., 1962.

FROMM-REICHMAN, FRIEDA: "Loneliness," *Psychiatry,* 22:1–16, 1959.

GLASER, BARNEY: *Awareness of Dying.* Chicago: Aldine Publishing Co., 1966.

GOLDSMITH, WILLIAM, and ZEITLIN, MAURICE: "Don Quixote and Dr. Caplan," *Exchange,* November/December, 1937, pp. 3–7.

GOODMAN, LOUIS S., and GILMAN, ALFRED, eds.: *The Pharmacological Basis of Therapeutics,* 4th ed. New York: Macmillan Publishing Co., Inc., 1970, p. 1546.

GORMAN, WARREN: *Body Image and the Image of the Brain.* St. Louis: Warren H. Green, 1969, p. 104.

Group for the Advancement of Psychiatry, Committee on Aging: *Toward a Public Policy on Mental Health Care of the Elderly,* Vol. 7, Report #9, 1970.

HAVIGHURST, ROBERT J.: *Human Development and Education.* New York: Longmans, Green and Co., 1953.

————: "The Leisure Activities of the Middle-Aged," *American Journal of Sociology,* 63:152–62, 1957.

————: *Summary of Social Security Amendments of 1972 as Approved by Conferees,* Washington, D.C.

JOHNSON, ADELAIDE M., FALSTEIN, E. I. SZUREK, S. A., and SVENDSEN, MARGARET: "School Phobia," *American Journal of Orthopsychiatry,* 11:702, 1941.

KASTENBAUM, ROBERT: *New Thoughts on Old Age.* New York: Springer, 1964, p. 318.

KAYSER-JONES, JEANIE: "Care of the Institutionalized Aged in Scotland and the United States: A Comparative Study," *Western Journal of Nursing Research,* 1:3:190–200, 1979.

KENISTON, KENNETH: "Drug Use and Student Values," in Hollander, Charles, ed.: *Background Papers on Student Drug Involvement,* United States National Student Association, 2115 S. Street, NW, Washington, D.C., 1967.

————: "Psychological Development and Historical Change," in Rabb, Theodore K., and Rotberg, Robert I., eds: *The Family in History: Interdisciplinary Essays.* New York: Harper & Row, Publishers, 1971, p. 152.

KOHLBERG, LAWRENCE: "Development of Moral Character," in Hoffman, Martin, and Hoffman, Lois Wladis, eds.: *Review of Child Development Research.* Vol. 1., New York: Russell Sage Foundation, 1964, pp. 383–431.

KREPS, JUANITA M.: The Allocation of Leisure to Retirement," in Carp, Frances M., ed.: *The Retirement Process,* Washington, D.C.: Superintendent of Documents, 1968, pp. 137–45.

KRIS, ERNST: "Notes on the Development and on Some Current Problems of Psychoanalytic Child Psychology," in Eissler, Ruth, et al., eds.: *The Psychoanalytic Study of the Child,* Vol. V. New York: International Universities Press, Inc., 1950, p. 31.

LANGER, B. J., and RODIN, J.: "The Effects of Choice and Enhanced Personal Responsibility for the Aged: A Field Experiment in an Institutional Setting," *Journal of Personality and Social Psychology.* 34:191–198, 1976.

LEVINE, RHODA: "Disengagement in the Elderly—Its Causes and Effects," *Nursing Outlook,* 17:10:28–30, October, 1969.

LEVINSON, DANIEL J.: DARROW, CHARLOTTE N.; KLEIN, EDWARD B.; LEVINSON, MARIA H.; and McKEE, BRAXTON: *The Seasons of a Man's Life.* New York: Alfred A. Knopf, 1978.

LIEBERMAN, MORTON A.: "Psychological Effects of Institutionalization," *Journal of Gerontology,* 23:343–53, July 1968.

_____: "Psychological Correlates of Impending Death, Some Preliminary Observations," in Neugarten, Bernice L.: *Middle Age and Aging.* Chicago: The University of Chicago Press, 1968.

_____: "Relationship of Mortality Rates to Entrance to a Home for the Aged," *Geriatrics,* 16:515–19, 1961.

LINDEMANN, ERICH: "Symptomatology and Management of Acute Grief," *American Journal of Psychiatry,* 101:141–48, 1944.

_____ and DAWES, LYDIA G.: "The Use of Psychoanalytic Constructs in Preventive Psychiatry," in Eissler, Ruth, et al., eds.: *The Psychoanalytic Study of the Child,* Vol. VII. New York: International Universities Press, 1952, pp. 425–28.

MAHLER, MARGARET S.: "On Child Psychosis and Schizophrenia," in Eissler, Ruth, et al., eds.: *The Psychoanalytic Study of the Child,* Vol. VII. New York: International Universities Press, 1952, pp. 286–305.

_____: "On Sadness and Grief in Infancy and Childhood," in Eissler, Ruth, et al., eds.: *The Psychoanalytic Study of the Child,* Vol. XVI. New York: International Universities Press, 1961, p. 338.

MENNINGER, KARL: *The Vital Balance.* New York: The Viking Press, 1963.

NEUGARTEN, BERNICE L., and GARRON, D.: "The Attitude of Middle-Aged Persons Toward Growing Older," *Geriatrics,* 14:21–24, 1959.

National League of Nursing Education: *A Standard Curriculum for Schools of Nursing.* Baltimore: Waverly Press, 1917.

NIEBANCK, PAUL L.: "Knowledge Gained in Studies of Relocation," in *Patterns of Living and Housing of Middle-Aged and Older People.* Washington, D.C.: Superintendent of Documents, 1966.

OBERLEDER, MURIEL: "Emotional Breakdowns in Elderly People," *Hospital and Community Psychiatry,* 20:7:191–96, July 1969.

POTTER, RALPH: Notes taken from lectures on "Growth and Development from the Psychoanalytic Point of View," Napa State Hospital, Imola, Calif., 1962.

PIAGET, JEAN: *Genetic Epistemology.* New York: W. W. Norton and Co., Inc., 1970, p. 77.

_____: The Child and Reality: *Problems of Genetic Psychology.* New York: Grossman Publishers, 1973.

QUERIDO, PROFESSOR A.: "Mental Health Provisions in the Netherlands," National Federation for Mental Health, 1961.

RIBBLE, MARGARETHA ANTOINETTE: *The Rights of Infants,* 2nd ed. New York: Columbia University Press, 1965.

ROHWER, WILLIAM D., AMMON, PAUL R., and CRAMER, PHEBE: *Understanding Intellectual Development: Three Approaches to Theory and Practice.* Hinsdale, Ill.: The Dryden Press, 1974, p. 120.

ROSEN, JACQUELIN L., and NEUGARTEN, BERNICE L.: "Ego Functions in Middle and Later Years: A Thematic Apperception Study of Normal Adults," *Journal of Gerontology,* 15:1:62–67, January 1960.

SCHAFER, ROY: "The Loving and Beloved Superego in Freud's Structural Theory," in Eissler, Ruth, et al., eds.: *The Psychoanalytic Study of the Child,* Vol. XV, New York: International Universities Press, 1960, pp. 163–88.

SCHWAB, GUSTAVE: *Gods and Heroes.* New York: Pantheon, 1946.

SHANAS, ETHEL: "Family Help Patterns and Social Class in Three Countries," in Neugarten, Bernice: *Middle Age and Aging.* Chicago: The University of Chicago Press, 1968.

SMITH, WALLACE F.: *Preparing the Elderly for Relocation.* University of Pennsylvania, Institute for Environmental Studies, 1966.

SPENCE, DONALD L.: "Patterns of Retirement in San Francisco," in Carp, Frances M., ed.: *The Retirement Process.* Washington, D.C.: Superintendent of Documents, 1968.

_____: Notes taken from lecture "Psychiatric Problems of Aging," Mendocino, California, 1969.

SPITZ, RENE: "Hospitalism. An Inquiry into the Genesis of Psychiatric Conditions in Early Childhood," in Fenichel, Otto, et al., eds: *The Psychoanalytic Study of the Child,* Vol. 1. New York: International Universities Press, 1945.

State of California—Health and Welfare Agency: *California Mental Health Services Act.* Sacramento: California Office of State Printing, 1974.

STEVENSON, JOANNE SABOL: *Issues and Crises During Middlescence.* New York: Appleton-Century-Crofts, Inc., 1977.

SZALITA, ALBERTA B.: "Psychodynamics of Disorders of the Involutional Age," in Arieti, Silvano, ed.: *American Handbook of Psychiatry,* Vol. III. New York: Basic Books, Inc., 1966, pp. 69–74.

SZUREK, S. A., et al. in Szurek, S. A., and Berlin, I. N., eds.: *Training in Therapeutic Work with Children.* Palo Alto, Calif.: Science and Behavior Books, 1967, pp. 162–69.

Task Force of Prescription Drugs: *The Drug Users.* Washington, D.C.: U.S. Department of Health, Education, and Welfare, 1968.

TOWNSEND, PETER: *The Family Life of Old People.* Baltimore: Penguin Books, 1963.

TOYNBEE, ARNOLD: *Man's Concern with Death.* London: Hodder and Stoughton, 1968.

U.S. Bureau of the Census, 1970d. *Current Popu-*

lation Reports, Consumer Income. Washington, D.C.: U.S. Government Printing Office, p. 4.

———— 1970b. *Projections of the Population of the United States by Age and Sex.* Washington, D.C.: U.S. Government Printing Office.

————: *Statistical Abstract of the United States: 1973* (94th edition). Washington, D.C.:, 1973.

U.S. Department of Health, Education, and Welfare: Statistical Note 90. *Utilization of Psychiatric Facilities by Persons Under 18 years of Age,* United States 1971, Printed 1973.

————: Statistical Note No. 138. *Diagnostic Distribution of Admissions to Inpatient Services of State and County Mental Hospitals, United States, 1975.* Washington, D.C.: U.S. Government Printing Office, 1977, p. 1.

————: Statistical Note No. 148. *Changes in the Age, Sex, and Diagnostic Composition of Additions to State and County Mental Hospitals, United States 1969–1975.* Washington, D.C.: U.S. Government Printing Office, 1978, p. 1.

————: *FDA Drug Bulletin.* 9:1:2, February–March 1979.

U.S. Senate: *Developments in Aging, 1968. A Report of the Special Committee on Aging.* Washington, D.C.: Superintendent of Documents, 1969.

VICKERY, FLORENCE B.: *Creative Programming for Older Adults: A Leadership Training Guide.* New York: A.C.S.W. Press, 1972.

White House Conference on Aging, Washington, D.C., 1971: *Toward a National Policy on Aging: Proceedings.* Washington, D.C.: U.S. Government Printing Office, 1973.

WILNER, DANIEL M. WALKEY, ROSABELLE, and SHERMAN, SUSAN: "Psychological Factors in Housing for the Aged," in U.S. Department of Health, Education and Welfare, *Mental Health Program Reports No. 2,* Public Health Service Publication No. 1743. Washington, D.C.: U.S. Government Printing Office, 1968.

WILTSE, KERMIT: *Group Methods in the Public Welfare Program.* Palo Alto., Calif.: Pacific Books, 1963.

Suggested Readings

BENSON, EVELYN: "Care for the Elderly in Yugoslavia," *International Nursing Review,* 121:2:55–56, 1976.

————: "Observations on Health Care for the Elderly in the USSR," *Journal of Gerontological Nursing,* 4:5:18–20, October 1978.

BENSON, EVELYN R., AND MCDEVITT, JOAN Q.: "Know Your Community Resources," *Journal of Gerontological Nursing,* 4:2:20–24, June 1978.

BURNSIDE, IRENE MORTENSON, ed.: "Developmental Reactions in Old Age," in Kalkman, Marion E., and Davis, Anne J.: *New Dimensions in Mental Health Psychiatric Nursing.* New York: McGraw-Hill, 1974, pp. 177–200.

EBERSOLE, PRISCILLA PIERRE: "Reminiscing and Group Psychotherapy with the Aged," in Burnside, Irene Mortenson, ed.: *Nursing and the Aged.* New York: McGraw-Hill, 1976, pp. 214–230.

ERIKSON, ERIK, ed.: *Adulthood.* New York: W. W. Norton and Co., 1978.

GOULD, ROGER L.: "The Phases of Adult Life: A Study in Developmental Psychology," *American Journal of Psychiatry,* 129:5:521–531, November 1972.

————: *Transformations.* New York: Simon and Schuster, 1978.

LEAF, ALEXANDER: "Getting Old," *Scientific American,* 229:3:45–52, September 1973.

LOWENTHAL, MARJORIE FISKE, THURNHER, MAJDA, and CHIRIBOGA, DAVID: *Four Stages of Life: A Comparative Study of Women and Men Facing Transitions.* San Francisco: Jossey-Bass Publishers, 1975.

MOSES, DOROTHY, and LAKE, C. S.: "Geriatrics in the Baccalaureate Nursing Curriculum," *Nursing Outlook,* 16:4:41–43, July 1968.

NEUGARTEN, BERNICE L.: "Time, Age, and the Life Cycle," *American Journal of Psychiatry,* 136:7:887–894, July 1979.

VAILLANT, GEORGE E.: *Adaptation to Life.* Boston: Little, Brown and Co., 1977.

2

The Family

LEARNING OBJECTIVES / Persons studying this chapter should be able to:

1. Define the term family; name six dimensions of a family
2. Identify current changing trends in families; identify factors contributing to the change
3. Describe Spiegel's role theory including five sources of strain, the characteristics of role induction, and the process of role modification in families
4. Identify criteria for positive mental health of the individual
5. Identify eight basic conditions for survival, continuity, and growth of the family
6. Describe and discuss family develop-

ment, including eight stages of the family life cycle and developmental tasks for each stage
7. Define homeodynamics
8. Describe the following concepts as they relate to disturbed families:
   - Scapegoating
   - Marital schism and marital skew
   - Double-bind hypothesis
   - Pseudomutuality
   - Schizmogenesis
   - Schizophrenogenic mother hypothesis
   - Phantom family member
9. List major elements of data collection and assessment in family visits

Although other professionals have been concerned for many years with family work, it is only within the past twenty-five years that psychiatrists and psychiatric nurses have been involved in working with families. In order to be able to identify interaction within the family group, it is helpful to learn about healthy families. One way to do this is by getting involved with families without deviant members and studying them closely over an extended period of time. In family-centered nursing, it is essential to have a clear understanding of the constituents of health; the healthy family is the model that the family with mental disorder is attempting to achieve. Nursing students who learn current theories relating to processes within

families as well as that of individuals will be more effective practitioners.

The majority of people in the U.S.A. live in families. In 1977, of the 214,126,000 civilian population, approximately 76 percent were members of husband-and-wife families and 13 percent were members of other types of families (Metropolitan Life, 1978). The most significant change in living arrangements within the decade is the increase in households of persons living alone or with unrelated persons. The average household size declined from 3.14 to 2.86 in 1977. These changes reflect varying life styles and social attitudes of the era.

A family is defined as a group of two or more persons residing together and related by blood, marriage, or adoption. The family is composed of two or more generations and one cannot escape the generational boundaries. The family is also composed of persons of two genders who form a coalition as parents (Lidz, 1974). The child grows into and internalizes aspects of family and culture and is influenced by the ways that parents themselves have developed, accomplished their developmental tasks, and taken their places in society and their cultural group.

There are at least six dimensions of a family: (1) It is composed of individuals, each of whom has needs and expectations. (2) It is a group and must be viewed also in this dimension—the action of one individual has an effect on the entire family. (3) It is a primary group and as such is (usually) small, with considerable emotional involvement and shared goals. (4) It is the basic unit of society and thus must be studied in the context of the total social system. (5) It is a medium for transmission of values of the social system of which it is a part. (6) It has a geographical and occupational status, as is evidenced by the differences in urban and rural settings (Kluckhohn and Spiegel, 1954; Parsons, 1952 and 1964).

During 1970 to 1977 households headed by a family member declined from 80 percent to 76 percent. Husband-wife families increased by 8 percent; other families headed by a male decreased by 10 percent. The number of families headed by a female rose by 37 percent (Metropolitan Life, 1977).

Approaches to the Study of Families

The *developmental life cycle* approach to the understanding of healthy families is described by Duvall (1971). In this approach, expectations and tasks of the family as a group are presented.

The study of family process is important to the understanding of those conditions responsible for the mental health or mental disorder of its members. Some major approaches to the study of family processes are:

1. *Psychological*—Here, the family is considered from the viewpoint of the individual; the individual is helped through developing insight into the other members. Undergirded by psychoanalytic theory, Ackerman's work (1958, 1963, 1966) exemplifies this approach. Another view, i.e., learning theory, advocates working with the manifest behavior in the family group; behavior is changed through dealing with the "here and now" (Stuart, 1972).

2. *Communicational*—In this approach, communication patterns within the family group are considered independent of the individual members; for example, the communication theory of the double-bind (Bateson, 1956, 1958), and the theory of pseudomutality (Wynne et al., 1958).

3. *Ecological*—In this approach, the psychological aspects of individual family members are linked to the larger social and cultural systems; for example, in the work of Howells (1971) and Minuchin (1974).

4. *Symbolic Interaction*—This approach is based on the idea that a study of families must begin with the family members' perception of themselves. Analysis of family phenomena on the basis of internal processes, roles, status, relationships, communication, stress, and decision making is done through intensive interviews (Knafl and Grace, 1978, p. 11). Dating, courtship, married life, and parenting are examined in this approach. For example, multiple role expectations, ambivalences, management and control of social roles for the professional woman, and motherhood are examined (Cox, 1978).

5. *Transactional*—In this framework, the structural parts of a social system are viewed as a system of roles. This approach integrates the cultural, psychological, and sociological, and biological approach in a unified theoretical framework (Papajohn and Spiegel, 1975). The assumption is made that processes in these fields affect the individual and that change in one field is related to change in the other. Intrapsychic conflict thus can relate to social-role conflict and cultural conflict. In this framework, particular attention is given to the importance of varying cultural values, especially in relation to ethnic families. Important to the unified framework is role theory given in the following pages.

ROLE THEORY

Life-style refers to the ways in which families cope with needs, conflicts, and crises. Depending on how they resolve it, some families emerge from a crisis stronger; others become weaker. When the family as a group is threatened with disruption, there are several processes that restore the equilibrium. Spiegel (1957, 1971) delineates the following aspects of conflicts and restoration of equilibrium of the family group.

A frame of reference is necessary for the systematic observation of processes within families. In this section, some concepts related to role theory are introduced. The concepts are useful to study family processes.

ROLES

Role theory is based upon the assumption that a person inherently seeks relationships with objects and strives throughout life both consciously and unconsciously to develop a sense of personal identity. A fundamental idea in the study of the family system refers to description of the behavior of a person in his relations with others. Every role ties in with the role of another. In the nuclear family, there are fewer roles than in the extended family.[1] The basic roles of the nuclear family are mother, father, lover, child, spouse, brother, and sister. Role concepts may vary markedly within different cultural groups. The young Philippino woman in modern American society, expected by her parents to delay her marriage until the older sister is married, may experience considerable role and cultural conflict.

Complementarity is necessary for role integration. For any one person who holds a particular role in a group, there is a role partner. An example of the role of performer and the role of the listener follows: A grandmother invited her family to her piano concert. They gathered around her living room; she played some unpublished Schubert and just before the end of the

[1] The nuclear family refers to the smaller family of contemporary society in which there are at most two generations with conjugal parent–child and sibling relationships. Extended family refers to the two-generation nuclear family, plus either a third generation or relatives such as uncles and cousins.

piece, everybody began talking. In a loud voice, she exclaimed. "Quiet! *I'm* still the main person!" and restored the complementarity. All behavior in interpersonal relations has this idea of complementarity built into it. If complementarity is not maintained, disruption occurs within the family. Since no family remains the same for very long, it is likely that complementarity changes.

Following Spiegel (1957, 1971), value and role conflicts are connected with the acculturation process in families and family psychopathology. Observation in research and clinical work with families tie together the part that each person has to play in the family according to its cultural heritage and demonstrates that these roles have a potential for mental health or mental disorder.

In Spiegel's theory, role complementarity maintains the equilibrium; however, if the underlying conflict is avoided, complementarity is destroyed and *role distortion* occurs, which has two subcategories: (1) *role induction,* which evades the actual conflict, and (2) *role dislocation,* which shifts to each other or someone else the role that is the seat of the conflict. In order for complementarity to be restored, *role modification* must occur.

Sources of strain are the same in normal families as in disturbed families. Normal families tend to resolve conflict by role modification but disturbed families tend to use role distortion. In the study of families we attempt to identify what forces establish, maintain, or disrupt complementarity. Spiegel has described five sources of strain:

Cognitive. Individuals cannot carry out roles unless they know what is expected of them. Parents have to learn how to interpret cues from the child and to learn what to expect as children develop; likewise, the child also learns expectations as he matures. Knowledge of life's crises and what each phase has in store can help the individual within his family. Courses in marriage and family life, and parenting, for example, can assist in a smoother transition from familial limbo to the married state. Family conferences at periodic intervals also help individual members.

Conflict in Goals. Roles enable one to work toward goals, and if different goals are being pursued, conflict occurs and complementarity is lost. Agreement on mutual goals restores the equilibrium. Biological deficiencies and limitations also affect pursuit of goals, as do genetically determined and other handicapping conditions such as poverty, fatigue, and malnutrition.

Differences in Culture. How one is to behave as a husband or wife or parent may be different depending on the cultural background of each. Some parents plan ahead so much that a bank account is opened for an infant before it is born. We have been said to spend so much energy on planning for the future that we cannot enjoy the present. In the United States, cultural conflict is widespread. The American bride who expects to do the grocery shopping is surprised to find that her Persian husband insists that it is his job.

Instrumental. This strain is very marked in our money-oriented society if such necessities as money and transportation are lacking. Food, clothing, shelter, furniture, and money are necessary in our consumer society for individuals to carry out roles.

Allocative. In this scheme, roles are distributed throughout the family. Other major divisions of family roles are: (1) *formal,* (2) *informal,* and (3) *fictive.* Formal roles are stylized, visible, and easily identified by others; informal roles are not so visible and not so easily identified; and fictive roles are imaginary.

ASCRIPTIVE.   These roles are fixed as in age and sex (Parsons, 1964). No one can get out of an age or sex role without conflict. An older person cannot act young or a child act old without violating certain sanctions. Although surgery now permits some individuals to change their sex and transvestism is rather common, the conflicts can remain. In the ascriptive roles, there is no choice or control and these roles are formal.

ACHIEVEMENT.   For example, a person prepares himself for an occupation. This role requires effort, recognition of it, and it is a formal role.

ADOPTED.   In this instance, the person takes the role but does not have to do it. No one asks permission to do it. This is

an informal role. The older brother who adopts the role of protector toward a younger sibling is an example. If he can protect the sibling and be the hero in the action, he has both achieved and adopted the two roles.[2]

ASSUMED.   These roles are taken in jest or in play or as the result of a defect in reality testing. This is a fictive role. Play and jest relieve strict reality whereas delusions are defects in reality testing. Assumed roles have a vital part in family equilibrium because through play, cues can be responded to and tested out in moving toward change.

In role theory, equilibrium maintenance occurs via two major processes: role modification and role distortion. Role modification leads to healthy conflict resolution whereas role distortion does not. Role modification involves a mutuality of effort of the interacting partners to face their basic conflicts. It is based upon insight of the underlying conflict and involves a change in both parties to the conflict, whereas role distortion occurs when one person induces the other to conform to his expectations, i.e., role induction, or to shift his role, i.e., role dislocation. In role distortion, one of the other family members agrees with, submits to, or goes along with the role; one takes the complementary role without a change occurring and superficial equilibrium is restored. Role distortion is based upon manipulative techniques. It avoids the basic conflict and the conflict is therefore likely to reappear.

The following are grouped together as characteristic of role induction.

1. *Coercing.* One person forces the other to accept roles by threats or punishment. It may be neutralized by defiance.
2. *Coaxing.* Asking, promising, pleading, and begging. This involves the manipulation of rewards and may be neutralized by refusal.
3. *Evaluating.* Praising, blaming, shaming, approving, and disapproving. Some elements of this may be influenced by a per-

---

[2] See Haley, Alex: *The Autobiography of Malcolm X.* New York: Grove Press, 1964 (p. 24) for a vivid example of these roles.

fectionistic childhood of parents. "Stop behaving like you were born in a barn" and "In you former life, you must have been a pig" are typical comments. The specific neutralizing technique is denial.

4. *Masking.* Correct information is withheld or some other incorrect information is substituted. It includes behavior such as pretending and evading; unmasking is the neutralizing element. Spiegel (1957, p. 558) notes the belief that masking is as significant to the function of the social system as repression is to the function of the personality.

5. *Postponing.* Time permits changes to take place that solve the conflict. During this time, intrapsychic processes reduce tensions that bring about a change in attitude. "I'll think about it" is an example as is the old adage, "When in doubt, do nothing." Provoking is the specific neutralizing technique and incites the conflict to emerge.

6. *Role Reversal.* This can be the transitional point to role modification. One person puts himself in the position of the other and sees the other's point of view.

Because role induction is primarily defensive, the same conflict can occur repeatedly. it is like a process that treats the symptom instead of the disease. On the other hand, role dislocation can occur when the role partners try to solve the conflict by shifting to each other or someone else the role that is the basis of the conflict.

Role modification, which leads toward insight, begins with (7) *joking;* (8) *referral to a third party;* (9) *exploring* (this is the testing phase and describes the work of the helping person who is involved in assisting the family to find solutions to conflicts); (10) *compromising,* the phase in which parties to the conflict perceive the need for a change of goals; and (11) *consolidating,* learning how to make the compromises work. Roles are modified through redistribution of goals.

If role conflicts are present at the time of marriage, there is a greater possibility of role distortion occurring in the family instead of role modification. Role distortion is connected with psychopathology in a family member. It is difficult to discern and it may also affect the personalities of the others in the family unit.

The foregoing frame of reference provides a method for systematic observation of processes within families that may otherwise go unobserved. Miller's (1963) study of family dynamics was based upon these processes. Her primary emphasis was upon *masking,* which seemed to be the technique most often present in the family studied. In her paper, a dramatic picture was drawn of the deleterious effects of masking upon the mental health of the family.

In our present rapidly changing pluralistic society, roles and values have assumed a new importance and need to be understood by nurses working with families. No longer is the therapist confined to understanding intrapsychic conflicts; society and culture also have to be understood in relation to the conflict.

Family Dynamics

HOMEODYNAMICS

The change, interaction, growth, and adaptation to new conditions in interpersonal relations is referred to as *homeodynamics* (Ackerman, 1966). It refers to the addition of certain healthy dimensions to the self-image on a continuous basis. In contrast with homeostasis it is not aimed at the maintenance of a steady state but is directed, instead, toward a fluid state. In this context, intrapsychic and interpersonal patterns of organization are interrelated.

CONFIRMATION–DISCONFIRMATION

Related to the concept of homeodynamics is the concept of confirmation of the "self-other." It is the idea that people need people, that the person is a social being, and that we are what we are partly in terms of how others view us. In this context, Chagall said that one of his greatest sorrows is the fact that his parents were no longer around to see his success. Even after the death of parents, children are influenced by them in terms of what they would think of an idea, action, or situation were they still alive. Children often do things that they think their dead parent or parents would have preferred. Disconfirmation, on the other hand, does not permit the person to be himself. It refers to being denied existence by others. Family members have a powerful influence upon each other through the dynamic process of confirmation and disconfirmation. In disturbed families, children are often not called by their real names. Instead, they may be referred to as "pig," "stinkpot," or "a human garbage pail," which practice disconfirms the self.

MENTAL HEALTH OF FAMILIES

Families serve to provide reproduction, socialization of offspring, values, roles, tension management, emotional support, and communication. However, emotional neglect or emotional exploitation may occur. *A healthy family provides perception of needs of others, respect accorded to these needs, and satisfaction of them.*

MATERNAL DEPRIVATION

Today it is generally accepted by those working with families that one of the essential ingredients for mental health of the individual is ". . . that the infant and young child should experience a warm, intimate, and continuous relationship with his mother (or permanent mother-substitute) in which both find satisfaction and enjoyment."[3] A situation in which the child does not have this relationship is called maternal deprivation. Deprivation can be partial or rather complete; it can also occur in the presence of the mother.

Ainsworth et al. (1962), in a review of findings and controversy over what constitutes maternal deprivation and its effects, summarized the findings as follows: The effects of deprivation are now thought to be more reversible than they were in 1951, but cases of long-standing deprivation have

limited improvement. The conclusion remains that early deprivation is of such magnitude that all efforts should be made toward prevention. In Bettelheim's (1967) work with Joey, an autistic boy, it was discovered, after several years, that behind Joey's anger at his parents was not the bad things they did to him but the fact that they had not even cared enough to be "bad" (p. 259). At Joey's birth, his mother was so terrified at the new responsibility that all her emotions were bound up in controlling her anxiety. She did not want to see Joey because she felt he was more than she could manage. Although parental deprivation as with the case of Joey is possible, emphasis is placed upon the mother figure because she is most likely to be the one to care for his needs in our culture.

Two cases of extremely isolated children demonstrate the effect upon an individual of lack of social influence. Both children were illegitimate and had been hidden away and given little attention from anyone for about six years. Both acted like infants and were without speech (Davis, 1948).

BASIC NEEDS OF INDIVIDUAL MEMBERS

Many of the basic needs of individuals are met in families. Levels of need have been classified by Maslow (1954), who put basic needs into the following hierarchy: (1) physiological, (2) safety, (3) love and belonging, (4) self-esteem, and (5) self-actualization. Another function of the family is to provide for the mental health of its members. The need to be secure can be provided by the family unit. Every child needs to learn to love and to be loved, something he can be taught within his family.[4] He can also gain a sense of belonging and can achieve impulse control from his family. Impulse control may be one of the most difficult things to teach disadvantaged children. They find it very difficult to delay gratification because of their many experiences in which they never had anything unless they took it when they first saw it.

The growing child needs to be accepted

---

[3] Bowlby, John: *Maternal Care and Mental Health.* Geneva: World Health Organization, 1952, p. 11.

[4] A provocative account of peer-group influence within the kibbutz and without the constant attendance of family members has been given by Bettelheim (1969).

for what he is at all phases of development and must receive personal recognition, both of which can be provided within the family. The need for expansion or achievement can be observed and commented upon, and facilities and materials can be provided for the child to develop his potentialities. Encouragement, approval, and other forms of emotional support can be given. Children need to belong to a group in which they share their experiences; the family can constitute such a group. Ego integration depends on awareness of one's own identity and self-assurance in knowing who one is. The family is the group that provides roles to carry out, tasks to perform, and reflection of the mirror-image self, all important in the identity maintenance that is the mainstay of mental health. It is thought by many mental health professionals that a secure childhood provides the individual with the necessary psychological armor for the remainder of this life.

CHARACTERISTICS OF POSITIVE MENTAL HEALTH

In assessing positive mental health of the individual members of a family, Jahoda's list of indicators is useful (1958). She synthesized psychological theory into six major points. How these characteristics are developed in the individual in infancy and childhood affect his life behavior. The first indicator of positive mental health relates to *the attitudes of an individual toward himself.* An objective view of the self, an acceptance of self including the high points and the shortcomings, and a sense of identity are included under this heading. Erikson's (1963) eight ages of the person include the crisis of identity versus identity diffusion (see Chap. 1, this book). The behavior of the individual, the phenomenal self, gives clues to the assessment of this characteristic. The child who knows who he is and who is secure in his family constellation will manifest this characteristic of positive mental health.

The second indicator is the individual's style and degree of *growth, development, and self-actualizing* as expressions of mental health. The psychosocial developmental milestones of the person described by Havig-

hurst (1953) and Erikson (1963) are measuring sticks for this indicator. Nonattainment of developmental tasks may result in maladaptation. The attention, interest, love, and other ingredients of a healthy family aid the individual child toward an adequate self-concept, which is a strong component of this characteristic. Conditions within the family can help each individual member meet his need for expansion and reach his highest potential.

The third indicator of positive mental health is a central synthesizing function or *integration* incorporating some of the two preceding aspects. Integration emphasizes an equilibrium of intrapsychic forces, a philosophy of life, and an ability to resist stress and tolerate anxiety.

The subsequent indicators are all a part of reality orientation. *Autonomy,* the fourth indicator, refers to the individual's independence from others. Although in infancy and early childhood the individual is totally dependent on others for sustenance and life, he moves rapidly toward independence. Autonomy refers to the ability to make a choice between different factors within situations. Autonomy versus shame and doubt has also been described by Erikson (1963) as the second stage-specific crisis that the person encounters. Singling out the person's degree of independence from social influences is most revealing of the state of his mental health; it is the ability to manage for oneself. The autonomous person is self-directed.

As the fifth indicator, mental health is also expressed in the *adequacy of the individual's perception of reality.* Perception of his environment as it is without distortion and supporting what he perceives are included under this heading, along with empathy or social sensitivity. Jahoda (1958) states that "the major requirement of the healthy person in this area is that he treat the inner life of other people as a matter worthy of concern and attention."[5] Moving from the real world to the unreal world is an indicator of mental disorder. Perception of reality is strongly influenced by culture, which must be included in the assessment of each

[5] Jahoda, Marie: *Current Concepts of Positive Mental Health.* New York: Basic Books, 1958, p. 52.

individual's mental health in relation to himself, his family, and to the social system to which he is attached.

The sixth criterion of positive mental health is *environmental mastery.* Inherent in this indicator is the ability to love and adequacy in love, other interpersonal relations, work, and play. The ability to meet the situational requirements of life, to adapt, adjust, and solve problems effectively are all aspects of this characteristic. Three dimensions of healthy problem solving are (1) an individual goes through the process and all the stages, (2) maintains an appropriate feeling tone, and (3) directs an attack on the problem. In a technological, industrial society, this indicator may become more and more complex. For example, toward the end of life, what does environmental mastery mean to the individual who is in retirement? The basic need to do purposeful work remains, yet there are many years left without employment for hundreds of thousands of older people in their retirement years. Retirement enforces a reduction in striving and therefore a redistribution of energy from work to new purposes.

SOME CHARACTERISTICS OF FAMILIES

The role of the family in the maintenance of mental health is crucial. In contemporary society, there is a downgrading of the authority of parents, currently referred to as the "generation gap." There is also a move toward an egalitarian family: More wives are working at public work than ever before and the traditional roles of men and women are merging. Men no longer return home after a day's work to evenings of leisure; they are expected to participate in recreation with children, help to care of them, and do housework. Margaret Mead said that husbands are so tamed domestically that they are losing their sense of adventure. There is a relative decrease in the authority of the father in the modern family. Economics play a part where women are educated, are working, and are financially independent as contrasted with a depressed economy where education and employment are scarce. In our money-oriented society, where the symbol of power is the dollar, the father often turns over all his earnings

to his wife to manage and carries only a few dollars in his pocket. The suburban husband is simply not present most of the time to discipline the children; thus, mother becomes the moral authority in the family. Even when he is present, there is now a deemphasis on discipline; both the parents and the children are "nice." Parental uncertainty is widespread, and there is hesitancy to set limits.

Students of the ecological revolution now advocate a shift from emphasis on procreation as a function of the family to the smaller or childless family. Many factors have contributed to our zero-population growth: changes in the role of women, contraception, legal abortions, a tendency toward childbearing at later ages, and a concern with overpopulation (U.S. National Commission for UNESCO, 1977). Knowledge of the effects of influences and changes within the smaller family remain for the future.

Because nursing students have their own opinions about what constitutes family life, attitudes toward unconventional living arrangements may interfere with objectivity. The nonjudgmental attitude of the professional does not develop overnight but has to be acquired gradually before one can be of much assistance to patients and families.

During my experiences with nursing students and their child psychiatric patients, some have been profoundly moved coming into contact with children who are unwanted by their parents, who may be suffering from the battered-child syndrome, or who evidence other types of neglect and abuse. New knowledge arises from contact with both nonconforming families and those exhibiting deviant behavior. Knowledge of the ways of life of different groups within one's own social system as well as those of other cultural groups aids in identification of healthy components of families as well as deviant behavior. Discussion with others also helps to foster self-understanding.

The decrease in importance of the grandparents is new in this society; the nuclear family often has no place for older people. Box houses, labor-saving devices, the pace of modern living, and facilities outside the home providing social and recreational activities for different age groups instead of group family activities contribute to lack of place for older family members. The time budget, so highly valued in our society, often does not include the older person. Vertical and horizontal mobility[6] tend to leave out the grandparents.

War has increased distances between people. In their travels, servicemen meet people wherever they are, and some marry and locate in a distant area instead of nearer to their own homes. The career military man and his family move many times from country to country, often at great distances from grandparents. These factors all contribute to the absence of interaction during ceremonies, holidays, and other times important to all, especially for the young; to the failure to establish family identity; and to the loss of a sense of connection with the past. For the older person, love, acceptance, belonging, and aid in meeting crises may not be so readily available as they can be for the young.

Interdependence, Independence, and Dependence. Although in the nuclear family older people may not live under the same roof as their children, patterns of mutual help and assistance remain as they exist in the extended family, where the generations live near each other. The family that does not have proximity to the older generations often forms peer-group associations in which members of other families become substitutes and are even exchanged temporarily (as in husband and wife swapping).

A national study of patterns of help to the elderly within families was found to relate to family size, structure, and living arrangements (Shanas, 1968). Shared living arrangements of older individuals differ by social class; middle-class white-collar parents in the United States are likely to live independently of and at some distance from their children.

The kinds of mutual aid given relate to general assistance during illness and other emergencies. Older people help by giving gifts, assisting with grandchildren, doing home repairs, gardening, and yard work,

and helping with the housework. In turn, the children help their parents by giving economic support, personal care, transportation, gifts, outings, and assistance with household chores (Shanas, 1968, p. 304).

In an earlier national study, it was found that less than 3 percent of persons over sixty-five preferred to live in institutions (Shanas, 1962). It was also found that almost all older people feared and were hostile to a move to an institution because it signified (1) loss of independence, (2) a prelude to death, and (3) rejection by children. On the psychological effects of waiting for institutionalization, the central position of the family in the world of the older person is supported (Prock, 1969). A cluster of characteristics of the waiting-list group was found to show that what had been termed "effects of institutionalization" actually occur before these people become residents of institutions. Helplessness, powerlessness, low interaction with others, depressed mood, low self-esteem, little hope for the future, disorganization of experience, low ego energy, tension, and anxiety were evidenced by the waiting-list group. Comparison of persons on and off a waiting list showed that for the waiting-list group "the intimacy and mutuality of family ties were decidedly weaker . . . ." (Prock, 1969, page 1841). This suggests an intrafamily disequilibrium and complements the work of Lieberman (see Chap. 1, this book) that the critical period of need for the older person who is to be institutionalized is within the six months or more preceding the institutionalization itself. Not only does the older person himself need help with his feelings, but the family must be helped to combat feelings of guilt, anger, ambivalence, helplessness, and powerlessness.

The contemporary family is a dependent consuming unit, different from the independent economic unit that existed in the past. The emphasis now is not so much on making something one's self (e.g., a toy or a garment) but to make enough money to buy these articles. Families are no longer held together by the necessity of cooperation in the maintenance of a life-style. More and more facilities are being developed that draw individuals away from family activities, thereby fragmenting togetherness.

---

[6] Vertical mobility refers to movement from one social class to another. Horizontal mobility is the movement from one place to another.

Since members of families are now mouths to feed instead of each contributing to the economic unit of the family, grandparents may also be viewed as consuming members. Children no longer have economic responsibilities in the family and thereby also assume the consumer role.

Family Developmental Tasks. To help the family with mental disorder, one needs a parallel concept of the healthy family. Psychological disruptions in families must be compared and contrasted with the functions, developmental tasks, and interactions of healthy families. Assessment, interaction, and communication therefore become the foci for the nurse.

Duvall (1971, p. 149) cites eight basic conditions for survival, continuity, and growth of the family: (1) *"physical maintenance; (2) allocation of resources; (3) division of labor; (4) socialization of family members; (5) reproduction, recruitment, and release of family members; (6) maintenance of order; (7) placement of members in the larger society;* and (8) *maintenance of motivation and morale."* In Duvall's developmental approach, tasks are growth responsibilities for eight stages of the life cycle and are shown in Table 5.

Alienation. In the contemporary middle-class family, there is an emphasis upon being sensible, talking things through, and being tolerant. Rebellion toward such a family is not easily accomplished. Therefore, new forms of rebellion have appeared, e.g., campus demonstrations, freer sexual practices, abuse of drugs, and dropping out of the

Table 5. Stage-Critical Family Developmental Tasks Through the Family Life Cycle*

Stage of the Family Life Cycle	*Stage-Critical Family Developmental Tasks*
1. Married couple	Establishing a mutually satisfying marriage Adjusting to pregnancy and the promise of parenthood Fitting into the kin network
2. Childbearing	Having, adjusting to, and encouraging the development of infant(s) Establishing a satisfying home for both parents and infant(s)
3. Preschool-age	Adapting to the critical needs and interests of preschool children in stimulating, growth-promoting ways Coping with energy depletion and lack of privacy as parents
4. School-age	Fitting into the community of school-age families in constructive ways Encouraging children's educational achievement
5. Teenage	Balancing freedom with responsibility as teenagers mature and emancipate themselves Establishing postparental interests and careers as growing parents
6. Launching center	Releasing young adults into work, military service, college, marriage, etc., with appropriate rituals and assistance Maintaining a supportive home base
7. Middle-aged parents	Rebuilding the marriage relationship Maintaining kin ties with older and younger generations
8. Aging family members	Coping with bereavement and living alone Closing the family home or adapting it to aging Adjusting to retirement

* Duvall, Evelyn Millis: *Family Development,* Philadelphia: J. B. Lippincott Co., 1971, p. 151, by permission.

culture that highly values "making it." What could irritate middle-class parents more than such behavior?

Our culture is marked by discord between the individual and the larger society—alienation, identity confusion, and the search for self through conformity. One effect of this is that the individual now depends more on the family group for self-renewal, acceptance, sense of self, and belongingness. Alienation from the larger society requires more tenderness and closeness from the nuclear family. To keep in touch with the psychic pulse of each of its members is an added task for the modern family. Is it able to provide for these needs?

Togetherness is a familiar topic; we hear about it everywhere. But when the family gets together on a Sunday, it is very tense. Accustomed to individual activities, its members find doing things together difficult.

In urban areas, large numbers of families live in close proximity without knowing each other. The lack of support from others within the immediate community affects family relationships. New suburban housing estates may also contain similar elements of anonymity where kinfolk do not precede families in long residence to help bridge the gap between the nuclear family and the wider community. This situation requires that more psychological glue be given to each individual from the family itself. The disharmony between rural and urban life is exemplified below:

The W. family recently moved from the bayous of Louisiana to a large urban area. They knew no one around their block, and their only acquaintances were the minister, the teachers, and the visiting nurse. When the mother hung her clothes out to dry, they were stolen. She feared letting the children go out of the house or to summer camp because of the possibility of trouble. One of the current acts of vandalism was breaking windshields with baseball bats, and she was determined that her children would not do that. The husband, who worked at construction out of the city, left home very early in the morning and returned late at night. He worked long hours and as many days per week as possible during the dry season, because he was out of work when the rains came. The house in which the family lived was condemned and better housing was unavailable at what they could afford

to pay. The move from a rural area to an urban area was a difficult adjustment to make. Superficial adaptation had been made, but the whole family felt lonely and out of place.

Because the values, beliefs, and social relations of the city are vastly different from those of the country, the use of psychic energy is required in the adjustment and adaptation process.

When the equilibrium of the family interrelationships is upset, emotional isolation occurs. Tenderness is gone and the family seeks equilibrium in conformity; there is an unusual preoccupation with issues of control and discipline. Security, gratification, and family unity are not present. Attempts to solve intrafamilial conflicts revert to enforced family group activities, compulsive care of children, moving, or the use of alcohol or drugs. Roles may be so circumscribed that role complementarity is absent; for example, a parent may be more like a child than an adult. Adults who have not learned how to be parents perhaps have the most difficulty in learning to communicate with children, accepting their changes as they mature, separating from them at school age, and accepting rejection and building a new life for themselves at the empty nest phase.

Familial Limbo.[7] Although most people in the United States live with families, many do not. In 1977, nonfamily household residents were 10 percent (22 million) of the total civilian population (Metropolitan Life, 1978). Later marriages have contributed to the increase in nonfamily households. When teenagers break the ties with their family of orientation, there may be a period of many years before they establish their own families. After establishing their own families, there are more years for many people in which they live alone due to either separation, divorce, or the death of a spouse. Little attention is given in the literature to the effect upon individuals involved in these particular situations of familial limbo. Often, substitute family members are secured, particularly if there are no living members of the original family. On the other hand, when family members live at a great distance from each other, substitutes are found

[7] This term is borrowed from Cumming (1959).

in their home communities and mutual assistance patterns formed. Communes, popular in the nineteenth century, are again popular; other rather loose living arrangements are frequent. Stop now and think of the members of your own family. If you are away from home or without a family, who are the substitutes? Compare your findings with those of others in your situation.

IMPACT OF DISEQUILIBRIUM

Healthy families complement rather than tear apart each other's thoughts and feelings. Criticism of others can be rationally made without loss of emotional control, and each family member is clear about his position within the group. The environment of the healthy family aids in the process of each individual member carrying out his required developmental tasks and those of the family as well. Members of healthy families are supportive to each other and have a respect for the needs and manifestations of the different generations. Variations in multiple cultural backgrounds of the American family make it an impossible task to describe criteria and standards for the mental health of any one family; each family has to be assessed against its own patterns. Spiegel's approach provides a systematic way to view realities within their psychological, sociological, cultural, and ecological units. The new specialty of transcultural nursing provides definitive ways for the study of culture and its impact upon health (Leininger, 1977).

At the time of illness of one family member, the equilibrium of family interaction is disrupted and new adjustments and adaptations are required. *Behavior expressed by any one member of a family is related to the state of the whole family.* An example is given as follows:

The patient, Mrs. A., was admitted to the inpatient psychiatric services six weeks after the birth of her son. A very attractive, well-dressed, and well-groomed woman, she exhibits superficially sweet affect, expresses some paranoid ideation, is preoccupied and impulsive. The precipitating factor for her psychotic break is cited by her psychiatrist as the reemergence of her own oedipal conflict upon the birth of the child. The husband, age thirty, is a handsome South American and an executive in a large shipping firm. Proud of his beautiful wife and new son, he is stunned by the calamity of the condition of his wife and the fact that the son is bereft of the mother while she is in the hospital. He expressed fear of what effect her illness would have on the development of the child. Living fifty miles away in the expensive suburbs with no relatives available to help, he is suddenly required to be mother in addition to his usual roles and the new role of father. After seeing Mr. A. in an evening appointment when he came to visit Mrs. A., the nursing student later conferred with the psychiatrist and supported his view that Mrs. A.'s parents should be requested to come from the East Coast to help.

Pathogenic Relating

Scapegoating. Scapegoating[8] may be observed in some disturbed families where they do not want the extruded family member in the fold because he is thought to be the one that caused all the family quarrels. In disturbed families, the weakest, most defenseless member, a child, or the more docile of the marital partners may be the one first to see the psychiatrist. The family may thereby use the primary patient to screen their own problems or to hide them altogether. One father brought his daughter for inpatient psychiatric treatment and left her alone in the lobby to manage her own admission. Families may also blame their problems on someone outside the family. The following is an example of a small child who was the scapegoat in his disturbed family.

Mr. and Mrs. J. lived in the ghetto. There were five children: Catherine, ten; Edward, eight; Curtis, six; Clarence, three and a half; and Julian, two. Curtis had shown aggressive behavior in school, disrupted the class, and had also kicked his pregnant mother in the abdomen several times. Subsequently, he was admitted to the children's service of the local state hospital. In his absence, he was cited by the children and the mother as the cause of all the family quarrels; no efforts were being made either to visit him

[8] Scapegoating refers to "the action or process of casting blame for shortcomings or failure on an innocent or at most only partly responsible individual or group." *Webster's New Collegiate Dictionary.* Springfield, Mass.: G. & G. Merriam Co., 1977.

or to take him back into the family unit. This family was dealing with its emotional problems by scapegoating and temporarily maintained itself by excluding the "acting out" member.

Scapegoating may be conscious or unconscious. It may be found within the group or outside the group. Whole families may displace their hostility onto one of their members as did the J. family onto Curtis, or they may find something or someone outside the family to serve the same purpose. Confusion, irritability, and other aspects of insecurity may result in scapegoating. Parts of a family may team up and use other members as scapegoats. Scapegoating is common among adolescents. Other groups undergoing stress and conflict may find a scapegoat to hide behind instead of resolving the conflict.

If the J. family could have been seen as a family before the aggressive behavior of one member was directed toward the pregnant mother, perhaps it could have been helped to resolve its many problems.

Problems of mental disorder may either be hidden from the visiting nurse or be difficult to discern. Depression, for example, is not always obvious, and it is not uncommon for depression—even of the type leading to suicide—to go undetected by family members and the uninitiated nurse.

Some of the following theoretical concepts about families were developed from the study of families with schizophrenic members.

Marital Schism and Marital Skew. Disturbed families show a pattern of *marital schism* where one spouse constantly undercuts the other and there is severe, long-standing discord (Lidz, 1973). One spouse seeks to win the children to his side or the child may become a substitute for the spouse. Many schizophrenic patients report their experiences of being depended upon by one parent as though they were a spouse. Disturbed families with the *skewed* pattern demostrate overt harmony between the parents but underneath, the psychopathology of the dominant parent is passively accepted by the other. Thus, serious conflict is masked and conflicting messages are passed on to the children. The masking creates an

unreal atmosphere for the child because what is verbalized is different from the feeling. Disturbed families may withdraw from each other where their home simply becomes a filling station to tank up for supplies and to follow their solitary pursuits; emotional isolation results. One family with several children, living in a large two-story house in a suburban town, had gotten to the point where each person came in and out of the house via his own individual entrance and exit. Disturbed families are deficient in parental nurturance; they fail to socialize the child and to transmit other basic aspects of culture; thus, the parents transmit their irrationality to their children (Lidz, 1960, 1963, 1965, 1968, 1973, 1974).

Double-Bind Hypothesis. This concept is best phrased in terms of people caught up in an ongoing system that creates different definitions of the relationships; it results in distress to the participants. It emerged from research on communication and was arrived at deductively from work with schizophrenic patients (Bateson et al., 1956, 1968). It is not an explanation of the etiology of schizophrenia, but it is an inevitable part of schizophrenic communication. Ingredients of the double bind involve a repeated experience between two or more people in an intense relationship that is long-lasting and gradually becomes habitual. Learning is based upon avoidance of punishment instead of reward and the content of a message given carries with it a secondary injunction conflicting with the first at a more abstract level, usually nonverbal. The receiver of the message cannot escape the field. If the message is perceived correctly, the receiver is punished for correct perception and therefore his self is disconfirmed. For example, a parent may say to a child, "Go to bed, you are tired and have to get up early in the morning," when the parent actually means, "Get out of my sight, I am sick of you," and communicates this message nonverbally. Thus, the parent is defining how the child feels. Parents of a family system with the double-bind communication may, in fact, answer questions directed toward their children related to their activities and what they think and feel instead of waiting for the children to answer for themselves. In this system, when the child responds to overtures of affection from the parents, they become anxious and may punish the child or state with certainty that the child's demonstrations of affection are simulated. Therefore, the child becomes uncertain about his own feelings and is unable to discern feelings, to differentiate one feeling from another, and the result is development of a wall between the child and the parent with regard to intimacy and security. If the child attempts to indicate love, he is punished and he is punished if he does not.

Pseudomutuality. This concept emerged from a long-range research program on the families of schizophrenics. It was developed independently of the double-bind hypothesis and is conceptualized as a major feature of families where schizophrenia develops but is not itself the etiology of schizophrenia. In normal families, there is mutuality or complementarity, whereas in deviant or disturbed families, pseudomutuality takes over (Wynne et al., 1958, 1978).

Pseudomutuality requires that the individuals involved try to maintain a sense of relatedness and emotional fulfillment to and with each other. In this situation, relationships can neither be abandoned nor allowed to grow. Differences are viewed, in these families, as causing disruption and are therefore suppressed. Subsequently, when differences are avoided, growth is impossible. Not only are differences submerged but perceptions of situations where divergence is possible are camouflaged.

In pseudomutuality, contradictions are concealed but are labeled the same. For example, parents may both make positive remarks about something that one of them does not believe; they do not comment on their differences and the children learn them through modeling. Therefore, the ego of the child fails to discern the meanings of participation and experience.

Mechanisms that maintain pseudomutuality are (1) *myths, legends,* and *ideology* highlighting the terrible consequences of family members acting in different ways. For example, if one member of the family wishes to do something different, it may be "the death of me." Or, as one family described

it, "We have had twenty years of married life and we have never had a fight. Our daughter never did anything we didn't want her to do. She was always good, never disobeyed us; we never had any problems with her. She had music and dancing lessons and was happy and normal. We can't understand why she is ill." The teenage daughter had just shot her sister. This violent disruption is characteristic of how some children break out of the family system. Family therapists who see parents who believe that "marriage is made in heaven; we have no fights" look for a disturbed child. (2) *Bland, indiscriminate approval* where the attitude is "we want you to do what you want to do". Parents, for example, may approve of an early marriage for their daughter but privately discourage the fiancé. (3) *Secrecy* is marked in some families with regard to situations outside the family. If the parents cannot approve of divergent behavior, they do not talk about it, but try to find out about it secretly. One father kept a journal about the behavior and activities of his son. (4) *Formalizing experiences* is another mechanism and is seen where certain topics are designated for discussion and argument but no other topics are permitted exploration within the family. One child who kept complaining about the younger sister's recent birthday party was required to write down all her complaints. (5) *The use of intermediaries* is a common operation with families where pseudomutuality exists. For example, one set of parents arrived one Sunday afternoon at the psychiatric unit, wearing some of their finest clothes, to take their son out to dinner. John was dressed in slacks and T-shirt and had not shaved. The parents wanted the nursing staff to make their son shave and dress in a suit and tie so *they* could go to Trader Vic's. Nurses are often unwittingly put into the role of the intermediary. The intervention here was to require the parents to make their own arrangements with their son.

The pseudomutuality hypothesis purports that the overall family role structure is internalized and that ego functions are thereby constricted. It also purports that an acute psychotic schizophrenic break is a breakdown of pseudomutuality and a miscarried attempt toward individuation.

Other Concepts. *Silence* affords the family member the opportunity to gather power by simply being silent and the positions of all members thereby become deeply set. *Silencing* where one family member assumes the role of admonishing others to be silent thereby encourages compliance and conformity. *Babbling* occurs in disturbed families where some members talk a lot but do not actually say anything; they say nothing or next to nothing. *Threats of physical violence and physical violence* are commonly employed in disturbed families as ways of relating and maintaining the status quo. Battered children and battered spouses are often the result. *Schizmogenesis* occurs where there is polarization of feelings with regard to the extended kin. Some disturbed families involve the extended kin in their conflicts and are quite sensitive to the influence of their extended kin. The polarization of feelings often occurs with the giving of a gift from one side of the family to the other. The gift may become a symbol for something else and feelings spiral upward as a result. Coalitions form as family members take sides and disruption is inevitable. One part of the family thereby holds itself in one piece at the expense of another part.

Schizophrenogenic Mother Hypothesis. This hypothesis concerns itself with the idea that certain characteristics of the mother are associated with the etiology of schizophrenia. Coldness, rejection, and overprotection are viewed as characteristics that set into motion an emotional withdrawal in the child that results in psychosis. A study of sixty-seven families using Bales's Interaction Process Analysis confirmed that mothers of schizophrenics were cold and withdrawn (Cheek, 1964). In essence, this study confirmed the theory of the double-bind but also posed the question as to whether the child may have made the mother that way.

Phantom Family Member. The *phantom* family member still exists in which others are forbidden to speak of the member, to each other, to the children, or even to involved professionals. This seems the most extreme example of disconfirmation. This person may be the "black sheep," the family skeleton, and/or its mentally disordered member. Many people who are phantom family members live in institutions and residential care homes and receive no communication from their families in the form of presents, letters, or cards; in fact, their very existence is denied by the very group essential for their recovery. Others with rich parents are maintained in distant cities or countries in posh residential hotels under constant psychiatric care. Other family members, especially children, who see this happen to one of their group must surely think, in horror, that it may sometime happen to themselves.

Family factions, splits, and conflicts are painful. There is great comfort when conflicts are resolved. Family therapy may be the modality for the removal of the pain.

Family Therapy

BACKGROUND

Child-guidance clinics, developed in the twenties, involved mothers in the problems of their children even though the mother was likely to be required to wait outside the physician's office while the child was being interviewed. For the most part, nurses were not involved in child guidance clinics. Public-health nurses have been involved in working with disturbed families for many years. They, like most of the helping professions, worked on an empirical basis without a theoretical frame of reference; they used eclectic approaches in attempting to help families, some of which helped and some of which did not.

After World War II, child patients were hospitalized more and more and the parents were seen in psychotherapeutic sessions by different therapists, often psychiatric social workers. Admission of a child to one inpatient psychiatric unit occurred only after elaborate intake procedures to determine the commitment of the parents to treatment themselves. In fact, agreement to enter treatment was a prerequisite for admission of the child. Nurses were involved in the twenty-four-hour care of the child, and the child, in addition, would receive treatment from a physician or psychologist. The primary therapist of the child was officially a physician but often unofficially was one of the nursing staff. At periodic intervals, all the staff came together in a conference to review the problems and progress of treatment. This was referred to as *collaborative treatment.*

During 1952, John E. Bell was on sabbatical in Scotland and heard of the work with families conducted by Jack Sutherland and John Bowlby. The reader is referred to the practice begun in 1948 at Cassel Hospital, England, of admitting children with the mothers in order to avoid separation problems (Main, 1968). The use of milieu therapy in family-centered nursing is portrayed at Cassel Hospital, England. Grounded in psychoanalysis and group dynamics, nurses work with whole families within the institutional setting (Barnes, 1968). Even today not enough attention is given to the separation of mother and child when the mother is admitted to a mental hospital. Meanwhile, Ackerman (1958) began seeing families, and during the midfifties the movement of anthropologists and sociologists into the study of psychopathology gave a new dimension to the study of families. Jackson (1968) studied normal families and looked for patterns of behavior within normal families but instead found a diversity of patterns. He coined the word "conjoint" to describe family therapy sessions where family members were seen together as a group in psychotherapeutic sessions. Virginia Satir (1964) gave demonstrations of the technique of conjoint family therapy to a wide variety of professionals. Communication theory was being developed, for example, by Ruesch and Bateson (1951, 1961). Therapeutic community concepts were influencing mental hospitals to become more open systems. William Caudill (1952), an anthropologist, did a research study in which he was admitted to a psychiatric unit as a patient. He received psychotherapy and lived on the wards for eight weeks. Stanton and Schwartz's (1954) study described pathogenesis in a mental hospital system. By this study it was demonstrated that *disturbance in behavior of patients was related to conflicts among staff.* These studies added to the knowledge of human behavior in groups

and thus of family systems. The practice of housing mental patients in remote hospitals automatically removed them from the environs of their families. Prescribed visiting days in these institutions further isolated mental patients from their families. The stigma of mental disorder often resulted in families covering up the fact from friends, acquaintances, and even the helping professionals.

During the 1950s and early 1960s, psychiatric nurses were struggling for professional status in the large public mental hospitals as well as other areas. Part of the struggle related to getting qualified as group therapists. In addition, psychiatric nursing became the first clinical specialty. Now psychiatric nurses are getting their qualifications in family therapy and some are in private practice.

DEFINITION IN FAMILY THERAPY

The emphasis is on the family group as a single unit and the family is treated simultaneously on a periodic and continued basis. Behavior and symptoms are therefore viewed as a result of processes within the family that have an interchangeable relationship with each family member's intrapsychic life. The assumption underlying such therapy is that mental disorder in one member of the family may be an indication of dysfunction within the total group.

Ackerman (1958) said ". . . the family becomes a source of sick emotional contagion."[9] Psychiatric patients, he added, ". . . come from disordered families, and the first family member referred for psychiatric care may prove to be the most or the least sick member of the group."[10]

WHAT FAMILY THERAPISTS DO

A principal impetus for referral for treatment is conflict within the family, not symptoms of mental disorder per se. When mid-

[9] Ackerman, N. W.: *Psychodynamics of Family Life.* New York: Basic Books, Inc., 1958, p. 101.
[10] Ackerman, ibid., p. 104.

dle-class families get to the point of no return, one parent often goes to an encounter group. Since the openness sought for in encounter groups then applies to only one parent, further conflict may ensue within the family.

Several variations or techniques of treatment are used, with the trend being toward including the nuclear-family members. Some family therapists, however, also include others. After several joint sessions, the children may be dropped while the parents continue. The principal focus is toward knowing the interactions among the various family members in the best way possible to aid them with their problems. Collaborative therapy has been used in some institutions for many years. This technique refers to the parents of hospitalized patients being seen in individual treatment by different therapists. On a periodic and continued basis, all therapists of the family members then hold conferences about the problems, needs, and interactions within the family group. *Conjoint therapy* in which all the family members meet together as a unit was developed at the Mental Research Institute, Palo Alto, California (Jackson, 1968, first published 1961). *Network therapy* is used by Fleck (1967) and others. In this treatment, as many as thirty to forty people, including relatives, neighbors, police, clergy, and others as well as family members may be involved in one session. Several families may also be seen together in groups for treatment. In some instances, families are admitted to inpatient psychiatric services for treatment.

Because members of families are individuals with self-concepts, when family members give out messages that do not fit with the individual's definition of himself, it destroys the self-concept; he is therefore *disconfirmed.* Since children are different every day, whatever parents do, they confirm and disconfirm their children. People can be taught to see a different world by introducing to them a new concept. Family therapy can introduce a new concept into the family group, and the family members get the idea that they themselves control behavior. For example, one family complained that their fourteen-year-old son was always late to school. The therapist suggested that

they make him more late, and as a consequence, the tardiness stopped.

For the most part, women make the initial contact for family therapy. If there is antagonism between the wife and husband, then one cannot expect the wife to bring the husband in for therapy.

If there are more than two people in the family, at least one and one half hours are needed for the first session. The average length of treatment is four to six months although six to ten sessions may help some families. Patients who come for treatment usually want to stop doing something or they want to be able to do something they have not been able to do. Therapists themselves have to be active and assertive to work with families. Openness all the time is not the goal for the family. Sometimes cruelty is justified as authenticity. The therapist has the responsibility for helping families be better. It is imperative that the therapist trace clearly the dynamic relations between specific trends of family conflict and the intrapsychic conflicts within individual members. It is easy for the therapist to get caught up in the pathology of the family. Objectivity in family therapy is of utmost importance.

With regard to the question as to who should come for therapy, some therapists insist that all family members come for the assessment interview while others do not. The work situation of the family may prevent all of them coming at once. Ackerman advocated the home visit as being ideal for the diagnostic interview. He also liked to keep the children involved in therapeutic sessions whereas other therapists do not. Some therapists talk with each family member alone in the initial interview, and at other times during therapy. Patients have a right to give private information to the therapist.

Many family therapists do not insist that every family member be present at each session. Parents may be seen together without the children, for example. Some therapists advocate the therapeutic value of the parents discussing the covert nature of their marriage contract. In marriage itself, maintaining separateness and togetherness is a main problem. What therapists do in working with families is influenced by their theoretical orientation, their own abilities, experiences, and cultural value orientation. Although it is not the purpose here to include the universe of family-therapy techniques, some current practices are described in this section.

Some families never stay together long enough to talk, and therefore, the therapist may put all the family members in a room with a one-way mirror and go to the adjacent room to observe. The therapist and the family may never agree on the problem within the family but in the process of getting together, talking, and interacting, the family gets better. The therapist uses drama, humor, tact, ambiguity, and ceremony and helps people save face. Ambiguity is part of healthy communication; when communication is crystal-clear, it is likely to be hostile. Where there are different premises in people's minds about a situation they are both in, the result is conflict. Some therapists ask each family member in turn for comments; the families most often have not had this experience before and it can be most illuminating to those concerned to hear their perceptions about each other. The therapist may question, model, and summarize at the end of the session.

TECHNIQUES

Behavior exchange may in a very direct way be contracted between the therapist and the family for different behaviors. The behaviors may be tried out in the session or practiced outside the session.

Regrouping of family members may be carried out where triangulation[11] occurs. For example, the therapist tries to restructure to parent–child functioning.

Focusing on a member other than the identified patient may assist in the development of new behaviors.

Positioning within the therapeutic session may aid communication. A family member, for instance, may be requested to view the others through a one-way mirror.

[11] Triangulation refers to a situation where each parent demands the child to side with him against the other parent (Minuchin, 1974, p. 102.)

Tasks are assigned by the therapist. For example, if a parent is scapegoating a child, the parent may be assigned to complete a task with the child. If a child is consistently late to school and the family complains, the whole family may be assigned to make him late.

Sculpting may be used to portray the sculptor's perception of members of a group and their relationship to each other. In sculpting, group members are asked, in turn, to position other members of a group according to their perception of their interpersonal relationships (Mealey, 1977).

Bargaining is another technique in which the therapist aids the family members in their agreements, negotiations, and understanding of the family process (Padberg, 1975).

Treatment in the home involves combined elements of group therapy, activity therapy, and role playing (Francis, 1968). The use of this psychiatric nursing technique with the urban poor emphasizes concern with the family as a whole unit within the home. The therapist brings play materials that the family can use together to help elucidate their conflicts. During the session the therapist acts as a catalyst to pinpoint conflicts, intervenes if necessary, and demonstrates other ways family members can relate to each other.

The concept of the nurse as a primary agent in home treatment, assisting with supervision of patients on pharmacotherapy, conducting individual and family therapy, and supervising the general needs of patients and families, is outlined by Weiner (1967). Orientation of the nurse to the giving role helps in reaching individuals and families where approaches by other professionals may fail. Nurses are now gaining expertise in family therapy in graduate programs.

Application of the concept of interdependence within families is presented by Hover (1968) in her work with a family with many problems. Her first impression was the need for hospitalization of one member. Subsequent visits involved assessing the total needs of the entire family, making a diagnosis of the family problems, setting priorities, and providing help. Busch (1968) describes the use of the home visit with a child and mother in follow-up care after hospitalization and in collaboration with the child psychiatrist and the school nurse. Special techniques used in therapy were operant conditioning and role playing.

The effect upon a family of hospitalization of the mother with emphasis on how the father manages has been studied by Merrill (1969).

The systems approach in family therapy, in which the nurse works with the "here and now" interactions in every family interview, is applied by Anderson (1969). In this approach the behavior of the individual is perceived in its relationship to other members of the family and discussed in this context. The nurse–family relationship is emphasized in the report by Kovacs (1966) of her work with an acutely disturbed man whom she followed, together with his family, through hospitalization and aftercare.

HOME VISITS

One of the challenges that confronts the nurse is how to collect meaningful data in identifying the needs of families. There is no substitute for the home visit; facades are often unveiled by the family when it is in its familiar setting. Nurses perhaps more than any other professionals are accepted in the homes of their patients. They may carry their own case load of families and in some areas work on outreach teams where initial assessments are made of the condition of the identified patient. If necessary, in my own county, designated nurses sign patients in for seventy-two-hour involuntary observation. Currently it is most likely that the nurse works in collaboration with others on the mental health team: a psychiatrist, a psychologist, a social worker, and the family physician. There may be still others, depending upon philosophy and availability. Therefore, data collected are usually combined with information taken by the other members of the clinical team. Problems are shared and team members consult with each other. One of the unique facets of home visiting is that it is relatively

unstructured; it is informal, direct observations can be made, and the professional is in the territory of the family. The following information from a home visit speaks for itself:

The patient, Tom S., twenty-eight years old, a former post office employee, is now on disability due to a back injury. He has been in psychotherapy for two years on an outpatient basis and is now admitted to a private psychiatric hospital with a diagnosis of depression. On a home visit to assess the family situation, the nursing student learned that the patient's "wife," Maria, is three months pregnant, that they are not married, and that the ailing mother of Tom with whom she lives strongly disapproves of the whole relationship. In addition, Maria is not a citizen, speaks only Spanish, and has made no attempt to gain citizenship or learn English. Furthermore, she has had no prenatal care. The student also learns that Tom had just moved out of the mother's house before hospitalization.

The identified patient, Tom, accepts help from professionals and agencies. This ability to accept help was noted to be a strength. Maria, despite all the conflicts with Tom's mother, has stayed with him. The mother, although overprotective and disapproving of Tom's relationship with Maria, was originally the one who insisted that Tom go to the psychiatrist.

The student communicated with the family physician, who had treated Tom for several years and who welcomed assistance. Information about the family was brought back to the hospital psychiatric team and recorded in the patient's record. A high priority was to get Maria into prenatal care. The student explored several possibilities with those concerned and wound up going with Maria to the prenatal clinic of the county hospital, which automatically put the family in touch with a public-health nurse.

The conditions and conflicts within the family were unknown to the psychiatric team until the home visit was made. The role of the student centered around assessing the family situation, communicating findings to those individuals already involved, and getting the family into additional supportive systems. It was recognized that this was a family with many problems that would not be quickly resolved.

Students who have visited a family will

probably have less anxiety in subsequent family visiting than the highly skilled professional who has never made any home visits. The best time to visit a family to assess its interactions is during a meal, because this is probably the only time that the whole family is together (except for Sundays, which are usually not used for visiting). To study family-interaction patterns, it is necessary that all members be present. The nurse acts as a participant observer. Note taking is not done because it takes attention away from observation.

Some work can be done beforehand with regard to the ecological unit of the neighborhood and the larger community. Cities are divided into census tracts with data available about the demography of the tracts and the city itself.[12]

A cursory survey of the immediate block in which the family lives may yield valuable data. It is important to build upon the census tract data, which, for example, do not deal with mobility within neighborhoods subsequent to the census count; neither do they describe the quality of the life within a particular community, which itself influences well-being. The human aspects of life in a neighborhood should be added to the census figures. Individuals and families may live in a congested area but still suffer from social isolation.

Before going out into the city alone, nurses should make certain preparations. As the American city becomes more and more uncomfortable as a place to live, individual safety is a factor. Nursing students may never have been alone in the interior of a big city or in a ghetto area; many come from nonmetropolitan areas. The first thing to do is to know where you are going, the transportation schedule, how to get there, and how to get back. A good city map with block numbers is a must. If you know where you are going you will not only feel purposeful, but you will convey self-assurance. Carry some dimes in a pocket for telephone calls, and do not forget to carry your professional calling cards. Spot the places within the areas you are visiting where there are telephones: the grocery store, gas station,

---

[12] This book does not purposely omit problems of rural areas. Focus is upon the urban/suburban setting because that is where most people live now and where many more will live in the future.

drugstore, or bar. If you are to be in the neighborhood regularly, get acquainted with others: firefighters, for example, or local business people.

There are many ways to structure home visits to aid in collection of data and assessment of needs.

In making home visits it must be remembered that unless rapport is established very little will be accomplished. One way to begin a home visit is by stating or restating who you are, how it is that you are there, and presenting your card. The family may then be asked to identify what is troubling them.

DATA COLLECTION AND ASSESSMENT

Although one rarely can gain as much information as one needs in the first visit, major points on which information is needed are:

1. A full description of the presenting problem.
2. Description of the ecological unit of the family. This includes:
   - A short description of each member of the household (including pets), living arrangements (space for sleep, work, play, and privacy), safety hazards, developmental tasks, education, cultural background, and health assessment (including nutrition, use of medications, and abuse of drugs).
   - The family as a group (interactions, communication, role behaviors, values, developmental stage, and developmental tasks); occupation of members; and economic status.
   - Interfamily and community relationships: social network (relationships with other families, friends, etc.); activities shared; memberships in church, school, and other community groups; and dependence on community agencies.
   - Communications: the use that the family makes of television, radio, newspapers, magazines, films, and books and their influence on the family.
3. Elements of culture affecting self-concept and health status, for example, ideology, caring behaviors and acculturation status.

4. Strengths within the family.
   - Gives emotional support, affection, and security for its members.
   - Provides basic biophysical supplies.
   - Complementarity of roles.
   - Healthy communication within and outside the family.
   - Mutual respect for individual members.
   - Provides experiences that promote growth.
   - Degree of cooperation and cohesiveness.
   - As a group, the family has goals and works toward them.
   - Provides for tension management.
5. Needs of the family.
6. A brief sequential summary of the elements of the visit.

Assessments of culture of the individual are now receiving attention in nursing. Although a definitive assessment of culture is surely the domain of experts in anthropology and specialists in transcultural nursing, nurses need to develop their cultural awareness in order to be more effective practitioners. One cultural inventory tool for assessment of health-care needs of individuals includes "language and symbolic systems; concepts of health and disease; folk health practices and other health coping mechanisms; social norms; values; and socioeconomic, religious and political history."[15]

Although some of the points given here may overlap, they are presented as a guide. Because much of the nurse's work with families centers around some problem or crisis, strengths within the family may not be immediately evident due to the fact that so much attention is focused upon the problem or crisis. However, assessment of strengths of the family should be part of every contact with them.

INTERVENTION

Most important is that the family come to its own aid. Ask the family to restate the problem and identify what aspects they wish to change. Families can and do solve many of their own problems once they are

aware of them. In goal setting, assisting the family to be aware of its strengths and use of them may be the only intervention needed. In mutual goal setting, the nurse and the family need to agree on realistic goals that they will work on together. Where conflict occurs, psychological, social, and cultural conflict should be differentiated. The new cultural pluralism in American society focuses on the uniqueness and strengths of ethnic groups. Cultural value orientations of families have therefore assumed a new importance. Where cultural conflict occurs, pluralism can aid acculturation. If the goal is acculturation, awareness of the differences between values of the ethnic group and the larger society is essential for both the family and the nurse. If the goal is to merge with the ethnic group, the nurse can assist the family to identify strengths, and resources within the ethnic group. Because conditions in families are in constant change, the goals are also in constant change and need to be renegotiated from time to time.

Because specific recall fades rapidly, the written report should be made as soon as possible after the visit. Evaluation and use of relevant data and information about families are important parts of family diagnosis. Another aspect is the assessment of problems presented by the family that require assistance. No family can be expected to do much work on its interrelationships if resources such as food, shelter, and clothing are lacking. It is the work of the helping person to assist with needs on a priority basis conducive to the total health of the family. No program of mental-health services is effective unless it is supported by multiple health and welfare resources.

The skills of the nurse who may carry out the goals for the family set by the mental-health team require assessment. Students are often torn between meeting the demands of the curriculum and meeting the needs of particular families with whom they are involved. The abilities to set realistic goals, time interventions, carry out specific techniques, recognize one's limitations, know when the family needs others, be aware of one's own reactions, and withdraw when the needs are met are not learned all at once. Each nurse, each home visit, and each family is different. There are no

---

[15] Orque, Modesta S.: "Health Care and Minority Clients," *Nursing Outlook,* 24:5:313–316, May 1976.

formulas for action; each situation requires individual assessment, action, and evaluation.

Summary

This chapter deals with some aspects of families in the United States. Emphasis is made upon ways that nurses can systematically study families. Role complementarity within families is described in equilibrium maintenance. Mental health of families is presented in terms of the role of the family group in influencing itself as a group and also of its effect upon its individual members. Some characteristics of the contemporary family are described, including alienation and familial limbo. Developmental stages and tasks are outlined. The concept of interdependence is discussed in terms of the impact of illness. Theoretical concepts relating to family dynamics and pathogenic relating in families are presented. Some aspects of family therapy and the involvement of nurses in work with families are described. The importance of cultural awareness in working with families is emphasized.

References

ACKERMAN, NATHAN W.: *Psychodynamics of Family Life.* New York: Basic Books, Inc., 1958.

————: "The Family as a Unit in Mental Health," *Proceedings of the Third World Congress of Psychiatry.* Toronto: University of Toronto Press, 1963, Vol. 3, pp. 109–12.

————: "Family Therapy," in Arieti, Silvano, ed.: *American Handbook of Psychiatry.* New York: Basic Books, Inc., 1966, Vol. 3, pp. 201–12.

————: *Treating the Troubled Family.* New York: Basic Books, Inc., 1966.

AINSWORTH, MARY D., ANDRY, R. G., HARLOW, ROBERT G., LEBOVICI, S., MEAD, MARGARET, PRUGH, DANE G., and WOOTEN, BARBARA: *Deprivation of Maternal Care—A Reassessment of Its Effects.* Geneva: World Health Organization, 1962.

ANDERSON, DOROTHY B.: "Nursing Therapy with Families," *Perspectives in Psychiatric Care,* VII:1:21–27, 1969.

BALES, ROBERT F.: *Interaction Process Analysis.* Cambridge, Mass.: Addison-Wesley Publishing Co., 1950.

BATESON, GREGORY, JACKSON, DON D., HALEY, JAY, and WEAKLAND, JOHN H.: "A Note on the Double-Bind—1962," in Jackson, Don D., ed.: *Communication, Family and Marriage.* Palo Alto, Calif.: Science and Behavior Books, 1968, Vol. 1, p. 55.

————: JACKSON, DON D., HALEY, JAY, and WEAKLAND, JOHN H.: "Toward a Theory of Schizophrenia," *Behavioral Science,* 1:4:251–64, October 1956.

BETTELHEIM, BRUNO: *The Empty Fortress.* New York: The Free Press, 1967.

————: *The Children of the Dream.* New York: Macmillan Publishing Co., Inc., 1969.

BOWLBY, JOHN: *Maternal Care and Mental Health.* Geneva: World Health Organization, 1952.

BUSCH, KAREN D.: "The Use of the Home Visit by the Child Psychiatric Nurse," *American Nurses' Association Clinical Sessions.* New York: Appleton-Century-Crofts, 1968, pp. 352–57.

CAUDILL, WILLIAM, REDLICH, F. C., GILMORE, H. R., and BRADY, E. B.: "Social Structure and Interaction Processes on a Psychiatric Ward," *American Journal of Orthopsychiatry,* 22:314–34, 1952.

CHEEK, FRANCES E.: "The 'Schizophrenogenic' Mother in Word and Deed." *Family Process,* 3:1:155–77, March 1964.

COX, NORMA TRAUB: "Creating a New Role: The Professional Woman and Motherhood," in Knafl, Kathleen Astin, and Grace, Helen K., eds.: *Families Across the Life Cycle: Studies for Nursing.* Boston: Little, Brown and Company, 1978, pp. 223–32.

CUMMING, JOHN H.: "The Family and Mental Disorder. An Incomplete Essay," in *Causes of Mental Disorders: A Review of Epidemiological Knowledge.* New York: Milbank Memorial Fund, 1959.

DAVIS, KINGSLEY: *Human Society.* New York: The Macmillan Co., 1948.

DUVALL, EVELYN MILLIS: *Family Development,* 4th ed. Philadelphia: J. B. Lippincott Co., 1971.

ERIKSON, ERIK H.: *Childhood and Society.* New York: W. W. Norton, 1963.

FLECK, STEPHEN: "The Role of the Family in Psychiatry," in Friedman, Alfred M. et al., eds.: *Comprehensive Textbook of Psychiatry.* Baltimore. Williams & Wilkins, 1967, pp. 213–24.

FRANCIS, TONI M.: "Treatment in the Home as a Psychiatric Nursing Technique," in *American Nurses' Association Clinical Sessions.* New York: Appleton-Century-Crofts, 1968, pp. 286–95.

HALEY, ALEX: *The Autobiography of Malcolm X.* New York: Grove Press, 1964.

HAVIGHURST, ROBERT J.: *Human Development and Education,* London: Longmans, Green and Co., 1953.

HOVER, DOROTHEA EITEL: "The Theory of the Interdependence of Family Members and Its Application in an Emotionally Disturbed Family," in *American Nurses' Association Clinical Sessions.* New York: Appleton-Century-Crofts, 1968, pp. 46–52.

HOWELLS, JOHN G., ed.: *Theory and Practice of Family Psychiatry,* New York: Brunner/Mazel, 1971.

JACKSON, DON D., and WEAKLAND, JOHN H.: "Conjoint Family Therapy; Some Considerations on Theory, Technique and Results," in Jackson, Don D.: *Therapy, Communication and Change,* Vol. 2, Palo Alto, Calif.: Science and Behavior Books, Inc., 1968, pp. 222–48.

JAHODA, MARIE: *Current Concepts of Positive Mental Health.* New York: Basic Books, Inc., 1958.

KLUCKHOHN, C., and SPIEGEL, JOHN P.: "Integration and Conflict in Family Behavior," Report No. 27, *Group for the Advancement of Psychiatry,* August 1954.

KNAFL, KATHLEEN ASTIN, and GRACE, HELEN K., eds.: *Families Across the Life Cycle: Studies for Nursing.* Boston: Little, Brown and Company, 1978, p. 11.

KOVACS, L. W.: "A Therapeutic Relationship with a Patient and Family," *Perspectives in Psychiatric Care,* 4:2:11–21, 1966.

LEININGER, MADELEINE: *Transcultural Nursing: Concepts, Theories and Practices.* New York: John Wiley & Sons, 1978.

LIDZ, THEODORE, and FLECK, STEPHEN: "Schizophrenia, Human Integration and the Role of the Family," in Jackson, Don D., ed.: *The Etiology of Schizophrenia.* New York: Basic Books, Inc., 1960, pp. 323–45.

_____: *The Family and Human Adaptation, Three Lectures.* New York: International Universities Press, 1963.

_____: CORNELISON, A., TERRY, D., and FLECK, S.: The Transmission of Irrationality," in Lidz, T., Fleck, S., and Cornelison, A.: *Schizophrenia and the Family.* New York: International Universities Press, 1965.

_____: *The Person.* New York: Basic Books, Inc., 1968.

_____: *The Origin and Treatment of Schizophrenic Disorders.* New York: Basic Books, Inc., 1973.

_____: "The Family: The Developmental Setting," in Arieti, Silvano: *American Handbook of Psychiatry.* New York: Basic Books, Inc., 1974, Vol. I, pp. 252–63.

MAIN, T. F.: "Mothers with Children on a Psychiatric Unit," in Barnes, Elizabeth: *Psychosocial Nursing.* London: Tavistock Publications, 1968, pp. 119–36.

MASLOW, A. H.: *Motivation and Personality.* New York: Harper and Bros., 1954, pp. 80–106.

MEALEY, ANN R.: "Sculpting as a Group Technique for Increasing Awareness," *Perspectives in Psychiatric Care.* 3:XV:118–121, 1977.

MERRILL, GEORGIA: "How Fathers Manage When Wives are Hospitalized for Schizophrenia," *Social Psychiatry,* 4:1:26–32, 1969.

METROPOLITAN LIFE: *Statistical Bulletin,* 58, May 1977.

_____: *Statistical Bulletin,* 59:4, October–December 1978.

MILLER, SALLY: "A Study in Family Dynamics," *Perspectives in Psychiatric Care,* 1:3:9 ff, March–April 1963.

MINUCHIN, SALVADOR: *Families and Family Therapy.* Cambridge, Mass.: Harvard University Press, 1974.

ORGUE, MODESTA S.: "Health Care and Minority Clients," *Nursing Outlook,* 24:5:313–316, May 1976.

PADBERG, JOAN: " 'Bargaining' to Improve Communications in Conjoint Family Therapy," *Perspectives in Psychiatric Care,* 2:XII:68–71, 1975.

PAPAJOHN, JOHN, and SPIEGEL, JOHN: *Transactions in Families.* San Francisco: Jossey-Bass, 1975.

PARSONS, TALCOTT: "The Transmission of Values," *Psychiatry,* 15:1:15–25, February 1952.

_____: "Status and Authority," in Coser, Rose Laub, ed.: *The Family: Its Structure and Functions.* New York: St. Martin's Press, 1964, pp. 251–66.

PROCK, VALENCIA N.: "Effects of Institutionalization; A Comparison of Community, Waiting List and Institutionalized Aged Persons," *American Journal of Public Health,* 59:10:1837–44, October 1969.

RUESCH, JURGEN: *Therapeutic Communication.* New York: W. W. Norton, 1961.

RUESCH, JURGEN, and BATESON, GREGORY: *Communication: The Social Matrix of Psychiatry.* New York: W. W. Norton & Co., Inc., 1951.

SATIR, VIRGINIA: *Conjoint Family Therapy.* Palo Alto, Calif.: Science and Behavior Books, 1964.

SHANAS, ETHEL: *The Health of Older People; A Social Survey.* Cambridge, Mass.: Harvard University Press, 1962.

_____: "Family Help Patterns and Social Class in Three Countries," in Neugarten, Bernice L., ed.: *Middle Age and Aging.* Chicago: The University of Chicago Press, 1968, pp. 296–305.

_____: TOWNSEND, PETER, WEDDERBURN, D., FRIIS, H., MILHOJ, and STEHOMWER, J.:

Older People in Three Industrial Societies. New York: Atherton Press, 1968.

SPIEGEL, JOHN P.: "The Resolution of Role Conflict Within the Family," in Greenblatt, Milton; Levinson, Daniel J., and Williams, Richard H., eds.: *The Patient and the Mental Hospital.* Glencoe, Ill.: The Free Press, 1957, pp. 545–64.

———: "Cultural Strain, Family Role Patterns, and Intrapsychic Conflict," in Howells, John G., ed.: *Theory and Practice of Family Psychiatry.* New York: Brunner/Mazel, 1971, pp. 367–89.

STANTON, A. H., and SCHWARTZ, MORRIS S.: *The Mental Hospital,* New York: Basic Books, Inc., 1954.

STUART, RICHARD B.: "Operant—Interpersonal Treatment for Marital Discord," in Sager, E. J., and Kaplan, H. S., eds.: *Progress in Group and Family Therapy.* New York: Brunner/Mazel, 1972, pp. 498–508.

UNITED STATES NATIONAL COMMISSION FOR UNESCO: *Report on Women in America.* Washington, D.C.: U.S. Government Printing Office, 1977.

Webster's New Collegiate Dictionary. Springfield, Mass.: G. & C. Merriam Co., 1977.

WEINER, LEONARD, BECKER, ALVIN, and FRIEDMAN, TOBIAS T.: *Home Treatment. Spearhead of Community Psychiatry.* Pittsburgh: University of Pittsburgh Press, 1967.

WYNNE, LYMAN C., RYCKOFF, J. M., DAY, J., and HIRSCH, STANLEY J.: "Pseudomutuality in the Family Relations of Schizophrenics." *Psychiatry,* 21:205–20, 1958.

Suggested Readings

ACKERMAN, NATHAN W., and BEHRENS, MARJORIE L.: "Family Diagnosis and Clinical Process," in Arieti, Silvano: *American Handbook of Psychiatry,* Vol. II. New York: Basic Books, Inc., 1974, pp. 37–50.

ASCH, STUART S., and RUBIN, LOWELL J.: "Post-partum Reactions: Some Unrecognized Variations," *American Journal of Psychiatry,* 131:8:870–74, August 1974.

BULBULYAN, ANN AGAVNI: "The Psychiatric Nurse as Family Therapist," *Perspectives in Psychiatric Care,* 7:2:58–68, 1969.

DAVIS, ANNE J.: "Social Factors," in Kalkman, Marion E., and Davis, Anne J., eds.: *New Dimensions in Mental Health—Psychiatric Nursing.* New York: McGraw-Hill, 1974, pp. 503–19.

DE YOUNG, CAROL D.: "Nursing's Contribution in Family Crisis Treatment," *Nursing Outlook,* 16:2:60–63, February 1968.

DUMAS, RHETAUGH: "This I Believe . . . About Nursing and the Poor," *Nursing Outlook,* 17:9:47–50, September 1969.

FOA, E. B., and CHATTERJEE, B. B.: "Self-other Differentiation: A Cross Culturally Invariant Characteristic of Mental Patients," *Social Psychiatry,* 9:119–22, 1974.

GARDNER, L. I.: "Deprivation and Dwarfism," *Scientific American,* 1:76–83, 1972.

HALL, JOANNE E., and WEAVER, BARBARA R.: *Nursing of Families in Crisis.* Philadelphia: J. B. Lippincott Co., 1974.

HARRINGTON, MICHAEL: *The Other America.* Baltimore: Penguin Books, 1963.

HENRY, JULES: "Family Structure and the Transmission of Neurotic Behavior," *American Journal of Orthopsychiatry,* 21:800–818, 1951.

JONES, SUSAN L.: "The Double-Bind as a 'Tested' Theoretical Formulation," *Perspectives in Psychiatric Care,* 4:XV:162–169, 1977.

LEAVITT, MARIBELLE: "Discharge Crisis: The Experience of Families of Psychiatric Patients," *Nursing Research,* 24:1:33–40, January–February 1975.

LEDERER, WILLIAM J., and JACKSON, DON D.: *The Mirages of Marriage.* New York: W. W. Norton & Co., Inc., 1968.

LEININGER, MADELEINE: "Changing Foci in American Nursing Education; Primary and Transcultural Nursing Care," *Journal of Advanced Nursing,* 3:2:155–166, March 1978.

LEWIS, OSCAR: *Five Families.* New York: Basic Books, Inc. 1959.

———: *The Children of Sanchez.* New York: Alfred A. Knopf, Inc., 1961.

LIEBOW, ELLIOT: *Tally's Corner,* Boston: Little, Brown & Co., 1967.

MEZZROW, MEZZ: *Really the Blues.* New York: The Dell Publishing Co., 1946.

NYE, F. IVAN, and BERARDO, FELIX M.: *The Family: Its Structure and Interaction.* New York: Macmillan Publishing Co., Inc., 1973.

RUSSELL, BERTRAND: *Marriage and Morals.* Liveright edition published October 1929, New York: Bantam Books, Inc., 1959.

SIEWON, MARK I.: "Family Subsystem: Working with School-age Children Experiencing Psychosocial Stress," in Longo, Dianne C., and Williams, Reg Arthur: *Clinical Practice in Psychosocial Nursing: Assessment and Intervention.* New York: Appleton-Century-Crofts, 1978, pp. 289–318.

SMOYAK, SHIRLEY, ED.: *The Psychiatric Nurse as a Family Therapist.* New York: John Wiley & Sons, 1975.

SHAINESS, NATALIE: "The Effect of Changing Cultural Patterns Upon Women," in Arieti, Silvano, ed.: *American Handbook of Psychiatry,*

Vol. 1, New York: Basic Books, Inc., 1974, pp. 467–81.

WEAKLAND, JOHN H., FISCH, RICHARD, WATZLAWICK, PAUL, and BODIN, ARTHUR M.: "Brief Therapy: Focused Problem Resolution," *Family Process,* 13:2:141–68, June 1974.

WINSTEAD-FRY, PATRICIA: "Family Theory and Application," in Haber, Judith et al., eds.: *Comprehensive Psychiatric Nursing.* New York: McGraw-Hill Book Company, 1978, pp. 161–176.

WHITLEY, MARILYN PEDDICORD, and MADDEN L. (SISSY): "Encountering Dysfunction in the Family System" in Longo, Dianne C., and Williams, Reg Arthur, eds.: *Clinical Practice in Psychosocial Nursing: Assessment and Intervention.* New York: Appleton-Century-Crofts, 1978.

3

Social Psychiatry

Although the orientation of this book is toward social psychiatry, this chapter includes specific concepts in the field toward which current programs are directed. Social psychiatry is the field of psychiatry that is concerned with sociocultural and ecologic factors that affect maladaptive behavior; it also is concerned with involvement of the patient, the family, and the community in prevention and treatment. Social psychiatry is often used synonymously with community psychiatry. This chapter relates to some of the sociocultural and ecologic factors associated with the living experiences of psychiatric patients in institutions, other services, and to the potential patient in the wider society.

Epidemiology of Mental Disorder[1]

Mental disorder is America's major health problem. The list of the ten leading causes of death includes suicide but omits mental disorder per se. Yet, the incidence and numbers of suicides are considered to be one barometer of the mental health of a population. The epidemiological approach identifies populations at risk within communities and detects origin of diseases and the ways they spread. The distribution of mental disorder is studied in relation to ". . . time,

---

[1] The study of the mass aspects of mental disorder.

space, or the distinguishing characteristics of individuals or social groups affected."[2] Once the history of mental disorder within a population has been determined, preventive methods are established. The uses of epidemiology are (1) to assess changes in incidence, prevalence, and mortality from disorders, (2) to conduct community diagnosis, (3) to estimate individual risks of acquiring various mental disorders, (4) to assess the actions of the health facilities, (5) to identify syndromes, (6) to solidify the clinical picture and describe the onset and progress of chronic disorders, and (7) to provide clues to etiology (Morris, 1964).

For the past two decades, psychiatric professionals have been taking a broader view of mental disorder. Not only are they concerned with the intrapsychic dynamics of individuals, but they are focusing as well on the family and the community.

We need to know more about the dynamic interconnections of individual, family, and community. Where there is a family, mental disorder is thought to be regularly preceded by interpersonal conflicts within the family group. Therefore, the more that is known about family development, family dynamics, and the interrelationships of culture, the better we will be able to identify etiology of mental disorder. Nurses who practice in these settings can add data to the much-needed research in this area.

CLASSIFICATION OF MENTAL DISORDERS

A classification is needed to study epidemiology. The first classification of mental disorder was made by Emil Kraepelin toward the end of the nineteenth century (Deutsch, 1937), although a division into two main groups of mania and melancholia had been made previously by Hippocrates. Kraepelin described two entirely new groups of patients with mental disorder: manic depressives and what were later termed schizophrenics by Bleuler (1971). Kraepelin's classification, introduced into

the United States in 1896, provided the basis for the classification used today.

Any science requires a system of classification; therefore, the adoption of a classification of mental disorder was a move toward development of a science of psychiatry. It provides a method of studying the spread of mental disorder in a specified population. Some of the interconnections between the population—its biological, demographic, psychological, and socioeconomic aspects—and mental disorder lead to the study of etiology. It also aids the clinician to provide appropriate treatment measures for the patient.

The data of classification are also useful in assessment of preventive and treatment services. Despite the late start of psychiatry in medicine, it adopted a standard nomenclature in 1917 and cooperated in the establishment of the *Standard Nomenclature of Disease*, published in the thirties. Most psychiatric problems encountered in World War II did not fit the old nomenclature, so the Veterans Administration, the Army, and the Navy each devised its own system. After World War II, a new classification was made[3] by the American Psychiatric Association; this was revised in cooperation with the *International Classification of Diseases*, eighth revision.[4] An international committee worked together to reach consensus on the diagnostic groupings. The *DSM II* coincided for the most part with the international classification, although there were some differences. Some changes were made for national use, which did not, however, interfere with the broad international divisions.

DSM III was introduced in the United States in 1980 (see Appendix C). Many changes have been made in the new *DSM III*. Neurotic disorders formerly under their own heading are now included in Affective, Anxiety, Somatoform, Dissociative, and Psychosexual Disorders. Psychophysiologic disorders no longer appear in the nomenclature. Psychosomatic reaction takes the place of psychophysiologic disorder and this category can be used to indicate psychological

[2] Reed, D. D.: *Epidemiological Methods in the Study of Mental Disorders.* Geneva: World Health Organization, 1960, p. 8.

[3] *Diagnostic and Statistical Manual of Mental Disorders.* American Psychiatric Association, 1952.

[4] *Diagnostic and Statistical Manual of Mental Disorders, II.* American Psychiatric Association, 1968.

aspects of any physical disorder or condition, for example, ulcers as well as diarrhea. In addition to the changes in the list of clinical syndromes, operational criteria and a multiaxial approach to diagnosis are unique features of *DSM III.* Each patient is evaluated on five axes:

"I. Clinical psychiatric syndrome(s) and other conditions
II. Personality disorders (adults) and specific developmental disorders
III. Physical disorders
IV. Severity of psychosocial stressors
V. Highest level of adaptive functioning, past year"[5]

In this revised classification, criteria for diagnosis take considerable time and thought to use. The multiaxial scheme provides for multiple categories to be coded for any one patient. All mental disorders appear in either Axis I or Axis II. Psychosocial stressors are evaluated on the basis of, for example, none to catastrophic. Evaluation of adaptive functioning is based upon role performance, social functioning, self-care and autonomy. Recognition of the importance of stress, social system, and the developmental life cycle in the life of the individual is evidenced by the use of the Axes III, IV, and V in the evaluation process. Strengths of the individual therefore become a part of each evaluation. The convergence of sociology, anthropology, and psychiatry has perhaps been responsible, in part, for the new nomenclature of *DSM III.* However, because *DSM III* is at variance with the *Manual of the International Statistical Classification of Diseases, Injuries, and Causes of Death* (World Health Organization, 1977), this fact itself indicates problems in international understanding of the diagnostic categories.

A long-range epidemiological psychiatric study has been conducted by the World Health Organization in nine countries of varying cultures: Colombia, Czechoslovakia, Denmark, India, Nigeria, Taiwan, U.S.S.R., United Kingdom, and the United States of America. It is known as the *Interna-*

tional Pilot Study of Schizophrenia, an international, transcultural study of 1202 patients, 80 percent of whom were followed up and reassessed after two and five years (Sartorius, 1976). A striking finding was that the rates of recovery without social impairment were higher in developing countries with their larger family groups than in developed countries with their nuclear families. Social relationships were considered to play a key role in a favorable outcome (Strauss et al., 1977). Three variables stand out as key predictors of two-year and five-year outcome: (1) social contacts, (2) work functions, and (3) duration of hospitalization prior to evaluation (Strauss et al., 1977).

International mental health has had minimal discussion for several years in the Health Assemblies of the World Health Organization. Recently, a new mental health program has been developed with three principal objectives:

- "To prevent or reduce psychiatric, neurological, and psychosocial problems, including those related to alcoholism and drug dependence
- To increase the effectiveness of the general health services through appropriate utilization of mental health skills and knowledge
- To develop strategies for intervention based on an increased awareness of the mental health aspects of social action and change"[6]

ECOLOGY OF MENTAL DISORDER

Within the last two decades emphasis in psychiatry has turned toward the study of the person in relation to his environment. This approach is now added to the consideration of the intrapsychic self. Knowledge about the self or the patient and the effect the person has upon another person is fundamental to the understanding of patients with mental disorder. Although there are many aspects of ecology that can contribute to mental disorder (e.g., genetics and the *Treponema pallidum),* this book limits its emphasis to some of the sociocultural concepts.

[5] American Psychiatric Association: *Diagnostic and Statistical Manual of Mental Disorders, III.* Washington, D.C.: Amerian Psychiatric Association, 1980.

[6] Sartorius, N.: "WHO's New Mental Health Programme." *WHO Chronicle.* 32:2:60–62, February, 1978, p. 60.

MIGRATION AND RELOCATION[7]

These two aspects of finding a new home do not necessarily result in mental disorder, but they do add stress to the family unit. A disrupting event such as migration can bring about stress and emotional reactions that can result in a variety of mental problems. The father's change in jobs, loss of job, discrimination in the labor market, the family's change in life-style, and loss of friends may result in adverse reactions. Immigrants face learning a new language and establishing an economic standard of living.

The relationship between migration and mental disorder varies with the characteristics of the migrants, the sending and receiving communities, and the situation of the migration (Kantor, 1969). In a study of hospital admission rates, it was found that rates of first admissions to mental hospitals in New York were higher for migrants than for nonmigrants (Malzberg and Lee, 1956). In a later paper, Lee (1963) found that widowhood was more likely to be followed by institutionalization in migrants than in nonmigrants. Opler (1959) cites sociocultural stress as one of the prominent explanations for higher rates of mental disorder in migrants. The study of Faris and Dunham (1960) showed that most of the foreignborn in Chicago had higher hospitalization rates for schizophrenia than the native-born. Malzberg (1969) analyzed the reports on high rates of first admissions to mental hospitals of the foreign-born. He found that when the factors of age, sex, and urban–rural distribution differentials were considered, the rates of first admissions to mental hospitals were almost equivalent for native-born and foreign-born, although the foreign-born are reported uniformly as having higher rates. Migration is now changing character because the population in the central cities is declining and nonmetropolitan areas are growing the fastest. Murphy's (1959) studies of migration and mental disorder of migrants to Singapore showed that the Chinese extended family seemed to give more protection against mental disorder in old age whereas a high incidence of involutional melancholia was found in the *kongsi*[8] dweller.

Migration tends to increase the distance between older people and their children and decrease responsibility.

In migration, the attitude toward the change is important in the adjustment of the family members. Disintegration of patterns of communication, cooperation, help, and support has occurred. New patterns must be developed if mental health is to be maintained. In families who are prepared to move and have a favorable attitude toward the move, adjustment and adaptation are perhaps better than for those who are not. Favorable attitudes of parents can influence the children. In the case of relocation, the primary prevention is clearly to assist families to be prepared to make the move. Migrants of low socioeconomic status are perhaps harder hit than those in the higher status group. Changes in status sometime accompany migration and may be perceived as a threat to the ego, thereby adding to the stress.

Relocation has been found to result in a sense of loss with intense grief reactions (Fried, 1965). The varieties of problems affecting isolated older persons in relocation have been presented by Smith (1966), who pointed out that the greatest deficiency in community resources was the link between such people and the services themselves. Self-help groups such as the Salvation Army have long recognized the needs related to migration and relocation and are organized to provide some of the material aid required at these times; various other organizations also assist.

Relationships and forms of communication within a community take time to develop. In some instances after migration and relocation they may never be developed, and alienation and other problems will emerge. Nurses in community mental health can aid in prevention of mental problems by (1) case finding (knowing who these families are), (2) helping them to

[7] *Migration* refers to a change of residence from one community to another, whereas moving is simply a change of residence within the same community. *Relocation* refers to forced moving, usually thought of in relation to urban renewal conversion of apartments to condominiums or some other event such as disaster.

[8] *Kongsi* refers to a system of residential clubs for adults.

know their community and its resources, (3) helping them get needed help, (4) organizing regular community meetings in relation to the needs of a community, (5) referral, and (6) provision of emotional support. Forced migration or relocation as at the time of a disaster involves local, state, and federal aid and the assistance of many agencies. These agencies are generally not functioning well, if at all, in a country torn by war, and the suffering endured by those fleeing battle zones is severe.

POVERTY

Although many studies have shown the adverse effects of poverty on the health of human beings, few have considered why the majority of slum dwellers grow up without mental disorder (Sartorius, 1978). Because one is poor does not mean that he will become mentally disordered although the researchers have shown that the risk is higher for the poor. Schwab and associates (1978) cite lower socioeconomic status as high risk for both mental disorder and physical illnesses. The high incidence of mental disorder among the poor has been studied and documented by the classic study of Hollingshead and Redlich (1958). In the Midtown Manhattan Study's Home Survey, a sample population of 1660 individuals, somewhat more than 80 percent, were found to have some kind of psychiatric symptoms. The best mental health occurred in persons whose parents were in high socioeconomic status groups, and relatively poor mental health was found in persons whose parents were of low socioeconomic status (Srole et al., 1962, Chap. 12). More people in the low status groups were exposed to disintegrative influences (Leighton et al., 1963). Poverty adversely affects the mental health of our nation's children (Joint Commission on Mental Health of Children, Inc., 1970).

Although the implementation of the concept of available mental health services for poor and rich alike has resulted in better distribution of services, a better quality of life afforded by adequate employment, housing, education, and delivery of general health care has yet to be achieved for the poor. Until a better quality of life is available for the American poor, they will continue to be high-risk groups for mental disorder.

CULTURE AND MENTAL DISORDER

A major problem associating culture and mental disorder is the all-inclusiveness of a definition of culture, for example, from practices of parenting to choices of housing. Culture thereby becomes a multivariate entity (Sartorius et al., 1976). However, the use of this approach confirms that there are common, basic forms of psychological disturbance across cultures and that they may be manifest in different ways. Patterns of behavior among Irish and Italian men who were schizophrenic established this point of view where sharp contrasts appeared in the expression of emotions; for example, the Italian group acted out their feelings whereas the Irish group tended toward fantasy life (Opler, 1957).

In any study of culture one must be careful to avoid stereotyping any specific group. The importance of recognition of individual differences within a specific ethnic group therefore cannot be overestimated.

Striving and interference with the striving are both related to mental disorder (Leighton, 1966). Horney (1936) considered the problem of competition to be a central issue in individuals with neurotic conflicts, and that, in the American culture, those who have met the demands of competition to a high degree may be more subject to neurotic conflict.

Cultural conflict between the parental culture and the American culture is an important consideration as a psychosocial stressor in mental disorder. It is widely accepted that membership in a cohesive family that offers group support can act as a cushioning effect against life's stresses (World Health Organization, 1976). Large social networks tend to help overcome the stresses of cultural conflict. A major sociocultural force of the times is a strong emphasis upon reaffirmation of ethnicity, the search for roots, study of ancestors, and traditions. Highlighted by the Black identity movement and later the Asian-American, Hispanic, and native American, the list continues to grow. This reaffirmation of ethnicity among varied groups is the new cultural pluralism, and represents a search for a sense of belonging and self-esteem (Giordano, 1973). Where merging with the wider society of the American culture is not considered desirable, reaffirmation of ethnic identity aids many individuals to find satisfactions, comforts, security, enhancement of self-concept and other ingredients of positive mental health.

Racism[9] was cited by the Joint Commission on the Mental Health of Children as a health hazard:

. . . the racist attitude of Americans which causes and perpetuates tension is patently a most compelling health hazard. Its destructive effects severely cripple the growth and development of millions of our citizens, young and old alike. Yearly, it directly and indirectly causes more fatalities, disabilities and economic loss than any other single factor.[10]

Researchers have in the past perhaps studied international cross-cultural societies rather than the cultural diversity within the United States, although this is now changing. The ethnic identity movement is also resulting in a reaffirmation of ethnicity among all groups. More research is needed on the influences of the sociocultural aspects of society on the mental health of its members. Willie and Associates (1973), stated that the present knowledge about racism and mental health is conflicting and, for some, confusing.

Profound social changes are underway throughout American society concerning the traditional roles of women as housewives and childbearers. *Sexism*[11] serves as a barrier for women to realize their full potential as human beings.

Social isolation is another factor. The inner American city is likely to be populated with older persons who live alone, prostitutes, schizophrenics, alcoholics, and drug addicts. All, in some sense, suffer social isolation

and alienation from the wider society and are thereby subject to multiple crises.

There is a heightened appreciation in psychiatry that mental disorder does not result from a single agent but is multidetermined. Although the precipitating event may truly be, for example, automation resulting in loss of job, money, and therefore loss of status and security, the stresses of war, or forced migration, such episodes do not occur in isolation from the usual ways of reacting or from the cultural background of the individual and of the family. There are many other cultural conditions that can lead to crises.

A disruption of the basic needs of the individual and of the primary functions of the family can result in a crisis. The principal focus of nursing is related to helping individuals and families to meet such needs and functions or to find suitable substitutes for them.

Reform and Locus of Care

In 1955 the number of patients (558,-992) in state and county mental hospitals was at its peak (Talbott, 1978). A dramatic reduction of the resident population of state and county mental hospitals has occurred. Resident patients decreased from 475,999 in 1965 to 191,391 in 1975, a decrease of 60 percent (U.S. Department of Health, Education, and Welfare, 1978). Of the 385,200 persons admitted to state and county hospitals in 1975, over 34 percent were schizophrenic and 28 percent were alcoholic; 12 percent were diagnosed as depression (U.S. Department of Health, Education, and Welfare, 1977a).

DEINSTITUTIONALIZATION

Deinstitutionalization in its common usage refers to a process that avoids state mental hospitalization for care of mentally disordered persons and expansion of services in the community for these individuals. Another aspect of deinstitutionalization is sociopolitical reform (U.S. Department of

---

[9] Racism is "a belief that race is the primary determinant of human traits and capacities and that racial differences produce an inherent superiority of a particular race." (*Webster's New Collegiate Dictionary*, 1977).

[10] Joint Commission on Mental Health of Children: *Crises in Child Mental Health: Challenge for the 1970's*, New York: Harper & Row, 1970, p. 216.

[11] *Sexism* is "prejudice or discrimination based upon sex" (*Webster's New Collegiate Dictionary*, 1977).

Health, Education, and Welfare, 1977b). Central to this reform were the underpinnings of sociopsychiatric and other studies, which lead professionals to believe that any form of treatment was better than an institution.

During the 1950s the influences of sociopsychiatric, anthropological, and sociological studies were keenly felt by practitioners. Interaction of staff and patients in psychiatric institutions became a focus for research. Caudill and associates (1952) used the technique of concealed participant observation, the anthropologist playing the role of the mental patient. Caudill's study re-emphasized the importance of informal group living in a psychiatric ward upon the clinical course of the patient.

A classical study in the field of psychiatric nursing reflects the importance of nursing intervention (Tudor, 1952).

A three-year study of a psychiatric institution, using formal and informal participation in the life of the institution as methods of study, described the origins of disturbances in patients as related to conflicts among staff and among patients (Stanton and Schwartz, 1954). Main (1946), Jones et al. (1953), Opler (1956), Goffman (1961), and Leighton (1966) and others added the sociocultural approach to psychiatry. How nurses communicate and relate with patients and how they understand and help them was described (Schwartz and Shockley, 1956). The patient's point of view of interactions among patients was contained in a study at a small teaching hospital (Carter, 1959), and, at a later date, a larger study was made as a recommendation of the earlier study (Carter and Davis, 1963, and 1964). Effective behavior of psychiatric nursing personnel from the patient's point of view was described (Fatka, 1958). A renewed humanistic concern occurred in which the mentally disordered person was viewed not only as an individual with intrapsychic conflicts but as a person in an environment that may have contributed to his condition. Psychiatric wards that had been locked for over a century opened their doors and thereby restored some freedom to patients, and psychiatric staff began to interact with patients in different ways. Psychiatric nurses doffed their uniforms in an effort to de-emphasize status. Group therapy, psychopharmacology, the therapeutic community, and establishment of rehabilitation departments in state mental hospitals with the wide use of volunteers aided in the new reform. For accreditation by the National League for Nursing, schools of nursing were required in the early 1950s to provide experience in psychiatric nursing for their students (NLN, 1977). As these students and their instructors moved into state hospitals, their work, perceptions, and criticism contributed to more humane conditions for patients. The rise of psychiatric units in private general hospitals made community care possible for those who could afford it. A new field arose called social psychiatry and the first meeting of the International Association of Social Psychiatry was held in London, August 17–21, 1964.

In 1955, 77 percent of patient-care episodes were provided in inpatient facilities and 23 percent in outpatient facilities. In 1975 a different picture emerged: Twenty-four percent of patient-care episodes were provided in inpatient facilities; 47 percent of patient-care episodes were provided in outpatient facilities; community mental health centers provided 29 percent (see Fig. 1.)

Central to this drastic change has been the community mental-health movement enabled by the Mental Retardation Facilities and Community Mental Health Centers Construction Act of 1963 (Public Law 88–164), and the subsequent amendments. The federally funded community mental-health centers include inpatient and outpatient services. Community mental-health centers have shown increasing importance in psychiatric care in that the proportion of patient-care episodes in the inpatient and outpatient services of community mental-health centers more than doubled between 1967 and 1969 from 4 percent in 1967 to 9.9 percent in 1969 and almost doubled again between 1969 and 1971, comprising 19 percent of all episodes in 1971, and 29 percent in 1975. A most significant change has occurred in the state mental hospitals, which provided 49 percent of all services in 1955 and nine percent in 1975.

The enabling legislation—Public Law 88–164—the Mental Retardation Facilities

Figure 1. Percent Distribution of Inpatient and Outpatient Care Episodes in Mental Health Facilities by Type of Facility, United States 1955 and 1975.[a]

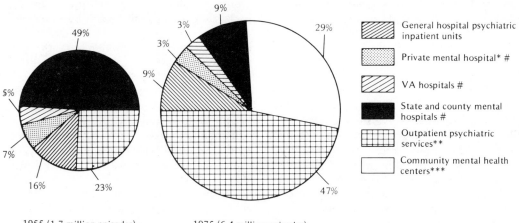

1955 (1.7 million episodes)   1975 (6.4 million episodes)

Legend:
- General hospital psychiatric inpatient units
- Private mental hospital* #
- VA hospitals #
- State and county mental hospitals #
- Outpatient psychiatric services**
- Community mental health centers***

  * Includes residential treatment centers for emotionally disturbed children

  \# Inpatient services only

  ** Includes free–standing outpatient services as well as those affiliated with psychiatric and general hospitals

  *** Includes inpatient and outpatient services of federally funded community mental health centers

  [a] Source: President's Commission on Mental Health, *Task Panel Reports,* Vol. II, Appendix. Washington, D.C., U.S. Government Printing Office, 1978, p. 54.

and Community Mental Health Centers Construction Act of 1963 has made community care of patients with mental disorder a reality. Former President Kennedy signed it into law October 31, 1963. PL 88–164 provided funds for construction of community mental health centers and staffing on a declining basis with the expectation that states and local communities would eventually pick up the cost. Central to the provision of services was the idea of the catchment area—a population of 75,000 to 200,000 people for whom each center was designated to serve.

The Act required that the centers provide five essential services: (1) *inpatient care,* (2) *outpatient care,* (3) *emergency services,* (4) *partial hospitalization,* such as day care, weekend care, and night care, and (5) *consultation and education* services to community agencies and professional personnel and information services to the general public.

For a fully comprehensive service, five additional services are: (1) *diagnostic,* (2) *rehabilitative,* including vocational and educational programs, (3) *precare and aftercare* services in the community including foster home placement, home visiting and halfway

houses, (4) *training,* and (5) *research and evaluation.*

Subsequent amendments to PL 88–164 were passed to authorize more funds for construction and support of staffing. In addition, alcoholic and narcotic-addict rehabilitation programs were funded and for the first time, alcoholics were to be treated as patients instead of being sent to jail.

In addition to extending earlier legislation, still more legislation was passed to provide needed mental health services for underserved populations, for example, children. Poverty areas then became a priority for funding.

Under Public Law 94–63 (1975) all new and existing mental health centers were required to offer the essential services, and in addition, a variety of new services were made compulsory and some old services given new guidelines. Services for older persons and for children were made compulsory, including diagnosis, treatment, liaison, and follow-up services. All patients were to be screened by the mental health centers and alternatives to hospitalization found where possible. After-care services were made mandatory. PL 94–63 also required that services be organized to overcome cultural, linguistic, and economic barriers and required citizen participation in agency policy making. It also made mandatory a quality assurance program and improvement in medical-record systems. These socio-political changes have resulted in a great impact on patient care and consequently on nursing.

Although much progress has been made, many persons still receive inadequate care. The President's Commission on Mental Health (1978), cited racial and ethnic minorities, the urban poor, migrant and seasonal workers and the chronically mentally ill as among those who are underserved. Among many problems addressed by the Commission, special attention was called to alcohol-related problems, the abuse of psychoactive drugs, and mental retardation.

Many factors contributed to the shift in locus of care for mental patients. The dehumanizing conditions in many state hospitals following World War II must not be forgotten. Deutsch (1948) and others exposed these bad conditions to the public. Many of these institutions were not hospitals in the true sense of the word but custodial places for large numbers of people who were unwanted elsewhere. Thousands of patients spent most of their lives in state hospitals. The state hospitals were underfunded and therefore had to rely on the free labor of the patients in order to function. I have known many patients who had never seen a modern traffic light or a modern kitchen. One patient whose initial diagnosis was "mentally defective" and who had spent thirty-eight of his fifty years in state hospitals saved the life of an attendant who accidentally locked himself in the morgue freezer.

Other factors that have made the move to community care possible are: psychopharmacology, Medicare and Medicaid, and federal aid to the mentally disabled, for example, Aid to the Totally Disabled and in 1974, the Supplemental Security Income under Social Security.

A new philosophy of care arose that state hospitals were no longer treatment centers, and that institutionalization in these places added to mental disorder instead of improving it. The cruel and inhuman conditions

in some of these institutions made people feel that anything was better than a state mental hospital. The reform of the care-giving system was to take place by legislation that provided funding and consultation and the organization and implementation were to be carried out by local governments in cooperation with citizens. Many people in communities were accustomed to the state mental hospitals being faraway places where people with mental disorder were safely incarcerated. Resistances to establishment of mental health services in neighborhoods became widespread and the progressivism slowed down. Although over two thousand community mental-health centers were expected to be built in the eight years following the enabling legislation in 1963, fifteen years later only five hundred were in existence.

Closing the bad state mental hospitals and making a better life for persons with mental disorder within the community seemed to be related to a new sociopolitical reform seeking self-determination of smaller units of government. Instead of depending on state government for care, protection, and nurturance, mental patients were to be cared for in their home communities. Fed-

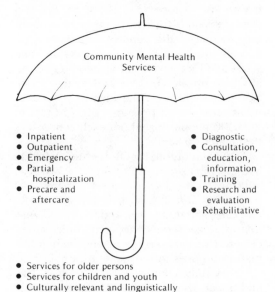

- Inpatient
- Outpatient
- Emergency
- Partial hospitalization
- Precare and aftercare

- Diagnostic
- Consultation, education, information
- Training
- Research and evaluation
- Rehabilitative

Community Mental Health Services

- Services for older persons
- Services for children and youth
- Culturally relevant and linguistically appropriate services
- Citizen participation
- Services overcoming economic and geographic barriers

Figure 2. Community Mental Health Services.

eral assistance to counties was to be phased out over a period of eight years. Funds formerly used for patients in state mental hospitals were expected to be allocated to the counties for their care. Thus, a de-emphasis on large impersonal institutions with custodial care was to be carried out (see Fig. 2). The state governments that had provided minimal care for persons with mental disorder expected to hand over the problem to the counties as county government had left it to them for so many years.

LOCKED FACILITIES

Persons unable to live in Board and Care Homes or other residential places may be sent to locked facilities where minimal treatment is provided. These locked facilities seem to be the same custodial places, only smaller, less visible to the public, and operated by private enterprise (Carter, 1977). In my community, they are located *out of the county* due to: (1) politics, (2) economics (i.e., the owner of locked facilities can make more profit in a remote, less expensive area), and (3) community opposition.

Locked facilities, hotels, streets, parks, and board and care homes are now places where many patients live who formerly (1955) would have been in state mental hospitals. The locked facilities and board and care homes have been referred to as "hidden institutionalization" (California, State of, 1978). The number of people per one hundred thousand in mental hospitals and residential treatment centers has decreased from approximately four hundred in 1950 to approximately two hundred in 1970. However, people in homes for the aged and dependent increased from 196 per one hundred thousand in 1950 to 456 per one hundred thousand in 1970. (President's Commission on Mental Health, Vol. II, 1978, p. 65.) One can assume that homes for the aged and dependent have many of the patients who would have formerly been sent to state mental hospitals.

URBAN TRANSIENTS

Although probably not counted by the 1970 census or categorized into any institutional group, a large number of mentally disordered young people wander through cities sleeping in parks, laundromats, under freeways, subway entrances, bus stations, rooftops, and abandoned buildings. In my community, they are referred to as "no locals," having no local address and often no address at all. They often lack education, vocational skills, family support, and constitute perhaps the most marginal of the vagrant subculture (Segal et al., 1977). Mental health services do not adequately address the needs of these individuals who may become a new dependent group. One young man refused financial aid, prided himself by not ever sleeping on the street (he actually slept on a mat placed on the street), ate his meals from garbage cans, and spent much of the day in the nearby church. These individuals are often brought into the psychiatric services by the police upon the insistence of shopkeepers and others. Sometimes they arrive at the bus station or airport without a penny in their pocket, someone having provided them with a ticket to the West. Other street people refer to them as "space cases" (Segal et al, 1977) and consider them a liability. Having few resources and no plans to make for continuity of care, it is a challenge for professionals to find ways to help. Some are covered with lice, and scabies and with such badly matted long hair and beards that shaving is necessary. One young woman found incoherent in an alley near a night club was brought into the hospital by the police. Her long hair and body were full of lice. In addition, her clothes were rags and she had extensive scabies. Current psychiatric departments may not have been designed for isolation of patients with communicable diseases. Therefore, these conditions challenge the ingenuity of the nursing staff not only to treat the patient but to protect the other patients as well as themselves. At least one state hospital and one *new* psychiatric unit have reinstituted a delousing procedure.

Services to this group are usually available in terms of General Assistance and/or Supplemental Security Income. However, to get General Assistance, an intent to reside must be stated. Proof of current residence such as a statement from a landlord establishes residence. For Supplemental Security Income, proof of disability with dates of hospitalization and therapists are required. This group of urban transients often panhandle for cash, preferring freedom to financial assistance from the government. They appear in the free-meal lines with untreated wounds and are sometimes persuaded to get treatment in the free clinics.

OTHERS

Another group, more organized, but disabled, use and depend on Supplemental Security Income. They live in the cheap downtown hotels, may use the outpatient psychiatric services and/or private therapists paid for by Medi-Cal (in California). They use health and welfare services, know where all the free meals are distributed, may attend local day-treatment programs and take courses in the local community college. These individuals are often robbed of their few dollars and other possessions and their subsequent distress comes to the attention of someone, for example, the hotel manager who refers them to the psychiatric services.

RESIDENTIAL CARE HOMES

These homes, referred to as Board and Care Homes, are run by private enterprise. In my community they are most likely to be large Victorians in the poorer sections of the city. Although the idea of board and care is expected to provide a homelike setting for those mentally disordered persons who do not need hospitalization but need some supervision, in fact, many persons have been placed in homes where this has not occurred. Board and Care Homes house individuals from the ages of eighteen to sixty-five and may also take in veterans. Some homes are small, housing as few as six but others are large (in my community, housing as many as eighty-five). Board and care homes cost much less than hospitalization. Supplemental Security Income provides approximately $465 per month. Of this amount, approximately $425 goes for room and board, leaving $40 each month for all other expenses of living. Clothing, cigarettes, make-up, toothpaste, soap, razor blades, and all other personal items have to be purchased. Little money is left over for recreation, eating out, or taking a trip anywhere out of town. Often, the person

needs assistance to handle the cash. Some spend it all the first few days of the month and then beg cigarettes, etc., for the rest of the month.

People who live in these homes often need assistance with taking their medications, not only for their mental condition but for other problems as well. Many need assistance with personal hygiene, such as bathing. Lice and scabies are two problems in some of these homes. General health and medical supervision may be at a low level due to many factors some of which are the following: (1) unrecognized problems, (2) reluctance to seek it, (3) hesitancy on the part of some physicians to have these individuals in their office, (4) inability to follow the therapeutic regime, (5) lack of coordination between involved agencies such as health and welfare, (6) untrained and unsupervised staff attempting to provide the care, (7) anxiety due to relocation from structured, controlled psychiatric hospitals to a different milieu, and (8) lack of transportation.

Safety. Communities are struggling for and with regulations for these homes to make them safe places to live. Communities that have strict fire regulations and enforce them are likely to be safer. However, the recent fire at Farmington, Missouri, where the building had no sprinkler system and where many patients died attests to a lack of concern for safety measures. Nine mental patients died in a fire in a halfway house in Washington, D.C. Although licensed by city housing officials, the house did not have a *fire escape* or *smoke detector* (*San Francisco Chronicle,* 12 April 1979). The recent robbery and rape of individuals in a Board and Care Home in San Francisco calls for additional safety measures.

During the past ten years some three hundred thousand persons have been discharged from mental hospitals (Sokolovsky et al., 1978). Because financial responsibility for them has now shifted to the federal government in the form of SSI, no other segment of government seemed to want responsibility for their other needs. One conclusion is:

Responsibility for the care of these individuals must be designated and a system of coordinating the diverse array of services for them must be designed and implemented.[12]

Title I of President Carter's proposed Mental Health Systems Act sent to Congress 15 May, 1979 addresses the needs of persons with chronic mental disorder. It proposes specific coordinated services for this group. Barriers to care are to be identified, competency of mental-health personnel improved, and the public educated about the needs. It also proposes that each patient have a coordinator of services.

The Department of Housing and Urban Development is providing funds for housing (new and/or rehabilitated) in group homes for up to twelve persons or small apartments up to ten units for chronically mentally disordered patients eighteen years of age or more.

The increase in nursing home beds and a drop in the number of persons over sixty-five in state and county mental hospitals have great implications for nursing and planning at a community level. The number and proportion of older persons with mental disorders in nursing homes have increased, and under the benefits of Medicare and Medicaid they will continue to rise. The Social Security amendments of 1965 provide insurance for the care of the older person with a mental disorder. Section A of Title XVIII encourages the use of general hospitals, extended care, and home health services. This change in care and residence of older persons with mental disorders is planned to provide better care at a local level. For example, for nursing homes to be licensed, definite standards must be met and the provision of qualified nurses and nursing care plans, formerly unknown in some large public mental hospitals, is mandatory. However, in many instances, the institutions that now house individuals who would formerly have been in state mental hospitals are the new "human warehouses."

TRENDS: PRIVATE SECTOR

An important trend to notice is the recent change of the care of mentally disordered persons in the private sector. The number

of private psychiatric hospitals has increased during 1968–1975 but not at a uniform rate. During 1968–1972, church-operated hospitals decreased by 24 percent, individual- or partner-operated hospitals decreased by 30 percent whereas fifty-five new for-profit corporation hospitals were established (*Schizophrenia Bulletin*, 1978).

These trends demonstrate the decrease in the number of patients treated in mental hospitals. Outpatient treatment doubled since 1955 and treatment in community mental-health centers is increasing. Community mental health services are planned to continue this pattern. The recent movement of the care of mentally disordered persons into the private sector and the shift from inpatient to outpatient care have significance for those persons and for program planning and for education and practice of professionals.

Therapeutic Community

Perhaps no other concept had such a widespread effect to humanize large authoritarian public mental hospitals as the therapeutic community. Introduction of therapeutic community concepts into large state mental hospitals in the 1950s resulted in the open-door policy and introduction of new roles and responsibilities for both staff and patients.

The therapeutic community has three major facets: (1) a place where milieu therapy is used, (2) an orientation toward bridging the gap between psychiatric hospitals and community life, and (3) full use of social organization and interaction in the treatment of the patient. It can be described as a social organization involving teamwork including every person in the treatment unit working cooperatively toward the patient's growth and recovery. Probably the best known example of a therapeutic community was developed by Jones et al. (1953) at Belmont Hospital, England. At Belmont one hundred patients and thirty staff were involved in the treatment program; the patients had personality problems or acting-out disorders. Work therapy was a central part of Belmont's inpatient program and

[12] President's Commission on Mental Health, *Report to the President.* Vol. II, Washington, D.C.: U.S. Government Printing Office, 1978, p. 371.

Resettlement Officers from the Ministry of Labour assisted in job placement upon discharge. Group meetings were held one hour daily by a psychiatrist and nursing staff for groups of ten patients. The small group meetings were run on psychoanalytic lines and techniques varied with the orientation of the psychiatrist. At Belmont, the single therapeutic goal was the adjustment of the individual to social and work conditions outside the institution (Jones, 1956).

Current therapeutic community programs differ according to the philosophy, experience, capabilities of the staff, availability of resources, the patients in the treatment program, and their length of stay. The environment of the therapeutic community includes: (1) a democratic social organization, (2) permissiveness, (3) a spirit of inquiry and helpfulness, (4) a culture that values verbalization of feelings and sharing these feelings, and (5) reality confrontation.

COMMUNITY MEETINGS

The community meeting represents a function of the therapeutic community. Open communication between staff and patients is desired and regular community meetings where all staff and patients are in one room together provide a place and time for anyone to bring up subjects that affect each other. The community meeting is a kind of clearing-house for current problems. Sometimes a whole meeting centers around a particular individual. Problems specific to a smaller group such as a psychotherapy group may be referred to that group for later discussion. Community meetings may be held daily in the morning and two to three times per week on the evening shift and at any other time when an extraordinary event occurs. The group usually elects its leader and recorder. In some instances, where turnover of patients is rapid, a staff member acts as co-leader for the purposes of support and continuity.

AUTHORITY AND RESPONSIBILITY

The concept of the therapeutic community does not mean that everyone does what he pleases. Through the therapeutic community, patients are encouraged to use their initiative and share responsibility for the purposes of increased self-esteem, recovery, and growth. Patients are expected to help themselves and to help each other. This does not mean that the staff abrogates their professional authority and responsibility. Clear designation of decisions that can be made by the patients and those that are made by the staff tends to minimize distortion, although in practice it is often difficult to make these designations. I have seen a therapeutic community program where all decisions were made by majority vote; the result was chaos. Problems arising when staff relinquish their responsibilities have been described by Fischer et al. (1971) and Kincheloe (1973).

Important in the therapeutic community is the caring attitude of the senior staff toward other staff. This caring attitude sets the tone for the atmosphere of the unit.

A major agenda item in a community meeting relates to *tensions*. Tensions within the unit probably receive the most attention in a community meeting. Some examples are: (1) complaints of being ignored by staff on other shifts, (2) conflicts between roommates, (3) complaints of patients who wander around into other patients' rooms and beds, (4) sexual activity, (5) begging, and (6) theft. Housekeeping, personal hygiene, planning activities such as outings, announcements of daily events, and other items may be on the agenda. Reality confrontation, setting limits, and negotiating contracts between individuals involved in conflict are some techniques used by the group. Task assignment is usually done in the community meeting, for example, patients who will orient all newcomers to the psychiatric unit. The following set of rules was developed by a locked short-term treatment unit in a general hospital in a metropolitan area. These rules are posted on the unit bulletin board and included in each patient's orientation brochure:

RULES

1. No physical or verbal assaultive behavior. Such behavior will lead to immediate removal from the situation and appropriate action by staff.
2. Personal space will be respected.

No intrusive touching
No sexual activity
No stealing
Respect of each other's bed space
3. All patients are expected to participate in unit activity.
(See Daily Schedule)
4. No drugs, alcohol, or weapons allowed on the unit.
5. Smoking only in dining room and day room—no smoking in bathrooms. Matches maintained at front desk.
6. Patients demonstrating responsible behavior in the community may become eligible for passes designated by their team physician. Passes are for a specific purpose and specified length of time.
7. All visitors check in at the front desk. Daily visiting hours for adults: 2:00 P.M. to 8:00 P.M. Visitors under fourteen years of age are allowed on the unit only upon request of the patient's team. Inappropriate visitors will be asked to leave.

THIS IS YOUR THERAPEUTIC COMMUNITY AND FOLLOWING THE ABOVE RULES MAKES IT A PLEASANT AND WORKABLE COMMUNITY FOR EVERYONE.

In psychiatric units where a rapid turnover of patients occurs, the community meeting is a place where all staff and patients can be introduced to each other. It also serves as a medium for staff to get in touch with the immediate group atmosphere, especially after weekends and holidays.

Patients and staff are expected to arrive on time and remain during the entire session.

Referred to as a re-hash, following each community meeting, staff usually meet to review how the meeting went, the themes of the meeting, the behaviors observed, and the meaning of the interactions and implications for the patient. A tendency occurs for the re-hash to be long and drawn out unless a definite time limit is set. Sharing of observations is expected by all staff members. Nursing students often express that their psychiatric mental-health nursing experience is the first time that their observations and ideas are valued by an interdisciplinary team.

Through intensive social interaction in the therapeutic community, patients can increase their awareness of the effects of their behavior upon others and develop a sensitivity to the needs of others. Enhancement of self-esteem, recovery, and growth are expected to occur.

To facilitate communication, blackboards for posting rapidly changing data and events are helpful. Bulletin boards and posters are useful areas for posting unit schedules, administrative regulations, and rules set by the community itself. Some recently built psychiatric units and remodeled old ones have open nurses' stations, thereby facilitating communication between staff and patients.

TRANSITIONAL SERVICES

To bridge the gap between hospital and community life, an array of transitional services has emerged within the last two decades; for example, therapeutic social clubs, halfway houses, day, night, and weekend treatment centers. Residential care homes and satellite housing represent two types of living arrangements.

THE ROLE OF THE NURSE IN THE THERAPEUTIC COMMUNITY

In a therapeutic community, nurses often lead the community meetings or work in close cooperation with the patient–leader. Some large institutions have a therapeutic community council where representatives from all units meet periodically in one large group to discuss problems and issues that affect the total population. Nurses keep in touch with the discussions and recommendations of the council. Nurses can also be supportive to patients who are reluctant to speak up in community meetings, for example, by helping them get their subject on the agenda. Nurses are also involved in working together with patients to actualize their desired activities such as bowling, walks, and shopping. Problems in implementation of planned activities are usually dealt with by the nursing staff. Nurses have to be in touch with changes in patients that necessitate changes in plans decided on by the group.

Because nursing staff are with inpatients

twenty-four hours per day, they are in a position to know more about the behavior of the patient than other members of the psychiatric team. Systems of communication in which reports and records are made provide data about the patients covering the twenty-four hours. Oncoming shifts may receive written, tape-recorded, and/or verbal reports from the previous shift. At Belmont, England,[13] the ward nursing report was read at the 8:00 A.M. community meeting where all patients and staff were present. Another form of open communication used in some therapeutic communities is the open report where the nurse's verbal report to the oncoming shift may be given in the day room and any patient may attend. Access to the rand where medications, privileges, and the like, and the nursing care plan are posted is another variation. The use of a communications book, available at the nursing station for all community members to read, where nurse–patient and team assignments and other information are posted is another variation.

Nurses are also usually responsible for seeing that the psychiatric unit is run efficiently, for example, that patients have ample and appropriate food, that needed repairs are completed, and that supplies are readily available.

Responsibility for administration of and monitoring of medication falls to the nurse. Nurses also observe for signs and symptoms of physical illness and give nursing care for patients who are physically ill. Impacted bowels, self-inflicted wounds such as cuts and burns, head injuries, infected feet, pneumonia, chronic diseases, and malnutrition appear frequently in inpatient psychiatric services. When patients are ready for it, nurses have an enormous responsibility for health teaching.

Nurses also have a public-relations role with visitors, now that many citizens are involved in community mental-health services. If the psychiatric unit is part of a general hospital, the public-relations role extends to other departments, and the nursing staff from the other clinical divisions. Psychiatric departments and staff are often derogated by staff from other sections of a general hospital and much can be done by the nursing staff and others as well to promote better understanding. Nurses also have a supervisory and teaching role with other nursing personnel in a therapeutic community.

Nurses who have been educated in and who have practiced in authoritarian roles may have difficulty with the democratic process of the therapeutic community. If so, they may need consultation and supervisions themselves to accept and to learn the new roles. To establish and maintain a therapeutic community requires democratic leadership and recognition of the value of each person's contributions.

Milieu Therapy

It is widely accepted by the health team that the nurse is responsible for the milieu in psychiatric treatment. Milieu therapy is presented here in reference to the conscious use of the social setting or environment in the treatment of psychiatric patients. It is concerned with physical environment, atmosphere within the psychiatric setting, attitudes, interaction among staff and patients, interaction among patients, and social organization. It adds use of the social system[14] to individual therapy. In milieu therapy, the patient becomes an active participant instead of passively receiving treatment. His strengths are emphasized together with those areas in which he needs help; he is recognized as a part of a community that has a culture of its own.

Slavson (1955) experimented with the use of principles of a therapeutic milieu with delinquent boys and girls in 1935. Aichorn (1939) was working with youth on this same principle in Vienna about the same time. Bettelheim and Sylvester (1949) and Redl and Wineman (1951) were also pioneers in the use of the therapeutic milieu for young people.

[13] Site visit by the author, November 1961.

[14] Two major approaches to the study of social systems are: (1) the study of functions, requirements for the functions of the system, communication, and role structure and (2) the study of interaction within the social system. The latter is more frequently used in the psychiatric field.

Milieu therapy emerged from and is a part of the therapeutic community concept formulated by T. F. Main (1946), Joshua Bierer (1960), and Maxwell Jones (1948, 1953).

In the use of milieu therapy, the environment is modified to facilitate more satisfactory patterns of interaction; full use is made of the social environment and social interaction as part of treatment of the psychiatric patient.

ATTITUDES

Attitudes of helpfulness and permissiveness are of very great importance in milieu therapy. The patient is accepted for himself, but expectations are held for behavior at the highest level of the potential of the individual. Milieu therapy should be flexible enough to provide for the needs of the patients within it. Important in milieu therapy is the confidence and ability of staff to help patients who are out of control to gain control. It should help those who do not know how to identify feelings, those who are mute as well as those who are emotionally expressive and impulsive. It should provide support for those who need it, a place where the suspicious patient can feel secure as well as confrontation and limit setting for others. Staff members are expected to participate in treatment planning and to implement the plan decided upon for the individual patient. When disagreements and anxieties occur among the staff, they are expected to be resolved because they also create disturbances among the patients.

SOCIAL ORGANIZATION

A milieu program that is well planned and organized includes provisions for patients and staff to make decisions on matters concerning themselves through the medium of community and small-group meetings. Group therapy and patient-centered activities, including recreation, that are planned and carried out by patients are essential to a complete program. Work therapy or vocational rehabilitation is also an integral part of milieu therapy. It receives more attention

in the Soviet Union than in the United States; the philosophy guiding Soviet citizens and patients is "If you don't work, you don't eat." Provisions for informal interaction are also important. Patients need rest from the intensity of a highly organized social structure. At evening nourishment time, in the kitchen, or around an open fire are places where some fears and anxieties get sorted out, for example.

The importance of the milieu is that it provides a place in which problems can be dealt with as they occur in the activities of daily living. Use of the life-space interview assists in helping the patient deal with problems as they appear, not a week later in an office interview when the events are distant (Bettelheim, 1974). The purpose of the milieu is to assist the patient toward positive mental health.

Decision making in a therapeutic milieu is done by those with the familiarity or insight into a particular situation, not by professional rank. There is a leveling of status hierarchies in which autonomy is respected by those involved, i.e., psychiatrist, psychologist, psychiatric nurse, psychiatric social worker, psychiatric aide, and mental health worker. It does not mean that the patient is being treated by the least skilled individual but it does mean that the knowledge and expertise of all staff are committed to the treatment of the patient.

Bettelheim believes that the structure of a therapeutic milieu should be described as *social solidarity.*[15] That is, there is a commitment to what the institution stands for (philosophy); it includes disagreements and arguments about issues and the ethos of the institution, and therefore solidarity is strengthened by the openness of staff to disagree with each other.

INTERACTION

In milieu therapy, intensive interaction, both verbal and nonverbal, occurs between staff and patients. Verbalization is highly valued in the milieu but nonverbal communication carries a lot of impact. Patients who are quiet are sought out, expected to be

---

[15] Bettelheim, Bruno: *A Home for the Heart.* New York: Alfred A. Knopf, 1974, p. 245.

present at all events, and efforts made to assist them to follow the proceedings and to participate actively.

Patient–Patient Interaction. The therapeutic potential of the patients for each other is one of the pillars of milieu therapy. One major aspect of this potential relates to *caring for each other,* for example, who needs someone to listen, who needs assistance with eating, bathing, clothing, supplies from outside the unit, a buddy to accompany someone who does not have a pass or who wants company on a pass. These needs may be agenda items for the community meeting. In some instances, staff may indicate individuals who are on precautions for suicide, assault, and elopement and patients volunteer to help these individuals. A description of therapeutic patient–patient interactions experienced by patients diagnosed as schizophrenic was made by Carter and Davis (1963). By use of the critical incident technique (Flanagan, 1954), two acute treatment wards that had established milieu therapy were used for the study. Patients gave their observations through recorded interviews. Five hundred and seventy-eight incidents were grouped into five major categories developed from the incidents and defined in terms of behavior:

1. *Emotionally supportive.* Behaviors in this group expressed friendship, closeness, empathy, and acceptance of fellow patients, by making an effort to understand another person's problems, comforting another by listening and/or reassurance, sharing mutual feelings, ideas, or general experiences.
2. *Fulfillment of physical needs.* This category consisted of interactions associated with grooming, feeding another patient, serving food, sharing snacks and personal items, massaging, guiding, directing, and assisting patients.
3. *Promotion of reality testing.* All behaviors that assisted or actively supported the patient in broadening his perspective, enhancing self-image, facilitating recall, and assisting to make decisions were placed in this category.
4. *Facilitation of socialization.* Socializing events or activities of living with a group

is the major focus in this group. It included interactive behaviors directed toward movement from pairing to activity involving others in the social spectrum ranging from spontaneous groups, recreational groups, to the more formal unit meetings.
5. *Promotion of mature role expectations of patients.* Cooperation in the performance of daily tasks with respect for the rights of others included behaviors that demonstrated team work, relaying information, application of democratic rules, and interest in the improvement of the physical environment of the unit.

These behaviors are perhaps not those that specifically define a turning point in the patient's therapy, but represent adaptive behaviors in the daily life of the patient on the unit. Recognition by the nursing staff of the helpful, caring behaviors of patients can provide a stimulus for their continuance. Patients have been frequently observed to take the cue from the caring behaviors, adopt the behaviors and expect this interaction for themselves. Nurses and patients thereby act as role models. Therapeutic patient–patient interaction has long been known and used in other nursing practice areas, for example, for patients with laryngectomies, ostomies, and mastectomies.

R. D., a twenty-two year-old mute, blond young man was brought to the admissions unit by the police, who had found him wandering barefoot in the middle of a busy downtown street. In the milieu therapy program, he came to the dining room for meals but required assistance with bathing, changing clothes, oral hygiene, and other aspects of daily living. In treatment planning, the nurse who was primary therapist for R. D. discussed his withdrawal and a plan was made for daily one-to-one sessions with him in addition to the group meetings. Soon after that, an older Black female patient took an interest in him, sought him out for all meetings, and so on, learned that he liked milk and saved her portions for him, for example. Gradually R. D. became more responsive, both verbally and nonverbally and able to care for himself. After one month, he was discharged improved to a residential care home. It was the clinical judgment of the staff that all aspects of interaction in the milieu had contributed to his improvement.

PHYSICAL ENVIRONMENT

A clean, aesthetically pleasing environment conveys to the patient using it that he is of some value. Comfortable, durable living-room-type furniture that does not easily burn gives a day room a homelike appearance. Plants, low tables, good lighting, and tables on which to play games should be available in the day room. Patients should have access to magazines, books, and a daily newspaper. Walls that are painted with soft, warm, light colors are pleasing to most people. Original art work of quality can transform the walls of a day room. Wall space for exhibiting art work of patients is important. Space needs to be designated for posting the daily ward schedule, rules, policies, changes, and nurse–patient assignments. Although an orientation to the unit on admission is helpful to some patients, for others the anxiety level is so high they do not take in the information and need it posted for later reference. In California, by law, rights of patients must be posted both in English and in Spanish, although this law does not address the needs of those unable to read English or Spanish, for example, some Asians.

Rooms of patients should have comfortable furniture, clean surroundings, curtains, daylight, and cabinets in which to keep personal articles. Toilets and bathing facilities should provide for privacy and be kept clean and well supplied. Space on the unit for television viewing, dining, piano playing, group meetings, record playing, smoking, for quiet and solitude, and visiting need to be designated. A wall cigarette lighter is useful when patients are not permitted to carry matches. A small kitchen stocked with nutritious snack foods such as cereals, fruit, and milk and where patients can cook and make preparations for parties is desirable.

Because of the symbolic importance of food, meals should be plentiful, palatable, attractively served, and, of course, nutritious. Tablecloths, flowers, and holiday decorations provide a festive touch to dining.

Laundry and ironing facilities are important for encouragement of self-care. Where clothing is a problem, nurses should contact local volunteers for assistance.

The nurse is responsible for seeing that the patient has linen on his bed and fresh towels. Soap, shampoo, toothpaste, toothbrushes, combs, deodorants, sanitary napkins, shaving materials, paper towels, tissues, and toilet paper are necessary supplies in our Western society.

Nurses need privacy for talking with patients, for treatments and preparation of medications, charting, rest areas, areas for educational conferences, and lockers for personal materials.

A nurses' station that is open so staff can be easily approached by patients increases communication. The nurse's white uniform—symbol of the sick role to the patient, symbol of *non compos mentis,* hospitals, and helplessness—is disappearing in psychiatric nursing. Although children's services discarded uniforms many years ago, the practice did not readily spread to adult psychiatric services.

If we are to emphasize the well part of the patient who is mentally disordered, to look for his strengths, and to build upon them, we must consider all aspects of the environment surrounding the patient, including the uniform. After substitution of street clothes for nursing uniforms in one institution, the treatment environment was judged more therapeutic by patients and staff (Brown and Goldstein, 1967–68).

Since staff members act as role models for patients, it is accepted as part of milieu therapy that their appearance influences the patient. An attractive, vitally alive staff carries much nonverbal impact.

SAFETY AND PROTECTION

The therapeutic milieu must offer some protection to the patient until he is able to cope with the problems haunting him; it is therefore not a custodial place where the *status quo* is maintained and no attempts are made for the recovery of the patient. We all know of many patients who have adjusted to the environment of a psychiatric hospital and who are terrified of moving out.

A safe environment for persons with mental disorder varies probably according to experience, philosophy, kind, and amount of nursing personnel and the behavior of patients admitted. In some cases, a swing back to locked units has occurred with sophisticated security operations. Attention should be given to the handling of keys so that their presence is not overemphasized. Keys should not be jingled, swung in a circle, or lost. They should be kept in a pocket or attached to the nurse.

Shatterproof window glass or windows with safety screens, and durable furniture that does not easily burn are safety features. Facilities for seclusion of disturbed patients should be built with the safety features of wall lighting safely covered with unbreakable glass, durable walls and floors that are easily cleaned, elimination of electrical wall outlets, and a bed bolted to the floor in case the patient has to be restrained. A small window in the door to the room is required for frequent observation. Bath and toilet facilities should be nearby.

Procedures to be followed in case of fire, suicide attempts, seizures, physical assault, and other emergencies need to be worked out by staff and thoroughly understood by all personnel. Up-to-date and functioning emergency equipment needs to be on hand, including appropriate medications.

A safe place for the valuables of the patient must be provided. If at all possible, valuables should be sent home with family members. Patients need protection from outsiders, for example, in large institutions where patients are on passes out on the grounds. Psychiatric institutions now have security guards to protect the patients from the public.

Work Therapy

The importance of performing a purposeful activity such as a job cannot be overemphasized in our technological society where one's identity is closely connected with work. The idea that one is productive in the work world and is respected and approved by fellow-workers fosters self-esteem. For the hard-core unemployed, the recently jobless, and institutionalized individuals, the lack of a job is dehumanizing. More attention needs to be given to the psychosocial effects of joblessness. Work meets one of the basic needs—*to achieve and to do something purposeful.* It does not neces-

sarily mean work for pay, although paid work enables one to buy the goods of our consumer society. Economic recession is consistently correlated with increased admissions to mental hospitals (Brenner, 1973). Our urbanized, automated, technological society should at least provide each individual with the right to work.

Counseling centers are needed that provide vocational counseling and rehabilitation. Computerized vocational testing is now a reality and should be more widely available.

Work therapy was an integral part of the therapeutic community developed at Belmont, England. It is a major part of the rehabilitation of the mental patient in Holland and in other parts of England. Patients in mental hospitals in the Soviet Union are expected to work and I have seen regressed, schizophrenic patients making beautiful flowers and large baskets for harvesting sugar beets, all made for the market and *for which the patient was paid.* It is not uncommon for a former patient to be in charge of supervision of work of a particular production room. Poland likewise uses work therapy for mental patients who make useful and decorative objects from scarce materials. Praise for a job well done is ego building for almost everyone. The knowledge that the nurse has of the patient and his particular situation can be of great aid to the psychiatric team in helping the patient obtain and hold a job. The nurse is likely to know the patient's stress points, some of his strengths and weaknesses, and ways to bolster his ego and to help him deal with problems encountered at work. The motivation of patients with institutional recoveries is particularly challenging for the nurse, for it is often difficult for them to leave the security of the hospital, or their community residence, for the work world.

In some mental hospitals in the United States a few jobs are available for patients; however, the trend is for the staff to do all the work of keeping the institution functioning. At the Colony of Gheel in Belgium, mental patients do agricultural work.

Discharged patients who cannot compete in the labor market may be able to work in a sheltered workshop where some guidance and supervision are provided, if the community has these workshops available.

Team Relationships

Most of your work as a nurse is in relation to other people on a team. Team relationships may exacerbate unresolved conflicts in your own family. Some problems arising in team relationships are *scapegoating,* where team members readily focus their aggressions and frustrations upon one of their members. Unconscious aggression in others may then be aroused and focused on the same members. Sometimes this person resigns, is moved to another work assignment, or goes into psychiatric treatment; the team regroups and the process may repeat itself.

In a situation where there are nursing students and other students, the role assigned to the learner may not exactly coincide with the goals set up by the team. Clarification of roles, objectives for learning, and treatment goals for the patient and his family may help the team move toward the *needs for professional learning* as well as professional competence for the patient.

Transference relationships appear on the team as well as in the treatment situation. Team members with ambivalence toward their parents may react to the team leader in a distorted fashion. Where there is sibling rivalry, destructive competitiveness may emerge and the defenses against these feelings disrupt the work of the team. Polarization of the team inhibits productive action.

Narcissism may interfere with the work of a team. The power-hungry individual who needs to control others, to have status and prestige, to clown, and to otherwise show off makes for difficulty in getting teamwork done.

Nurses are expressing themselves more about the components of effective care of patients and families; the challenge now is to implement comprehensive nursing care.

THE TEAM IN ACTION

The area of focus is an eighteen-bed inpatient psychiatric unit in a community mental-health center. The approach is called rounds, where all team members sit down around a table every morning. Patients are young adults and middle-aged and older persons who came from a catchment area of the center of a city emcompassing skid row, cheap hotels, Chinatown, a population living on the streets, the bus station, the airport, and other areas.

The team is composed of nursing personnel, psychiatric social worker, occupational therapist, nursing students, psychiatrist, and the patient.[16] The patient is brought into rounds and sits at the table with the team, is interviewed, can ask questions, and make requests known to the whole team. The primary goal of the team is to holistically assess the patient's situation, to provide crisis-oriented treatment, and to help the patient make plans for the future. All team members are free to express their ideas about the patient although the primary therapist[17] of the patient is responsible for presentation of the patient to the team. The atmosphere of the team is permissive although lengthy discussions of theory are discouraged. The conference itself opens lines of communication among staff. If bad decisions are made about a patient, this, too, is analyzed in the conference.

The team at rounds acts as a formal area of communication but when the pressure is off, informal communication flows. It is important to realize that all problems of patients are not solvable by any team and that the team itself can act as a source of support and learning for its members.

The following is an example of how the team functioned for the care of one patient:

The patient, P. G., was a thirty-seven-year old woman admitted on a seventy-two-hour observation from a downtown hotel where she had checked in after a cross-country flight. Her appearance was disheveled: she was dressed inappropriately. She was constantly in motion. Her gait was interrupted by choreic jerks and she had choreiform movements of all extremities. She was agitated, fearful, suspicious, evasive, illogical, her affect was labile, her speech was slow and slurred and delivered in a high-pitched whining monotone. She was unable to subtract seven from one hundred and her immediate memory was poor. The patient stated, "There's no cure

---

[16] Families are seldom physically present because the patients are alienated from their families or have otherwise lost touch with them.

[17] In this unit, the primary therapist is one of the nursing personnel on the day shift. This person is responsible for relating to the patient, collecting data about the patient, and implementing the team's plan of action.

for it. My mother and sister had it." She was diagnosed as having agitated depression with Huntington's chorea. Antidepressants and ataractic drugs were ordered. The primary therapist developed trust with P. G. and began collecting data. The patient, a former schoolteacher, had drawn all her savings out of the bank for her trip to the Coast. It was learned that she had a friend back East; so the friend was contacted who then gave the address of the patient's father. Both the mother and sister of the patient had died of Huntington's chorea and the father had not seen his daughter for ten years. Moreover, he did not wish to see her now or to take any responsibility for her. The patient then decided to fly back East and one of the nursing personnel planned to go with her. At that time, the friend refused to meet her at the airport or to otherwise be further involved with her.

In the meantime, the patient became more and more agitated. The team reassessed the situation and tried to get the patient admitted to the local rehabilitation unit, which refused her because of her mental state. After two weeks, the patient was transferred to a local state mental hospital.

Team members were openly affected by the tragedy of this patient. Frustrations and feelings were shared. No interventions could alter the course of this patient's problem. Therefore, efforts were made to maintain the safety and comfort needs of the patient and thus the team acted in a supportive sense.

COLLABORATION

Whereas the traditional role of the nurse involved compliance and conformity, the contemporary nurse is concerned with collaboration. Collaboration means working together with others and taking responsibility for the results of the mutual efforts. It cannot occur with nurses dressed up like nineteenth-century chambermaids, thinking of themselves as saints in the traditional submissive handmaiden role. For several years, psychologists, psychiatric social workers, psychiatric nurses, and psychiatrists have been taught psychodynamics, psychotherapeutic intervention, and community organization. This has resulted not only in overlapping of roles but in overlapping of responsibility as well. Collaboration requires confidence in one's own professional

ability and that of other team members. It requires flexibility, integrity, and a willingness to work with others.

Rights of Mental Patients

Recent aspects of rights of mental patients are discussed in this section. Up until recent times, mental patients were often legally held in hospital without access to telephones, voting rights, their own clothes, and other personal materials. The era of civil rights has brought forth legislation and litigation with regard to rights of mental patients.

CIVIL COMMITMENT

Since the Middle Ages children and adults deemed unable to make decisions for themselves have been protected by the state. This doctrine, *parens patriae* (substitute parent) is the power of the state to act on the behalf of those individuals who cannot make decisions about their own needs. The state also has the power to protect the community from dangerous persons. Recently, challenges to the doctrine of *parens patriae* have occurred, for example, the *Donaldson v. O'Connor* case in Florida, in which a patient who had been confined for fifteen years sued the state hospital psychiatrist, resulted in damages being awarded. Federal District Judge William Stafford in Tallahassee, Florida, ruled that Kenneth Donaldson was entitled to reasonable attorney's fees from defendants. The Supreme Court, in a unanimous decision, judged that a state cannot constitutionally confine a nondangerous mentally ill person who is capable of surviving on his own. The U.S. Supreme Court thus held that a mentally disordered person who is thought not to be dangerous to himself or others and who is not being treated must be released at his own request (422 U.S. 563, 1975). Ken Donaldson's fifteen years at Chattahoochee are described in his own words (Donaldson, 1976). In 1978 he received the Clifford W. Beers Award from the National Mental Health Association for his work on behalf of mentally disordered persons since his discharge.

Challenges are now being made to the power of the state to protect the community from those individuals deemed to be dangerous on the basis that prediction of dangerous acts is impossible and that persons should be committed only on the basis of a dangerous act.

RIGHT TO TREATMENT

The recent right to treatment litigation in Alabama, the famous case of *Wyatt* v. *Stickney* (then *Wyatt* v. *Hardin* and *Wyatt* v. *Aderholt*) was heard by Federal District Judge Frank M. Johnson, Jr., and holds that a patient in an institution has a constitutional right to adequate treatment in addition to custodial care. This order refers to both mentally ill and mentally retarded patients. It also lists minimum standards of mental treatment: (1) an individual treatment plan, (2) adequate staffing and training, and (3) a humane physical and psychological environment. The Mental Health Law Project of Washington, D.C., brought the class action suit against state hospitals in Alabama. This was the first right-to-treatment suit brought forth on behalf of civilly committed patients. The *Wyatt* order also designated that persons released from Alabama institutions would get appropriate transitional care and the right to the least restrictive setting for treatment. Because the state of Alabama has not complied with the standards set down by the right to treatment decision of the *Wyatt* order, Judge Johnson ordered the state institutions to be placed in receivership and required those in charge to file specific steps for compliance as of January 1980.

Dixon v. *Weinberger* was a class-action case in which patients at St. Elizabeth's Hospital brought suit against the U.S. Department of Health, Education, and Welfare and asked them to develop alternatives to hospitalization and treatment under the least restrictive conditions. This case was heard by Judge Aubrey Robinson of the U.S. District Court for the District of Columbia. The right to treatment in the least restrictive setting is now being recognized by state legislatures.

RIGHT TO PROTECTION FROM HARM

The constitutional right of mentally handicapped persons to protection from harm has been established by *New York State Association for Retarded Children* v. *Carey,* ratified by Federal District Court Judge Orrin Judd, 5 May 1975. It is referred to as the Willowbrook case and forbids corporal punishment, routine use of restraints, and other practices deemed harmful.

These historic cases have established the propriety of the role of the courts in psychiatry.

RIGHT TO REFUSE TREATMENT

Legislation now exists in many states providing for the right to refuse ECT and psychosurgery. Some states provide procedures for informed consent of patient, family, or guardian to psychosurgery. The administration of ECT in California requires documentation by the attending physician, approval by a medical committee, and consent by the patient or responsible relative or guardian. A few states provide for the right to refuse drugs. For example, the state of Iowa provides the right to refuse drugs and the specific consent by next-of-kin or guardian is needed to administer them, in case the patient refuses them.

OTHER

Laws are spelled out for each state in relation to the rights of mental patients and must be known by professionals for the states in which they practice. There is a trend toward increased state regulations regarding psychosurgery, drug therapy, and electroconvulsive therapy. Confidentiality and release of information with regard to mental patients are current issues in the era of centralized data banks.

Patients in mental hospitals are no longer expected to work without pay, and this abolishment of institutional peonage is credited largely to the persistence of one person, F. Lewis Bartlett, M.D., of Haverford State

Hospital, Pennsylvania. Freedom above everything else is the antithesis of the ethics of the helping professions and is perhaps the far end of the legal scale. The current trend to hospitalize persons with mental disorder only on the basis of physical harm to self or others may deny the patient the right to treatment because of need. Professionals must be especially alert to the needs of mentally disordered persons for treatment. A rigid overconcern for rights of patients overbalancing treatment had led, in some cases, to situations where patients died (Treffert, 1974).

The Welfare and Institutions Code of the State of California sets forth the following:

Each person involuntarily detained for evaluation or treatment under provisions of this part, each person admitted as a voluntary patient to a state hospital, a private mental institution, or a county psychiatric hospital, and each mentally retarded person committed to a state hospital pursuant to Article 5 (commencing with Section 6500), Chapter 2 of Part 2 of Division 6 shall have the following rights, a list of which shall be prominently posted in English and Spanish in all facilities providing such services and otherwise brought to his attention by such additional means as the director of Health may designate by regulation:

(a) To wear his own clothes; to keep and use his own personal possessions including his toilet articles; and to keep and be allowed to spend a reasonable sum of his own money for canteen expenses and small purchases.

(b) To have access to individual storage space for his private use.

(c) To see visitors each day.

(d) To have reasonable access to telephones, both to make and receive confidential calls.

(e) To have ready access to letter writing materials, including stamps, and to mail and receive unopened correspondence.

(f) To refuse shock treatment.

(g) To refuse psychosurgery. Psychosurgery is defined as those operations currently referred to as lobotomy, psychiatric surgery, and behavioral surgery and all other forms of brain surgery if the surgery is performed for the purpose of the following:

• Modification or control of thoughts, feelings, actions, or behavior rather than the treatment of a known and diagnosed physical disease of the brain;

• Modification of normal brain function or normal brain tissue in order to control thoughts, feelings, action, or behavior; or

• Treatment of abnormal brain function or abnormal brain tissue in order to modify thoughts, feelings, actions, or behavior when the abnormality is not an established cause for those thoughts, feelings, action, or behavior.

(h) Other rights, as specified by regulation.

RIGHTS OF CHRONICALLY MENTALLY DISORDERED PERSONS

The following is a suggested bill of rights:

1. The right to live in the community without suffering further stigma.
2. The right to live in an atmosphere free from constant fear of physical assault, arson, and theft.
3. The right to live in a home where organized behavior is expected.
4. The right to have access to and participate in purposeful activity as in the larger community, such as a job, sheltered workship, recreational and work programs for the handicapped.
5. The right to have one primary therapist, not multiple agencies and multiple workers.
6. The right to have accessible, responsive, and professional crisis intervention available twenty-four hours per day and seven days per week.
7. The right to have access to alternatives to hospitalization.
8. The right to have access to mental health services that are appropriate for my language and culture.
9. The right to have access to frequent, regular, and appropriate medical, dental, and psychiatric treatment.
10. The right to have a periodic physical examination.
11. The right to be examined periodically to determine if maintenance antipsychotic drugs are needed.
12. The right to have general health supervision, especially supervision of medications, sexual counseling, and health teaching.
13. The right to treatment in the least restrictive setting.

ADVOCACY

Advocacy refers to the process of pleading the cause of another. The rights of mental patients movement has resulted in varied approaches for systems of protection. As used here, advocacy refers to the protective systems for rights of mental patients, including access to appropriate and adequate services. Protective services for individuals fall under the following general headings: (1) guardianships, (2) conservatorships, (3) trusts, (4) protective agencies, (5) informal supports, (6) formal supports, such as an official advocate, and (6) combinations of these services (Wolfensberger, 1977).

The *ombudsman,* pioneered in Sweden, is an official within government who investigates complaints from citizens about the way they have been treated by departments of government. The *ombudsman* is one approach to a formal system of advocacy; others are the use of lawyers or patient-representatives. Other approaches are a committee that trains and pays private attorneys, or the use of nonlawyers and rights advisers. Because specific formal, separate systems of advocacy for mental patients are new, experiences with the various models will tell us more about their usefulness in the future. One part of an advocacy program is the use of representatives for patients to inform them of their rights; legal advocates are needed at another level and an *ombudsman* functions at the department or state level (Wilson, 1977).

In keeping with the individualism of this society, over the long run it is probably better for persons to solve their own problems; however, the existence of protective services speaks to the need for them.

Psychiatric mental-health nurses (and others) who become advocates need special training for the advocacy role.

Social Action

Perhaps in no other field is the social-action role of the nurse more important than in psychiatric mental-health nursing. Here, social action refers to the efforts to modify sociopolitical policies, legislation, and regu-

lations for the purpose of improvement of psychiatric services on a community-wide basis to those individuals who are in need. In a wider sense, social action refers to the efforts within a community to improve the health and welfare of its members and to assist them in coping with their crises of life (Evans, 1968). Nurses, as individuals as well as through the collective action of their professional organizations, can have great influence on legislative bodies at all levels of government. Citizen groups, for example, the National Mental Health Association, are also influential in this work. Citizen participation in health-care planning is now provided by government regulations. For the nurse's voice to be heard and contributions to be made, involvement in these citizen boards is desirable. More nurses need to be aware of and involved in psychiatric mental-health issues in their communities. Political aspects of delivery of psychiatric mental-health services should be a high priority in the activities of the psychiatric mental-health nurse.

Social isolation, stigma, and alienation of persons with mental disorder have not been overcome. Whole communities rise up in opposition to establishment of local psychiatric services to treat members of their own community. Nurses have a responsibility through their social action role to assist in overcoming this rejection.

Summary

In this chapter an attempt has been made to present some aspects of social psychiatry. In the study of epidemiology, the necessity for a classification of mental disorder that extends to all countries is shown. Discussion of the new classification of mental disorders is included and the classification itself is given in Appendix C. Some aspects of ecology of mental disorder are discussed, with emphasis upon migration and relocation, poverty, and culture. Reform and locus of care are described with an emphasis upon deinstitutionalization. Concepts of the therapeutic community and milieu therapy are presented and the role of the nurse outlined. Rights of mental patients and advocacy are discussed. The social-action role of the psychiatric mental-health nurse ends the chapter.

References

AICHORN, AUGUST: *Wayward Youth.* New York: Viking, 1939.

AMERICAN PSYCHIATRIC ASSOCIATION: *Diagnostic and Statistical Manual of Mental Disorders.* Washington, D.C.: American Psychiatric Association, 1952.

_____: *Diagnostic and Statistical Manual of Mental Disorder, II.* Washington, D.C.: American Psychiatric Association, 1968.

_____: *Diagnostic and Statistical Manual of Mental Disorders, III.* Washington, D.C.: American Psychiatric Association, 1980.

BETTELHEIM, BRUNO, and SYLVESTER, EMMY: "Milieu Therapy: Indications and Illustrations," *Psychoanalytic Review,* 36:3:54–68, January 1949.

_____: *A Home for the Heart.* New York: Alfred A. Knopf, 1974, p. 245.

BIERER, JOSHUA: "Social Experiments in Social and Clinical Psychiatry in Great Britain," published by the Committee on the Celebration of the 60th Birthday of Professor S. Naka, Japan, 1960.

BLEULER, EUGEN: *Dementia-Praecox.* Leipzig and Vienna: F. Deuticke, 1911.

BRENNER, M. HARVEY: *Mental Illness and the Economy.* Cambridge: Harvard University Press, 1973.

BROWN, JULIA S., and GOLDSTEIN, LESTER S.: "Nurse–Patient Interaction Before and After the Substitution of Street Clothes for Uniforms," *International Journal of Social Psychiatry,* 14:1:32–43, 1967–68.

CALIFORNIA, STATE OF, ASSEMBLY PERMANENT SUBCOMMITTEE ON MENTAL HEALTH/DEVELOPMENTAL DISABILITIES: *Improving California's Mental Health System: Policy Making and Management in the Invisible System.* Berkeley, Calif.: Teknekron, Inc., Health and Human Sciences Division, December 1978, p. 20.

CAUDILL, WILLIAM, REDLICH, FREDERICK C., GILMORE, HELEN R., and BRODY, E. B. "Social Structure and Interactive Processes on a Psychiatric Ward." *American Journal of Orthopsychiatry* XXII:314–332, April 1952.

CARTER, FRANCES M.: "The Critical Incident Technique in Identification of the Patients' Perception of Therapeutic Patient–Patient Interaction on a Psychiatric Ward," *Nursing Research,* 8:207–211, Fall 1959.

_____: *Report to the President's Commission on Mental Health* (typewritten, 19 June 1977).

CARTER, FRANCES M., and DAVIS, JOSEPH C.: "Therapeutic Patient–Patient Interactions on a Psychiatric Ward," presented at the One Hundred and Nineteenth Annual Meeting of the American Psychiatric Association, St. Louis, May 10, 1963.

_____: "Therapeutic Patient–Patient Interactions on a Psychiatric Ward," presented at the First International Congress of Social Psychiatry, London, August 21, 1964.

CARTER, FRANCES MONET, and HEALY, WILLIAM: *Report of the Committee on Board and Care Homes of the Mental Health Advisory Board of the City and County of San Francisco* (typewritten, 16 December 1974).

DEUTSCH, ALBERT: *The Mentally Ill in America.* Garden City, N.Y.: Doubleday, Doran and Co., Inc., 1937.

_____: *The Shame of the States.* New York: Harcourt, Brace, and Co., 1948.

DONALDSON, KENNETH: *Insanity Inside Out.* New York: Crown Publishers, Inc., 1976.

EVANS, FRANCES MONET CARTER: *The Role of the Nurse in Community Mental Health.* New York: Macmillan Publishing Co., Inc., 1968.

FARIS, R. E. L., and DUNHAM, H. W.: *Mental Disorders in Urban Areas.* New York: Hafner Publishing Co., 1960.

FARMBOROUGH, FLORENCE: *Nurse at the Russian Front: A Diary 1914–18.* London: Constable, 1974, p. 148.

FATKA, NADA: *Critical Requirements of Psychiatric Nursing Personnel as Determined by Selected Psychiatric Patients* (Master's thesis, University of Colorado, 1958).

FISCHER, AMES, and WEINSTEIN, MORTON: "Mental Hospitals, Prestige, and the Image of Enlightenment," *Archives of General Psychiatry,* 25:7:41–48, July, 1971.

FLANAGAN, JOHN C.: "The Critical Incident Technique," *Psychological Bulletin,* 51:4:327–358, July, 1954.

FRIED, M.: "Transitional Functions of Working Class Communities: Implications for Forced Relocation," in Kantor, Mildred B., ed.: *Mobility and Mental Health.* Springfield, Ill.: Charles C. Thomas, 1965.

GIORDANO, JOSEPH: *Ethnicity and Mental Health.* New York: Institute on Pluralism and Group Identity, 1973.

GOFFMAN, ERVING: *Asylums: Essays on the Social Situation of Mental Patients and Other Inmates.* Garden City, New York: Doubleday and Company, Inc., 1961.

HOLLINGSHEAD, AUGUST, and REDLICH, FREDERICK C.: *Social Class and Mental Illness.* New York: John Wiley & Sons, 1958.

HOLMES, MARGUERITE J., and WERNER, JEAN A.: *Psychiatric Nursing in a Therapeutic Community.* New York: Macmillan Publishing Co., Inc., 1966.

HORNEY, KAREN: "Cultural Neurosis," *American Sociological Review,* 1:221–30, 1936.

JOINT COMMISSION ON MENTAL HEALTH OF CHILDREN, INC.: *Crisis in Child Mental Health: Challenge for the 70's.* New York: Harper & Row, 1970.

JONES, MAXWELL: "The Concept of a Therapeutic Community," *American Journal of Psychiatry,* 112:8:647–650, February, 1956.

_____: *Beyond the Therapeutic Community,* New Haven, Conn.: Yale University Press, 1968.

_____, BAKER, A., FREEMAN, THOMAS, MERRY, JULIUS, POMRYN, B. A., SANDLER, JOSEPH, and TUXFORD, JOY: *The Therapeutic Community.* New York: Basic Books, Inc., 1953.

_____ and TANNER, J. M.: "Clinical Characteristics, Treatment and Rehabilitation of Repatriated Prisoners of War with Neurosis," *Journal of Neurology, Neurosurgery and Psychiatry,* 11:53–60, 1948.

KANTOR, MILDRED B.: *"Internal Migration and Mental Illness,"* in Plog, Stanley C., and Edgerton, Robert B., eds.: *Changing Perspectives in Mental Illness.* New York: Holt, Rinehart and Winston, Inc., 1969, pp. 364–93.

_____ *Mobility and Mental Health.* Springfield, Ill.: Charles C. Thomas, 1965.

KINCHELOE, MARSHA: "Democratization in the Therapeutic Community," *Perspectives in Psychiatric Care,* **XI**:2:75–79, 1973.

LEE, EVERETT: "Socio-Economic and Migration Differentials in Mental Disease," *Millbank Memorial Fund Quarterly,* 41:249, 1963.

LEIGHTON, ALEXANDER H.: "Psychiatric Disorder and Social Environment," in Bergen, Bernard J., ed.: *Issues and Problems in Social Psychiatry.* Springfield, Ill.: Charles C. Thomas, 1966, pp. 155–97.

LEIGHTON, DOROTHEA C., HARIND, JOHN S., MACHLIN, DAVID B., MACMILLAN, ALLISTER M., and LEIGHTON, ALEXANDER H.: *The Character of Danger:* The Stirling County Study, III. New York: Basic Books, Inc., 1963.

MAIN, T. F.: "The Hospital as a Therapeutic Institution," *Bulletin of the Menninger Clinic,* 10:3:66–70, May 1946.

MALZBERG, BENJAMIN, and LEE, E. S.: *Migration and Mental Disease.* New York: Social Science Research Council, 1956.

_____ "Are Immigrants Psychologically Disturbed?" in Plog, Stanley C., and Edgerton, Robert B.: *Changing Perspectives in Mental Illness.* New York: Holt, Rinehart and Winston, Inc., 1969.

MORRIS, J. N.: *Uses of Epidemiology.* Edinburgh and London: E. & S. Livingston, 1964.

MURPHY, H. B. M.: "Culture and Mental Disorder in Singapore" in Opler, Marvin K., ed.: *Culture and Mental Health.* New York: The Macmillan Company, 1959, pp. 291–316.

NATIONAL LEAGUE FOR NURSING: *Criteria for Appraisal of Baccalaureate and Higher Degree Programs in Nursing.* New York: National League for Nursing, 1977.

OPLER, MARVIN K.: *Culture, Psychiatry, and Human Values.* Springfield, Ill.: Charles C. Thomas, 1956.

_____: "Schizophrenia and Culture," *Scientific American,* 197:2:103–112, August 1957.

_____: *Culture and Mental Health.* New York: Macmillan Publishing Co., Inc., 1959.

PRESIDENT'S COMMISSION ON MENTAL HEALTH: *Task Panel Reports.* Vols. I, II, Washington, D.C., U.S. Government Printing Office, 1978.

REDL, FRITZ, and WINEMAN, D.: *Children Who Hate.* Glencoe, Ill.: The Free Press, 1951.

REID, D. D.: *Epidemiological Methods in the Study of Mental Disorders.* Geneva: World Health Organization, 1960.

San Francisco Chronicle, 12 April 1979.

SARTORIUS, N.: "WHO's New Mental Health Programme" *WHO Chronicle,* 32:2:60–62, February 1978.

SARTORIUS, N., and JABLENSKY, A.: "Transcultural Studies of Schizophrenia." *WHO Chronicle.* 30:1281–485, December 1976.

Schizophrenia Bulletin, 4:1:77, 1978.

SCHWAB, JOHN J., TRAVEN, NEAL D., WARHEIT, GEORGE J.: "Relatiohships Between Physical and Mental Illness." *Psychosomatics,* 19:8:458–463, August 1978.

SCHWARTZ, MORRIS, and SHOCKLEY, EMMY LANNING: *The Nurse and the Mental Patient: A Study in Interpersonal Relations.* New York: Russell Sage Foundation, 1956.

SEGAL, STEVEN P., BAUMOHL, JIM, and JOHNSON, ELSIE: "Falling Through the Cracks: Mental Disorder and Social Margin in a Young Vagrant Population," *Social Problems,* 24:389–400, 1977.

SLAVSON, S. R.: *Re-educating the Delinquent Through Group and Community Participation.* New York: Harper & Row, 1955.

SMITH, WALLACE F.: *Preparing the Elderly for Relocation.* Philadelphia, Pa.: Institute for Environmental Studies, University of Pennsylvania, 1966.

SOKOLOVSKY, JAY, COHEN, CARL, BERGER, DIRK, and GEIGER, JOSEPHINE: "Personal Networks of Ex-Mental Patients in a Manhattan SRO Hotel," *Human Organization,* 37:1:5–15, Spring 1978.

SROLE, LEO, LANGNER, THOMAS S., MICHAEL, STANLEY T., OPLER, MARVIN K., and RENNIE, THOMAS A. C.: *Mental Health in the Metropolis.* New York: McGraw-Hill Book Co., Inc., 1962.

STANTON, ALFRED H., and SCHWARTZ, MORRIS S.: *The Mental Hospital: A Study of Institutional Participation in Psychiatric Illness and Treatment.* New York: Basic Books, Inc., 1954.

STERNLIEB, GEORGE, and HUGHES, JAMES W.: "The Changing Demography of the Central City." *Scientific American,* 243:2:48–53, August 1980.

STRAUSS, JOHN, and CARPENTER, WILLIAM T.: "Prediction of Outcome in Schizophrenia. III. Five-year Outcome and Its Predictors: Follow-up Data on the U.S. IPSS Patients." *Archives of General Psychiatry.* 34:1:159–163, February 1977.

TALBOTT, JOHN A.: *The Death of the Asylum: A Critical Study of State Hospital Management, Services and Care.* New York: Grune and Stratton, 1978.

TREFFERT, DAROLD A.: "Dying with Your Rights on," paper presented at the 127th meeting of the American Psychiatric Association, Deboult, Michigan, 7 May 1974.

TUDOR, GWEN E.: "A Sociopsychiatric Nursing Approach to Intervention in a Problem of Mutual Withdrawal on a Mental Hospital Ward." *Psychiatry: Journal for the Study of Interpersonal Processes.* 15:2:193–217, May 1952.

U.S. DEPARTMENT OF HEALTH, EDUCATION, AND WELFARE: *Statistical Note No. 138.* DHEW Publications No. (ADM) 77–158, August 1977a.

———: *Deinstitutionalization: An Analytical Review and Sociological Perspective.* Washington, D.C.: U.S. Government Printing Office, 1977b. DHEW Publication No. (ADM) 77–351.

———: *Statistical Note No. 146.* DHEW Publication No. (ADM) 78–158, March 1978.

Webster's New Collegiate Dictionary. Springfield, Mass.: G. & C. Merriam Company, 1977.

WILLIE, CHARLES V., KRAMER, BERNARD M., and BROWN, BERTRAM S.: *Racism and Mental Health.* Pittsburgh: University of Pittsburgh Press, 1973.

WILSON, JOHN P., BEYER, HENRY A., and YUDOWITZ, BARNARD: "Advocacy for the Mentally Disabled" in U.S. Department of Health, Education, and Welfare; *Mental Health Advocacy: An Emerging Force in Consumer's Rights.* Washington, D.C.: Government Printing Office, 1977, pp. 3–15.

WOLFENSBERGER, WOLF: "A Model for a Balanced Multicomponent Advocacy/Protective Services Scheme," in U.S. Department of Health, Education, and Welfare: *Mental Health Advocacy: An Emerging Force in Consumer's Rights.* Washington, D.C.: Government Printing Office, 1977, p. 20.

WORLD HEALTH ORGANIZATION: "Psychosocial Factors and Health," *WHO Chronicle,* 30:8:337–339, August 1976.

———: *Manual of the International Statistical Classification of Diseases, Injuries, and Causes of Death.* Ninth Revision. Geneva: World Health Organization, 1977.

Suggested Readings

ALLEN, PRISCILLA: "A Consumer's View of California's Mental Health Care System," *Psychiatric Quarterly,* 48:1:1–14, 1974.

BAKER, FRANK: "From Community Mental Health to Human Service Ideology," *American Journal of Public Health,* 64:6:576–82, June 1974.

BASSUK, ELLEN L., and GERSON, SAMUEL: "Deinstituitionalization and Mental Health Services," *Scientific American,* 238:2:46–53.

BELLAK, LEOPOLD, ed.: *A Concise Handbook of Community Psychiatry and Community Mental Health.* New York: Grune & Stratton, 1974.

CARTER, FRANCES MONET: "Community Mental Health Services in the U.S.S.R." *Nursing Outlook,* 20:3:164–68, March 1972.

CAUDILL, WILLIAM: *The Psychiatric Hospital as a Small Society.* Cambridge, Mass.: Harvard University Press, 1958.

COLEMAN, JULES V., and DUMAS, RHETAUGH: "Contributions of a Nurse in an Adult Psychiatric Clinic: An Exploratory Project," *Mental Hygiene,* 46:3:448–53, July 1962.

COLES, ROBERT: *Children of Crisis.* Boston: Little, Brown & Co. 1964.

DAVIS, ANNE J.: "Economic Factors," in Kalkman, Marion E., and Davis, Anne J., eds.: *New Dimensions in Mental Health—Psychiatric Nursing.* New York: McGraw-Hill Book Co., 1974, pp. 483-502.

DAVIS, JOHN E.: "The Rights of Chronic Patients," *Hospital and Community Psychiatry.* 29:1:39, January 1978.

DAVIS, KINGSLEY: "The Migrations of Human Populations," *Scientific American,* 231:3:93–105, September 1974.

DEVOS, GEORGE: "Cross-Cultural Studies of Mental Disorder; An Anthropological Perspective," in Arieti, Silvano, ed.: *American Handbook of Psychiatry,* Vol. II. New York: Basic Books, Inc., 1974, pp. 551–71.

DELOUGHERY, GRACE W., GEBBIE, KRISTINE M., and NEUMAN, BETTY M.: *Consultation and*

Community Organization in Community Mental Health Nursing. Baltimore: Williams & Wilkins Co., 1971.

DIX, GEORGE E.: "The Alabama 'Right to Treatment' Case: An Opportunity Not to be Missed," *Community Mental Health Journal,* 12:2:161–167, Summer 1976.

ENNIS, BRUCE, and SIEGEL LOREN: *The Rights of Mental Patients.* New York: Avon, 1973.

GROUP FOR THE ADVANCEMENT OF PSYCHIATRY: *The Chronic Mental Patient in the Community.* Vol X:102, May 1978.

JONES, MAXWELLL: "Nurses Can Change the Social Systems of Hospitals, *"American Journal of Nursing,*78:6:1012–1015, June 1978.

KINCHELOE, MARSHA, and HOGAR, LORRAINE: *Out of the Back Wards' Door.* 1974 (no publisher given), available from Marsha Kincheloe, 130 East 4th Street, New York, N. Y. 10003.

KLERMAN, GERALD L.: "Better, but Not Well: Social and Ethical Issues in Deinstitutionalization of the Mentally Ill," *Schizophrenia Bulletin,* 3:4:617–631, 1977

LEAF, PHILIP:*"Wyatt* v *Stickney:* Assessing the Impact in Alabama," *Hospital and Community Psychiatry,* 28:5:351–355, May 1977.

LEIGHTON, ALEXANDER H.: "Social Disintegration and Mental Disorder," in Arieti, Silvano: *American Handbook of Psychiatry,* Vol. II. New York: Basic Books, Inc., 1974, pp. 411–24.

MALZBERG, BENJAMIN: "Internal Migration and Mental Disease Among the White Population of New York State, 1960–1961," *International Journal of Social Psychiatry,* 13:3:184–91, Summer 1967.

NUSSBAUM, KURT: "Psychiatric Disability Determination Under The Social Security in the U.S., *"Psychiatric Quarterly.* 48:2:63–72, 1974.

OPLER, MARVIN K.: *Culture and Social Psychiatry.* New York: Atherton Press, 1967.

OSBORNE, OLIVER H.: 'Anthropological Issues in Mental Health Nursing," in Leininger, Madeline M., ed.:*Contemporary Issues in Mental Health Nursing.* Boston: Little, Brown & Co., 1973, pp. 39–61.

QUERIDO, ARIE: "The Shaping of Community Mental Health Care," *International Journal of Social Psychiatry,* 7:5:300–311, May, 1969.

RACHLIN, STEPHEN, GROSSMAN, SAUL, and FRANKEL, JAY: "Patients Without Communities: Whose Responsibility?" *Hospital and Community Psychiatry,* 30:1:37–40, January 1979.

ROBERTS, PEARL R.: "Human Warehousing: A Boarding Home Study," *American Journal of Public Health.* 64:3:277–282, March 1974.

RUBIN, RONALD S.: "The Community Meeting: A Comparative Study," *American Journal of Psychiatry,* 136:5:708–712, May 1979.

STRASSER, JUDITH A.: "Urban Transient Women," *American Journal of Nursing,* 78:12:2076–2079, December 1978.

STUBBLEBINE, JAMES M., and DECKER, J. BARRY: "Are Urban Mental Health Centers Worth It?" *American Journal of Psychiatry,* 127:7:909–12, January 1971.

SWEARINGEN, DOLORES, and THOMPSON, JULIA M.: "What Does the Patient Think? An Evaluation of a General Psychiatric Ward." *Hospital and Community Psychiatry.* 29:3:182–184, March 1978.

THOMAS, ALEXANDER, and SILLEN, SAMUEL: *Racism and Psychiatry.* New York: Brunner Mazel, 1972.

TYBERG, DELORES A.: "Creating an Intermediate Care Facility," *American Journal of Nursing,* 79:7:1236–1239, July 1979.

WALLACE,ANTHONY F. C.: *The Death and Rebirth of the Seneca.* New York: Vintage Books, 1969, pp. 184–236.

WITTKOWER, ERIC D., and PRINCE, RAYMOND: "A Review of Transcultural Psychiatry," in Arieti, Silvano, ed.: *American Handbook of Psychiatry,* Vol. II. New York: Basic Books, Inc., 1974, pp. 535–50.

4

Therapeutic Communication

LEARNING OBJECTIVES / Persons studying this chapter should be able to:

1. Describe cultural components of communication: ethnocentrism, time, waiting, and territoriality; compare and contrast with your point of view
2. List three main purposes of interviewing
3. List four aims of the therapeutic nurse–patient relationship
4. List three phases of the nurse–patient relationship, describe the major components of each phase, and the nurse's responsibilities
5. Describe five major parts of the mental status examination and the components of each
6. Discuss the purposes of the Problem-Oriented Medical Record; describe each of its four components
7. Describe self-awareness, empathy, cathartic listening, leverage, touch, and their use in the therapeutic nurse–patient relationship
8. Define transference, resistance, and countertransference and their importance in therapeutic process
9. Describe cognitive dissonance
10. Define halo effect, stereotype, constant error, variable error, and discuss the role of each in the interviewing process

Alone is a nice word
Sometimes
My hands feel Shakey
Because eyes are
secretly, subtly watching
So they'll know a word or two
to write (in) their reports
Of how you seem
What you say
What you do
all weirdness unreal
feeling to be in a hospital again.
Unrealness touching
making sure matter is real
or if this is purely illusion
let me out
in and out
Rather be out

a place, people paid to help
how they want—speaking of
Where they will go for dinner
after the shift—
Who and what am I doing here?

By an Anonymous Patient

Communication with patients requires the use of the ordinary words of daily life, with their multiple meanings. Therefore, effective communication requires work from the professional level—an ability to analyze behavior both of the patient and of self—and an interest in the patient under your care. It also requires that all the senses of the nursing student be intact.

In order to consider the holistic needs

of the person, it is important to be comfortable in one-to-one relationships with patients where the emphasis is upon communication.

In face-to-face communication, there is a sender, a message, and a receiver (see Figs. 3 and 4). Both the nurse and the patient assume the roles of sender and receiver at different times. Listening is the principal task of the receiver. The sender (speaker) should know what he wants to say and be able to say what he means. There are several aspects to each message: what the sender wants to say, what he really says, what the receiver hears, and what the receiver thought was said, all referred to as metacommunication (Reusch and Bateson, 1951). Since the mind works faster than the mouth, the thought processes have a jump on words. The reciprocal behavior of the receiver is necessary for communication and allows for verification of the effectiveness of communication.

Although nurse–patient relationships have elements of other types of interpersonal relationships, they differ in their conscious application for a specific purpose related to promotion, maintenance, and restoration of health, and prevention of disease. Communication skills may be practiced with persons other than patients in order to effect higher levels of professional competence. Students report that their communication skills with friends improve after concentration on this aspect of nursing.

Kinds of Communication

It is through behavior, both verbal and nonverbal, that people communicate. Verbal behavior refers to spoken words; nonverbal behavior may consist of written words, signs, symbols, and other behavior, i.e., affect, perceptions, dreams, moods, fantasy, thoughts, and body language (intonations, facial expression, and gestures). Behavior includes overt actions of individuals and the more intangible psychological processes of the mind such as learning, perception, and dreams.

Cultural Components of Communication

The new cultural pluralism, a major sociocultural force of the times, has resulted in the expectation that our health services will be accepting of, knowledgeable about, and sensitive to the needs of a pluralistic society (Carter, 1978). In turn, national planning now includes provision for culturally relevant health services for the patient. Culturally relevant services refers to services that preserve human dignity, that are practical, acceptable, and accessible to the diverse ethnic groups who need them. Communication is an integral part of every contact with a patient.

Emphasis upon what the nurse brings to the interaction with patients is of great importance in communication. What is the mirror-image self? The cultural background of the nurse is asserted nonverbally. Imposing one's likes and dislikes on the patient, for example, because this is important to the nurse, may violate the mores of the patient. Communication must go both ways

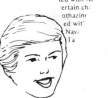

Sender (nurse)   Receiver (patient)

Figure 3. Face-to-Face Communication.

but the responsibility for opening channels of communication, keeping them open, and showing care and concern lies with the professionals.

ETHNOCENTRISM

Nurses who are able to relate to all kinds of people are better practitioners than those who may have prejudices or idiosyncrasies related to working with certain age and cultural groups. In nursing, one should be familiar with one's own country, and its diverse cultural groups. The social screen between the nurse and the patient who is from a different class or culture can be overcome, although some discomfort may be incurred in the process. In some cultures the helping professional is a last resort and is accepted first by the patient as a member of his national group and secondly as a person. Choosing patients who are different from yourself for your assignments and studying everything you can see about them, including your own reactions, is one approach. Travel and study within your own country and others is another way to become more objective about your own culture.

TIME

Time represents one of the most significant cultural components of communication in this country. Think of the fantastic timing, down to the millisecond, of the astronauts in their lunar orbits. We tend to schedule every minute of our waking hours, striving for efficiency of effort and achievement (DeGrazia, 1962). Roth (1963) emphasizes the stress incurred by the hospitalized individual who tries to make up a timetable

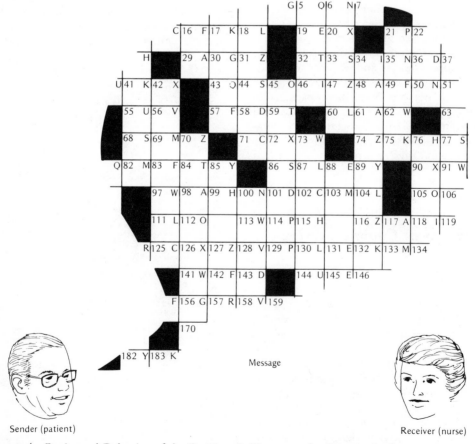

Figure 4. Reciprocal Behavior of the Receiver Is Necessary for Communication.

of his own progress or regression. Share your hospitalized patient's schedule with him as a courtesy to him and his time budget.

In hospitals, times of events that we usually control ourselves are often not known to the patient, e.g., delivery of mail and mealtimes. It is not uncommon to visit a convalescent home and find that patients confined to their rooms have no clocks or calendars. I once visited an elderly friend in the local county hospital where all the patients were in one large room, with twenty five beds on each side. Over the doorway to the ward entrance hung a large clock. My friend, whose old eyes could not see the clock, asked the time of day from the orderly, who replied, "What do you wanna know for? You're not going anywhere!" Ways of determining the time of day and night, the date, and the year are necessary for the well-being of patients. Those who are hospitalized spend a lot of their waking hours discussing time. In a mental hospital, dates of entry and exit are compared and contrasted; many queries are made to others with regard to departure dates.

Patients try to determine the usual amount of time that patients stay in the hospital and try to set their own dates. Marking the halfway point eases the tension; often days and hours are ticked off in anticipation of reaching a time goal. Patients in a mental hospital need time to think, deliberate, and clarify what is happening to them and should not be expected to involve themselves in a sixteen-hour day flurry of activities with no time left to think about their problems.

WAITING

In our culture, waiting communicates a great deal. It is unfriendly to keep people waiting. No one seems to like to wait very long for anything. Punctuality is important in our culture, and lateness should be avoided at all times in your contacts with your patients. To keep patients waiting increases their frustration and decreases their sense of worth. Notification of delay is essential to the maintenance of trust in your nurse–patient relationships.

TERRITORIALITY

Territoriality is important to most of us, particularly if we have not been reared in a collective or in some other type of communal living arrangement. We have our own houses, rooms, and cars; comforts are often given up when we enter hospitals as patients. The impact of one's territory being constantly invaded by strangers in a hospital unit has an effect on patients that should be recognized by the nurse.

Several different types of space are relevant to nursing practice. Thermal space is the area immediately surrounding a person. Our thermal detectors in the skin, olfaction, and visual images all inform us when we are within the patient's thermal space. One human being feels the warmth of another when they are in close proximity. When there is a fast turnover of patient population in a hospital unit, nurses often refer to "keeping the beds warm." In fact, we make sure that all traces of preceding patients are removed from a hospital room that a new patient will occupy.

Hall (1966) identified four principal categories of space distances: intimate, personal, social, and public, symbolizing each with a bubble. Nursing involves all these distances, with particular emphasis upon the first three. Visual, kinesthetic, tactile, and thermal aspects of the patient are affected by his environment, and feelings of wellbeing or irritation can be evoked depending upon how the nurse enters into his space distances. If the patient can have some control over his territory, he will be better able to maintain his identity. Territorial rights of those in mental hospitals have long been ignored, and the lack of such rights has contributed to the dehumanizing of the mental patient. Legislation in California[1] requires institutions to provide for individual storage space, for example, in recognition of the importance of this concept in therapeutic care. The patient without control over his own territory may become irritable and defensive.

[1] The Lanterman-Petris-Short Act, effective July 1, 1969. This act is primarily concerned with the patient who is mentally disordered and who is being involuntarily held in a treatment facility for his own protection or for the protection of others.

Rest from this constant invasion is a necessity for some people. If the patient in a ward constantly pulls his curtains around him, find out why. He may not be withdrawing at all; he may be asserting his territorial rights! The need for retreat to one's intimate space bubble should not only be provided for within the nursing care plan but scrupulously honored by the nurse.

Perception

Perception, which relates to what is taken in through the senses, also refers to the process that occurs between sensing and thinking. It uses the immediate sensory experiences and experiences from the past; one sense is modified by the other. Nursing is concerned with the elimination of misperception; if we want to help our patients, we have to perceive each one as a human being. Nursing is also concerned with understanding sensory defects and deprivation and their effects upon patients. Preceding events influence us and must be considered in ourselves as well as the patient. The individual's biological needs are factors in perception. It is well known that experience influences perception. Some other factors influencing perception are intactness of the sense organs, direct suggestion, intelligence, surroundings, anxiety level, culture, and the influence of others. Perception usually involves symbolic and emotional processes. During an exciting event, for example, we do not usually think of details. Perception and interaction are reciprocal; therefore, the patient also perceives the nurse in his own way. Preceding knowledge may have created a perceptual set. *Perceptual set* refers to the expectations we have of a sensory experience similar to a previous experience, even though the two may involve different circumstances or people. For example, in the process of grief and mourning, the bereaved widower, accustomed to hearing his recently deceased wife's footsteps on the garden walk, hears the nursing student's approach and asks, "Betty, is that you?" Be aware that previous experiences affect perception, and keep your senses ready for new and different perceptions; be open to new experiences with different patients and under varied circumstances.

PROFESSIONAL ATTITUDES

The attitudes you bring with you affect the outcome of your patient contact. Bermosk and Mordan (1964) cite as essential the professional attitudes of warmth, acceptance, objectivity, and compassion. As a professional student you are responsible for what you do with your patients and families. You learn your limits and stay within these limits, and seek assistance when it is needed. Appearance is also important when you meet your patient. A neat, well-groomed appearance may be appropriate for gaining the confidence of your patient. The odor of cigarettes about the nurse negates the impact of health teaching about giving up smoking. The overweight nurse carries little impact in attempts to teach patients to lose weight. Being as natural as you can aids development of rapport; sit back in your chair. Inattention, boredom, constantly checking the time, talking about one's self without refocusing on the patient, note taking, and other distracting behavior may indicate a lack of interest in the patient. Talking with others who may be within earshot instead of with your patient may increase his anxiety.

A therapeutic relationship requires the use of the self as the instrument for understanding and helping the patient. Knowledge of human behavior, including self-understanding, is the core component. Achievement of objectivity in the therapeutic relationship can occur only through experience.

Interviewing

Although nurse–patient relationships are as old as the profession of nursing itself, interviewing in nursing is relatively new. In this era of transitory relationships in life as well as in nursing, interviewing has a strong emphasis.

Interviewing is a principal assessment and therapeutic tool in nursing practice. It is primarily the verbal communication within the interaction between the nurse and the patient, family, or other members of the health team that is directed toward the maintenance, promotion, or restoration of health (Bermosk and Mordan, 1964). Interviewing is conversation with a purpose.

The interview is the first meeting of the nurse and the patient. Your initial contacts with patients are often made after someone else has assessed the condition of the patient, although this is now changing in some areas of practice where nurses do intake interviews and therefore are the first ones to see the patient and to make an evaluation.

Much of psychiatric nursing in inpatient and day treatment centers is concerned with the life-space interview, which provides assistance to the patient in the daily events of life (Redl, 1959). In addition, it provides psychiatric first aid at the time that it happens; feelings are thereby dealt with immediately, support is given, and communication is maintained.

Although nurses must be aware of organic problems in patients, this chapter deals primarily with psychosocial data; here, also, interviewing and therapeutic communication are considered inseparable.

Therapeutic communication differs from other communication in purpose. As a professional, your responsibility is to help others. In therapeutic use of self, the secret of caring for your patient is *to care* about him; the techniques used in therapeutic communication draw from methods of communication that we use every day. Therapeutic communication is not limited to the couch of the psychoanalyst; it can occur at home, at the bedside, in the outpatient clinic, on the street, or at work. If you are yourself with your patient, you encourage him to do the same. As a nurse you incorporate the idea of therapeutic communication into your role concept. Listening and ego-strengthening behaviors exhibited by the nurse are two major components of nursing practice.

Interviewing includes the interaction (behavior and other communication, i.e., symbols, cultural components) between the nurse and the patient and is an integral part of every contact the nurse has with the patient and his family. Three main purposes of interviewing are (1) to gain information, (2) to give information, and (3) to motivate.

To gain more information about the patient, the nurse may interview a newly admitted patient for a history, which is then placed on the patient's record for use by all professionals, or used to help in establishing the nursing care plan. Information required from patients entering crisis clinics may be secured by the nurse member who may then give assistance or make an appropriate referral.

Many examples of nurse–patient interaction—help with diet, preparation for surgery, lectures on mental health to teachers and mothers—show the purpose of giving information. Orientation of patients to the hospital or to new services offered is giving information, as is health counseling.

Interviewing for the purpose of motivation involves some aspects of both giving and gaining information. Encouraging one's patient to schedule a yearly health examination or to have hope of recovery is part of the nurse's work. Motivating the regressed schizophrenic patient toward recovery is also included under this heading, along with one-to-one nurse–patient relationship therapy.

The impetus for better interviewing technique has come from psychoanalysis; nursing is therefore concerned with the dynamics of rapport, empathy, transference, countertransference, and resistance. Emphasis is upon relating to the patient and understanding his phenomenal self and that of the nurse rather than cataloging behavior.

In the process of interviewing, basic aspects of the teaching–learning experience relate to the thoughts, feelings, and perceptions of both the patient and the nursing student. Through relating to patients in a goal-seeking way, the nursing student undergoes a human experience that is more successfully achieved in this manner than through formal lectures given by the instructor. The formal content is not omitted but is better retained and used in a more creative manner when it is learned in relation to a perceived problem. There is an attempt through social interaction with patients to try to achieve a quality of reciprocal influence that improves the learning of student and patient. Since learning also involves changes in people's thoughts, feelings, and perceptions, analysis of nurse–patient interactions is one of the most effective ways to become conscious of the feelings involved in learning and to discover ways to help others.

Interacting with a patient enables the nursing student, with guidance, to reflect upon actions, perceptions, thoughts, and feelings and thereby increase one's own reactions to an event. The most effective content to begin with is the feelings that the student is aware of experiencing. Relationships with patients and families offer the nursing student the opportunity to feel the process of finding meaning in the experience and to learn new ways of looking at one's own place in the profession and in the universe. Literature, music, and drama also add to this learning process.

Therapeutic Process: The Nurse–Patient Relationship

Therapeutic process is conceptualized here as the communication between the nurse and the patient directed toward being beneficial or helpful. From a practical point of view the aims of the therapeutic nurse–patient relationship are: (1) to assist the patient to resolve the immediate problem, (2) to focus on causes of the present problem, to clarify issues involved, (3) to help the patient improve future adjustment and growth, and (4) to emphasize prevention.

Nursing interventions are aimed toward helping the individual, family, and community maintain health status and move toward positive mental health, and those that help the patient regain health are all included in therapeutic tasks and interventions. The science lies in the knowledge of human behavior, the art in the ways of helping people solve problems. Learning therapeutic process, however, requires supervision by or consultation with an experienced person. In some instances, seeing a person through whatever he is undergoing requires years. The way in which most nurses work *at this*

time requires termination either at the end of the curriculum for students or at the discharge of the patient to his home or another agency.

It is important to understand that although not all contacts with patients are therapy, each has the potential of being therapeutic, promoting interpersonal growth, changing behavior, or benefiting the patient in some other way.

Phases of the Nurse–Patient Relationship

Every relationship has a beginning, a middle, and an end. The nurse–patient relationship has an *establishing phase*, a *maintaining phase*, and a *terminating phase*. These phases are not clearly demarcated from each other; as you and your patient go through each phase, you will find some aspects of the other two phases contained in it. The strategy and tactics of the contact with your patient depend upon his needs. There are no formulas, no programming, no predetermined roads to follow; what happens in that contact is effected by you.

Establishing Phase

Purposes and goals of interviewing in the helping professions are different from those of other types of interviews in that you can only have a general objective before your contact; it has to be acted on as it happens. This calls for a great deal of flexibility and alertness–what Theodor Reik (1956) called listening with the third ear. It is not so much hearing the actual words of your patient as *what he is trying to tell you.*

In addition to the maintenance and restoration of mental health, the general aim of the therapeutic nurse–patient relationship is to assist the patient in the change of behavior through growth, not a sudden transformation. In this phase of the relationship, data are collected for assessment purposes from all available sources and systematically recorded in the patient's record. The patient's problems are identified, goals determined, priorities set, and plans made to achieve the goals. Goals should be subject to revision at all times. Therapy begins when the nurse–patient relationship extends beyond the exchange of information to subjective content underlying behavior.

The purpose of the first contact is to get acquainted and to begin the working relationship.

Structuring your interaction reduces ambiguity. Structure is established by the nurse who finds a comfortable private place to talk, listens, helps the patient feel safe, is empathetic, understanding, and as a result the patient has a feeling of being helped. Spending time together and working toward mutually set goals are parts of the structure.

It is important to state clearly who you are, why you are there, and how long you will stay. During this first contact you also begin to prepare your patient for termination. It is here that you set the limits of the relationship by noting the time span that you will be with the patient. Is it just for one morning? Is it three times a week for two weeks? Is it for the full length of his hospital stay? Is it for the full academic year, or for as long as help is needed? At this time you and your patient agree on when you will see each other. It is important not only to define the time limit of the relationship right from its beginning, but to discuss termination openly during the relationship. (Do not use the word "termination" itself with your patient; it has a different meaning for him!) During this phase of the relationship, the establishing phase, you set the tone of subsequent contacts. To be effective in your communication skills, you control the time, complexity, and amount of communication.

Particularly in a first interview the patient may think you expect him to tell you everything about himself and, afterward, feel guilty or resentful over saying too much. If you limit the contact to one hour and set a time and place for you to continue at a later date you will maintain the rapport. Significant changes in patients do not often occur with one contact. Express your concern and willingness to continue seeing the patient.

In nursing, contacts with patients may be prolonged or they may be very transitory.

If we value continuity of nurse–patient relationships, it is the responsibility of the nurse to ascertain something about the duration of the relationship with each patient and family under her care wherever this is possible. Manifestations of a suicidal attempt, broken relationships, loss, extrusion from social setting, excessive hostility, suspicion, withdrawal, stresses of life, physical illness, and injury require capable care. Acutely disturbed patients resistive to psychiatric treatment, hysterical, and drug-dependent individuals represent some of the human problems dealt with in nursing. These behaviors and problems are too deeply rooted to change by one contact.

In most instances in nursing, the patient does not choose the nurse[2] who will be caring for him. This may help clarify a finding of Duff and Hollingshead (1968) that patients did not get as much satisfaction from the nursing care they received as the nursing personnel did from the care they gave. The fact that the patient in most instances does not choose his nurse makes it particularly important during the first contact for the nurse to state who the nurse is, why present, what the nurse and the patient will do together, and so on. Nothing should be taken for granted; patients are often unaware of the expressive symbols of the profession and require exact information as to what is expected of them and what the nurse intends to do. If someone else has preceded you in the care of your patient, it is important for you to define your relationship with him.

Stating your purpose of contact and how you happened to come to the patient also gives him and his family a chance to clarify their position. If you have been preassigned, asking your patient to tell you why he thinks you are there may be helpful. One community patient thought the nurse had come to help her with the housework; another thought the nursing student would be his "girl friend" who would go to Chinatown with him every Friday for lunch. Another patient thought the student had been assigned to spy on him. One patient considered that the presence of the student meant that she was becoming more helpless and

[2] Patients may employ private-duty nurses, and if a patient does not like the nurse, he can dismiss her and ask for another until he gets one who is compatible.

on a downhill course. Another patient, who was in a manic state, met the student with the greeting "my little nurse" and expected her to wait on her that day. Mr. H., a patient in day treatment, thought he had to pay an extra fee because a nursing student spent time with him. If there are other patients in the hospital units who do not have students assigned to them, it is important for them to be informed of the purpose of the student–patient assignments so that they do not feel left out or think that their illness is a stigma that makes them inaccessible to the students.

Privacy. Always do whatever you can to assure privacy when interviewing your patients. If you are in a hospital ward, pull the curtains and speak in a low voice to him when the other patients in the room are occupied. Do sit down with your patient instead of standing poised as if to fly out of the room. In other settings, if possible, choose a quiet room with two chairs. If in a busy day room, pull two chairs off to a corner. In a home when others are around, you may want to go outside into a garden or ask the person to come with you into the kitchen for a few minutes. In a mental hospital, you could go out with your patient for a walk or use a conference room. In some crowded situations, you may have to use a corner of the ward or the day room.

Rapport and Trust. Rapport is the feeling of mutual interaction, respect, and willingness of the patient and therapist to work together. It may be quickly and easily established or it may never be achieved. It may be easier for the student to accept the patient than it is for the patient to accept the student. Showing interest and concern for the patient, persistence, and consistency aid in establishing rapport. Trust is placing one's confidence in and reliance on someone. The feeling of trust and rapport enables the patient to more fully reveal his troubling thoughts and perceptions. The patient should be addressed by his formal name. Nothing can be quite so infantilizing as to be addressed by one's first name by strangers.

The therapist in many instances must, like a mother, introduce the patient to the idea of trust. Without rapport and trust, little progress occurs. Although all nurses do not develop positive relationships with all patients, usually in an inpatient psychiatric unit, there will be at least one of the nursing personnel who has a positive relationship with the patient.

Observation and Appraisal. In the establishing phase there are mutual observation and appraisal. One of the most important skills of the nurse is observation. What is perceived?

The patient appraises the motives and sincerity of the nurse, and the nurse appraises the patient. In observing the patient, the nurse should look directly at him but avoid staring. The uninitiated may tend to think that locking gazes is intended; however, this intensity makes people uncomfortable. Relinquishing one's gaze to focus on other objects for a few moments and then returning to the patient is desirable.

Mental Status

The *mental status* is useful in the assessment of patients and is a long-accepted aspect of psychiatric examination; it is an integral part of assessment. A complete examination includes a physical and neurological study. In addition, a psychiatric history is obtained, which includes the reason why the patient has come in for treatment, the statement of the problem, a careful identification of the present episode with the reason why the patient came at this particular time, a personal history, and a family history. Any specifically traumatic events should also be elicited. A lethality rating and homicidal assessment are made.

Some patients with mental disorder may have severe physical impairment and never mention it; therefore, this fact must be remembered in the initial assessment as well as in subsequent contacts. The mental status is useful as an assessment tool in all areas of nursing practice and is presented as follows:

1. *General appearance*
   - *Facies or demeanor:* Sad, serious, happy, smiling, masked, immobile, hostile.

- *Grooming/Hygiene:* Neat, clean, skin color and condition, unshaven, body odor, halitosis, scabies, pediculosis. Now that large numbers of people live on the streets in central cities, the importance of attention to the physical aspects of the patient must be reemphasized. Nurses have the responsibility to inspect the body and clothes of the patient for lice. Infestations occur on the scalp, other hairy parts of the body, even the eyelids, or on the clothing, especially along the seams of the inner surfaces. Medications for eradication are available both on prescription and over the counter.
- *Dress:* Colors, adequate, appropriate or bizarre, jewelry, makeup, condition of clothes.
- *Prostheses:* Eyeglasses, contact lenses, cane, dentures, hearing aid.

Comments re: appearance.

2. *Expressive aspects of behavior:* This section relates to the general activity of the patient, for example, as follows:
- *Body movement:* Slow, quick smooth, jerky, immobile, statuesque, agitated, wringing hands, mannerisms, stereotypy, gestures, stuporous, *cerea flexibilitas,* convulsive, athetosis, compulsions, echopraxia, chorea, hyperactive, hypoactive, grimacing, impulsiveness, combativeness, posturing, tics, tremor, and agitation.
- *Posture:* Stooped, erect, slumped, slouched, horizontal, seated.
- *Gait:* Walks with a cane, shuffles, limps, fast, slow, akathisia.
- *Scars and other marks:* Birthmarks, warts, scars, wounds, needle marks, tattoos, bruises, rash, pustules, decubitus.
- *Speech:* Excessive, pressured, slowed, clear, slurred, stuttering, accent, silent.
- *Voice:* Loud, monotone, mumbling, whispering, soft.
- *Attitude during interview:* Irritable, demanding, hostile, evasive, passive, aggressive, negativistic.
- Comments re: behavior.
- *Affect and mood:* What is the affect of the patient? "How are your spirits?" is the traditional question asked to determine affect. Is the patient breezy, capricious, euphoric, gay, cheerful, pleasant, labile, flat, anxious, apathetic, sad, hopeless, despondent, dejected, depressed, inappropriate, angry? The intensity of the mood is determined as well as fluctuations and duration.

Comments re: feeling.

3. *Thinking*
- *Process:* Note is taken here of the characteristics of the thought processes; for example, flight of ideas, loose associations, blocking, indecisive, circumstantial, tangential, and perseveration.
- *Content and mental trend:* Depersonalization, dereistic, ideas of guilt, worthlessness, helplessness, preoccupation with poverty, somatic complaints, suicidal, homicidal, obsessions, phobias, preoccupation with sex, excessive religiosity, ideas of reference, delusions of grandeur, persecution, influence, nihilism, systematized delusions.
- The patient may be asked to write an account of his life to determine mental trend.

Comments re: thinking.

4. *Perception:* Here the determination of the presence of illusions and/or hallucinations is made. If the patient assumes a watchful or listening posture and attitude, it is suggestive of hallucinations. Disorders of perception may affect any of the senses.

Comment re: perception.

5. *Cognitive functioning*
- *Orientation:* Is the patient oriented to time, place, and person?
- *Consciousness:* Here, one notes the sensorium of the patient. This area denotes his mental clarity. When the patient is aware of his surroundings, his sensorium is said to be clear. If not clear, it is clouded. Can the patient concentrate?
- *Memory:* When the patient is asked to give a chronological account of his life, his remote memory can be assessed as he relates it. Memory for recent events can be assessed by asking about events in the recent past. If memory for the recent past is impaired, determine the presence of confabulation and/or retrospective falsification. Retention and recall is assessed by giving the patient several consecutive numbers and ask-

ing him to repeat them. Amnesia should be assessed.

- *Intellect:* Here the patient may be given serial sevens (i.e., starting at 100 and subtracting serially). Proverbs may help in determining abstracting ability. While interacting with the patient, a few questions about current events will help determine the patient's fund of information.
- *Judgment:* This area refers to the ability to make comparisons of thoughts and events, understand the relationships, and draw valid conclusions. It is a central aspect of an integrated person. An inquiry into the daily life events of the patient will help evaluate this aspect of functioning.
- *Insight:* Is the patient aware that he is ill? Many patients describe their disorder as being "nervous" or as a "nervous breakdown." Does he know why he is in the hospital? Does he blame others? Is he motivated for treatment? True insight refers to not only the awareness of the patient that he has a problem but the understanding of the underlying motivation as well. Many patients develop an intellectual insight but lack an insight on the affective level.

Comments re: cognitive functioning. Psychological testing is also often done as part of the examination of the patient.

Additions to the initial assessment are made by daily observations in inpatient and day-treatment facilities as well. A brief mental-status exam should be made often, including the following points: appearance and behavior; speech; mood; thought content; perception; and orientation with regard to time, place, and person.

As you develop working relationships with patients, additional knowledge about him unfolds and is added to the initial assessment data to aid in treatment planning and thereby in the progress of the patient. Where the patient is, in terms of his cultural background, positive mental health, psychosocial growth and development, as well as physical growth and development, is important to know. (Refer to Chap. 1 for the aspects of positive mental health, developmental tasks, and psychosocial stages.)

In the process of relating to patients, students often have difficulty perceiving the phases of the nurse–patient relationship. It must be understood that there is no clear line separating the phases; they are interrelated.

If you are interviewing a patient for information, as in a screening process for determination of his emotional problem or for hospital admission, specific questions will be asked and data sought as in the following suggested outline.

A Suggested Outline for History of a Patient

Name	*Date*	*Address*	*Telephone:*	Home: Work:

Identifying Data: age, marital status, economic status, ethnicity, employment status, religion, Medicare or Medicaid numbers (if any).

Individual or Conjoint Interview: (if conjoint, what is the relationship of the other person to the patient?)

Presenting Problem: why is the patient presenting himself for treatment—"What brings you here today?" "Who suggested you come for treatment?" (referral source)

1. *Symptoms:* onset, duration, severity, person's history of complaint—how is ability to function affected?
   - How has the patient dealt with such symptoms in the past?
   - Why are coping mechanisms ineffective now?
2. *Precipitating Stress:*
   - Loss (job, death, or separation from significant other, extruded from social setting).
   - Threat to survival needs (robbery, eviction, no finances, assault).
   - Challenge (promotion, first job, etc.).
   - Signs of stress—insomnia, diarrhea, anorexia, unable to concentrate, and so on.

History of Previous Mental Disorder and Treatment: Complaint, method of treatment (hospitalization, medications, outpatient psychotherapy, and so on.), duration of treatment, when, where, by whom? Results? "Have you ever gone to anyone for psychiatric treatment before?"

Present Living Situation:
1. Available support system.
   To whom do you go if you need help?
   Is the person(s) still there?
   Who are your friends?
2. Changes in immediate past.

General History: include birth to family of origin, procreation, and up to the present.
Points to discuss:
1. Siblings? Patient's order in family, relationships with siblings.
2. Relationship with parents, spouse, children, significant others and co-workers. Age and circumstances of death of family members and significant others.
3. Relatives with emotional, neurological, and substance abuse problems.
4. Marital history—separations, divorces, pregnancies, number of children.
5. Educational background; employment.
6. Physical problems—medication, other treatment, drug use and abuse, allergies.
7. Current involvement of significant others (and social agencies).
8. Developmental stage and developmental tasks achieved.

Brief Mental Status: (establishes tentative diagnosis).
1. General appearance and behavior.
2. Orientation (time, place, person).
3. Affect—appropriate, inappropriate, anxious, depressed.
4. Speech—pressured, clear, slurred, slow, accent.
5. Thought content—mental trend, delusions, ideas of reference?
6. Perception—hallucinations? Illusions?
7. Intellectual functioning—memory, recent and remote; ability to abstract, i.e., use of proverbs; judgment; mathematical ability (serial sevens—ask the patient to begin at 100 and subtract 7 serially).

Developmental:
1. Birth and infancy: zero to fifteen months. Wanted or unwanted, birth (normal?), developmental milestones, separations, crises.
2. Childhood and latency: fifteen months to ten years. Relationships with parents, siblings, and peers. Separations, performance in school, crises.
3. Adolescence: ten to eighteen years. School and vocational development, sexual development and sexual orientation, crises.
4. Adulthood: life-style, present life-style, vocation, jobs (duration, reasons for leaving them), stress losses, military experience, disability (for what reason?), crises.

Impulse Control:
1. Suicidal—history of suicidal attempts; fear of harming self, lethality rating.
2. Homicidal—fear of harming others, history of assaultive behavior, possession of weapons, current homicidal threats and plans.

Psychodynamic Explanation: what in the patient's background helps explain his problem?
Diagnostic Impression: (using the nomenclature of the American Psychiatric Association).
Summary and Recommendations:

It is important for the nurse to enquire of the patient if he has any questions about his condition and take time to answer them fully and accurately.

Contract. Early in the interaction the nurse should request from the patient his view of the reason for the meeting. Unless there is agreement about the starting point,

the interview could end without the participants ever understanding what it is all
about. It is also necessary to agree on the
end point with respect to time as well as
objective. This agreement, whose purpose
is role clarification, is called the contract.
Secured *verbally,* or written, the contract can
also designate goals, what the nurse will do,
and what the patient will do while they are
together. Contracting involves mutual responsibility, for example, designating a time
and place to meet, consideration of alternatives, keeping appointments, exploring
problems, maintaining confidentiality, and
re-evaluating at any point in the relationship. The contract provides reassurance of
continued care and concern for the patient.

Be careful not to use *jargon* with your
patients. You are asked to transpose what
you have learned in theory to other expressions, much like the musician takes a page
of music and transposes it into another key.
The melody will be the same but it comes
through with different sounds. Your contract may be only for one contact if your
patient is in a crisis center or it may be for
several months or the duration of the patient's disorder, according to the philosophy
of treatment and the roles of the professionals in the treatment situation.

Rivalry.   In your contacts with patients,
there is social give and take. There is also
rivalry. Rivalry may be encountered by the
nurse whose patient or family takes the initiative in each contact, thereby keeping the
nurse from achieving goals previously set
for the contact. A firm but unaggressive direct manner by the nurse may be necessary
to effect goal achievement. One nurse in
a situation where the patient's mother arrived every day to visit her son, after visiting
hours, found herself bypassed by the mother
as she met her at the doorway of the psychiatric unit. Finally, screwing up her courage,
the nurse took the initiative before the
mother could say anything and got her point
over. It took a lot of role playing for the
nurse to take the initiative.

Facilitating.   If the nurse remembers that,
in the establishing phase, the primary task
is to learn what the patient has on his mind,
it will be easier to assist him. The ideas and
affects expressed by the patient may evoke
similar reactions in the nurse, who must
curb these reactions if the patient is to be
helped. It is one thing for nurses to help
patients discuss what is on their minds and
another for patients to be told what is on
the nurses' minds. The reciprocal relationship involves some giving of self on the part
of the helping person but not a complete
history of one's own life.

Techniques within the nurse–patient relationship are adapted to the goals of the interview. The use of direct questions, open-
ended questions, nonverbal techniques, and
reflective and restatement responses requires practice. Premature reassurance is in-
sincere, does not meet the need of the patient, and closes off communication.

Questions

Direct questions can be liberally used
where necessary. Some nursing students
who are anxious themselves may handle
their anxiety by asking many questions in
sequence or by overloading with two or
three questions asked of the patient before
the patient has had time for a response.

Think of someone you know who does
this. If you have this reaction, try another
approach in your next patient contact and
evaluate its success.

For example, if your patient is in pain,
you can be very direct, as follows:

Where is your pain?
Describe your pain.
Show me where it hurts.
When did it begin?
Have you had it before?
How long did it last?

Or, if you find your patient with his wrists
cut, your first question may be: "What did
you use to cut your wrists? Where is it?"

Such questions, words, and phrases as
who, what, where, when, why, how, describe, show me, and tell me are indispensable to the nurse.

The open-ended question is useful in determining how a patient thinks and feels.
It gives the patient a more relaxed framework within which to reply and provides

for freer responses. Some examples of open-ended questions are as follows:

Tell me about yourself.
Tell me about your family.
Tell me about . . .
What do you think about that?
I'm not sure I understand what you mean.
Is there anything else?

On the other hand, closed questions usually elicit a rather terse response. For example, asking, "How many children do you have?" and "How old are you?" runs the risk of stopping the patient at the numerical answer. Closed questions may give you valuable information, but you will get little, if any, elaboration.

Nonverbal Communication

Therapeutic communication involves both verbal and nonverbal interaction. Being there, pausing now and then to allow both you and the patient to collect your thoughts, leaning forward, and showing an alert expression of interest and concern communicate to the patient that you care for him as a person. Maintaining some eye contact and sitting near the patient are also helpful.

A twenty-nine-year-old woman on the psychiatric unit was having a tantrum because of some limits set by the staff. She was screaming, crying, and pounding the couch. A staff member hurriedly walked over to her, took her by the arm, and walked her to her room.

Spontaneous human reactions are very important; they do not always have to be put into words. The tone and inflection of your voice communicate many messages to the patient. For the patient who does not verbalize, activities may be the medium of communication.

Nondirective Technique

A nondirective technique in therapeutic communication may be required to enable some patients to express themselves better. The nondirective technique, originated by Rogers (1942, 1951), refers to an interac-

tion in which the interviewer does not decide the subjects to be discussed or the goals or solutions of the client.

In using the nondirective technique, paraphrasing the content (the restatement response) of what the patient says and employing the reflective response are dominant. Paraphrasing aids in the clarification of what you do not understand. The restatement response lets the patient know that he has been understood and encourages him to continue:

A twenty-nine-year-old man with a history of multiple suicidal attempts and chronic alcoholism went AWOL from the psychiatric unit and was found about to jump from the eleventh floor of a downtown hotel. Returned to the hospital, he was placed on a two-week involuntary admission and requested a judicial review.

Patient: I hope the judge doesn't hold me in contempt of court.
Nurse: Contempt of court?
Patient: When I tell him off for not letting me go.

The patient continued to talk about his anticipated court appearance, to agree not to tell the judge off, and to discuss plans for day treatment after discharge.

The *reflective* response tells the patient you understand his feelings and encourages him to elaborate on them. In using this response, the nurse reflects feelings that the patient is expressing. This technique immediately coordinates your perceptions with those of your patient. An example is as follows:

The patient is a thirty-one-year-old man on the psychiatric unit who is a paraplegic resulting from a suicide attempt.

Patient: I've been here two months and I don't feel any different. They're not doing anything for me (eyes downcast, solemn facial expression).
Nurse: D., you sound discouraged . . .
Patient: I am discouraged. I cannot live alone. I've tried it. The nurse has to come in to help me. Someone else has to do the shopping. There are just too many things I can't do for myself. The Center for Independent Living has too many on their waiting list. I think I'll go to the state hospital.

The patient continued on to review what he could and could not do for himself and the nurse described the state hospital services and the local rehabilitation unit in an effort to help him make plans for the future.

A *tangential* response may be evoked in the nurse who is anxious or has not thought through what to say to the patient. Nontherapeutic, it is a response to be avoided. An example follows:

Patient: I feel really nervous today. At group meeting this morning everybody got a chance to talk for the first time in a week. Johnny interrupted us and Billy took up more time than anyone else. I just can't stand Vincent; he is always asking too many questions.
Nurse: You don't like Vincent . . .

(This response ignores the basic feeling expressed by the patient as being "really nervous today."

Such a response cuts the patient off from the human communication that he is crying for and does not know how to get. The patient's cue to his feelings has been ignored, and his need to discuss his feelings has not been met. He may feel further isolated from human contact, feel increased anxiety; mounting tension could ensue. A reflective response would be more therapeutic in this case.

Premature or false reassurance is a response often assumed by the uninitiated nurse. Patients who are fearful of medical procedures and surgical interventions may seek reassurances from the nurse. The nurse can acknowledge the seriousness of such events and help the patient prepare for them by giving accurate information about the procedures and outlining some of the things the patient can do to help.

Nurses in their contacts with patients hear many complaints, fears, and uncertainties expressed by patients about their physicians and the institutions to which they are attached. It is not helpful to the patient for a nurse to react by defending them, but it will help to sit down and listen to what he has to say and indicate that you understand his feelings. The *reportorial approach* here would be of value. "Reportorial" refers to relating to the patient experiences the nurse has observed other patients undergo in similar situations. It is an important aspect of nursing practice; it helps the patient to know that many other patients have gone through

similar experiences and reassures him that he, too, will make it. It also fills in for the patient what to anticipate and what may be expected of him in his particular situation. In using this technique, the experienced nurse may say to the patient, "Before this kind of procedure, patients often feel like you do. I have seen many patients take this safely. Now you can do this and help." If we are having a problem, we all wish to know whether or not someone has taken that road before and, if so, what it was like for him.

In talking with patients it is often easy to veer from the main topics, especially if the patient "turns the tables" and focuses on the nurse. The nurse then finds a way to quickly and definitely refocus on the patient.

Hundreds of reactions and feelings come up in the therapeutic process; all are not focused upon—the nurse should stay with the core problem.

MAINTAINING PHASE

In the *maintaining phase* or middle phase, the stage has been set by the initial agreement or contract about goals, structure, and end point. This phase is the period of problem solving, where the most work is accomplished. It is here that interventions are carried out. All nurse–patient relationships are not problem solving but they have the potential of being so. Of all the conditions, circumstances, and situations encountered by the nurse, it is in this phase that one focuses on specifics. The nurse and the patient find out what they can accomplish. If the student can be assigned to a patient and family over a long period of time, the longitudinal view itself can be valuable in learning about problems that people face, how they cope with them, and how to help them cope. The student has a better opportunity to carry out long-term goals, and the patient may also have more of a chance for interpersonal growth through the experience.

In this phase of the nurse–patient relationship the patient will most likely feel secure and will quite openly discuss topics that he was unwilling to communicate in the earlier phase of the relationship. On the other hand, if rapport has not been established, much restatement of the purpose of the relationship may be necessary.

Working Through. Working through refers to the exploration and solution of a problem by the patient and the nurse. Progress depends on many factors; the complexity of the problem, the motivation of the patient, and the skill of the nurse. Hurrying the patient or trying to reach unattainable goals will only lead to being discouraged. The patient should not be pressed to reveal more about himself than he is ready to give.

Spacing of nurse–patient contacts gives the patient time to think and work out what has been discussed; therefore, positive influences can be felt and growth can occur between contacts. Working through helps the patient clear up painful feelings, for example, crying like a child may be a new experience. Systematic confrontation is important for the patient to deal with painful feelings, for example, anxiety, guilt, shame, and fear. Final solutions are not formulated or found all at once; working through is an incremental process. Ask the patient directly if progress is being made, if he is being or has been helped, and what it is that helped him. This reaffirms that the help he receives is important.

Summarizing. Summarizing briefly from time to time what has taken place so far and asking the patient if the summary represents what has been covered can aid in clarification of issues and enhance mutual understanding.

It is in this phase that the gratification or psychological reward of communication will be at its peak. Satisfactory communication leads to growth in interpersonal relationships for both student and patient.

TERMINATING PHASE

The ending of a nurse's relationship with patients and families may occur after a long period of time, or it may come abruptly. Until changes are made in the provision of health care that will make it possible to follow patients and families until their basic needs are met or until it is politic to withdraw and refer them to someone else, short-lived relationships between the nurse and the patient are likely to continue. Students' relationships with patients and families end with the dates set by the curriculum.

Although sociologists term this an era of transitory relationships, I have observed patients, upon subsequent admissions to the same hospital, request the same unit and room in order to be around nursing staff they know and with whom they feel secure. One patient with multiple admissions to a mental hospital preferred the staff of the "disturbed" unit and, therefore, in order to get the admitting personnel to send her to the disturbed unit, threw her coffee onto the floor during the admission procedures. The opposite occurs with patients who have had unsatisfactory relationships with nurses known to be in a certain unit.

Termination begins at the first contact with patients as the nurse clarifies her professional role and the duration of the nurse–patient–family contact. Naturally, production-line care or curb-service nursing does not lend itself to the therapeutic use of self. However, even when the nurse functions as a steady, secure, and constant person to the patient, distorted reactions of fear, hate, and guilt may be encountered. When the patient loses the person upon whom he has learned to depend he may be hit with the impact of his own emotional needs for that person, unless he has been adequately prepared for termination of the relationship.

At the time of termination, if the patient feels insecure and unloved, he may regress. Since termination may provoke stress, knowledge of coping behavior and defense mechanisms and sensitivity to the individual needs of patients are all important at that time. There is a loss of a real relationship. Anxiety may occur with regard to the upcoming independence. There may be a reenactment of feelings of separation from the family of origin and feelings of guilt and depression may occur. The patient may act out the crisis, run away, or attempt suicide. "Forgetting" appointments, destroying objects, and physically attacking others may be expected, particularly in younger patients. Other losses the patient has experienced come into play. It is a time for the nurse to help the patient with unfinished grief work and to complete it. Deaths that have occurred years before may be discussed or more recent deaths of significant others mentioned. The patient may discuss departure of previous professionals as well as other separations that he has experienced. If he has had contacts similar to the one that is ending, he may be better prepared for what to expect. Patients wonder what the next nurse will be like, and they may verbalize wishes that the next one will be "just like you."

Tapering off the amount of contact is one approach to termination. However, for a patient whose anxiety level is high at termination, intensive contact will be necessary to help him work through his feelings. Hostility and anger may also be expressed before or after the terminating date; much depends on the intensity and quality of the transference. Physical symptoms may develop during the last few contacts, or the patient may catalogue the old ones as though they might indicate to the nurse that he cannot be left in this bad condition. Giving the patient a way to contact you, even though you are transferring him to another therapist, is often all that is necessary. Patients most often do not contact the departing professional but feel secure with the knowledge that they can. Unless the patient is prepared for termination and can adapt to giving up the nurse, he may continue to mention this person repeatedly to the professional who takes over.

Summarizing with the patient the events of the relationship is part of the technique of termination. Verbalizing feelings of loss is one approach in preparation for termination, e.g., "I am sorry we will not be seeing each other after next week." Identification of your own feelings about termination is another important aspect of the process. Relating to the patient some of your gains from the relationship may enable the patient to do the same. Problems encountered in the relationship is one way to begin; for example, start the conversation by saying, "We've been meeting now for a month . . ." and go on to review what you talked about and accomplished. Termination is like a "little death" and the dynamics involved in grief and mourning apply. You may now wish to read the sections in this book on grief and mourning and depression (see Chap. 6).

Evaluation. Although evaluation is continuous throughout the therapeutic process, the end point becomes a time not only for determining the progress made but for reassessment, and revision of plans.

Gifts. Despite rules made to the contrary in some institutions, gifts make their appearance. Although the temptation may be strong to take a gift, the motivation behind the offer must be considered in each case. Students sometimes feel that refusing a gift from a patient will hurt the patient; they accept it to avoid causing pain. It is wise not to accept an expensive item, a family heirloom (other family members may covet the item), or a present that is intimate. The need of the patient to be remembered can be met by your saying, "I'll think of you when . . ." Although gifts are unnecessary as tokens of remembrance, students and their patients often exchange small gifts or cards at termination.

The Nurse's Reactions. A nurse's reactions to termination generally fall into one of the following categories: (1) anger, (2) relief, or (3) grief. Students may be especially angry with the agency staff, the instructor, or the university. Recognition of the source of the anger usually enables one to handle one's feelings. If students are angry, they may say that it is not right to get involved with a person and then leave him, that it is unethical and not their idea of nursing.

Relief may be freely expressed by the student leaving the patient. It is my opinion that those who feel relieved usually have not gained much depth in their nurse–patient relationship, have been highly uncomfortable with their patients, or have reached an impasse in the relationship.

Students have termed grief reactions "termination pangs." They are usually of short duration, the intensity of the grief depending on the intensity of the relationship. Those who have moved frequently have experienced previous separations and may take termination in their stride. If the student is prepared to expect some personal reaction to termination and can talk freely to the instructor and peers about the relationship that is ending, it is usually easily understood. Group support from peers who may also be experiencing similar reactions can be of help to the sufferer. There may be an intense wish to continue seeing the patient past the time set by the curriculum. Students need help in accepting the reality of termination themselves, to perceive that they do move on to other experiences, that their patients survive quite well and find other relationships, and that life itself is a series of goodbys.

The use of holidays and semester breaks as "little terminations" or "little separations" helps both student and patient prepare for ending the relationship. Although the student may wish to prolong it, acknowledgment to the patient of this feeling and that it is impossible to do so may help the patient in subsequent relationships to perceive that his world will not collapse and that there is something to be gained from every person.

Both students and patients grow and learn from each other during their contact. Focusing on what each of you has gained from the relationship is helpful in your terminating phase. In long-term relationships following which patients and/or nurses will leave the area, the emotional relationship may end before the actual terminating date. The work of termination therefore should precede the last nurse–patient contact. After termination is accomplished and the pain is gone, both the patient and the nurse have places in their memories for each other.

CONFIDENTIALITY, RECORDING, AND RESPONSIBILITY

The basic guideline is that all information and records obtained in the course of providing services to any patient are confidential. Patients need to know that their confidences will be honored. This does not mean that you withhold information from other members of the health-care team, or your instructor, or that you are committed to secrecy. Informing your patient that a general record is made of nurse–patient contacts and assuring him that recordings are for purposes of teaching and learning and are read only by your instructor are usually enough. Give the general purpose of recording, withholding details. The use of professional calling cards with your name, address, and telephone number is important in a nonin-

stitutional setting. Ethics and legal considerations in nursing are exemplified in the *Nightingale Pledge,* the *Code for Nurses* of the American Nurses' Association, the *Code for Nurses* of the International Council of Nurses (refer to appendixes F, I, and J) and the statutes of the various states.

Privileged communication is defined as the patient's privilege of silence in regard to confidential matters on the part of his nurse; it has been extended for the most part to include hospital records. According to the ethics of the profession, the nurse is not allowed to divulge confidential information about the patient without his consent or unless required by law in some instances to do so. It is stated in the *Code for Nurses* as follows:

The nurse safeguards the client's right to privacy by judiciously protecting information of a confidential nature.[3]

The concept of privileged communication indicates that communication between a professional and the patient will be protected from disclosure in court unless the patient gives consent.

Nurses in all areas of practice make some kind of record of their interactions with patients. It must be understood by every nurse that this record may be subpoenaed in some instances and that all recordings are made succinctly and to the effect that they cannot be misconstrued in court. Therefore, all recordings should be based upon fact, not conjecture. The names of other patients should not appear in the patient's record unless there is a specific event requiring their use; this respects the privacy of the other patient. Nurses have the responsibility to inform themselves of the specific guidelines in their states providing for confidentiality. Now that there is overlapping of roles with other professionals, especially in psychiatric practice, nurses should be particularly alert to the laws relating to confidentiality in their state. As students, for the purposes of learning, you may write up interactions with and case studies of patients. Although these are not hospital records, they should be treated with the utmost confidentiality, i.e., no identifying data should be on these write-ups,

[3] American Nurses' Association: *Code for Nurses,* 1979. (See Appendix F.)

and they should be handled in a confidential manner. Audio recordings and photographs for the purposes of research and study require special permission.

Basically, confidentiality means that any personal information conveyed to the nurse is given with the implied agreement that it will be held there. There are certain exceptions such as guardians, conservators, and family members. Other exceptions are if there is a danger to the patient or others or if the nurse is compelled by law. In some instances, knowledge gained in confidence is essential to patient care and must be shared with other professionals. One must weigh carefully the information given over the telephone so as to ascertain what one should divulge and to whom. It is important for you to avoid getting caught in the bind of promising a patient that you will not tell anyone of what goes on between the two of you. Patients often are able to speak freely to nursing students when they have not confided in anyone else. Perhaps this is due to the fact that the student tends to spend more time with them and is not viewed as having authority over them. Information pertinent to understanding and the treatment of the patient must be shared with other professionals involved in the care of the patient.

The intent of the enabling legislation that established community mental-health centers was that necessary information about patients move freely with them as they are referred to different agencies. In previous years, in some states, lists of patients known to have threatened the governor and/or the President were made known to law-enforcement authorities. Murders triggered telephone calls to state hospitals asking for information as to whether or not there were any escaped patients answering to specified descriptions. New statutes in some states protect mental patients from this kind of practice.

The Problem-Oriented Medical Record. The problem-oriented medical record (POMR) is a method of documenting the findings of the clinician, the impressions of the findings, the diagnosis and treatment of the patient. It has four parts: (1) data base, (2) problem list, (3) a plan for each problem, and (4) progress notes. The POMR promotes separation of data collection from the assessment process.

For the psychiatric patient the data base is composed of the history, physical examination, neurological examination, mental status, and laboratory tests. As additional data are collected, problems may be changed.

A problem is something that concerns the psychiatric team and the patient. The problem list is made after collecting data and is the responsibility of the clinician. Problems are numbered sequentially on a master list and a plan made for each; orders are then written. Creation of a meaningful problem list requires the expertise of the total psychiatric team. The problem list may be incorrect if there is an inadequate data base or if the data base is interpreted incorrectly. To be useful in problem solving, the problem-oriented system must be kept up to date. As each problem is resolved, it is checked off on the problem list.

With the introduction of the POMR, progress notes are written and indexed according to the problem list: (1) problem number, (2) subjective, (3) objective, (4) assessment, and (5) plan—referred to as SOAP.

- *Subjective* (S): Here, what the patient says about himself in relation to the enumerated problem is recorded. It can be in quotations, summarized, or a combination.
- *Objective* (O): In this section, what the team member perceives in the behavior of the patient is recorded.
- *Assessment* (A): Here are included the ideas, hypotheses, and speculations that the team member has about the subjective and objective aspects.
- *Plan* (P): As a result of the process of thinking through the subjective, objective, and assessment aspects, the plan of what to do for the patient is made and carried out.

The following is one example of the use of the POMR in its initial stage. In this example, a shortened data base is presented:

Data Base: The patient is a twenty-two-year-old Caucasian man who slashed his left wrist the previous evening and was admitted to the psychiatric inpatient service. The psychiatric history revealed that his birth was unplanned, unwanted, and his father died when he was one year old. At the age of eighteen his girl friend was killed in a car accident and died in his arms. Subsequently he joined the Marines but has been AWOL for six months. For the past three months he has been living communally in San Francisco and hustling. Because his hustling was no longer lucrative, he was extruded from his living quarters yesterday evening. He is sad, speaks softly, his mood is severely depressed, his thoughts center on guilt, helplessness, and hopelessness. Cognitive functioning is not impaired.

The following is an example of an initial problem list and treatment plan for this patient:

contract that patient will inform staff if he feels suicidal. Encourage catharsis. Help patient feel hope. Keep bed in hallway near nurse's station. Twenty-four hour observation. Continuous assessment of lethality.

Problem #2: Laceration (L) wrist.
Subjective: "It doesn't hurt; it just feels a little, sore."
Objective: Dressing is clean and dry.
Assessment: Change of dressing not needed now.
Plan: Instruct patient to keep dressing dry. Provide patient with plastic covering for left arm when taking a shower. Inform patient of date of suture removal.

Problem List and Treatment Plan

Date	Date of Onset	Problem (by number)	Treatment Plan	Date Resolved Redefined
11–26–79	11–21–79	#1 Suicide attempt. #2 Major depressive episode, unipolar, first episode. #3 Lacerated (L) wrist.	#1 Suicide precautions. #2 Establish one-to-one supportive psychotherapeutic relationship. #3 Change dressing; remove sutures 12–1–79.	

Initial orders written by the physician were: (1) admit to psychiatric inpatient services, (2) routine lab, (3) regular diet, (4) suicide precautions.

The following progress notes were made by the nurse on the day shift. Progress notes are written by a nurse for each shift. All members of the psychiatric team may write progress notes on the same patient, in sequence.

PROGRESS NOTES (SOAP CHARTING)

Problem #1: Suicide attempt.
Subjective: "I have no place to go, and lost my friends, Nina died in my arms, there's nothing left for me to do but kill myself."
Objective: The patient is preoccupied, withdrawn, and refuses breakfast. Upon approach he readily verbalizes his feelings. Facial expression is sad; patient speaks in almost a whisper. Sits in day room with his head in his hands.
Assessment: Suicidal ideation. High lethality due to recent losses, unresolved grief, and mourning, for girl friend, and feelings of hopelessness and helplessness and a downhill course.
Plan: Develop one-to-one relationship. Secure

When problems are resolved, they are checked off the master list in team conference. As treatment of the patient progresses, additional problems (or redefined problems) may be added to the problem list.

Written Nurse–Patient Interactions. Widely used in the teaching/learning process, a written nurse–patient interaction is a verbatim, sequential reconstruction of the patient's verbal and nonverbal communication, the nurse's responses, rationale, summary, and evaluation of the interaction. Verbatim reconstructions greatly aid in learning the nuances of the helping relationship. Some students may choose to use a tape recorder if the permission of the patient is secured and such a practice is within the policies of the agency. However, finding time to listen to tapes and having them transcribed present problems. Reconstructions of nurse–patient interactions can be written immediately after contact; key words are quickly jotted down in a pocket notebook after the nurse–patient contact is closed and are later translated into a full report (see Appendix K for a format of a written nurse–patient interaction).

These kinds of data, which should include verbal and nonverbal behavior, provide the basis for analysis of nurse–patient interaction. The recording gives the instructor, who guides the student in the nurse–patient relationship, a comprehensive view of the interaction and can be used in individual conferences with the student with regard to the analysis of communication and the rationale for nursing action. It can also be very helpful to the student who keeps a copy and reads it over before conference or reads it in a group for critique.

Nonverbal behavior, such as gestures, inflection of the voice, and movement, should be included in the write-up of interactions with patients. If a long period of time has elapsed from the event of the nurse–patient contact and the conference with the instructor, much is lost because recall has faded. The best work is done by students through the following timing and sequence: (1) patient contact, (2) recording, (3) thinking it over, (4) evaluation, (5) discussing with instructor, (6) achieving new understandings, and (7) renewing patient contact.

Students often include nurse–patient interactions in their case studies. Students should keep these interactions for future reference.

Psychodynamics: Therapeutic use of Self

SELF-AWARENESS

A healthy awareness of the impact that the nursing student has on a patient is imperative. Willingness to see our patients through the vicissitudes of life with a constant awareness of the effects that other people's problems have on us can lead to objectivity in human relations. No one person can be everything to everybody. Self-awareness helps each professional become cognizant of his own limitations in addition to his strengths.

There is no easy path to self-awareness.

Students who have just been through adolescence may still be painfully self-conscious; they can quickly pick up and respond to feelings of patients such as loneliness, joy, grief, and despair.

Identification of feelings within yourself and others is the first step. Use of introspection, diaries, and sharing feelings in group and individual conferences can also aid in the development of self-awareness. These processes, as necessary for the experienced as for the uninitiated, continue throughout one's professional life. In the development of self-understanding, it is comforting to share thoughts with others and find that they too are experiencing similar feelings.

For beginning professionals to be able to assist their patients in fulfillment of their psychosocial needs, a healthy self-awareness is essential. One way to increase one's sensitivity to patients is through discussion of thoughts and feelings with peers and instructors. Meeting regularly throughout the year in small groups can aid the student to make the transition from student role to professional role and to be more effective as a professional person.

Small-group work can increase self-understanding, the understanding of other persons, and awareness of one's impact upon them and the influence of the group on the individual. It also aids one to understand group behavior and to be a more effective group member. An increase in learning and the development of skill in carrying out role functions in other situations occur. In this kind of work these learnings can best be accomplished by analyzing whatever happens in the group sessions themselves.

Feelings of inadequacy in all clinical areas are expressed by students even up to the last day of classes in the senior year. The thirst for information and the search for perfection are real to the student. There are also feelings of imposition upon the patient in which students perceive themselves as intruders until they gain enough self-confidence to feel comfortable in the myriad roles in which they find themselves.

At periods throughout their education, nursing students feel imposed upon or overloaded in their curriculum. So much giving of self to others often leaves students feeling drained and sometimes a bit angry. The impact of space-age technology has resulted in so much information and so many complexities in nursing that students desire to know and learn more about many subjects but feel themselves "bogged down" with assignments. Group discussions aid them to perceive how others are handling the input overload; methods and shortcuts in the learning process are frequently shared. Conflicts between participation in university activities and the ability to participate fully and adequately in the professional curriculum have to be faced by all students. Peers assist each other in setting up priorities for development of the broader aspects of life, getting rest and relaxation, and being effective as emerging professionals.

Contact with people of all ages and social strata in the crises of life helps mature the student. The intimate contact with life and death and with the internal workings of the human body and mind together with other new experiences often results in a student's feeling alienated from friends at home and in other fields. This separation is felt very keenly. Patients begin depending on the student for help, and students express excitement and joy at finding their goal in life; a simultaneous dampening of spirits may occur because there is not time to do everything. Students begin to feel isolated from old friends when they share confidences and find that the old friends cannot understand why their thoughts are on anatomy and physiology or on what they plan to do for their patient the next week, for example. Discussion with peers aids students to view what they are gaining as emerging professionals in addition to what they are giving up. Students fear getting "hard-hearted" and "hard-boiled" and comment on behavior of other professionals around them, e.g., the loud voices of nurses in the recovery room, the anesthetist who writes out his bills during an operation, and the physician in a clinic who matter-of-factly informs a mother that her child is probably mentally retarded. Discussing behavior of others in their milieu helps them to think of ways they themselves might behave as professionals in similar situations. Students realize they are in the vulnerable age group for mental problems and express fear of "cracking up" under the pressures.

An opportunity to meet in a small group over a year's time affords students the chance to observe changes and growth within members of the group. Fears and complaints that patients have are usually expressed to students, who ordinarily spend more time with their patients than do the staff. Daily contact with people who are lonely, fear death, and are helpless, who have financial problems, and who look to them for sustenance can give students a feeling of responsibility that aids in achieving the professional role. Recognition of frustration and anxiety in patients leads students to identify their own reactions such as confusion, worry, anger, fear, and resentment. For example, students who are in contact with patients who have debilitating diseases often feel that the same thing will occur to them.

Students beginning their psychiatric nursing experience fear they will say something that will hurt the patient. They often feel vulnerable to mental disorder, to insights about their own behavior, and that of family members. Students may, for example, see reflections of themselves in psychotic patients and suffer increased anxiety. Focusing on identification of anxiety in patients and ways to help resolve anxiety helps students handle their own feelings and use themselves therapeutically.

Situations encountered by nursing students in all aspects of clinical work and in the social system in which they receive their education are often stressful. The following are examples of incidents encountered by students:

A severely depressed thirty-two-year-old Caucasion woman, S.P., with hepatitis was transferred from one psychiatric ward to another. During the transfer, the nurse in charge of the psychiatric unit was not immediately informed of the hepatitis; therefore, isolation procedures were not implemented right away. Students and staff became very upset because of fear of infection. The patient became upset because the staff were afraid of her.

A student went apartment hunting with her eighty-year-old female patient, P.W., from the psychiatric inpatient service. The patient had lived in the Tenderloin area of San Francisco in a three-room apartment piled high with newspapers, and old empty food cartons, had not paid her rent for three months, refused to answer her door, and was evicted. When the student and P.W. walked by the area of her old apartment, they found some of her belongings in the trash can. This was very upsetting not only to the patient but to the student.

Discussion with others helped the students with their feelings about these situations and problem solving what could have been done to prevent these situations from occurring.

In small-group work, stress clues in fellow students can be identified and dealt with so that members learn something about their own limitations and ways to handle stress. Students are then better able to respond to the needs of patients and families. Instructors and other students demonstrate ways to weather and surmount anxiety and the stresses of life. There are some students who feel that small-group work itself is depressing because of its emphasis on problems; others comment on the strength gained from knowing that others feel the same way about things. Other comments relate to the benefit gained in the discussion of nurse–patient relationships and in assisting each other to solve problems. Students often feel closer to one another after discussing mutual problems.

EMPATHY

The therapeutic nurse–patient relationship requires the ability to empathize with the patient. Empathy includes the ability to feel what the patient is presently feeling, what he has felt in the past and what you hope the patient is going to be in the future; it also includes the ability to maintain an objective view of the patient. The process of feeling what the patient is experiencing, in part, and on a temporary basis, and thinking about it is a vital part of therapeutic process. Every nurse cannot be empathic with every patient; there are limits to each nurse's abilities.

CATHARTIC LISTENING

"Catharsis" comes from the Greek word for purification and was introduced to psychiatry by Freud. It is also called "ventila-

tion." Cathartic listening refers to the attitude of the nurse; it means availability to hear what the patient has to say in an endeavor to understand what is going on with him and his situation without interrupting, arguing, or telling him what to do. There is an inborn need to share information, and a person feels uncomfortable when he has to keep a secret. Usually he does not keep it too long. The best thing about a secret is that it can be told to someone else! Most people like to talk, particularly about themselves, and a concerned, persistent person will eventually get through to the most nontalkative person. It is quite common for a patient on first contact with a nurse to get everything off his chest in one session and then he may feel guilty about revealing himself so fully and frankly and avoid the next contact. The nurse may ask the patient, "Are you certain that you want to tell me all this today?" thereby making it clear that there are subsequent possibilities for contact. The problem of being present one day and gone the next and the condition of the patient may influence your decision.

Listening, not just for the words but for what the patient is really saying, requires great concentration on the part of the listener. Although beginning students may at first think that listening is passive, as their listening skills improve they will find that this is not true. Like the symphony conductor, you hear all instruments separately but also in combination. Verbalizing acts as catharsis for most Anglo-Americans. However, if your patient is Yaqui, you may not expect much verbalization! Ask yourself when you are working with your patient, "Of everything that I know about my patient and his family, what is he telling me now?" In the therapeutic nurse–patient relationship talking through and sharing feelings is a healing process itself. The clinician serves as a model and the patient learns that painful affects may be tolerated and expressed. Acceptance of the painful affects is then possible.

Common to all forms of therapeutic relationships is the decrease of feelings of being alone, that is, of remembering details, correcting inconsistencies, learning about the patient's life and listening.

There is a tendency for nurses to be oriented toward physiological needs of their patients in general hospitals. It is also easy to think that all complaints of patients in a psychiatric unit results from anxiety. However, nurses in both areas should be aware of the holistic needs of their patients. Physicians may also have this tendency, as was noted in the study that showed that underdiagnosis of mental problems and overdiagnosis of physiological problems of patients in a general hospital were sometimes made when a patient's problems were actually linked to his mental status (Duff and Hollingshead, 1968, p. 162). Recently, nurses in a general hospital were found to have negative attitudes toward patients with a psychiatric history (Brady, 1976).

If you as a nursing student incorporate into your role concept and professional identification the holistic view of your patients and families, you will listen more effectively to the complaints of your patients. Stop now and think of a patient and his family that you know well and identify all the needs that they have, which ones you met, which ones others on the health team met, what needs were left unmet, and what you could have done better in the same situation.

LEVERAGE

The leverage of the therapist can be exerted through three fundamental processes: understanding, acknowledging, and agreeing (Ruesch, 1961). Understanding involves establishing an accurate idea of the patient's behavior in your mind. Acknowledging refers to the specific responses to the patient's messages. Staying with pediatric patients who have no visitors during visiting hours is an example of nonverbal acknowledgment or, if you are in a psychiatric unit, helping to plan a Sunday outing for those unable to spend the weekend at home. If you ascertain that your patient is bothered by something, a direct question— e.g., "What's bugging you?"—acknowledges his nonverbal message. Agreeing implies the identification of certain aspects in the human experiences and establishment of similar views or opinions. These are three pleasurable responses and result in gratifica-

tion. Once the patient experiences the gratification of the interaction, he will be moved toward more communication and can begin to help solve his own problems.

TOUCH

Tactile communication is transitory, lasting only while it is being done. It is also reciprocal; nurse and patient touch each other. Touch, when used judiciously, can be very reassuring to patients. The right of the nurse to the "laying on of hands" carries with it a status hierarchy that should be understood both for its responsibilities and for its limitations. The idea of the "laying on of hands" comes from the touch of the king to cure illness and also from the medicine man's power in the healing process.

The tactile sense, most primitive of the senses, serves in the lower animals as a method for exploration of their world. The antennae of butterflies, crabs, and fish as well as the whiskers of the cat give information necessary for life. In humans, the receptors for touch are in the skin. People who are easily hurt are often referred to as thin-skinned. The importance of tactile communication in everyday life is clearly stated in such commonly used expressions as "I *feel*," "I am so *touched*," "She is a *warm* person," and *"tender,* loving care."

Although touch is now a current popular emphasis, care must be exercised in the use of touch with psychiatric patients. Fragmented, uncertain ego boundaries, mistrust, and fear of closeness require maintenance of distance by the helping person working with psychiatric patients.

SIGNALS, SIGNS, AND SYMBOLS

When a person touches a hot, cold, or rough object, there may be a signal for withdrawal because of pain. When he learns to associate these uncomfortable objects as *signs* of pain, he avoids them; in responding to the words "hot," "cold," "tender," and "rough" by protecting himself, he is acting symbolically. If a patient perceives roughness in nurse–patient interactions, he may refuse to talk to the next nurse, who *symbolizes* pain, even though the nurse may not be rough at all. If the patient perceives the nurse as cold in the interaction with him, the approach of the nurse may be the *signal* for him to turn his face to the wall. The appearance of any nurse might then act as a sign for the patient to avoid contact.

The contact comfort and motion stimulation so loved by the Harlows' (1962) monkeys also applies to the human animals who run to mother for comfort or who in later years may buy "vibrator machines."

TRANSFERENCE

Transference, a concept discovered by Freud (1958), refers to the phenomenon of the unconscious attribution to the therapist of characteristics of significant others in the early life of the patient. It refers to those intensely emotionally charged relationships where the therapist is of unique importance to the patient and where the patient depends on the therapist; therefore, it is a relationship in which the patient feels that he and the therapist exist in opposition to the rest of the world. The nurse, dealing with life-and-death relationships, moves in a very emotionally intensive environment with people. Sickness itself engenders fear and the search for assistance. Since all relationships do contain elements of earlier relationships, nurses are in constant contact with patients whose childhood perceptions are reactivated by the stresses they are undergoing. Transference occurs in all significant relationships to some degree and may be a transitory identification that the patient makes with the nurse. The intimacy of a nurse with patients affects and colors the intensity of the relationships. The nurse's experiences with the patient's bodily functions may easily arouse the transference relationship to parent. It is very common for patients to reply to nurses, "O.K., Mother," when asked to do something. Or, a child may ask, "Will you be my mother while I am here?" Likewise, the patient may also attribute to the nurse the parental role of authority usually ascribed to fathers. Transference transcends age and sex. Although your patient may be a forty-year-old executive, he may react toward you as if you were the parent. Older patients may say to you, "You remind me of my granddaughter" (or grandson, as the case may be).

Although the examples given here are conscious attributions, they are signals to the importance of unconscious behavior and clues to the attachments felt by patients for nurses. Transference can be either positive or negative. A positive transference may appear in the patient as being overly dependent or affectionate; negative transference usually involves hostility. It is important to differentiate between the negative transference and other uncomfortable situations. If the patient is hostile because his call light is out of reach, this is not negative transference. If transference is positive, the "working through" phase of the relationship is facilitated; if it is negative, the work may be more difficult but can still lead to growth.

Transference may frequently take on aspects of sibling relationships. A patient may perceive and act toward all older women nurses as though they are sisters. Although the life-space, face-to-face encounters in nurse–patient relationships tend to minimize distortions, they are, nevertheless, still present.

In a general hospital setting students were assigned to patients within a three-bed ward during their stay on this particular unit. One patient was not assigned to students for care because students were not studying her particular condition at that time. When the students were present, she became more and more demanding of their attention, asking for little things. It was noted, however, that the patient was able and willing to do the same things for herself when the students were absent. The patient had regressed to the role of child at the times when students, the mothering figures, were present.

USE OF TRANSFERENCE

The transference relationship is very powerful and must be held in trust and considered with great seriousness. The patient has placed himself in the hands of the nurse and is therefore in a most vulnerable position. Feelings of every kind are displayed in the nurse–patient relationship. Feelings that have not been previously expressed may arise, for example, the need for love from a mother who did not express feelings to her child. If the transference is negative, the nurse may be required to show the patient different aspects from those of the person who elicited these feelings in the patient originally.

Nurse–patient relationships involve more than just encouraging your patient to tell you all about himself. Theoretical knowledge helps you to understand the significance of what your patients confide in you. When a patient tells you upon first contact of "the cruel nurses" who took care of her father, you may be fairly sure that she needs to work through her feelings about his death.

Once the transference relationship is developed, it is often helpful to the patient to talk out his problems to the therapist while the therapist listens carefully, thereby conveying to the patient that he is a person worth listening to. Therefore, the patient is encouraged to bring out what he considers to be meaningful.

The transference relationship is used in nursing to help the patient work through problems he has on his mind. The nurse recognizes the role of the unconscious without necessarily interpreting unconscious material to her patient. To deny and ignore the existence and functioning of the unconscious in modern nursing is to negate attention to the whole person. You are not a sponge or ink blotter merely soaking up the dependency needs of your patients; you help them and their families deal with reality situations, socialize, groom themselves, solve problems, and move toward their highest potential.

Experienced psychotherapists are more skilled in interpersonal relationships than the beginning nurse. However, it is important for the beginner to develop skills to recognize the dynamic forces within interpersonal relationships that foster effective communication.

RESISTANCE

Resistance in psychiatry refers to the defenses that prevent repressed thoughts of the patient from being brought forth. In an operational sense, it refers to the reluc-tance of the patient or his inability to relate his thoughts, feelings, and memories to the therapist. Some signs of resistance in the patient may take the following forms: (1) being late for an appointment, (2) falling asleep during an appointment, and (3) verbalizing that there is nothing else to say. Jourard (1971) describes resistance also in the therapist and identifies some danger signals of its presence: fantasizing during contact with the patient without telling it to the patient, and withholding one's true feelings.

COUNTERTRANSFERENCE

To Freud (1957) also we owe the concept of countertransference. Countertransference refers to the conscious or unconscious emotional reaction of the therapist toward the patient. It is the attribution of characteristics of the patient to a significant person in the early life of the therapist. Here, it is discussed as the total emotional reaction of the nurse to the patient (Kernberg, 1965). A partial identification with the patient, it usually does not last long (Reich, 1951).

In nursing, countertransference is often paraded under the guise of personality clash. It is unrealistic to think that all professional relationships will be 100 percent compatible; however, a personality clash between a patient and nurse requires study and self-understanding, not a change of assignments. Other expressions that may indicate countertransference are "involvement," "overidentification," and "uptight." In many instances, countertransference has been thought of as not particularly helpful; however, it can enable you to further understand the patient as well as your own behavior. In nursing students who are in the process of breaking away from parents, the intense emotions of childhood and adolescence may be very near the surface and color their relationship with patients, particularly those in the age group of their parents. Students who are in their teens therefore may find it easier to relate to patients in age groups other than the parental ones. Kloes and Weinberg (1968) describe some aspects of countertransference as being related to willingness to accept a rejecting role, anger, and also loss of interest in the patient.

Other alerting signals of countertransference are situations where the therapist has very strong emotions about situations involving the patient, for example, when the therapist has feelings of hostility toward the patient or emotions resembling falling in love.

If you are obviously upset and cry when your patient undergoes painful procedures or experiences, you abdicate your expressive role. In such a case, each injection that you prepare and give to your patient or each limit that you have to set with him is painful to you and this is clearly visible to the patient.

One nurse found it very difficult to work with geriatric patients when, in fact, she was transferring to her geriatric patients, as a group, the undesirable attributes of her own grandmother. Subsequent conferences with her supervisor resulted in a change in her attitude toward her patients. Other situations involving older patients may evoke the same responses as if the patients were grandparents. Students taught to revere and respect their elders may find themselves immobilized in the presence of older patients and may temporarily be unable to take the necessary initiative in providing care. A young patient, Mr. D., resembled the estranged husband of the nurse caring for him on the psychiatric unit. The nurse avoided and feared this patient. When she became conscious of the triggering mechanism, she was able to work with him. An older patient, Mr. F., whom the student visited in his home, reminded her of her grandfather. The nurse visited too frequently and, at the time of termination of her visits, was in tears.

Situations where nurses become romantically involved with patients may demonstrate transference and countertransference. One student and a patient on the psychiatric service became inseparable. The patient was an attractive young man, meticulous in appearance, who had a wife and two children. He was given special privileges by the unit staff, e.g., visits to their homes. The patient confided in the student the story of his life's

difficulties and his rebellion against the Establishment. They attended the evening dances together as a couple. When confronted with her behavior, the student perceived that she had become overly sympathetic with her patient in her quest to help him.

Another patient, a handsome young man and the president of the patients' council on the unit, had a history of failures in coping with the demands of society. Observed to be the favorite of one of the older nurses, he also managed to get special privileges and appeared nattily dressed for events where he presided. Sometime later the patient and the nurse eloped to Mexico.

A mentally retarded young adult with a long history of disrupted family relationships was unable to adapt to rules within the psychiatric unit. He was perceived by one of the nurses as having had a life like her own. The nurse became very protective of him regardless of his behavior.

A word of caution must be given with regard to erroneously labeling all strong emotional reactions in the nurse–patient relationship as attributable to transference or countertransference. Each complaint of a patient should be duly considered by the team involved in his care. Cold meals, cold rooms, cold bedpans, and coldness from the staff do not necessarily result from countertransference.

COGNITIVE DISSONANCE

Festinger (1957) in his theory of cognitive dissonance purports that new cognitions that make individuals vulnerable to illness, infirmity, and changes in body image that are dissonant with their self-cognitions (being whole, well, and strong) may result in anxiety until new adaptations have occurred.

For example, an older person who has just decided, on the basis of being robbed several times in his neighborhood while going to the store, to sell his house and move into an apartment with a doorman may be consumed with afterthoughts about the decision and enumerate in great detail to you on every home visit the unattractive aspects of the move. Although the decision has already been made, doubts about it persist. The tension can be reduced in at least two ways. To reverse the decision and remain in the house, since apartment living seems so unattractive, is one way. If this path is taken, however, the original tension for initiation of the move continues, i.e., the possibility of being subjected to robberies. Another path is to change the cognition or information about the move. This may be done in several ways. One is for the nurse to point out the positive aspects of the move—that there is less worry about taxes, upkeep, proximity to transportation, and neighbors. Another is to use the reportorial approach that "this is what happens to some people when they make important decisions."

If a younger person is encountering a similar experience, you can point out the process of making a big decision and validate with the patient whether he thinks this is what is happening to him. It may be helpful to the person who is experiencing cognitive dissonances to discuss what is happening to him with someone else who has experienced a similar situation. It is often a comfort to perceive that others have survived quite admirably what one is experiencing oneself.

Interviewing as a Method of Measurement

In nursing, precise objectives cannot consistently be made before the patient is encountered. Only general purposes can be made from which more precise objectives will emerge during the interview itself, depending in turn on what happens in the interview. It is during the interaction with the patient that hypotheses develop about nursing interventions that can subsequently be acted upon. In interviewing, there is appraisal and, after the interaction, comparison and contrast with previous experiences with patients. Behaviors observed are translated into theoretical knowledge and compared with the observations of others. The interviewer is the measuring device in nurs-

ing; there is no slide rule, pH paper, or centigrade thermometer to measure the inner person. It is the hunch you have that leads you to explore the thoughts, feelings, and perceptions of another human being.

Observational ability includes affective, cognitive, and sensory aspects of the person. Some people observe more than others. Is this related to personality? If we try to protect our own image, are we likely to see ways in which people we dislike resemble us? If you dislike obese people or hairy people, how does this affect your nurse–patient relationship?

In the process of nurse–patient interaction, some of the practical problems need to be understood. Knowledge of the sources and kinds of biases[4] will help you to be a better clinician.

Errors common to any interaction may occur in the nurse–patient relationship, errors of observation, in the kinds of questions asked, in recording, and in recall. Some of these are discussed on the following pages. Random errors are chance variations; however, they are canceled out over a large number of contacts.

HALO EFFECT

Awareness of the possibility of the *halo effect*[5] is important; you must be able to look at different qualities of persons and rate them individually, instead of forming general impressions dominating the specific qualities.

The halo effect can be either positive or negative. It can be positive in the sense of, for example, a patient's being very complimentary and generous, a fact that overshadows any other behavior of his, e.g., chronic alcoholism. In a negative sense, when a patient is irritable and demanding one morning, he may subsequently be labeled by the nursing personnel as irritable and demanding during his entire hospital stay.

[4] Bias is the systematic piling of errors in one direction only.

[5] *Halo effect* refers to the inability to isolate a trait of an individual and form an opinion about it without being influenced by knowledge of the person as a whole.

STEREOTYPE

A stereotype is a supposed appearance or behavior of a certain ethnic, age, sex, class, occupational, or social group. Some common stereotypes of certain groups include: All Italians eat spaghetti every day; all people who talk about homosexuality are homosexual themselves. The stereotype may also be referred to as a group halo.

Some other factors affecting our relationships with patients are (1) *logical error*, (2) *variable error*, (3) *constant error*, and (4) *recall*. Logical error is intellectual; it is cognitive confusion. You think rather than feel that something is true when it actually is not. Combining the halo effect and the logical error results in *constant error*.

CONSTANT ERROR

Constant error occurs when desirable traits in individuals are given undue importance in assessment and are overestimated; less desirable ones are more or less ignored and therefore underestimated. For example, so long as a patient awaiting surgery makes few demands of you, you may overlook the fact that he spends two hours every day in the bathroom without bothering to learn the motivation underlying his behavior. It is important to separate facts *observed* from inferences resulting from observation. Confirming your observations with the patient or others may be especially helpful.

VARIABLE ERROR

Variable error represents a divergence of opinion held by different persons in regard to a characteristic in an individual. The frame of reference from which a person thinks, speaks, and acts greatly influences variable error. The following is an example:

A crunching sound by a neighbor's house followed by a child's scream led several people to the scene. A small boy had been hit by a car. The mother, a nun from the neighboring convent, and a nurse converged on the scene. The mother screamed, yelled hysterically to the child,

"I love you," the nun knelt and prayed, and the nurse called the ambulance and administered first aid.

ERRORS OF RECORDING AND RECALL

Because recall changes quite rapidly, some method of recording immediately after contact with the patient is important. Written verbatim reconstructions of the nurse–patient interaction are useful tools in teaching and learning. However, they are helpful only if written openly and honestly immediately after contact, and if omissions are indicated with ". . ." where memory fails. A tendency to complete patient's sentences is therefore avoided. The interaction put aside and returned to for rereading and evaluation can be very useful to the student in the application of interviewing principles and in the improvement of communication skills. It also provides a record for the student to observe growth in self as well as the interpersonal growth or change in behavior of the patient. Tape recordings, videotapes, or handwritten process recordings are sometimes used by nurses in learning interviewing techniques. However, I do not advocate the use of taped material because of the amount of time one may have to spend on it. Process recordings, by their very nature of being written during the nurse–patient contact, remove spontaneity. Taping interviews is also expensive and omits some nonverbal communication. Films or videotapes record more completely than other methods after individuals become accustomed to the fact that they are performing.

If it is impossible to reconstruct an interview immediately after holding it, then jot down skeletal notes, which, at a later date, will aid you by *recognition* to reconstruct the nurse–patient interaction. You should take care that the analysis of a nurse–patient interaction records what was said and done, not what ideally should have occurred or what could happen if one had it to do over again. After recording interactions with patients and families, the process through which one goes in thought and in discussions with instructors, supervisors, consultants, and others is an essential part of learning to evaluate one's interviewing techniques.

SOME COMMON PROBLEMS EXPRESSED BY STUDENTS

Common problems expressed by students in the helping process are as follows: (1) inability to evaluate the effects of therapeutic use of self; (2) misperception of use of nondirective interviewing methods as being devious, with subsequent feelings of guilt; and (3) resistance to analysis of nurse–patient interactions. Students may feel that they are invading the privacy of their patients as they assume their professional role. In the transition from nonprofessional student to professional, they may express frustration, despondency, and anger and feel it is unethical to look into the private life of their patients. Emphasis in nursing on the inner life of the patient may evoke anxiety and defensive reactions in the student. In working with people who have multiple problems, students often have intense feelings about the fact that changes for the better are not occurring very rapidly and may feel a sense of failure themselves. The feeling that time, interest, and effort put into the helping process have not effected a visible change in the patient is often discouraging. It is at this point that reassessment of the situation occurs and more realistic treatment goals emerge or the student gives up trying to help and moves on to something else.

Summary

The rites of passage from student to professional occur as nursing students enter their major field. In this chapter attention is given to aspects of therapeutic communication that aid in professional role identification. An ability to view the mirror-image self as it is reflected from the culture of the nurse is emphasized, and phases of the helping relationship in nursing with component parts are discussed. Some guidelines on confidentiality and written nurse–patient interactions are described. The Problem-Oriented Medical Record is discussed.

Psychodynamic concepts of therapeutic use of self are presented. Interviewing as a method of measurement with discussion of halo effect, stereotype, constant error, variable error, and errors of recording and recall is also included. The chapter concludes with some common problems in interviewing and therapeutic use of self as expressed by students.

References

AMERICAN NURSES' ASSOCIATION: *The Code for Nurses with Interpretive Statements.* American Nurses' Association, 1979.

BERMOSK, LORETTA, and MORDAN, MARY JANE: *Interviewing in Nursing.* New York: Macmillan Publishing Co., Inc., 1964.

BRADY, M. M.: "Nurses' Attitudes Towards a Patient Who Has a Psychiatric History," *Journal of Advanced Nursing,* 11:11–23, January 1976.

CARTER, FRANCES MONET: *Psychiatric Mental Health Nursing in Generic, Baccalaureate Programs Accredited by the National League for Nursing in the United States.* Doctoral Dissertation, University of San Francisco, 1978.

DE GRAZIA, SEBASTIAN: *Of Time, Work and Leisure.* New York: Twentieth Century, 1962.

DUFF, RAYMOND S., and HOLLINGSHEAD, AUGUST: *Sickness and Society.* New York: Harper & Row, 1968.

FESTINGER, LEON: *A Theory of Cognitive Dissonance.* Evanston, Ill.: Row Peterson, 1957.

FREUD, SIGMUND: *The Collected Papers.* London: The Hogarth Press, 1957, Vol. XI, pp. 144–45.

———: *The Collected Papers.* London: The Hogarth Press, 1958, Vol. XII, pp. 159–71.

HALL, EDWARD T.: *The Silent Language.* New York: Premier Books, 1959.

———: *The Hidden Dimension.* Garden City, N.Y.: Doubleday & Co., 1966.

HARLOW, MARGARET KUENNE, and HARLOW, HARRY F.: "Social Deprivation in Monkeys," *Scientific American,* 207:5:137–46, November 1962.

JOURARD, SIDNEY M.: *The Transparent Self.* New York: D. Van Nostrand Co., 1971.

KERNBERG, OTTO: "Notes on Countertransference," *Journal of the American Psychoanalytic Association,* 13:1:38–56, January 1965.

KLOES, KAREN B., and WEINBERG, ANN:

"Countertransference," *Perspectives in Psychiatric Care,* **VI**:4:152–62, 1968.

KOLB, LAWRENCE K.: *Modern Clinical Psychiatry.* Philadelphia: W. B. Saunders Co., 1973, pp. 150–62.

LANTERMAN, PETRIS, SHORT Act, 1969, in *California Mental Health Services Act.* Sacramento, Calif.: California Office of State Printing, 1979.

REDL, FRITZ: "A Strategy and Technique of the Life Space Interview," *American Journal of Orthopsychiatry,* **XXIX**:1–18, January 1959.

REICH, ANNIE: "On Countertransference," *International Journal of Psychoanalysis* 32:25, 1951.

REIK, THEODOR: *Listening with the Third Ear.* New York: Grove Press, 1956.

ROGERS, CARL: *Counseling and Psychotherapy.* Boston: Houghton Mifflin, 1942.

————: *Client-Centered Therapy.* Boston: Houghton Mifflin, 1951.

ROTH, JULIUS A.: *Timetables.* New York: Bobbs-Merrill Co., Inc., 1963.

RUESCH, JURGEN, and BATESON, GREGORY: *Communication, the Social Matrix of Psychiatry.* New York: W. W. Norton & Co., Inc., 1951.

———— and KEES, WELDON: *Non-verbal Communication.* Berkeley: University of California Press, 1956.

————: *Disturbed Communication.* New York: W. W. Norton & Co., Inc., 1957.

————: *Therapeutic Communication.* New York: W. W. Norton & Co., Inc., 1961.

————: "The Social Control of Symbolic Systems," *Journal of Communication,* **XVII**:4:276–301, December 1967.

THORNDIKE, E.: "Constant Error in Psychological Ratings," *Journal of Applied Psychology,* 4:25–29, 1920.

Suggested Readings

BEMPORAD, JULES R.: "Cognitive Development," in Arieti, Silvano, ed.: *American Handbook of Psychiatry.* New York: Basic Books, Inc., 1974, pp. 328–52.

BENEDICT, RUTH: *Patterns of Culture.* Boston: Houghton Mifflin Co., 1937.

————: *The Chrysanthemum and the Sword.* Boston: Houghton Mifflin Co., 1946.

BUBER, MARTIN: *I and Thou.* New York: Charles Scribner's Sons, 1958.

DiANGI, PAULETTE: "Barriers to the Black and White Therapeutic Relationship," *Perspectives in Psychiatric Care,* **XIV**:4:180–183, 1976.

ENELOW, ALLEN J., and SWISHER, SCOTT N.: *Interviewing and Patient Care.* New York: Oxford University Press, 1972.

FLESCH, REGINA; *Treatment Considerations in the Reassignment of Clients.* New York: Family Service Association, 1948.

FORSYTH, GARRYFALLIA L.: "Exploration of Empathy in Nurse–Client Interaction," *Advances in Nursing Science,* 1:2:53–61, January 1979.

GREENHILL, MAURICE H.: "Interviewing with a Purpose," *American Journal of Nursing,* 56:10:1259–62, 1956.

HALL, EDWARD T.: *Beyond Culture,* Garden City, New York: Anchor Books, 1977.

HAYAKAWA, S. I., ed.: *Lanugage, Meaning and Maturity.* New York: Harper & Row, 1954.

————: *Language in Thought and Action.* New York: Harcourt, Brace, and World, 1964.

HEIN, ELEANOR: *Communication in Nursing Practice.* Boston: Little, Brown & Co., 1973.

JACKSON, D. N., and MESSICK, S. J.: "A Note on 'Ethnocentrism' and Acquiescent Response Sets," *Journal of Abnormal and Social Psychology,* 54:132–34, 1957.

JOHNSON, FREDDIE LOUISE POWELL: "Response to Territorial Intrusion by Nursing Home Residents," *Advances in Nursing Science,* 1:4:21–34, July 1979.

JOHNSON, MARGIE N.: "Anxiety/Stress and the Effects on Disclosure between Nurses and Patients," *Advances in Nursing Science,* 1:4:1–20, July 1979.

JOHNSON, MAXENE: "Folk Beliefs and Ethnocultural Behavior in Pediatrics," *Nursing Clinics of North America.* 12:1:77–84, March 1977.

JOURARD, SIDNEY M.: *Disclosing Man to Himself.* Princeton, N.J.: Van Nostrand, 1968.

LEININGER, MADELEINE: *Transcultural Nursing: Concepts, Theories, and Practices.* New York: John Wiley & Sons, 1978.

MITCHELL, ANN CHAPPELL: "Barriers to Therapeutic Communication with Black Clients," *Nursing Outlook,* 26:2:109–12, February 1978.

NOBLE, MARY ANN: "Communication in the ICU: Therapeutic or Disturbing?" *Nursing Outlook,* 27:3:195–98, March 1979.

RUFFIN, JANICE E.: "Racism as Countertransference in Psychotherapy Groups," *Perspectives in Psychiatric Care,* **XI**:4:172–78, 1973.

SENE, BARBARA STANKIEWICZ: "Termination in the Student–Patient Relationship," *Perspectives in Psychiatric Care,* 7:1:39–45, 1969.

STEVENSON, IAN: "The Psychiatric Interview," in Arieti, Silvano, ed.: *American Handbook of Psychiatry.* New York: Basic Books, Inc., 1974, pp. 1138–56.

TRAVELBEE, JOYCE: "Intervention in Psychiatric Nursing: *Process in the One-to-One Relationship.* Philadelphia: F. A. Davis Co., 1969.

WHITE, ELEANOR M.: "Initial Patient Assessment and Evaluation," in Kalkman, Marion E., and Davis, Anne J., eds.: *New Dimensions in Mental Health—Psychiatric Nursing.* New York: McGraw-Hill, pp. 547–56.

5

Patients Under Stress

It is necessary to understand that there are many theories about the life process and its effects upon the human being. The intangible effects on the human condition of experiences in living are still only imperfectly understood. The study of human behavior is a relatively new science that is destined to have a great impact on the nursing profession, inasmuch as nurses are concerned with behavior brought about by the exigencies of life and are in a position to be of assistance during stress periods in the life arc. Engel defined stress as follows:

Psychological stress refers to all processes, whether originating in the external environment or within the person, which impose a demand or requirement upon the organism, the resolution or handling of which requires work or activity of the mental apparatus before any other system is involved or activated.[1]

Thus, stress is the introducer, not the effect, of an action. Engel also states that for a situation or process to constitute psychological stress, it must be perceived, in whole or in part, and it must also be capable of some type of psychic representation or expression, whether conscious or unconscious. In contrast, physical stress is brought about by such factors as poisons, physical trauma, and the like; it affects, first of all, the operation and function of the physiological systems in the person. For example, the action of *Treponema pallidum* does not meet the criterion of psychological stress, but the *idea* of syphilis does. A physical injury may be felt simultaneously as both psychological stress and physical stress. Daniel Hack Tuke (1878) wrote of the "overbrain work" of modern life and cited the case of a nineteen-year-old youth at Cambridge who had accomplished a lot of work in a short time and went "raving mad" requiring three people to hold him. Stress tolerance varies in individuals. The intensity and duration of stress affect how people respond.

Shell shock was the name given to the condition that individuals suffered who reached their breaking point during World War I. It was called combat fatigue and gross stress reaction in World War II. Gross stress reaction was widely accepted as a diagnostic entity and appeared in the first *Diagnostic and Statistical Manual: Mental Disorders* (American Psychiatric Association,

1952). It has reappeared in the new DSM III as *posttraumatic stress disorder,* acute and chronic, under the heading of anxiety disorders (see Appendix C). In the new DSM III, Axis IV—Psychosocial Stressors—indicates to the clinician the evaluation of significant psychosocial stressors contributing to the mental disorder.

Psychic Trauma

Psychic trauma can be described as occurring as a consequence of trivial matters or of catastrophe. What is trauma for one individual may be an adventure to another. Psychic trauma occurs as a result of a stimulus or a series of stimuli, usually external, termed the *traumatic event.* If the traumatic event is beyond the capacity of the ego's barrier or defensive capacities, a traumatic intrapsychic process ensues as a result of the event, leading to a *traumatic state* or emotional discharge, which, for example, may result in helplessness, as an example of a symptom (Rangell, 1967). Thoughts, feelings, and other behavior may become disorganized and physical symptoms appear. If the ego withstands the onslaught of the traumatic event, and reconstitutes, recovery occurs instead of symptom formation.

STIMULUS BARRIER

Fundamental to the trauma theory is the concept of the *stimulus barrier.* The stimulus barrier is defined as an ego function that protects against excessive bombardment or excitation (Gediman, 1971). It was first described by Freud (1920). It is thought to be gradually developed in the infant, who, at birth, is subject to all excitations, by the influence of the protective shield of the parents. For most people, the stimulus barrier protects the integration of the ego and the personality remains organized under stress. Psychic trauma occurs when the ego receives stimuli too overwhelming to cope with in the usual manner. After a traumatic event, if the ego fails to reconstitute or reorganizes in such a way as to leave the individual with hypersensitivities, he may be left with unrealistic fears or mechanisms main-

[1] Engel, G. L.: *Psychological Development in Health and Disease.* Philadelphia: W. B. Saunders Co., 1962, p. 264.

taining control over emotional expression. The meaning that the trauma has to the person, the relationship of the person to his environment, and the effects of his past experience all determine the outcome (Titchener et al., 1974). The following example delineates the meaning of psychic trauma for one person.

"I never thought it could happen to me," stated a man whose wife had just begun divorce proceedings. The next phase was indicated by the query "Why me?" and the next phase became an expression of "There must be something I have done to cause this" and was followed by self-condemnation and guilt.

A friendly, supportive environment in which the person has some control over daily events and other factors helps the traumatized person toward healthy reintegration of the ego, whereas a hostile environment does the opposite. Knowledge of the past experience of the traumatized person helps us to understand its manifestations: previous conflicts are often again brought to the surface by the trauma, which may in turn trigger previous helpless feelings of infancy (a common component of immobilized patients). Knowledge of the past traumas and ways of coping with them is important when assessing strengths and weaknesses of the individual.

The essence of nursing lies in recognizing the areas in individuals and families where coping mechanisms no longer work and using this knowledge to help them handle successfully the problems of life. Since the nurse is in constant proximity to the inner person, the more the student learns about human behavior, the more it will be possible to provide help where it is needed. The nurse has the responsibility to: (1) assist those who are well toward high-level wellness; (2) aid those newly in crisis to an early recovery; and (3) assist those who are mentally disordered to restoration of health.

Conflict, Tension, and Anxiety

Conflict, tension, and anxiety are constructs basic to the understanding of intrapsychic human behavior; therefore, some emphasis is placed here upon understanding their origins, effects, and interrelationships. These constructs cannot be measured precisely; rather, they are inferred from behavior. They may go unnoticed unless the nurse is alert to the phenomenological approach to patients.[2] Nurses who are procedure-centered rather than person-centered will probably not ascertain the inner lives of their patients. On the other hand, the relevance to nursing practice of the emotional temperature of the patient and his family. The psychic pulse, the affect, the psychic wounds, as well as the condition of the skin and the newly made surgical wound, cannot be overemphasized.

In the process of living one thing must always be given up for another. Therefore, conflict is an integral part of human life. The ways in which human beings resolve their conflicts may determine the difference between mental health and mental disorder.

CONFLICT

Conflict is the clash, largely determined by unconscious factors, between opposing emotions. Conflicts create intrapsychic tension, which can be reduced if the conflicts are resolved. When there is unresolved conflict, tension continues within the psyche and coping behavior is demanded of the person; repression may also occur. Experiences evoking shame, guilt, anger, or lowering of self-esteem are likely to be repressed. From repression, anxiety arises, and continued repression may lead to further problems. Indirect outlets of anxiety may result in the use of defense mechanisms. Repressed impulses maintain their intensity, are further reinforced daily beneath facades, and may emerge later in anxiety disorders, psychosomatic reactions, or psychotic symptoms (see Fig. 5). For example, the paralysis of an arm—as in a person with conversion disorder—may represent a conflict between the desire to masturbate and the prohibition against it (English and Finch, 1957). Whereas, the patient with a psychosomatic

---

[2] "Patient" here refers to an individual under the care of a nurse, whether in a hospital, outpatient, or home setting. This term includes the person under care and his family, regardless of absence or presence of mental disorder.

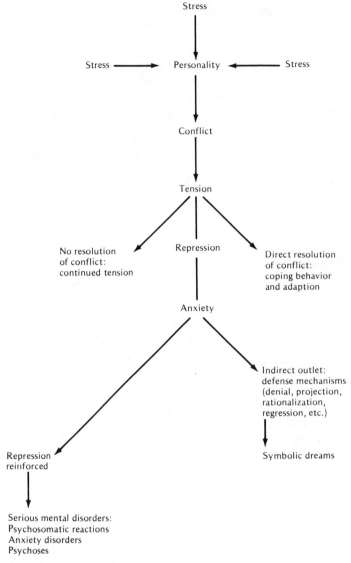

Figure 5. Reactions to Stress

reaction (e.g., essential hypertension) may be unconsciously angry, which keeps his blood pressure elevated. The symptoms of a manic-depressive disorder are thought by the psychoanalytic school to result from repressed trauma and unconscious wishes (Ayd, 1961).

TENSION AND COPING BEHAVIOR

Tension is a restlessness, a vague feeling that something needs to be done. The coping behavior of tension resolution is well known to most individuals, but it must be remembered that behaviors have more than a single purpose; those acceptable in some cultures may not be applicable to others. Coping behavior relieves stress, restores or maintains self-esteem, and assists the person under stress to solve the problems connected with the stress. What is acceptable to your society, culture, and age group? How do you cope with tension? The following list of coping behaviors is adapted from Menninger (1963).

1. Reassurance of touch, rhythm, and

sound. (These all recall the early comfortings of infancy—lullabies, rocking, cuddling, and patting.)

2. Eating and other oral behavior, such as smoking and chewing gum.
3. Use of alcohol and other drugs.
4. Laughing, singing, crying, and swearing.
5. "Goofing off."
6. Sleeping.
7. Thinking it through.
8. Talking it out—discussing one's problems with a sympathetic listener or even excessive verbalization.
9. Working it off in direct physical exercise, for example, running or other sports, cleaning, dancing, or working harder and later.
10. Pointless activity, such as walking up and down, pacing, scratching, finger tapping, and hand rubbing.
11. Retreating into fantasy and daydreaming, especially fantasies in which one's problems are solved or do not exist; excessive TV viewing and movie-going.
12. Boasting.
13. Asking questions.
14. Seeking new information and using it.

ANXIETY

Anxiety is primarily of intrapsychic origin in distinction from fear, which is the emotional response to a consciously recognized and usually external threat or danger. It is the apprehension or uneasiness that stems from the anticipation of danger; the source of the threat is largely unknown or unrecognized. Anxiety becomes pathologic when it occurs to such an extent that it interferes with effective living, the achievement of desired goals or satisfaction, or reasonable emotional comfort. Anxiety and fear are accompanied by similar physiologic changes (American Psychiatric Association, 1980).

Anxiety has also been described as a group phenomenon, which can result in riots, revolutions, and wars. Artists and writers have made it a main theme of their work, in content as well as style. The paintings and woodcuts of Edvard Munch, the ballet *The Burrow* of Kenneth Macmillan, Jean Paul Sartre's play *No Exit,* the writings of Albert Camus, the opera *Wozzeck* by Alban Berg, and *Peter Grimes* by Benjamin Britten are all dramatic portrayals of anxiety. The effect of this permeating theme has been to make the public quite conscious of the ideas and symbols of anxiety. It is a truism to call our time "the age of anxiety." This observation is as true for Europe as for America and perhaps holds for all countries with developing technologies.

Anxiety expresses itself in the loss of direction, the anomie of Durkheim (1951), and the feeling of alienation dealt with by the existentialists. Paul Tillich (1952) describes three major forms of anxiety, those of death, meaninglessness, and condemnation. Anxiety is always communicated interpersonally. It has been called existence by some theorists; others have said it is a threat to values: a threat of nonbeing, a threat of nonbelonging, or what one feels when suddenly confronted with freedom and the opportunity to do things previously forbidden (see Appendix H).

PHYSIOLOGIC CHANGES

Any threat to the ego causes anxiety. It is now known that anxiety, like fear, releases epinephrine; but because the threat is invisible in the former state, the results are in the nature of biochemical scarring and impairment of the physiological functioning. These effects depend upon the degree of anxiety; in general, mild and moderate anxiety heighten the use of an individual's capacities, whereas severe anxiety and panic paralyze or overwork the person. Increased heart rate, increased rate and depth of respiration, rise in arterial pressure, and rapid and extreme shifts in body temperature and blood pressure occur. The blood is diverted from the stomach and intestines to the heart, the central nervous system, and the muscles; processes in the alimentary canal cease; the spleen contracts and discharges corpuscles; and the adrenal medulla secretes its hormone. Symptoms ensue of "cold sweat," disturbances of menstrual flow, urinary urgency and frequency, dryness of mouth, anorexia, dilation of pupils, abdominal cramps, and release of sugar by the liver. An anxious person may feel weak in the knees, may have nausea and vomiting, vertigo, headache, insomnia, syncope; he may feel tightness in the throat, be tense and silent, complain of butterflies in his stomach, sigh, have diarrhea, turn pale, be unable to talk, tremble, say the same thing repeatedly, and have an urge to do something. Cannon was the first to pinpoint the significance of the physiological effects of intense feelings:

Fear has become associated with the instinct to run, to escape; and anger or aggressive feeling, with the instinct to attack. These are fundamental emotions and instincts which have resulted from the experience of multitudes of generations in the fierce struggle for existence and which have their values in that struggle.[3]

Cannon also noted that the responses of the body to intense emotions are designed to prepare the person for "fight or flight." The brain cortex sends a stimulus via the sympathetic branch of the autonomic nervous system to the adrenal glands. Epinephrine is secreted and induces deep respirations and accelerated heartbeats. The body is prepared to use the released energy or to act. Later workers found that the parasympathetic system is also involved during emotional stress; i.e., slowing of the heart rate and lowered blood pressure may also result from anxiety (Grinker and Spiegel, 1945). Selye (1956, 1973) described the *general adaptation syndrome,* focusing attention on the role of the pituitary-adrenocortical axis in the body's response to stress. He identified three states: (1) the alarm reaction, (2) the stage of resistance, and (3) the stage of exhaustion. According to Selye, the general adaptation syndrome comprises adrenal stimulation, shrinkage of lymphatic organs, gastrointestinal ulcers, loss of body weight, alterations in the body chemicals, and related changes. A *local adaptation syndrome* may occur—for example, at the point that microorganisms enter the body. Both of these syndromes are closely interconnected and work together to combat wear and tear within the body.

The reader should note that Selye's stress theory applies to a biologic unit and does not refer to the psychodynamic processes brought into play by specific intrapsychic threats to the ego. Psychological constructs are inferred from behaviors of individuals,

[3] Cannon, Walter: *The Wisdom of the Body.* New York: W. W. Norton Co., 1932, p. 227.

and there is as yet no known way to predict which of the coping behaviors and/or defense mechanisms will be brought into action when the ego is threatened. There are no microorganisms to observe for paths of entry to the human psyche or for triggering psychological defenses.

LEVELS OF ANXIETY

Anxiety occurs at different levels, ranging from mild forms to panic. To assist anxious patients, assessment of anxiety levels must occur first.

Mild Anxiety. A mildly anxious person is alert and has a heightened awareness of what is going on around him. Hearing is increased, communication is direct, and the person can carry out body functions.

Mild anxiety may be felt before taking an examination making a speech, or meeting a new patient. It is also felt by people making changes in their lives, entering a hospital, meeting a new physician or nurse, going for a checkup or undergoing a new diagnostic procedure. Visits of anxious friends and relatives may engender mild anxiety in the patient.

Moderate Anxiety. A moderately anxious person's perception moves toward a limited perceptual field. The person narrows his attention and pays no attention to other events but can notice them if they are pointed out. As anxiety mounts, ability to grasp ideas and learn decreases. The person feels more tense, upset, uneasy, and perspiration of palms, underarms, and feet may occur. Pulse and respiration increase and the person speaks rapidly. Moderately anxious persons may have tightness in the throat, "butterflies" in the stomach, nausea, and vomiting. A moderately anxious patient may hear only one thing that you say.

Severe Anxiety. A severely anxious person's perceptions are so decreased that they cannot take in the events around them. The attention span is very short and only very small details of a severely anxious episode can be recalled. Hearing is not possible for the severely anxious person. Perspiration may be profuse, urinary frequency, diarrhea, rapid, shallow respirations, body tremors, and repetitive speech may occur.

Panic. Small details are "blown up" out of proportion to reality, the person's attention cannot be drawn to notice events around him, and automatic behaviors occur. (See also catastrophic stress, this chapter.) Panicky persons may become so immobilized that they cannot walk or talk.

This kind of reaction may cause a person to ignore hurricane and tornado warnings, keep a person in a burning house or in the path of a flood. It must certainly have been one of the reasons that many Jews in Nazi Germany were unable to leave that country. There is a kind of emotional paralysis that leaves the victim unable to fight or to take flight, the final process of which is catatonia.[4] Others, however, may run over people to get into a lifeboat or fight those who are hospitalizing them.

A panicky person may shoot a gun if he has one, jump off a high building, attack others, or beat himself. He may yell at the top of his voice, run away, or wander about aimlessly. Persons in panic may be observed at the scene of an accident, as hostages, in the emergency room, and in disasters. Operations and treatments may precipitate panic, as may life encounters such as robberies, sexual trauma, heterosexual and homosexual overtures. Role-transition points may also bring on panic, such as leaving one job for another, going to college, marriage, and childbirth. Role-transition points in life are those in which changes are made in what others expect or demand of a person. Change of role may result in high levels of anxiety. Leaving familiar people, institutions, and patterns of behavior may present overwhelming conflicts to some individuals. Anxiety highly affects the individual's adaptation to new roles; each new role that a person has in life may demand different skills and new defenses.

Following is an example of an interaction with a very panicky patient in a psychiatric unit. The patient–nurse contact lasted for a period of one and one-half hours, but the critical time for assessment of the situation

[4] Here catatonia refers to immovable posture, inability to express feeling, and a lack of affective facial expression.

occurred during the first few minutes of contact.

Ecological Unit. The room of a patient in a psychiatric unit. The time is 4:00 A.M., and all other patients on the unit are asleep.

The Patient. The patient is a nurse, a very frail, pale young woman who is tall and thin. Her brown, closely cropped hair is tousled, she is barefoot, and she is wearing hospital flannelette pajamas. Her hands grasp the nurse's arm in a viselike grip. She is breathing heavily, her pupils are dilated, and there is an expression of terror on her face.

Nurse: Hello, Miss C.

Patient: Nurse, nurse, I'm so afraid. Something unusual is going on on this ward. That Tommy is going to surgery. (Peeks out from the door down the hallway.) They're going to do surgery on me too, I know. I want to see Dr. S. and the O.D. [officer of the day] right now. There is something funny going on around here. [She returns to her bed, closes her eyes, and rocks back and forth in a sitting position, moving her hands in bizarre gestures.] Are you a Catholic? [All of this is said with a great rush of words, some stammering, and quick, jerky movements as though very tense.]

Nurse: No, I am not Catholic. You remember me from last week? I'm Miss N. I work only part time. Dr. S. arrives at 8:30 A.M. and the O.D. is asleep. You are not going to surgery. You can talk to me.

Patient: I'm so afraid I'm pregnant, but Dr. S. says that I am not. But I've missed six periods. I have faith in this place and the nurses and the doctors, but I'm the sickest patient on the ward. You know what my trouble is? I take on too much, even here; I see too much of the other patients' symptoms. I'm worse since I got here. I don't like them [refers with gesture to other patients]. I can't stand Mary and Horace. Don't you think I'm the sickest patient here? [Her voice is calmer now.]

Nurse: Oh, Mary and Horace are okay [matter-of-factly]. I don't think of patients as being sick or sickest. Why do you think you're the sickest? [This is a statement of fact, plus an indication of interest in the patient's feelings.]

Patient: [Ignores question.] Well, I guess all of us are sick sometimes. I'm so upset. Look at me. [Trembles all over.] I'm a psych patient. I think I'm the center of the world. [Assumes a rather histrionic stance.] But I don't hear voices. [She covers her face with her hands and counts to six on her outstretched fingers.] Nurse, you're not listening. [The nurse had glanced away to look through the doorway at another patient who had gotten up.]

Nurse: Yes, I *am* listening. I just looked out at Mr. J. so he would know where I am if he needs anything. My name is Miss N. I will go make my rounds now and be right back.

How the Patient Felt. She was very tense, anxious, full of conflicts. She was suspicious of the hospital surroundings, although at the same time she said that she had faith in the hospital staff. She was probably trying to reassure herself; she had made the decision herself to come to the hospital. She verbalized this and also indicated it in her manner and movements. She had been acutely psychotic for two days. At this encounter, she was preoccupied with the thought of pregnancy and with sex in general. The patient was also testing the nurse to see if she would ring the O.D., call the supervisor, give more sedation, or talk with her. The patient was also claiming the nurse's full attention, except for the time she left the room to make rounds. In order to alleviate the patient's idea "that something funny was going on," the nurse asked the patient to walk with her up and down the hall, into the day room, and to help wash the coffee cups. The patient could see for herself that the day was like any other day, that the other patients were asleep, that the morning routine was the same, and that there was no preparation for surgery. The nurse's role was primarily one of listening and of reassurance.

Evaluation. The patient had a frightened facial expression, pressure of speech, and tense muscles, all of which attested to her anxious, suspicious, and conflicted feelings. She verbalized her concern and watched every move the nurse made to see if she was getting ready to give preoperative medications. Because most of the other patients were asleep, the nurse was able to devote her entire attention to the patient. The nurse repeated her name in an attempt to make the contact more realistic and personalized.

The nurse encouraged ventilation, used verbal reassurance, and listened. Exploration of the unit with Miss N. relieved the patient's anxiety about the pending surgery (as a nurse herself she knew what preoperative procedures would need to be done). Directing the patient's motor activity into such a routine thing as washing coffee cups was helpful. The nurse's presence as a non-anxious person helped allay the patient's anxiety.

The nurse was, however, unable to understand the bizarre hand movements of the patient and did not question her as to their meaning because the relationship had not developed to the point where the nurse felt comfortable about asking for meanings that might be heavily laden with emotion. The nurse's glancing out of the doorway while the patient was speaking was a mistake that the nurse immediately tried to rectify; otherwise, the patient probably would not have trusted the nurse. A need that was not met was an understanding of the source of the patient's anxiety.

FORMS OF ANXIETY

Anxiety denotes intrapsychic disequilibrium; different forms of anxiety may appear in the individual as follows:

- *Separation anxiety* refers to the consequence of the loss or the threatened loss of an outside agent. It continues throughout life.
- *Castration anxiety* refes to the threatened injury or loss (actual or irrational) of body parts. It therefore extends to both men and women and continues throughout life.
- *Id anxiety* refers to an ominous feeling of dread, ascending to panic, that one will lose all control of self. It often precedes a psychotic episode.
- *Superego anxiety* refers to the state that exists where the ego expects guilt due to the fact that the person has done something that the superego forbids and lives in dread of others learning about it (Nemiah, 1974).
- *Free-floating anxiety* is a severe generalized sense of dread felt directly without any apparent source.

DEFENSES AGAINST ANXIETY

The mental mechanisms are largely unconscious mechanisms and, since the time of Sigmund Freud, they have been central to the study of human behavior.

In human beings, behavior is integrated and indivisible. No behavior stands in isolation; all behavior is part of a developmental series; and all behavior is meaningful, multi-purposeful, and multidetermined. Behavior includes manifest actions and the psychological processes or activities of the mind: learning, perception, dreams, moods, fantasies, and affects. Psychological defenses are constructs and therefore intangible. Their existence is synthesized from observations of behavior and assessment of the personality. Constructs explain observable behavior but have no clear physical existence of their own. Although Freud thought of the defenses as irrational ways of dealing with anxiety, current psychiatry views them as necessary to existence and ego management. They may be viewed as reactions to the emotional pain of anxiety. When the defenses are no longer in operation for the defense of the ego, psychoses may occur.

Tension management is conscious, but mental mechanisms are largely unconscious. However, one may *become* conscious of one's own defense mechanisms. The level of intensity of use of defense mechanisms may be viewed as a continuum in which such things as hyperrepression and hyperprojection are progressively severe developments of mere repression or the use of coping behavior. If the ego is unable to overcome the punitive superego, depression results; or if the id behavior overcomes the superego, acting-out behavior may follow, culminating in asocial acts.

It is assumed in modern psychiatry that every person has his breaking point and that unusually stressful events may not be managed by the ego as adequately as the ordinary events of everyday life. Crisis theory relates to this concept and hypothesizes that there is a point at which the person requires help to defend the ego and thereby to adapt successfully to the stressful event. Intervention at this point may prevent serious mental disorder. If help is given at the critical point, healthy adaptation and growth may occur. If it is not given, however, the result may be maladaptive behavior.

The emphasis on the psychological needs of persons in this chapter does not negate the holistic approach to the assessment of each individual, by means of which his biological, socioeconomic, and cultural needs are also given due attention. Figure 6 is a mnemonic device to help place the patient in his social environment, with four key questions that help place him in his mental environment as well.

Since Freud proposed the original list of defense mechanisms, many others have been added. In this book, consideration is given to those reactions most commonly observed in nursing practice, particularly those that nursing students need help in identifying. Unless a student is able to recognize defense mechanisms in the patient, she will be of little assistance to him in anxiety-producing situations. Outstanding is the mechanism of denial, which is discussed in many of its forms in the following pages.

DENIAL OF REALITY

Denial is an intrapsychic defense mechanism by means of which consciously untenable wishes, needs, ideas, deeds, or reality factors are disowned by an unconscious refusal to admit their existence. What is consciously untenable is unconsciously rejected by a protective mechanism of unawareness. Reality is regarded as nonexistent, or it is transformed so that it is no longer threatening. The term "denial" as used in a psychiatric sense does not include a conscious attempt to repudiate or disown, as in malingering or lying.

The attitude of denial of a disorder is probably a lifelong pattern. Psychodynamically, denial of illness is probably determined in part by an inability to accept changes in body image or in role perception. Such a reaction to illness is also called anosognosia (when first used, this term referred mostly to paralysis). The function of denial is to defend the ego. When the defense occurs with people with minor disorders such as the common cold, it does not receive much attention; when, however, it is evident in people who have major disorders, it assumes a much greater importance. Denial, one of the most common mental mechanisms evidenced when people are under stress of diagnosis and illness, is almost a universal reaction to the diagnosis of cancer. It may be revealed either verbally or symbolically. Some patients may refuse to admit that they are ill or affected in any way. Verbal denials most commonly heard

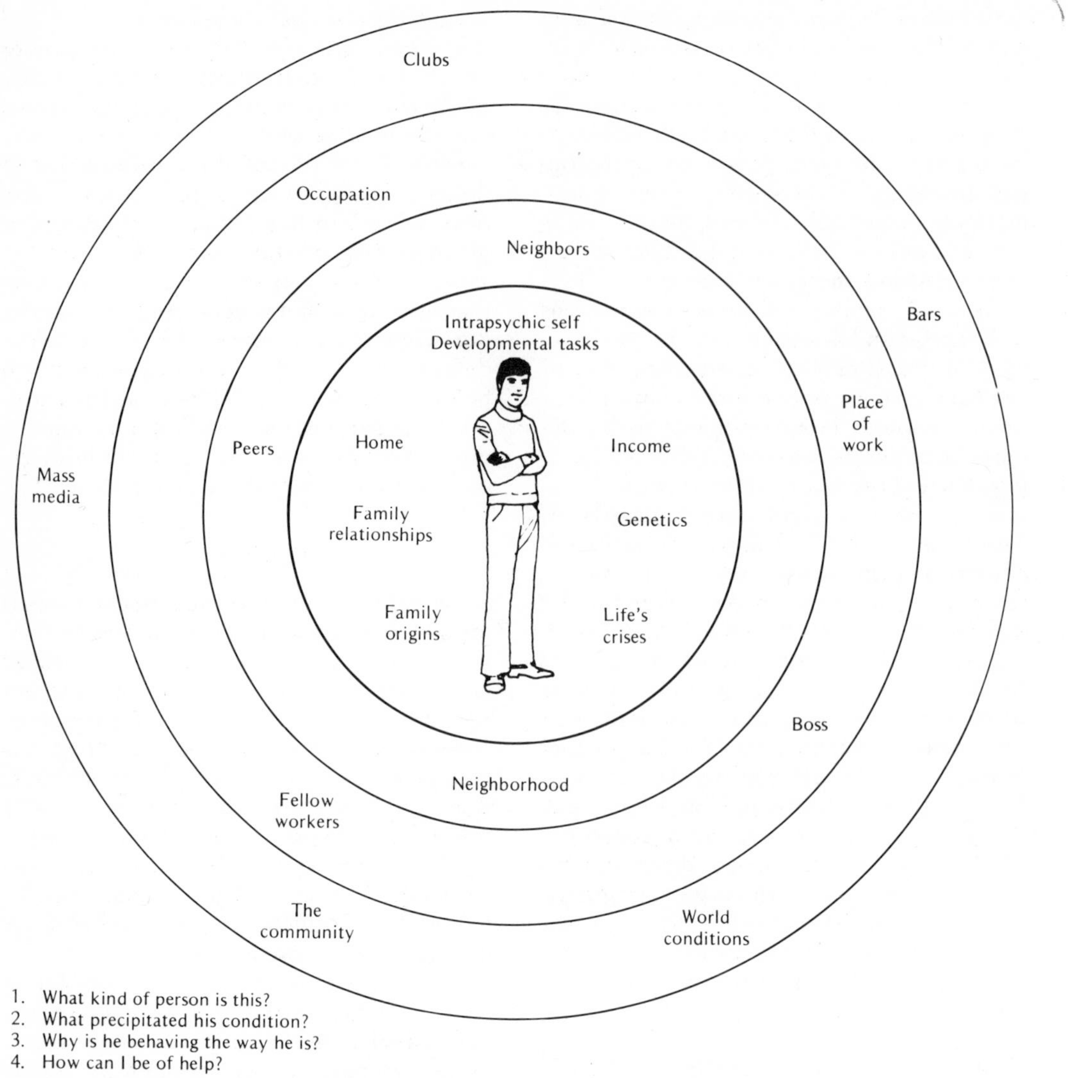
Clubs
Occupation
Neighbors
Intrapsychic self
Developmental tasks
Bars
Place of work
Peers
Home
Income
Mass media
Family relationships
Genetics
Family origins
Life's crises
Boss
Neighborhood
Fellow workers
The community
World conditions
1. What kind of person is this?
2. What precipitated his condition?
3. Why is he behaving the way he is?
4. How can I be of help?

Figure 6. The Patient in His Social Environment.

by nurses are "I am not a mental patient" and "I am just here for a rest." Other patients may refuse to admit a major disability but will complain of minor discomforts.

Following are five types of denial:

1. Nonverbal Denial. Some patients may refuse to admit that they are ill in any respect; others may deny illness by being overly compliant with therapeutic personnel but not making any references to their illness. Only close questioning will get them to verbalize that they are ill.

A patient with skin cancer, Mrs. H., was close to death but refused to accept her diagnosis although she had been transported from another state to the cancer-treatment unit. Every day when Miss B. changed the dressing over her entire back, Mrs. H. asked how the area looked and latched onto any observation by the nurse that could be interpreted as a hopeful improvement. Mrs. H. kept making plans to return to her home state. She was unable to verbalize that she had cancer to anyone.

2. Postponement. The almost universal denial that accompanies the diagnosis of cancer may continue for long periods, or it may be transitory. The affected individual's philosophy of life may greatly influence his psychological reactions. How his parents and other significant members of his family have reacted to stresses in their lives may also be an influencing factor. One of the most common forms of denial is seen when patients develop symptoms that make them suspect cancer.

A patient, Mrs. B., married, with two children and expecting a third, observed a lump in her breast for two months before mentioning it to anybody. Finally, she told her priest, who immediately sent her to her physician. A biopsy showed the lump to be a cyst.

Mrs. K. had been noticing some bleeding with her stool and finally, after months had passed, went to her physician for a checkup. He sent her to the hospital, where a GI series showed polyps in the colon. Exploratory surgery revealed carcinoma that had already extended to the liver. The surgeon informed Mrs. K. that she had cancer. In subsequent discussions, she said that the cancer had been removed and made plans for returning to work.

Another patient with newly diagnosed cancer of the GI tract said that she would wait and ask her physician in the Midwest about her condition when she returned there from the West Coast, although immediate surgery had been recommended to her.

3. Due to Harmless Cause. The third type is one in which the changes are said by the patient to be due to rather harmless causes; for example, the person who says that he was admitted to the mental hospital because of fatigue or the paralyzed person who says that he is just too lazy to move his legs.

Although a patient's arm or leg may be paralyzed, he will complain only of minor things such as headaches and constipation. (This phenomenon closely approximates *la belle indifférence*[5] of the patient with a conversion disorder.

A patient who has had a massive coronary may say that his "ticker" slowed down a

bit and that he will be back in his office the next month; or he will tell the nurse that he is glad his friends call so he can cheer them up.

4. Attributed to Someone Else. The fourth type of denial is that in which the disorder of the patient is attributed to someone else. For example, a patient in an acute psychotic episode refuses to leave her room for treatment, saying that there is nothing wrong with her, that it is her husband who is ill. Another aspect is that of displacement in time in which the patient who is obviously mentally disordered states that he was ill some years ago but made a full recovery. This type of denial may also resemble the mental mechanism of projection.

An example of projection is shown in the case of Mr. B., whose injured leg required amputation. Subsequently he placed the blame for the loss of his limb on his surgeon. By blaming another, the patient rid himself of unacceptable ideas, especially when neglect on his part resulted in the condition; his ego, therefore, was defended.

Another patient, Mrs. A., whose heart condition necessitated a pacemaker, insists that she does not need it and that "my doctor did it just to make money."

One patient, Mrs. D., had been hospitalized for fifteen years with a diagnosis of schizophrenia, paranoid type. In the hospital, she managed the kitchen and the feeding of eighty to ninety patients on the unit. Her maladaptive behavior evidenced itself in the writing of voluminous letters to the superintendent of the hospital and to the governor of the state denying that she was a mental patient or had ever been one and, furthermore, casting serious aspersions as to their characters.

5. Ignoring Disability. The fifth type of denial refers to ignoring or paying little attention to the severity of major disability. An example is the diabetic patient who refuses to adhere to his therapeutic regime, who eats what he pleases when he pleases and adjusts his insulin accordingly, or who skips doses.

Mr. W., retired and living alone, without any family left, was in the hospital for surgical removal of an ulcer. Although he also

---

[5] An inappropriate lack of concern.

had a severe heart condition, he defied the physician's instructions with regard to bed rest and climbed out over the bed rails at night to go to the bathroom, despite admonishment from his roommates. He died of a heart attack a few days later.

Ignoring the affected part of the body, such as a devastating scar or a particularly unwanted wound from an ileostomy or breast amputation, is another variant. The patient who does not look at his wound may be using denial; he may wish to have his eyes covered or will look in the opposite direction while his wound is being dressed; or he may joke about the wound so as to belittle its existence. Men who have suffered facial injuries may avoid shaving and thus the necessity to look into the mirror. One patient, Margaret A., in her late sixties was admitted to the psychiatric hospital for depression following a radical mastectomy for cancer. Massive denial now kept her from acknowledging the operation. In addition, she had frequent illusions that she carried a bad odor around with her and checked this out with her nurse. Adolescents may particularly ignore changes within themselves in order to meet long-awaited events; for example, they may pay no heed to the fever and malaise of mononucleosis in order to graduate with peers.

THERAPEUTIC TASKS

Since denial of disorder is a defense, if the situation is such that denial is the best solution for the individual patient and his family, the mechanism should be supported. Relatives may consider it providential, especially when the patient has cancer and it is uncomfortable for them to talk about it. Denial can help a patient cope with his situation in a way that otherwise would not be possible for him. Some nurses may feel that a patient should face up to reality even though, psychologically, the patient's use of denial may be saving him from a serious personality disorder or from suicide. Forcing the conflict to consciousness may be harmful. A sense of the right time to talk about what is happening to the patient is necessary in the art of nursing. Denial may be a momentary attempt to avoid reality. The need for time for the patient to work

through the shock of a serious or a fatal diagnosis should be recognized by the nurse, along with the fact that not everyone accepts illness and trouble in the same way.

The use of denial is more than a function of experience, knowledge, or intelligence. Just because your patient is a prominent "heart man" in the community does not mean that he does not use mental mechanisms when it comes to dealing with his own heart attack. Now that many patients spend less time in hospitals, it is even more imperative that nurses avoid jumping to conclusions that patients have bad attitudes simply because they are still denying aspects of their disorder upon discharge, after being hospitalized for two weeks. Denial will most likely continue until the patient has accepted the change in body image or in role. The nurse can (1) learn what part denial plays in the patient's patterns of adaptation, e.g., how he has previously reacted to stressful situations; (2) assess the underlying motivation of the patient (interventions to alter denial may not be appropriate); (3) assess the patient's particular level of anxiety and mental state at many points in time since the nurse is in continuous contact with the patient; and (4) act as a representation of reality to the patient through which he can "check out" his perceptions. Nurses can also learn more about the ways that people express denial and therefore be in a better position to help patients under stress.

If denial is manifestly harmful to the patient, as when he refuses to follow the therapeutic regime or runs away from the mental hospital, it is important to find out the exact motivation for his behavior. This usually requires the efforts of all members of the health team. If, for example, a previously described patient, Mr. W., who denied his severe heart disease and prescription for bed rest by climbing over the bed rails to go to the bathroom, dies soon thereafter (as he did), a psychological autopsy may diagnose cause of death as a subintentioned suicide.[6] Preventive techniques could perhaps have been employed with him had his motivation been known to the health team.

---

[6] The individual has played some role in hastening his own demise.

C. D., a twenty-two-old diabetic male, requires daily injections of insulin for his diabetes, which he denies having in spite of having been in a diabetic coma and close to death. C. D. is also schizophrenic and lives in a board-and-care home. Periodically he absolutely refuses his insulin and has to be hospitalized as a "danger to himself" so the insulin can be given. In spite of many team conferences, consultations, and efforts to intervene, none has been successful.

When the motivation of the patient is a wish to be admired for his strength and virtuosity, the task of the nurse and the health team is to help him adapt to other ways of winning approval—to help him develop ego strength that does not require such extremes of self-sacrifice. When fear is the motivation for denial, the least effective intervention is to frighten the patient into adherence to the therapeutic regime. Helping him review his assets so as to discover what he can do within the limits of his disability can be the first step to acceptance of his altered self-image. The nurse has an important role to play in encouraging the patient to accept help, whether it be vocational rehabilitation after a bout with schizophrenia or helping another family member to go out and work until convalescence is complete. Giving accurate information to the patient about his condition, without forcing the conflict of self-destruction, is of primary importance in the healthy recovery of the patient.

There is much psychic energy used up in the maintenance of mental mechanisms that can be used in more constructive ways once the ego is well defended and the patient can accept the changes in body image or role. Helping him identify with a friend or another patient who has successfully dealt with a similar problem can be supportive. The therapeutic potential of another person who has undergone a similar event and who has recovered should be tapped. It is vital that nurses in all areas of practice should be familiar with the various patients' organizations and the ways to put people in touch with each other who have adapted in healthy fashion to similar afflictions. Various clubs are now in existence for patients and families of patients to help each other. The Lost Chord Club for patients with laryngectomies has helped many persons through the despair of this surgery; Recovery, Inc., has a large number of clubs for mental patients in many states. The American Conference of Therapeutic Self help/Self health Social Clubs was founded in 1960 and publishes *Constructive Action for Good Health Magazine.* The international office of the United Ostomy Association, Inc., has many branches. All attest to the therapeutic potential of one person for the other.

Stress of Sensory Deprivation

Under the rubric of sensory deprivation are found other concepts; sensory restriction, sensory reduction, stimulus deprivation, sensory isolation, and perceptual isolation. Research with regard to sensory deprivation deals with experimental conditions aimed at reducing, altering, or by some means interfering with a person's normal stimulation from and interaction with his environment.

Brainwashing techniques and the isolation of individuals with mental disorder in seclusion rooms, in large remote public mental hospitals, and in nursing homes have some aspects of sensory deprivation and are therefore relevant to the field of psychiatric nursing. Seclusion is used by professionals for safety and protection of the patient when other techniques fail and at other times because of administrative failure to meet staffing standards. Helping patients to achieve internal controls of acceptable behavior is rarely aided by the use of seclusion rooms.

It is of interest to note here that in a sensory deprivation experiment (Schulman et al., 1967), 4 per cent of the subjects reported changes in body image. One person reported that several times his body felt heavy and numb; another subject had the feeling that he had two heads, the second separated from the first. Still another subject had the feeling of being out of his body, above it, where he could watch it lying on the bed. He also had the feeling that he and the room were rising and floating in space.

With the increased use of modern medical technology a new emphasis is required in nursing for application of principles derived from research on sensory deprivation. The hyperbaric unit and also the Life Island Isolator (Lunceford, 1965) for treating patients who are especially vulnerable to severe infection have implications for application of findings from sensory deprivation experiments. Common psychological problems found are: anxiety, depression, sleep disturbance, withdrawal, regression, and hallucinations (Kellerman et al., 1977).

Other types of apparatus, institutions, and processes used in the treatment of patients that necessitate changes in sensory input and output are as follows: institutionalization, oxygen tents, complete bed rest, respiratory treatment units, intensive-care units, body-splinting and immobilization of body parts, and isolation of patients (special precautions unit for communicable disease; seclusion).

THE RETICULAR ACTIVATING SYSTEM

The concept of homeostasis refers mostly to the vegetative actions in our bodies and does not credit the influences of the psyche, the brain, and the central nervous system in motivation.

Recent work in neurophysiology cites the importance of sensory input and output via the reticular activating system. The reticular formation is the lower brain stem, where the brain connects to the spinal cord. It is a "dense neurone network forming a central core which extends from the medullary of the lower brain stem to the thalamus of the diencephalon."[7] It contributes impulses upward to the cortex and downward with the automatic nervous system and the muscles. It receives a collateral branch from every channel or nerve connection between a sense organ and the cortex and interconnects extensively with systems of motor nerves. The reticular activating system can be thought of as a kind of control center for sensory input and output.

The two major sources of stimulation for the reticular activating system are considered to be sensory stimulation and cortical

[7] Schultz, D. P.: *Sensory Restriction.* New York: Academic Press, Inc., 1965, p. 15.

impulses. Stimulation from somatic, visual, auditory, olfactory, and visual sources can act somewhat interchangeably in activating the system. Excessive interaction may lead to complete blocking of the reticular activation of the cortex, resulting in disturbances in awareness and attention (Duffy, 1962). There are also marked behavioral disturbances under the opposing conditions of sensory restriction and sensory distortion. Behavioral effects can be explained in terms of the ascending reticular activating system (ARAS). Located where it can monitor the incoming and outgoing messages, it can influence alertness and attention, as well as serve a balancing function. It regulates sensory input and also provides a connection between the cortex and the reticular formation. Continued and persistent sensory variances may result in disrupted perception, distractibility, and boredom. Resulting behaviors may be stereotyped or maladaptive. Benjamin (1965) relates the reticular activating system to the concept of the stimulus barrier.

THE NEED FOR EXPERIENCE

The need for sensory variation, exploration, and expatiation of curiosity appears to have been added to the list of drives (Meerloo, 1964). Psychoanalytic and neurophysiologic research have indicated that the human organism requires a varied sensory input. Conclusions from current research show that *meaningful sensory input is necessary for psychic adjustment and that immediately unmeaningful stimuli often produce intense fear.*

Either too much sensory input or too little can lead to devastating mental states. The ego, the stimulus barrier, and the reticular formation are credited with being monitors of sensory input. The need for experience seems similar to the concept of heterostasis, moving away from the old and moving toward the new. The story is told of an animal experimenter who put a small monkey into an empty room in order to observe what he would do. The experimenter hastily closed the door on the monkey, then peered through the keyhole to see what it was doing, only to find a bright, brown eye staring right back at him.

The need for expansion or expansive creativity has been described by Buhler (1962) as reaching toward the realization of one's own potentialities. For example, at the age of eight months or so, a child chooses a toy that he can do the most with. In the older age group, the need may also be expressed as the wish to influence others as well as the desire to be remembered after death, a yearning for immortality that contributes concretely to the founding of institutions as personal memorials. The need for experience is observed in the activities of explorers, including astronauts and cosmonauts. In comparing the need for experience with that of homeostasis, it can perhaps be said that experience is a goal of the human organism, whereas homeostasis is a condition to which the organism attempts to return after disruptive events. Viktor Frankl has made one of the most relevant statements in defense of this reasoning:

Thus it can be seen that mental health is based on a certain degree of tension, the tension between what one has already achieved and what one still ought to accomplish, or the gap between what one is and what one should become. Such a tension is inherent in the human being and therefore indispensable to mental well-being. We should not, then, be hesitant about challenging man with a potential meaning for him to fulfill. It is only thus that we evoke his will to meaning from its state of latency. I consider it a dangerous misconception of mental hygiene to assume that what man needs in the first place is equilibrium or, as it is called in biology, "homeostasis," i.e., a tensionless state. What man needs is not a tensionless state but rather the striving and struggling for some goal worthy of him."[8]

SENSORISTASIS

A state in the human being in which there is optimum sensory input is called sensoristasis. It can be defined as a drive, "a state of cortical arousal which impels the organism (in a waking state) to strive to maintain an optimal level of sensory variation."[9] The reticular formation acts as a monitor in service to the sensoristatic balance. Other theorists, however, purport that the exploratory drive is nonhomeostatic in character (Buhler, 1962).

STRESS OF CONFINEMENT AND IMMOBILIZATION

Confinement refers to restraint or restriction of freedom on the activities of an individual or group by command, fear, or physical enclosure. It calls for adjustment to physical and temporal limits and adaptation to the changes perceived by self.

There is much in literature that deals with confinement, and these poems or stories are valuable to the nursing student as a means of deepening understanding of and empathy with the conditions of confinement and the feelings of patients.

The "little tent of blue which prisoners call the sky" in the "Ballad of Reading Gaol," written by Oscar Wilde,[10] who was jailed for homosexuality, is a particularly poignant and vivid description of imprisonment. The feelings of Hans Castorp in Thomas Mann's *The Magic Mountain* are also expressive of the conditions of confinement to a sanitarium for the treatment of tuberculosis. Two poems by Robert Louis Stevenson, who had tuberculosis, describe a reaction to sickness and the use of play and to confinement by command of parent.

The Land of the Counterpane

"When I was sick and lay abed
I had two pillows at my head
And all my toys beside me lay
To keep me happy all the day.

And sometimes for an hour or so
I watched my leaden soldiers go
With different uniforms and drills
Among the bed-clothes, through the hills;

And sometimes sent my ships in fleets
All up and down among the sheets
Or brought my trees and houses out
And planted cities all about.

I was the giant great and still

[8] Frankl, V. E.: *Man's Search for Meaning.* Boston: Beacon Press, Copyright 1959, 1962, by Viktor Frankl, pp. 106–107. (Also London: Hodder and Stoughton, Ltd.) By permission.

[9] Schultz, ibid, p. 30.

[10] Wilde, Oscar: "The Ballad of Reading Gaol," in Maine, G. F., ed.: *The Works of Oscar Wilde,* London: Wm. Collins Sons & Co., Ltd., 1948, p. 822.

That sits upon the pillow-hill,
And sees before him, dale and plain,
The pleasant Land of Counterpane."[11]

Bed in Summer

"In winter I get up at night
And dress by yellow candlelight
In summer, quite the other way
I have to go to bed by day.

I have to go to bed and see
The birds still hopping on the tree
Or hear the grown-up people's feet
Still going past me in the street.

And does it not seem hard to you
When all the sky is clear and blue
And I should like so much to play
To have to go to bed by day?"[12]

Factors of considerable import in affecting tolerance of confinement have been described by Ruff and Levy (1959) and Ruff and Thaler (1959) as follows:

• Activities undertaken by the subject
• Circumstances surrounding the confinement
• Characteristics of the subject: personality, motivation, education, and experience
• Extent of enclosure or restraint
• Sensory input (quantity, modality, and pattern)
• Degree of intercommunication
• Extent of "aloneness"
• Time
• Duration of confinement
• Degree of subject's control over confinement
• Subject's knowledge of expected duration of confinement
• Presence or absence of methods of measuring time

Confinement requires adjustment and adaptation of the individual. Adjustment is the establishment of a relationship between an individual and his meaningful environment. The stability of the mental state of a person depends on perception of the outside world. Adjustment criteria are external to the self-

[11] Stevenson, R. L.: *A Child's Garden of Verses.* New York: Charles Scribner's Sons, 1901, p. 5
[12] Stevenson, R. L., ibid., p. 21.

system. The patient, confined to a mental hospital, can be adjusted the psychiatric patient role, go to bed and get up at the expected hours, devote himself to meetings and activities, and carry on in the manner expected and still remain mentally disordered. A patient admitted postsurgery to an intensive-care unit who similarly goes along with the plan of the health team may never verbalize his longing for his loved ones or his abandonment of hope because of their lack of emotional support. Likewise, a patient who has been newly admitted to a nursing home, having given up hearth and home for institutional life, may go to meals as requested, be present when the physician makes rounds, have all physical needs adequately cared for, and give all appearances of adjustment to the change in ecological unit; but die because he has not really adapted himself.

Real adaptation requires intrapsychic changes that people must make to the social and cultural milieu in which they exist. Adaptation, learning to live in a particular way, involves coming to terms with one's inner self. A confined person must reorganize his territory in order to maintain control over his personal self; he also must seek alternative sources for satisfying his needs. Fantasies and dreams fulfill some needs not immediately gratifiable. The person must establish a new identity. He does this as a patient and through his desire to be known by personnel. Patients being readmitted ask for familiar staff members by name; they also ask if they themselves are remembered in order to establish identity. Sometimes gifts are given to nurses by departing patients as a way of being remembered. Patients who have formerly visited relatives and friends in a certain unit of an institution will often, when it is their turn to be admitted, request the same room.

The following vignette is an example of what effect confinement had upon one patient. It was possible to verify by personal observation the described conditions.

A patient, now past the acute phase of mental disorder and attending a fellowship club, told the group at one of its meetings about being placed in a seclusion room at his local county hospital. Since this hospital had no treatment facilities whatsoever for patients with mental problems, they were placed in some locked rooms just off the medical ward. Each room contained a bed and a toilet. The door had a window for observation of the patient and a slot for passing food and other necessities to him. He stated that since people were looking in at him as a "crazy" man, he decided to fulfill their expectations. He wrapped himself up in his sheets because he felt strange just wearing a hospital gown and started singing and dancing every time somebody came to the door. (At this meeting, other patients from the same county described similar experiences to such effect that the fellowship club decided to act as a group to try to remedy these poor conditions.)

The effect of confinement itself is profound, and in the cited instance it was probably influential in contributing to the patient's mounting anxiety.

Over a century ago a patient in an autobiography described his experiences with respect to his confinement in an asylum. He wrote that "it is in the busy haunts of men, not in the comparative solitude of the asylum, that the cure must be perfected."[13]

There does seem to be some correlation between the ability to endure pain and the ability to endure confinement. The possibility of synergistic effects of confinement plus other conditions must be considered in the care of patients. Confinement produces stress of a different type from that evident in experiments of perceptual and social isolation. In addition to psychological stress, there are also physiological effects, such as cardiac deconditioning, that result from reduction of physical exercise.

Prometheus eternally bound to the rock by Zeus suffered both social isolation and confinement. One of the most stressful situations for an organism to endure is to be tied down literally. The impact of immobility upon a child is rather severe and may lead to a pervasive and persistent *immobility fear*. It is now commonly seen in patients who had poliomyelitis in their childhood and who may suffer from reactivation of the immobility fear if they have to be reconfined. Patients with fractures or who are confined to bed for other reasons may have periods of anxiety due to earlier experiences.

[13] A Late Inmate of the Glasgow Royal Asylum for Lunatics at Gartnavel, 1847.

Think for a moment of the implications of the stress imposed upon patients by the use of physical restraints.

A patient, Miss D., now in her late seventies, was in a convalescent center. She had come from a distant state for retirement; all of her family had died, and her friends of forty years standing lived in a far distant state. Now in the convalescent center after a stroke, she refused to get out of bed. Instead, she turned from side to side in bed, constantly displacing her covers so that her body under the short hospital gown was fully exposed. In order to cover her up, the aide tucked a sheet snugly over her body, tying it tightly to the bed, and tied another sheet over the bed rails in a tentlike covering. The result was that the patient could not move from side to side and immediately began to cry, complaining that the nurses thought she had lost her mind and had tied her down. Hearing the crying, the aide came in and reprimanded the patient. The use of pajamas by the patient would have been a solution; she could have moved back and forth in bed without exposing her body. For this patient, restraint symbolized a loss of mental control and resulted in an increase of regressive behavior.

Intensive-Care Units: Sensory Overload

Sensory overload is thought to occur when the person can no longer handle bombardment from stimuli. Disruptive consequences occur in patients who suffer sensory deprivation at one extreme and sensory overload at the other.

The adaptation of patients to modern medical technology and to intensive-care units involves many changes in sensory modalities. In these units, only brief visiting may be permitted by relatives, and at times even this is done through a glass partition, without benefit of touch or smell, as in the case of heart-transplant patients. Some surgical intensive-care units are designed to exclude all visitors in the striving toward surgical asepsis. Body orifices may hold uncomfortable catheters, nasogastric tubes, and rectal tubes; patients may be receiving intravenous therapy, or they may have tracheotomy and be unable to talk. These various hookups with equipment may require staying in one position to avoid disconnecting them. Aside from visitors and care by the staff, the patient's visual field may be restricted to the ceiling. Noise, continuous light, frequent examinations, many injections, conversations of staff, and constant awareness of patients all around him and of what is happening to them may impinge upon the individual and contribute to his sensory input. Patients may also watch the cardiac monitors of other patients and vicariously suffer others' attacks. At this time, in some units little privacy is afforded, men and women patients may occupy adjacent beds, and there is inadequate provision for private care of natural body functions or for conversations with significant others about oneself.

Noble's (1979) study cites staff communications in the ICU as the largest single source of disturbance. Noble also relates "ICU psychosis" to increased mortality. From her study it was shown that the nursing staff in four intensive-care units did little to aid persons with perceptual distortions.

Visual illusions may first occur as patterns on the ceiling. Hallucinations and disorientation may follow. Derrick (1979) in a long letter to his nurses described how open heart surgery feels and the importance of staff helping him separate the unreal from the real as well as saving his life.

The Nursing Task: Prevention

SENSORY DEPRIVATION

The nurse's primary aim is prevention of psychological complications associated with sensory deprivation. The importance of establishing a specific nurse–patient relationship aimed at preventive intervention cannot be overestimated in the nursing care.

Although the patient should not be overwhelmed with *all* the details, cognitive aids of what is likely to occur during the course of his illness provides data for a mental rehearsal of what is happening to him. Unexpected events can be very anxiety producing. The patient needs time to ask questions and to ventilate fears. For example, if the patient knows his movements will be restricted and why, he will be better prepared to adjust to it when it occurs.

Where there is limited sensory input through one modality because of restriction of its usual function—such as in the use of eye patches, institutionalization, immobility resulting from the casting of broken bones, or central nervous system defects—consider how to substitute *meaningful* sensory input by means of the other senses and teach the patient and his family these modes of input. For a child, this meaningful sensory stimulation can prevent later immobility fear. Immobilization is in conflict with our life-style. We live in a technological society that is in constant rapid motion. To be immobilized is truly to be put out of action. Patients need to ventilate about earlier immobilizing events, if any, as well as the present ones. Meaningful stimuli reduce the disruptive effects of sensory deprivation upon the human psyche. Strangeness and unfamiliarity contribute to the development of confusion in patients.

Think of the blind person whose senses of hearing and touch become very acute. The modality of the input is not as important as that the input be meaningful to the patient. This factor must therefore be assessed carefully with each person. Merely flooding the room with sound or perfume is not the answer, but taking a bouquet of roses to a rose gardener is meaningful. For patients with broken bones, other limbs or areas of the body can be exercised. Reactions to sensory deprivation may be most severe at night and may occur with greatest intensity in those who are old and who have already suffered some degree of sensory impairment. Stress susceptibility is particularly high in foreign patients, whose reality testing may be verbally impaired. You may have to remind your patient of your identity, where he is, what day it is, and what has happened to him.

Getting something familiar for the patient, such as special foods to which he is accustomed at home, repeating the fact that he is in your care, showing yourself as an ally, inquiring about his thoughts, feelings, and fears—these acts of primary prevention will help him adapt more readily to his situation. Continuity of the same nurse can give the patient a sense of security. It is important to remain with your patient as long as possible. A family member, significant other, or a sitter can also give meaningful input. If you can, introduce him to others who may have recently been through what he is experiencing. To explain and describe to the patient what is happening to him, using the reportorial approach can also be helpful. There is an authenticity of reporting by the professional who has a broad experience and the scientific knowledge of what happens to patients, and this is listened to quite carefully by the patient. One might inform the patient as follows: "Patients who have their eyes covered may have different visual images. If you have them, tell me about them."

One of the problems in hospital nursing is the number of nurses and levels of nursing that come into contact with the patient without fully understanding what is happening to him. It is the responsibility of the nurse in charge to see to it that all staff are adequately informed of the needs of all patients and of the ways to meet those needs. The use of familiar objects, articles, and routines is helpful to the patient. It is therefore recommended that the patient use his own clothes (if he is in a hospital), his own radio, and the like, and that he follow his usual newspaper and morning routine insofar as this is possible. Darkness, silence, solitude, and interruption of usual habits and ways of meeting psychological needs may all be significant factors of stress. In a study of seventy-eight patients with eye surgery, averaging sixty-three years of age, the conclusion was made that "orientation, reassurance, and support that the nurse can provide can help the patient to cope with experiences that occur" (Ellis et al., 1967). Much more investigation is needed about the different reactions of people and the appropriate nursing interventions for the particular patient who is undergoing the experience of sensory deprivation. We learn from mistakes if we are able to analyze what went wrong and what should have been done to prevent the negative consequences. I am therefore including the followng case, which clearly delineates the effects of sensory deprivation and confinement. As you read it, think of all the nursing actions that you could have initiated on a preventive basis. Discuss your suggestions with your peers.

Mr. F. d'I., a patient in his sixties who speaks and understands little English, is now in his second postoperative day for eye surgery. He has both eyes covered and is in a ward with three other patients who have other kinds of surgical problems. He awakens early in the morning while the aide is taking TPR's and asks for a cheroot. Since it is hospital policy that patients cannot smoke in bed unless attended by a staff member, the aide refuses permission because she cannot spare the time to attend him. When informed of this, the patient becomes increasingly excited, tears off his eye bandages, gets out of bed, and gropes around for his clothes and cigars, announcing that he is leaving the hospital. Six people are required to put him back to bed and to hold him there. When the day-shift nurse, who came ahead of time, arrives, she gives the patient his cheroot, sends all the other staff out of the room, holds his hand, stays with him, and speaks comfortingly to him. By the time the physician comes, he is able to carry on a calmer conversation with him in Italian.

SENSORY OVERLOAD

The life-saving and life-sustaining technologies of modern medicine will continue to increase. The complexities of what patients experience in terms of these technologies are requiring adaptations never previously experienced. More important than ever before is the nurse–patient relationship in helping patients endure and adapt to the new treatments. Anticipatory guidance, respecting privacy, explanation, reassurance, the human touch, instillation of confidence, helping the patient differentiate the unreal from the real all contribute to successful recovery of the patient. "Talking to the walls" is an example of caring for an unconscious patient "when the walls listened" (Wisser, 1978). Because nurses are responsible for the milieu of the patient, their own actions in it can reduce sensory overload and influence others to do likewise, although the physical structure itself may remain the same.

Stress of Social Isolation

Social isolation is a condition resulting from few contacts with family, community, and significant others. All of the experiments and situations discussed in the section on sensory deprivation also involve social isolation to an extent. Social isolation or solitude refers to the separation in time and space from human contact. Hermits endure this kind of environment, as do subjects confined in a normal sensory environment either alone or with a small group of people. People in submarines, and at South Pole stations are familiar with the monotonous environment of small groups, as well as some degree of confinement. The early flyers who carried the mail from continent to continent, desert travelers, hostages, truck drivers, concentration-camp victims, astronauts, and night nurses encounter some aspects of this experience. Feelings of detachment from the usual rhythms of life that result from working at night and attempting to sleep during the day have implications for nurses who work the night shift. Being out of tune with the opportunity to attend social events that those working the day hours can participate in or going to such events anyway and having to leave early, for instance, demands special adaptation and adjustment by the nurse assigned to night duty.

The question arises as to whether the sexual drive is really as strong under the stressful conditions of social isolation as is commonly believed. There was uniform agreement on the disappearance of sexual feeling among the ordinary prisoners of the Nazi concentration camps—not among the privileged prisoners, however (Luchterhand, 1967). Pairing within groups without reference to sex was ubiquitous and so necessary to the survival behavior of the camp inmates that those who failed to make such alliances were the most likely not to survive.

. . . Much of the strength for survival—psychic and physical—seems to have come from "stable" pairing. With all of the raging conflicts in the camps, it was in the pairs, repeatedly disrupted by transports and death paradoxically restored in the general bereavement, that the prisoner kept alive the semblance of humanity. The pairs gave relief from the shame of acts of acquiescence and surrender. The pairs produced expertness in the survival skills known as "organizing.[14]

Although the foregoing is an example of extreme isolation complicated by many other factors, it can also serve to guide us in nursing. People who are socially isolated by reason of accident or against their wishes may have the most difficulty in coping. For example, the older person who lives alone may experience various degrees of social isolation. If he has a confidant with whom he can share his thoughts and feelings about the little things that happen every day, he may be able to cope better with the crises of aging. If his social relationships have narrowed to the point that he knows no one by name and his acquaintances are merely familiar faces in cafeterias, outpatient clinics, and church, his reduced sensory input from social relationships may result in fantasies, delusions, and hallucinations. It has become increasingly evident that the isolation of the aging in our culture contributes to the beginnings of mental disorder.

ISOLATION AND AGING

The following situation is an example of an isolated older individual who was visited by nursing students in successive classes for several years. The situation also includes nursing intervention.[15]

Mr. Houlihan, now retired for several years, left Ireland several decades ago and never returned. Although he says that he has brothers, they do not correspond. He worked for many years as an orderly and now lives in a boarding house with ten to twelve others in a neighborhood close to a hospital and the outpatient department where he gets his medical care. He is also very near his church and the bus line. Mr. Houlihan spends his days and some of his nights in church, helping to do whatever needs to be done. He has no hobbies. In one church,

[14] Luchterhand, Elmer: "Prisoner Behavior and Social System in the Nazi Concentration Camps," *International Journal of Social Psychiatry,* 13:259–60, 1967.

[15] Evans, F. M. C.: "Visiting Older People: A Learning Experience," *Nursing Outlook,* 17:3:20–23, March 1969. Copyright, The American Journal of Nursing Co.

his favorite, which is in the central part of the city, he ushers people out at night, locks up, cleans, and spends the night there to avoid the dangers of being on the bus late at night. He seems to have no significant others in life. However, he knows the people in the churches, the hospital cafeteria where he takes his meals, and the outpatient department where he gets his medical care by their faces but not by name. He feels secure in these places and seldom ventures outside them unless accompanied by the nursing student. He is a bachelor and an octogenarian.

Mr. Houlihan expressed much prejudice and at times borders on having somatic delusions and hallucinations. At one time he thought that an organ in his body had burst, created a bad odor in his nose that could be detected by those around him. When the student visited, they met in the hospital cafeteria over coffee. She aided him in reality testing by meeting him in his usual environment, commenting on the everyday occurrences as she saw them, listening to his thoughts and feelings, and stating that she did not detect any bad odors about him (when he brought up the subject). She would then go on to discuss subjects that were more reality-oriented. She did not push discussion of odors and prejudice (which he expressed quite pointedly). Instead, she focused on reality-oriented events.

The student aided Mr. Houlihan in reality-testing by her presence, calling him by name, and being a person herself with a name and interests to be remembered and with whom interaction was required. The memory requirement made of Mr. Houlihan by the student to note the time, place, and date of the visits was another aspect of reality-testing. A young person with whom he could relate over a continuing period of time gave him contact with the upcoming generation and a sense of connection with the present that he otherwise would not have experienced. With the student, he was able to sit down and check out his perceptions on different topics, which may have been one of the most important facets of reality-testing. Because he had worked as an orderly for a great part of his life, he felt free to discuss these former times with the nursing student, who, in turn, encouraged him to do so. The anticipation of the student's visit, the visit itself, and thinking about it afterward all required relating to the world outside of himself.

During the third year of visits by the nursing student, Mr. Houlihan agreed to visit a senior center, but only if the student accompanied him. Because the center is located in a maritime museum, they also visited the latter, where Mr. Houlihan grandly pointed out the type of ship that brought him to this country. The student was amazed to learn that he had never been in the museum before and, in fact, had not known of its existence.

For Mr. Houlihan, the contact with the student provides a sense of connection with the present. She aids him in reality-testing because she is one of the few persons he knows by name, and she attempts to expand his sphere of social relationships. By her presence and therapeutic use of self, she interacts in the relationship, which reduces his need for defensive reactions.

Although there could certainly have been other factors in the disappearance of the patient's symptoms, it is my view that the human influences of the nursing student were of central importance.

INSTITUTIONAL ISOLATION

Patients with communicable diseases who are socially isolated often complain of the monotony of their restricted environment, and especially about the few visitors encountered or permitted and the hasty entrances and exits of the staff. Nurses are often wrapped up so securely that all that is evident to the patient are their eyes and their hands. In remote mental institutions or infrequently visited units within institutions, the envelopment of the visitor by the patients may be evidence of the monotony of their environment. A similar phenomenon may be observed in the staff in these units, who often show a great need to verbalize.

Social isolation is one component of alienation, the others having been described as powerlessness, normlessness, meaninglessness, and self-estrangement (Seeman, 1959). While lifelong extreme isolation (i.e., the life of a hermit) is not in itself conducive to personality breakdown, because of adaptation patterns, lifelong *marginal* social adjustment very often contributes to the development of mental disorder (Lowenthal, 1968). Each of us has a social identity in addition to our personal identity, a sense of our own situation, a kind of continuity of character that is developed as a result of our various social experiences. Stresses affecting individuals can be both within and without the person. In the case of social isolation, the influence on the human organism may be directly damaging unless they are reversed.

Loss of personal liberty, imprisonment, solitary confinement, and being lost at sea or cast adrift constitute highly stressful experiences. The film *King Rat* gives a realistic picture of life in a Japanese prisoner-of-war camp during World War II and should be seen by every student of human behavior. The classic film on war, *Grand Illusion,* shows Eric von Stroheim as the manager of a war prison for officers in World War I, located in a remote castle. He becomes highly interested in a living plant, a lone geranium on the windowsill of the castle's turret.

Stop now and think of examples of isolation that you may have experienced. Put yourself in a quiet room for a few hours away from others and study the effects upon yourself.

Components common to experiences of isolation involve separation from familiar surroundings, objects, and persons, danger to life and health, severe restriction of quantity and variety of sensory experience, and limitations on the range of motor activity. There may be monotony, little opportunity to exercise, and a limited environment to explore, and one may be at the mercy of those in charge. If the person is lost at sea or in a snowstorm, he is helpless in the face of nature. In all individuals there is the need for sensory input and motor activity for psychic adjustment. In solitary confinement, the hunger for human contact is so great that prisoners welcome even interrogation by their captors.

The process of social isolation involves a difficulty in maintaining contact with reality, the emergence of vivid imagery, visual or auditory hallucinations, a tendency to misinterpret environmental stimuli, depersonalization,[16] and a decrease in rational thinking. Individuals may fight it by systematically reviewing their past experiences or making contact with animals. Patients in remote mental institutions or people who are otherwise socially isolated may feed stray cats and rats and become agitated when exterminators appear. If contact can

[16] Depersonalization refers to the feelings of unreality or strangeness concerning the environment, the self, or both.

be made with an animal, the isolation can perhaps be made more bearable. Sometimes a very isolated person can make such contact when he is unable to relate to available persons. The money spent yearly on pet food in this country attests to the importance of animals to people. I have observed long-stay patients in mental hospitals save parts of their dinners to feed the rats that gathered together at the proper time for their surreptitious handouts. Other patients gathered food and daily fed the cats that had gradually accumulated around the institution.

In every city park are socially isolated people who feed squirrels, pigeons, and other animals as a daily ritual, despite the admonished dangers of adding to the rat population. At least one person in a Nazi concentration camp kept his sanity through his interest in a rat. Other isolates become interested in insects, invent elaborate mathematical equations, recite poetry or the multiplication table, write, improvise games with pebbles or other materials, and count the features of the cell or room.

A game one person played was what she called the "mostest game." She was a university dean confined to her bed by a stroke. Although living with friends, she was far across the country from her place of work and many friends and acquaintances. She asked herself, "Of all the places I have been, what did I enjoy the most?" and went down the line with different places and events. Persons who do not have the capacity, experience, or opportunity to engage in mental play of this nature may become profoundly depressed or withdrawn, often experiencing periods of disorganized panic and dying prematurely.

The behavior of individuals under circumstances over which they have little or no control gives pertinent data for the study of human behavior and suggests possibilities for application of these concepts in nursing.

The age of the person undergoing social isolation may be a factor in his ability to withstand the isolation. If the aging process changes the nature and strength of the individual's attachment to the social system and the bonds are weakened, social isolation may ensue. For example, with a work-oriented generation of older persons such as we have today, retirement brings about a significant change in contacts with a familiar social system. In a youth-oriented society, where values are vastly different, the older person may be alienated from the larger social system and feel separated from his milieu. Decreased income upon retirement can result in a change in living arrangements that, in effect, greatly alters the contact with previous social systems. Illness decreases the person's ability to maintain his pattern of action and the life-style of his social system, as does poverty or the sudden stoppage of income. These catastrophes are most severe for an elderly person who lives alone. If the aging person's relatives cannot provide care for him, social isolation may occur rapidly, accompanied by mental changes.

With respect to those in other age groups, it should be noted that adaptation and adjustment to *confinement and social isolation* have been found to be easier than adapting and adjusting to the usual or normal environment *after confinement*. Awareness of the patient's problems when he returns home after hospitalization may help the health team to be of assistance to him. As one patient after a long hospitalization expressed it, "Convalescence is the most difficult part of getting well—it's so lonely and painful."

PREVENTIVE TASKS

Because isolation is stressful and anxiety-producing and can be potentially detrimental to the mental health of individuals, all actions for preventive care should be carried out after an assessment has been made of the needs of the particular individual who is being isolated.

An isolated patient should have visits from the nurse as often as is feasible for that particular patient. In addition to regular visits during meals and at the times for medication and treatment of hospitalized patients, who anticipate them eagerly, unscheduled visits are highly valued. Intercommunication systems are of great assistance here and should be used more effectively in hospitals in this age during which, it seems, communication is more easily accomplished between the earth and the moon than between the nursing station and the

patient. Machines can be put to excellent use to improve human relations.

Ways to keep in touch with *time* are necessary. Every good convalescent center and nursing home should have a wall calendar with the date of the month in bold black letters easily visible to old eyes. A clock is also essential, and radio and television will help. Institutional walls are often monotonous; the nurse can see to it that patients place some of their favorite objects around the walls. The nurse should also give attention to prompt delivery of mail and favorite foods to the patient.

Ways to overcome boredom may be found for the individual patient; what works for one may not work for the other. A thorough explanation should be made to the patient as to what is happening to him. For example, if a patient has contracted an infection during his stay in the hospital, he should be informed about the nursing preparations being made for a change in his care. Status hierarchies have no place in these interventions. However, if they are present, tact and skill are required in interpersonal relations. A nurse may feel guilty when the patient develops an infection when, in fact, the nurse may not have had anything at all to do with it. If a patient is to be transferred to an isolation unit, now euphemistically called special precautions unit in some hospitals, the physical layout of the isolation unit should be described to him. Informing him of the name of the chief nurse and of the special rules observed in the new unit may help him adjust to the change of environment. In short, he should be prepared in every way possible for the change.

If the patient is in a ward, some explanation of the transfer should be made to the other patients. They have a right to know, and some may even be enlisted to aid the patient being transferred by continuing communication with him afterward via the telephone.

To assist the patient's orientation to his new surroundings in an isolation unit, nurses can do the following: Give him his new floor and room numbers and inform the visitor's desk so that all visitors, messages, and telephone calls will be transferred promptly to his new location. A patient will wonder whether the new nurse will understand what medications he is to take. How will his physician find him? Will the nurses in the new unit know that he likes to have a bath at a certain time? It is a simple matter, but often forgotten in the hustle of transfer, to inform the patient that you will alert the nursing staff on the new unit of his needs and predilections and that the kitchen will send his special diet to the new room. Patients should be forewarned of the restrictions on visitors in the isolation unit.

In the isolation unit itself, the nurse informs the patient of the details of this special environment and the purpose of nursing action. Provision of an aesthetically pleasing environment is the responsibility of the nurse, for example, the arrangement of the room so that an ambulatory patient can move around freely and disposable decorations to break the monotony of the four walls. Seeing to it that the patient's room is clean is essential, particularly if the unit does not have a unit manager and/or a housekeeping department prepared for doing this work in isolation units. Solitary games and reading material should be made available. The preventive, restorative, and supportive potential of the family members should be tapped if the patient has an available family.

Preventive potentials of families for isolated members center around fulfillment of the need to belong to a group. If an isolated patient feels that he is truly still part of a family, he is more likely to be motivated to withstand the stresses of isolation. Therefore, the nurse can mobilize the family to show their concern, if they are not already doing so, with letters, cards, telephone calls, visits, and other signs and symbols of caring. Encouraging the family to talk about what is going on in the family itself can be restorative action to the isolated patient who temporarily loses his family role. The nurse can aid the family in supportive action toward the patient by keeping them informed of his condition and asking them to be helpful. Explanation can be given to them of the necessity of isolation, and they can be informed of ways to protect themselves so that they may be able to conquer their own fears and therefore be more accepting of the isolated member. If the isolation of the patient is to continue on a long-term basis, the need for catharsis may be met through talks with family members, telephone conversations with significant others, and venting feelings to the nurse and others who are available.

The opportunity to express thoughts, feelings, and perceptions about the experience of isolation itself can be helpful to the patient. Once they are shared, they become less of an emotional burden and the patient can be more objective about the question, "Why did it happen to me?" The nurse can also help the patient think through what he will do when he is released and has recovered by asking leading questions. When periods of isolation are known, the nurse can also assist the patient to note the midpoint and to celebrate that day and the day the isolation ends.

Stress of Changes in Body Image

The body image refers to the picture a person has of himself, his inner sense of identity, where he belongs, what he can do, and his assets and liabilities. It includes sensations from muscles and their innervations. Concerned with whatever originates within—voice, breath, odors, body discharges, and hair—it is a composite of feelings and perceptions each person has of his own body, its characteristics, functions, and limits.

DEVELOPMENT OF THE BODY IMAGE

The body image is intimately related to the development of ego functions with particular reference to reality testing and perception. The perceptions of sight and touch in the development of the ego are differentiated as follows:

Coming in touch with its own body elicits two sensations of the same quality and these lead to the distinction between the self and the not-self, between body and what subsequently becomes environment. In consequence this factor contributes to the processes of structural differentiation. Delimitation between the self-body and the outer world, the world where the objects are found, is thus initiated.[17]

In infants, the first perceptions are tactile. The ability to differentiate between the "me" and the "not me" is achieved through tactile experiences (Frank, 1958). The differentiation between the "me" and the "not me" by the infant is probably related to recognizing objects within his very specific environment. Objects experienced through tactile communication such as *my* rattle, *my* bottle, and *my* mother are recognized quite early. Later, the child replaces his specific world of "not me" objects with the concepts and symbols of the world in general. Auditory and visual cues and language add to the growth of concept formation. Therefore, transition is gradually made from the highly specific world of the child's "not me" to the world of symbols and adult concepts.

The postural model of the body plays a part in the building up of knowledge about the body (Schilder, 1950). Movement and dance change the postural model, as do sickness and maldevelopment. The horizontal patient has a different feeling about himself from having to stay in bed. The depressed patient feels differently about his body because of psychomotor changes and the older person because of sensory and motor changes. Kinesthetic stimuli are connected with a high level of cortical activity. The kinesthetic receptors are in the muscles, tendons, and joints. The labyrinthine receptors, which keep one informed as to position in space, are in the inner ear.

There seems to be a human need to build up some idea of the wholeness of a person, whether it be accurate or not, even if we use a medium that leaves out everything but that which can be observed during a single moment of perception. Draw part of a circle and the human mind completes it. We can see a photograph of someone just fleetingly and feel that we know something about that person. A TV performer may be a familiar visitor in our home, even though he is only a picture on a screen. We often feel disappointed when we meet a person whom we have previously known

only through an intervening medium. When we read a book and later see a play or a film based on it, we are frequently disappointed because our imaginings and fantasies are more satisfying to us than the interpretation projected by others. This also is true of our acquaintances, who can disappoint us because we have built up fantasies about them from the limited ways in which they appear to us; only through later experiences do we discover that they are more human and therefore more fallible than our original concept. We often feel that "they have let us down." Nursing students often experience these feelings with regard both to the profession of nursing and to physicians, if they have not had members of these professions in their families.

Parents do something similar with their children, as do teachers with pupils and nurses with patients. Nurses may judge their patients by an image that they themselves created of the "ideal patient" or the "good patient." There is a tendency to have a mental imge of patients and to place them into categories. The moment you are aware that this process is going on within you, get rid of the image and find the real patient, *not what you think the patient should be.* Nurses sometimes take it as a personal affront whenever they are forced to alter the first mental picture they have of a patient. This also applies to engaged couples, whose ideas of each other often change as they become better acquainted. The "halo effect" is real. All observations have some distortions. The tendency to give to the image of oneself should also be recognized; for example, parents often force on their children goods or experiences that they themselves would have liked.

In hospital nursing, we make our patients very much aware of their bodies by constantly asking what goes in and out of them. Innumerable questions must be answered by the patient with regard to his body. The examination by the physician that may have preceded entrance to the hospital has already alerted the patient to high body concern, and further examination by the interns and residents may have occurred. Determination of the temperature, pulse, and respiration, securing urine and blood for analysis, and the routine chest x-ray may

[17] Hoffer, Willie: "Development of the Body Ego," *The Psychoanalytic Study of the Child,* Vol. 5. New York: International Universities Press, 1950, p. 19.

contribute to the patient's mounting body concern. In the medical history the patient has to recall all the illnesses and operations he has ever had as well as the significant diseases of his ancestors to which he might be susceptible. Inasmuch as the event of hospitalization is itself a crisis, the patient should not be asked the same questions repeatedly by different nurses. One means of avoiding repetition is to have one nurse write up the patient's history and place it on his record for all to see.

Body image is also derived from those around us, our family, and our society. It may be transformed by clothes, jewelry, wigs, makeup, and false eyelashes. Some peoples put holes in their earlobes; others put them into their noses and lips and insert wood or metal into different parts of their bodies. Body image refers to the postural model of the body and to the emotions, attitudes, and sociocultural implications.

In some hospital environments patients are estranged from contact with family members and significant others; they are cared for totally by personnel dressed in white, the symbol of sickness, dependency, and death to many patients. Those with mental problems sometimes joke about being ready for the "men in the white coats." A movement is now current to eliminate the distressing symbolism of white uniforms in favor of wearing ordinary street clothes in nursing.[18]

STIGMA

Stigma[19] is a Greek term for the brand that was cut or burned into the body to advertise that the bearer was a slave. Later, in Christian times, stigma referred to bodily signs of physical disorder. Hawthorne, in *The Scarlet Letter*, records its use by the Puritans in this country to brand an adulteress. More recently, the Nazis used this method to identify Jews, criminals, and traitors.

Disease, mental disorder, and body imperfections may create in the individual the

---

[18] It is of interest to note that in the Soviet Union, where uniforms are otherwise quite prevalent, nurses and physicians wear street clothes over which they put on a kind of smock.

[19] A body sign designed to expose something unusual or undesirable about a person's moral status.

sense of bearing a stigma (whether immediately observable or not), with consequent feelings of shame and guilt. Whole families may be ashamed that one of their members has mental disorder or some debilitating disease. Huntington's chorea and other genetically determined diseases still stigmatize a family line.

Mental retardation is a classic example of stigma within families in this culture; however, Pearl Buck and the family of former President Kennedy, among others, have helped people in this country to perceive that it is no disgrace by talking freely about their own mentally retarded family members.

IMPAIRED BODY IMAGE

"Imperception of body impairment" refers to a frequently observed behavior in patients who do not seem to recognize the impairment. In major disability, such unawareness takes the form of denial, as discussed earlier.

It may occur with some hemiplegic patients who insist that a paralyzed arm is as good as the unparalyzed limb. Others pay no attention to their paralyzed arms, acting as if they do not belong to them. It has also been found that obese individuals increasingly overestimate their own body size during and following weight loss. This has been referred to as "phantom body size" (Glucksman and Hirsch, 1969).

The phantom experience of the person who has undergone an amputation can occur with loss of arms, legs, breasts, and other external body parts. It is chiefly represented by tactile, thermal, optic, and kinesthetic sensations although it has been reported in blind persons. There may be sensations of itching, pain in a part of the limb (heel or fingernail), burning, and throbbing of an amputated part. These sensations may show the wish to maintain the body's integrity.

Recently, a phantom experience not related to tissue disruption has been reported (Kane, 1977). Kane described a phantom urinary phenomenon in hemodialysis patients, a psychological response to loss of a physiological function.

The phantom experience is one of the

most dramatic examples of existence of a body image. Endocrine imbalances may also produce disturbances of body image. The psychiatric significance of the phantom represents an attempt at restitution of the missing part, a denial of its absence, or a somatic substitute for mourning over its loss (Gorman, 1969).

Surgical wounds may not be accepted by the patient as part of himself. Some patients may avoid looking at their wounds or washing them. Nurses can determine whether or not the patient has inspected his wound and instruct him to wash it just as he would any other part of the body, once the wound has healed.

THERAPEUTIC TASKS

In reference to patients with imperception of change in body image, nurses may make such comments as: "He does not admit that his leg is gone," or "She will not admit that she is fat." It must be recognized that such reactions are defenses. Tell the patient with phantom experience that you understand that he feels he still has his arm or leg or kidney and refer to the date of amputation or beginning of hemodialysis and the reality of the situation. When the time is right, inform him of the availability of prostheses and talk it over with him several times. With a paralytic patient, acknowledge the affected limb while bathing him, feeding him, and carrying out other nursing activities. Get him to touch the affected limb and use the senses of sight and movement to aid in reorienting his body.

A main objective to remember is to aid the patient in the defense of his ego. One of the most ego-strengthening devices for the patient is to have available all the materials necessary for the body arts.

ORGAN TRANSPLANTS AND OTHER COMPLEX TREATMENTS

Advanced medical technology that has made organ transplants and other complex treatments possible poses a new field for research on how these processes affect patients and families involved. For children undergoing change in body image, the bed may be included in the body boundaries (Smith, 1977). Sometimes the patient on hemodialysis imagines the machine as part of himself; frequently, nurses and technicians view the patient *and the machine* as one (Kemph, 1977). Heart, kidney, liver, lung, and pancreas transplants have now been carried out (Castelnuovo-Tedesco, 1971). The effects of internal transplants on the body image of the patient, the psychological factors affecting the rejection process, the live donor, the nondonor, and the families of the dead donor need definitive study and research.

Patients now make very complex decisions concerning their bodies: chemotherapy or radiation? If chemotherapy, which one? One that makes me sick one half the time or one that makes me sick all the time? Kidney dialysis or kidney transplant? If kidney transplant, who will be the donor? Simple mastectomy or radical mastectomy? Hormones or no hormones? Heart transplant or death? Same sexuality or transsexuality? Disfigurement or plastic reconstructive surgery?

Patients who receive organ transplants have usually been ill for a long time and welcome the decision for this change in body image by transplant. Some patients, soon after receiving organ transplants, often feel jubilant and the nurse shares in this joy.

Patients fear the rejection process. The uncertainty from day to day may result in anticipatory anxiety. Other effects are evoked during the rejection process that call for psychological sustenance for all those concerned. It is thought that the longer the transplant functions, the more intense is the reaction to rejection.

In a study of patients with renal transplants, it was found that eight out of eleven who died following their operations had felt a sense of abandonment by their families or had experienced a panicky state and a pessimistic feeling to a greater degree than those patients who survived (Eisendrath, 1969). It may fall to the nurse and others on the health team to motivate the patient to live. If other family members can be assisted with their feelings about what is happening to one of them, the patient will have a better chance for healthy adaptation. Deep and painful psychological wounds, on the other hand, may not be so readily manifest. The nurse's sensitivity to the interrelationships and psychodynamics of the individual and his family may elicit some of these wounds also for healing and reconstruction at the same time that the body is healing.

PERCEPTION OF CHANGE IN BODY IMAGE

Examples of recognition of change in body image are discussed under this heading, together with some of the implications for the nurse. No attempt will be made to cite all possible changes in body image, because it is an impossible task. However, some examples from the literature and nursing practice may be of help to students.

When I got up at last . . . and had learned to walk again, one day I took a hand glass and went to a long mirror to look at myself, and I went alone. I did not want anyone . . . to know how I felt when I saw myself for the first time. But there was no noise, no outcry: I did not scream with rage when I saw myself, I just felt numb. That person in the mirror could not be me. I felt inside like a healthy, ordinary, lucky person—oh, not like the one in the mirror. Yet, when I turned my face to the mirror there were my own eyes looking back, hot with shame. When I did not cry or make a sound, it became impossible that I should speak of it to anyone, and the confusion and the panic of my discovery were locked inside me then and there, to be faced alone, for a very long time to come.[20]

A similar feeling of shame must have been felt by a patient, Mrs. D., who was in a general hospital for a medical checkup and was so successful in hiding her deformed arm that the nursing staff did not notice it. An older woman, Mrs. L., now in her ninetieth year, said of her own changing body image:

I'm looking older and uglier. I used to be so pretty. Now look at me. I'm getting so old and ugly. My hair was so pretty and thick and now it is thin and gray and my arms are so thin.

[20] Hathaway, K. B.: *The Little Locksmith.* New York: Coward-McCann, 1943, p. 41. Copyright 1943, Coward-McCann Co.

Consider all the changes in body image of an octogenarian from birth to death and what they must have meant to the individual during the transitions. The developmental changes of infancy, childhood, and latency are well known and looked forward to by most children, who marvel at growing older and moving closer to the adults whom they admire. The infant moves from a horizontal to a crawling and then to a vertical position in this growth. At puberty there are hormonal changes with subsequent changes in body contour, hair growth, and sexual urges. Adulthood may be a kind of leveling-off period, and then comes the climacteric with decreased hormonal activity as well as other physiological changes. Continuing maturity and old age are usually accompanied by gradual changes in body image.

Smith et al (1977) describe four stages of re-establishment of body image in three children: (1) *global stage* in which one part is not distinguished from the other, (2) *stage of differentiation* where the child begins to distinguish between the changed body part from the rest of his body, (3) *stage of articulation* in which the child tests out the changed part, and (4) *hierarchic integration* in which the child views himself as whole once more. These authors think that re-establishing a child's body image parallels the development of body image.

CHANGE IN BODY IMAGE BECAUSE OF CANCER OF THE BREAST

If a member of your family has had a mastectomy, you may be keenly aware of the psychological impact upon her. Since cancer of the breast occurs more in middle-aged and older women who, at the same time, may be undergoing other changes, the nurse has much preventive work to do.

Breast cancer is the foremost site of cancer incidence and death in American women (American Cancer Society, 1979). Teaching regular breast self-examination is done by the American Cancer Society through the use of films and brochures. All women should be taught this simple technique and urged to perform it regularly. Girls of high-school age are now being taught this procedure. Ninety-five percent of all breast cancers are first discovered by the women themselves. Eighty-five percent of all patients with cancer of the breast will be free of any evidence of the disease after five years, if it is discovered while still localized and if it is treated properly (American Cancer Society, 1979). Patients who have radical mastectomies will have regular and frequent checkups and should be urged to make periodic examinations of the remaining breast. If a woman discovers a lump in her breast or elsewhere, nipple discharge, or other changes in her breasts, she should go at once to her physician. *The area should not be manipulated.*

After discovery of the lump, fantasies of body mutilation may be set in motion. The appointment with the physician, mammography, and the long wait for results often lead the patient to spend her waking hours thinking:

Will the cancer have already spread? If so, how long will I have to live? Should I make my will and otherwise prepare to die? What effect will my having cancer have upon my family? What will the scar look like? Or, will it heal? Will my husband ever look at me again? Will I be able to do my work?

The patient may review her life, looking at what she should and should not have done. She may have already prepared for death when the nurse arrives at her bedside with the preoperative medication. Waking up after surgery, the patient will instinctively examine the operative area to determine whether her breast is still there. Heavy dressings tightly taped omit some of the usual tactile clues to body image. Relaying "good news" to a patient is always a joy for the nurse, but informing a patient that her breast has been removed is painful. If the lump was benign, the patient's relief is immediate. If a radical mastectomy has been performed, the nurse prepares to assist the patient in adapting to the stress of diagnosis and to the change in body image. Patients suffer emotionally with a loss of feelings of femininity, a sense of mutilation, and fear of death (Jamison et al, 1978).

The affects of guilt, shame, and depression may occur. Depression is the most common (See Chap. 6 for therapeutic tasks). Patients with amputated breasts need time and privacy to sort out their thoughts and feelings. In a ward setting, patients are usually supportive of each other and respect each other's needs. If this is not the case, the nurse should enable patients to transfer to more suitable arrangements during this crisis.

Although the patient may be quite aged, widowed, or a great-grandmother with withered breasts, it is still her breast and body image. Nursing students are sometimes amazed to perceive that women in their seventies, eighties, and nineties whose breasts have served their function, so to speak, are greatly affected by a mastectomy. Of central importance in the nursing care is the recognition of the psychological reaction of the patient. One fourth of the patients studied by Jamison et al (1978) considered suicide.

Nursing Care. In addition to health teaching with regard to breast self-examination, the nurse may need to urge the patient to do something about the abnormal findings.

If surgery is to be done, the patient should be fully informed of the type of surgery that may be required and at all stages be encouraged to express thoughts and feelings. Simple mastectomies or lumpectomies are now sometimes done instead of the radical procedure. Patients should be informed of what to expect postoperatively.

One patient (Kennedy, 1977) looked at the wound during the first dressing change and was glad she did it. Husband and wife should look at the wound together *and* change the dressing (Wellisch et al, 1978).

Some equipment companies will send emissaries to the hospital with an assortment of prostheses. More often, with the rapid recovery rate common today, patients are returned to their homes before being fitted. Nurses can do a great deal while the patient is in the hospital to help her get ready for returning to her family and facing friends. Giving accurate information about the price of the prosthesis, the kinds available, and adjustments to be made in clothing are all necessary, but, for the patient, the actual purchase of the prosthesis may be difficult.

The following is an account of the work of a student visiting an older person in her home following mastectomy.

Mrs. B. had a radical mastectomy a few weeks previously. She lives with her daughter in the central city and is a member of a nearby senior center. The student learned that the patient had not been instructed about a prosthesis and did not know where to purchase one or how much it would cost. The student gave this item priority in her care; she telephoned the Social Security Office and asked if Medicare paid for it, which it did. She also did telephone shopping to determine which store had the best buy and accompanied her patient to purchase it. She learned through the surgeon that the patient had asked him to give her breast back. The student informed the surgeon and his office personnel that Medicare paid for the prosthesis (it can really be a big item in a monthly income under Social Security). Later, Mrs. B. returned to her senior center. She proudly told others, "My little nurse helped me to get a breast." The student, in addition to her instrumental role, also encouraged Mrs. B. to discuss her thoughts and feelings concerning the loss of her breast.

The prosthesis enables the patient with a mastectomy partially to restore her body image. Upon seeing family and friends for the first time, after removal of a breast, she is aware that their gazes drop immediately to the breast area. Consequently, some patients may not wish to receive visitors until they are "whole again." Psychological support by the nurse to the patient and her family is one of the most important aspects of the care of those with breast cancer.

OTHER EXAMPLES

Cancer patients who have multisurgery may suffer many changes in body image. It is not uncommon for some patients to have had hysterectomy, oophorectomy, mastectomy, and adrenalectomy (see Fig. 7). Note that the figure is neither male nor female. This diagram is used in a cancer-research center to mark the sites of cancer. Like the sexless diagram in Figure 7 the patient may feel like an "it" instead of a man or woman. Patients may state that they feel "cleaned out" and as if "there isn't much left." Depending on the site of the cancer, patients may require paracentesis, thoracentesis, bone-marrow studies, lymphangiograms, or other tests, all of which necessitate entry into the body. Chemotherapy may result in loss of body hair. Deper-

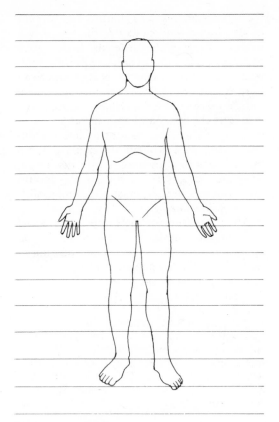

Figure 7. Diagram to Mark the Sites of Cancer.

sonalization may occur. Women patients who receive androgens may develop masculine characteristics, e.g., facial hirsutism and a deep voice. Men who receive estrogens, on the other hand, may be highly embarrassed at the development of their breast tissue. Discussion with the nurse of how the patient feels about himself can help him toward adaptation to the changes within himself.

Positive changes can also occur with changes in body image. Think of the changes in body image made possible by plastic reconstructive surgery. Patients who have burns and other disfiguring traumas suffer major and sometimes permanent changes in body image unless reconstructive surgery is possible. Scars acquired early in life may result in a child's avoiding any athletic or other activity that requires uncovering the scars—e.g., wearing a gym suit—unless he is assisted to make an earlier healthy adaptation. The nurse, at the time of the traumatic event, can aid the parents to look at the pretty features of a child with disfigurement and to then make plans for reconstructive surgery, if feasible. Operations for cleft palate are known to give an improved appearance, and someone dissatisfied with the shape of his nose can easily get a new profile. Those who wish to retain a youthful appearance may have their faces "lifted" and receive hair transplants.

Pregnancy. Pregnancy, which evokes universal concern with self-image (Bobak, 1969), is considered a crisis by Gerald Caplan (1964) and Highley (1963). In Bobak's (1969) work with parent-education classes, she found that the area of most concern to potential mothers was that of changes in body image. The following are typical complaints:

My body does not look the same and I do not like what I see in the mirror. My breasts are so big and ugly. The veins show terribly. I'm so out of shape! A butterball! My husband laughs at me.

A patient, Mrs. L., pregnant with her fourth child, was admitted to a mental hospital for the latter half of her pregnancy. This was a usual occurrence in her pregnancies. She had become so irritable and hostile to her husband and her family members that the situation was unbearable for them. In the hospital, she seldom verbalized her hostility but glared at the staff with such intensity that it made them very uncomfortable. After the birth of her child the hostility gradually disappeared and she was able to return home and care for her family. Some of the main points in the nursing care of Mrs. L. were to help her work off her hostility through daily walks and enable her to meet the basic needs of personal hygiene, nutrition, and rest. Psychodynamically, it was hypothesized that she had never resolved her Electra complex and adolescent identity crisis. With each pregnancy, the fact of being a woman was reemphasized and the old unresolved conflict brought again into the forefront.

Clinical disturbances of the mothering function are more likely to occur where the new mother does not have a well-established body image and when childbirth is seen as a loss (Main, 1968). Family-centered nursing focuses around recognition of one's own impulses and therefore being better able to assist mothers to tolerate and understand impulses within themselves. Unmarried nurses and those without children may especially be faced with recognizing their conflicts and impulses.

Sharing thoughts, feelings, perceptions, and actions within the treatment team can be of benefit to all. Since interpersonal crises may be more acute to you as a student when you are working with children and families who have new babies for the first time, look to others who are more experienced in this area for guidance and for support.

RECONSTITUTION

At times of stress, the defenses are often so involved with holding the psyche together that the libido is withdrawn and constricted from object relations, work, sex, recreation, and enjoyment in general. Anxiety, anger, and depression are some of the principal affects seen in patients under stress. Christine Beebe (1921) wrote of her psychiatric nursing experience: "It has taught us that some mental deviation from normal accompanies every form of physical ailment, that it must be studied and met as intelligently as possible, and that we do untold harm when we ignore." In the medical–surgical ward and in the family, human relationships affect how the psyche is put back together after traumatizing events. The depressed patient whose husband had been dead for one year, who denied the fact and was (incredibly) supported in the denial by her family, was obviously not assisted toward healthy reconstitution by them. Other resistances to reconstitution may occur, for example, secondary gain and lowering of self-esteem resulting from loss of a body part resulting in inability to help one's self except to take the role of an invalid. Communication, the form of object relations, and self-consciousness are all factors affecting reconstitution (Titchener, 1974). The nurse who is aware of the psychological trauma of patients as well as the physical trauma is in a position to help them regain self-confidence and trust as they experience the process of reconstitution. As individuals perceive the changes in their body images, the nurse can assist them in adapting to the new status by being available, assuming the listening and sustaining role, encouraging expression of feelings, and pointing out their assets. A pregnant patient can be given ego-strengthening support by a nurse who is able to describe what is happening in such a way that the patient can accept present body changes and look forward to their ultimate reversal. Suggestions can also be made to the husband and others to refer to the time of "getting her figure back" and to offer to buy a new dress at that time.

A fractured ego is not as easily repaired as a fractured bone; a patient needs time to adjust to changes and to incorporate the new image into his perception. Nurses can be supportive and do a lot of anticipatory guidance by helping the patient look ahead to the probable course of his condition until its ultimate resolution or termination.

Psychosomatic Reactions

Stress produces different reactions in the person according to the structure of personality, constitution, and experience. The nature of the stress is also a factor.

The disorders to be discussed under this heading represent the visceral expression of affect. Physiological and psychological effects of stress are interrelated, and the intermediary system between them is the autonomic nervous system (Weybrew, 1967). Where coping behavior and defense mechanisms no longer work for individuals, psychosomatic reactions may emerge. Psychosomatic reactions refer to those conditions caused by the physiological expression of chronic and exaggerated emotion, much of which is unconscious. It includes those conditions in which physiological and eventually pathological dysfunction is brought about by or exacerbated by a repressed emotional state in the individual. A functional etiology is proposed that involves a single organ system, usually under autonomic control. Psychosomatic reactions involve suppressed or repressed emotions

gaining expression through body organs and organ systems. An example of a young woman who was unable to express grief at her mother's death demonstrates the relationship. Every time her boyfriend sent her roses, she had an asthmatic attack. In a psychotherapeutic session, she recalled the roses on her mother's coffin. In this case, the asthmatic attacks were symbolic expressions of grief.

Theories of specificity with regard to the etiology of psychosomatic reactions are now questioned. Selye advocates the nonspecific theory (1956). We do not yet know whether the emotional constellations of patients with these problems have specific etiology. Because they are so prevalent in our society and nursing practice, some aspects of these conditions are discussed here. Students are advised to consult textbooks of medical–surgical nursing that emphasize the physiological needs of patients with these problems.

PATIENTS WITH PEPTIC ULCERS

Everybody has experienced the effect of emotions on the gastrointestinal tract. Nausea before an anticipated event or diarrhea is quite common. The transposition of feelings into words related to the organ affected are many—e.g., "You make me sick to my stomach," or "He makes me want to vomit"—and the imitation of the sound of vomiting is quite expressive in our culture. The familiar "butterflies" in the stomach before an examination or similar performance are a universal experience. The study of an infant with a gastric fistula showed that, with the appearance of food, his stomach became hyperemic and motile and secreted juices. It did the same thing when his favorite physician arrived. The hypothesis is made that environmental events can thus be either cognized or interpreted; they can be felt and responded to as if they were "gut" processes, which thereby involve the limbic system[21] or the visceral brain.

[21] The limbic system borders the part of the brain that has to do with olfaction. It consists of two rings of medially located cortex along the amygdala, hippocampus, and septal nuclei. The limbic system has several circuits; it is connected with the hypothalamus and is concerned with sex and emotions (Guyton, 1969).

One of the most frequent of the psychosomatic reactions is peptic ulcer. Studies of patients with gastric fistulas tend to support the impression that worry about business reverses and family quarrels affect the function of the stomach. At one time peptic ulcer was prevalent in women; now it is more frequent in men. The change in sex ratio is unexplained. Psychologically, the patient has developed a superego that forbids expression and gratification of his inner feelings and attitude of dependency. He overcompensates by giving the impression of being self-sufficient, competent, and industrious. Underneath the facade of self-confidence, however, he is a person with strong dependency needs.

HELPING THE PATIENT WITH A PEPTIC ULCER

Usually the dependency needs of the patient with a peptic ulcer are met in a very direct way. Rest and relief of stress and anxiety are recommended by the physician. Achieving these is accomplished in various ways within different individuals. A hunting or fishing trip, a vacation, or hospitalization may be prescribed. Psychosomatic reactions arouse dependency needs; whether the dependency needs are present because of illness or are the basis of it is not always clear. For the patient who is very dependent, and in hospital, the first goal to accomplish with the patient is to meet his dependency needs. If he requires a bed bath, give it to him. Meet the dependency needs so that he can then move gradually to independence again.

One of my patients, a prominent executive in high-tension work, promised his physician that he would come into the hospital if he could have a telephone in his room. The compromise was made, and instead of dealing all day with his usual business, he made one thousand dollars on the horses that week. Thus, this patient temporarily escaped his usual high-tension work but at the same time was not totally inactive, or dependent.

Patients with peptic ulcers frequently have tests done on the GI tract that require fasting. Considering the patient's comfort, the thoughtful nurse arranges for him to have these tests the first thing in the morning.

With regard to "no smoking," the nurse is often caught between the order of the physician and the wishes of the patient. Policing the patient is not the nurse's role. Cigarettes removed from the room of a patient who is not ready to quit will soon be replaced. An emotional contretemps between nurse and patient over the "no smoking" rule only aggravates the ulcerous condition. The nurse can reiterate the effects of smoking and perhaps help the patient give it up. Very little impact will be made on the patient if the nurse reeks of tobacco smoke.

The diet and medications ordered for the patient should be available and on time. In hospitals, bureaucracies and hierarchies may have to be confronted to provide needed supplies, for example:

Mrs. G. has been hospitalized for a bleeding peptic ulcer. Her physician ordered in-between meal feedings and informed Mrs. G. of the times for them. At the designated time, when the feeding did not come she enquired of the nurse, who said it was a policy of the hospital to *not* give in-between-meal feedings and telephoned the dietitian, who confirmed the policy. The patient had to telephone her physician to settle the issue of getting her own diet in a $200/day hospital room, and, in the meantime, bought her in-between-meal feeding in the hospital coffee shop!

The nurse is responsible also for the milieu of the patient and must be alert to noxious stimuli from the environment. If the patient is in a ward with other patients, constant analysis of interaction among the patients will aid in early identification of conflicts and tension, which perhaps can be handled.

Secondary gain[22] is sometimes a factor in delaying recovery. Fear of the unknown is of concern to all people. The nurse can educate the patient about his disorder and help eradicate fear. After the ulcer is healed, it may be difficult for some patients to give up their dependency gratifications.

Assessment and anticipation of needs,

[22] Secondary gain refers to the rewards derived from illness. Attention, disability benefits, and other rewards such as release from responsibility are not easily relinquished.

provision of supplies, supplying a therapeutic environment, and meeting dependency–independency needs add up to effective nursing care of the patient with a peptic ulcer.

PATIENTS WITH ULCERATIVE COLITIS

One of the interesting facts of history is that a medical student in the 1930s observed in his patients with ulcerative colitis a well-marked relationship between an emotional disturbance and the onset of symptoms (Murray, 1930). One of his patients had bloody diarrhea on the very day that she was secretly married. Patients with ulcerative colitis have the capacity to develop it in early life and the majority have a symbiotic relationship with the mother or mother substitute (Engel, 1975).

The changes in actions of the bowels may be sudden and associated with a well-defined stressful event or they may come on gradually. The person begins to feel unable to handle things, helpless, and gives up. The seriousness of the condition of the patient with a bleeding bowel must never be overlooked. In the course of treatment, the protection and support of a hospital may be necessary. Every patient with ulcerative colitis should have psychiatric consultation before any consideration of surgery. The psychiatrist may insist on no medication for the patient, the internist may prescribe many medications, and the surgeon may recommend an ileostomy.

Helping the Patient with Ulcerative Colitis

With every patient, the principal aim of nursing care is to give support. The establishment of a specific one-to-one relationship is a beginning. Patients with ulcerative colitis are extremely sensitive to the nuances of communication; therefore, assessment of needs, anticipation of needs, and making the patient comfortable are essential. Sensitivity to the changes of mood and interactions with others enables the nurse to help the patient discuss his thoughts and feelings. Unless trust is established, and a feeling of

hope emerges, the patient will probably get worse.

Dietary intake is important; special diets are usually provided from which the patient can make choices. The patient may be ambulatory, or complications may require bed rest; in the latter case, dependency needs take precedence. It is not uncommon for the patient with ulcerative colitis to have a psychotic breakdown, and all members of the health team should be alert ot this possibility. Each person is different, and there are no easy rules to follow. It is important to avoid getting into a power struggle with the patient over what he will eat and what he can eat, just for the sake of observing limits. Mistakes made in the diet kitchen can be corrected matter-of-factly and a real attempt made to get the food the patient can eat and to make it look attractive. Since food is the "original tranquilizer," it and the attitudes of the helping persons toward providing it are of central importance is conveying to the patient that you care.

S. J., an eighteen-year-old male, developed bloody stools after three months of constipation. Careful analysis of the chronology established that the change in bowel action occurred when his parents insisted that he go to college, which he did not wish to do. The surgeon recommended an ileostomy but S. J. refused. With the help of psychotherapy, family therapy, medical and nursing supportive therapies, S. J. recovered after a period of several months.

PATIENTS WITH ESSENTIAL HYPERTENSION

The effect of emotions on the heart and the blood vessels is symbolized in our culture by such expressions as "He'll give me a heart attack yet" or "She makes my heart ache." We also admonish angry people to "watch out for your blood pressure." The attention given to the heart emphasizes the importance of this organ. Any hint of trouble in the cardiovascular system itself may increase anxiety.

If a person is angry, one of the normal results is an increase in blood pressure. This occurs in everyone. However, some individuals who are inhibited in expression of feelings such as anger are thought to react

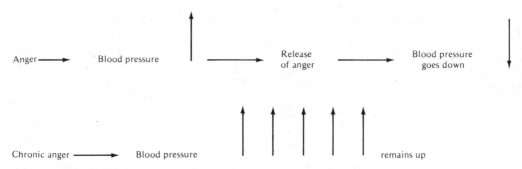

Figure 8. The Relationship Between Anger and Blood Pressure.

instead via the neuro-visceral route. Increased epinephrine flow constricts the blood vessels and increases the heart rate. The constricted blood vessels result in a patient's being "white with anger" and having heightened blood pressure. Essential hypertension is thought by some clinicians to occur after prolonged conflict in which emotions have not been expressed (see Fig. 8). Flare-ups of hypertension occur when the stress and conflicts break through the defenses.

THE ROLE OF THE NURSE

Assessment of the unique needs of each individual precedes nursing action. Because anger, anxiety, and hostility are the emotions most often identified as repressed in the patient with essential hypertension, assessment of these affects is important. Levels of anxiety, *i.e.,* mild, moderate, or severe, need to be assessed. Denial is one of the frequent defense mechanisms and should be recognized by the nurse. The reader is referred to earlier parts of this chapter for a more detailed discussion of this mental mechanism.

In the immediate surroundings of the patient in the hospital, a careful monitoring of the environment of the patient is necessary to assure rest and relaxation. With the numbers and kinds of personnel involved in hospital care, jurisdictional disputes often occur in a patient's room. The milieu has traditionally been the responsibility of the nurse. If the maid and the janitor have an argument in front of the patient, for example, you are not providing a therapeutic milieu.

The nurse can discuss ways of handling anger with the patient. Use of various methods to bring about self-assertion can be helpful. Physical exercise releases anger and can be encouraged by the nurse within the limits advised by the physician. Changing jobs may temporarily help relieve the stress of difficult situations. When professionals advise patients with hypertension to take it easy, they are not being very helpful. A patient with repressed and suppressed anger needs assistance in finding diversions. Peaceful walks and nature studies on a regular basis may be all that is needed. Family members may participate in provision of this diversion; enlist their aid. Genetic and mother–child relationships have also been suggested as etiological agents.

Although there is no unique personality pattern in the patient with hypertension, certain relationships are hypothesized and acted upon in treatment. Patients with essential hypertension have been described as aggressive but inhibited in the expression of it, dominating, rigid, perfectionistic, and very sensitive to rejection. In one study the hypertensive subjects did appear to be similar in their view of life, in their evaluation of events, problems, and challenges, and in the manner in which they deal with them (Wolf et al., 1955).

Following is a description of a patient with hypertension.

The patient, now in his sixties, was the oldest child in a large family. The father died when he was twelve, and he assumed the role of father and "husband" to the mother in the sense that he listened to her problems and those of the family members. During adolescence, he was not permitted the normal activities and expressions of rebellion and detachment from the family, because of heavy responsibilities—social, emotional, and work. One affect denied expression was anger. If things within the family had to be done—taking care of the pets, a stray dog, or a kitten; being sure that all the kids got their share at the table; being nice to siblings when he would prefer to give them a big wallop— he had the responsibility. This child with the highly developed sense of responsibility, not permitted to express anger, developed hypertension.

Treatment of the patient usually centers around long-term outpatient care in which a rapport between the patient and the clinician is of utmost importance. The use of various drugs, changes in environment, and supportive psychotherapy aid in the reduction of hypertension.

Because patients with essential hypertension frequently have rigid daily schedules, planning the daily hospital schedule together with the patient is essential.

Patients may need to be helped to think about and avoid stressful situations in their life. Changing jobs may temporarily help relieve the stress of difficult situations. When the patient is ready for health teaching, the importance of frequent blood-pressure checkups needs to be supported. If the patient has a prescribed physical fitness plan the nurse can be of assistance to the patient in teaching dietary requirements, and adequate physical exercise, for example.

PATIENTS WITH BRONCHIAL ASTHMA

Respiration is the only essential bodily activity under both voluntary and involuntary control (Wittkower and White, 1959). It is the first independent action of the newborn. Breath-holding attacks, characteristic of childhood, customarily disappear spontaneously between the ages of four and six. Attacks usually occur after a frustrating event that results in rage and crying. Crying stops with expiratory apnea, and recovery is spontaneous.

In bronchial asthma a reversible obstruction of the small airways occurs. The patient appears unable to breathe and wears a very panicked-frightened facial expression. An asthmatic attack can be dangerous and life-threatening; it demands immediate atten-

tion and treatment. Patients are therefore likely to be seen in outpatient departments, emergency units, and intensive respiratory-care centers of general hospitals. Some bronchial asthmas are due to high-allergic situations. Many patients, however, do not have strong reactions to allergy tests. There may be an undercurrent, deeply repressed, of a need for mother or a fear of estrangement from mother or from the mother substitute. Asthmatic attacks are tied up with the way in which the infant's cries brought mother; they can be viewed as symbolic cries for mother (French and Alexander, 1941). Other factors such as surgery, respiratory infections, marriage, pregnancy, separation anxiety, or a traumatic experience with water may activate the patient's unconscious conflicts, with the respiratory tract becoming the organ for somatic expression. A recent report (*San Francisco Chronicle,* 1979) described the death of a person with asthma while smelling a bouquet of roses. Her mother had died during similar circumstances.

A constellation of factors probably accounts for the etiology of asthma (Wittkower and White, 1959). Both children and adults tend to get asthmatic attacks during times of turbulence and anxiety. Midlife onset may run an acute, fatal course.

A change of environment, especially for children, has been shown to result in improvement with asthmatics, particularly away from the family. If the patient is treated with psychotherapy, medical allergic treatment goes along with it (Knapp, 1975).

The Role of the Nurse

Because psychosocial factors in etiology of asthma are so intertwined with biological factors, assessment of the interaction between the patient and his family is of major importance. Nurses can gain pertinent data from family visits where determination of ways that they handle frustration and anger can be made and suggestions for improvement outlined. A carefully made allergy history must be made available to all. In some institutions nurses take this history and post it on the cover of the patient's chart and on the rand. Particular attention must be given to this allergy history by all members of the treatment team. I have seen a case where the physician did not believe the patient was allergic to a certain medication, gave it to her, and she went immediately into a full-blown asthmatic attack. .

The nurse's presence helps allay anxiety. Staying with the patient during an acute asthmatic attack is important to provide security, one of the antidotes for a stressful situation. Special nonallergenic mattresses and pillows are usually available. Listening to the patient's description (and the family's and/or significant others) of the onset of the attack may be helpful to the treatment team in determining etiological factors, which, in turn, determine the long-term therapeutic modality.

TREATMENT

"In giving medications, we get evolution of the unexpected—the results—new poisons. We try to avoid medications. Instead, we take from Nature what we can."[23]

As a contrast with our treatment methods of patients with psychosomatic reactions, which make use of many medications, a different approach is used in the USSR. For example, a well-developed system of sanitaria along the Black Sea Cost as well as other areas of the USSR provide treatments for patients with psychosomatic reactions and other conditions as well.

A sanitarium often specializes in the treatment of one reaction, for example, respiratory disorders; others are diversified. One of the best known, the Ordzhonikidze Sanitarium at Sochi, was built in 1934. Ordzhonikidze was the Commissar of Heavy Industry. Built in the style of a nineteenth-century palace with tall, columned verandas, wide winding walkways, fountains, and plants, it has a sweeping view of the Black Sea. Inside, red-carpeted stairways and spacious lobbies add to the majestic splendor. Rooms, sparsely furnished, but with high ceilings, floor-to-ceiling windows, parquet floors, and colorful throw rugs provide a sense of grandeur for patients who probably live in very crowded areas at home due to the shortage of housing. At Ordzhonikidze

Sanitarium, balneological therapy (mineral, sun, air, sea, and mud baths), electrical treatments of various kinds (termed physiotherapy), suggestion, rest, diet, relaxation, prescribed exercises, and recreation are offered. For 810 patients, 27 physicians and 84 nurses provide the treatment.[24]

Patients with Neurotic Disorders

SOME DETERMINANTS

According to Freud, all neuroses originate in childhood from conflicts between the child and his parents. For example, the libido theory explains obsessive behavior in terms of regression to and fixation at an anal–sadistic level of organization without solving the oedipal conflict. If a girl has not solved her ambivalent feelings with regard to her mother (referred to as the Electra complex), she may, in later years perhaps as a nurse being supervised by a head nurse, reenact the earlier conflict.

Horney's (1936 and 1937) viewpoint on the pathogenesis of neurosis includes the conflicting demands of culture upon the mental life of the individual. In this theory, competition is a center of neurotic conflict in our culture. The process of competition includes a constant measuring up with others, trying to be the best of all, and the presence of hostility.

It is now thought that nuclear families produce more intense attachments with parents than do extended families and that this degree of intensity may be the basis for more intrapsychic conflict in the individual. Intrapsychic conflict and the ability to adapt and cope are all influenced by people around us and our culture, which in turn are internalized. We must be sensitive to this influence as we try to help individuals with mental disorder.

THE NEUROTIC PROCESS

The neurotic process is often described as representing the connection between normality and the psychoses. The neuroses

[23] Deputy Head Physician, Ordzhonikidze Sanitarium, Sochi, USSR, 21 August 1978.

[24] Site visit, 21 August 1978.

emerge from internal conflict and stressful situations that the patient is unable to master. Of the resulting disturbing psychological components, anxiety is generally regarded as the source. Repression no longer aids the individual to deal with uncomfortable situations; repetitious, symbolic functions appear based on affects of earlier stages of life; and the result is an inability to change (Kubie, 1974). The defense mechanisms commonly found in patients with neurotic disorders are regression, displacement, reaction formation, isolation, denial, rationalization, intellectualization, and undoing. Symptoms appear in the form of unrelieved anxiety, conversion, dissociation, phobias, obsessions, and compulsions. These symptoms express the internal conflicts symbolically and mask them.

SOME DIFFERENCES BETWEEN THE NEUROTIC DISORDERS AND THE PSYCHOSES

Some differences between the psychoses and neurotic disorders are thought to be a matter of degree and integration. In general, patients with psychoses have more severe symptoms than those with neurotic disorders. Reality testing is impaired in the psychotic person whereas there is no interference with reality testing in the neurotic person. In the psychoses, the ego is fragmented but is intact in neurotic disorders. In the psychotic person, the disorganization of the personality is severe and extensive. In the person with a neurotic disorder, behavior may be greatly affected but is usually socially acceptable; the personality is not disorganized. The neurotic individual can usually adapt to society whereas the psychotic person may have to be hospitalized. The principal symptoms of the neurotic disorders are: anxiety, conversion, phobias, obsessions, compulsions, and depression.

Patients with neurotic disorders usually receive treatment on an outpatient basis. Psychoanalysis and psychoanalytically oriented psychotherapy are the treatments of choice. Hypnosis and narcosynthesis have been used in the past and hypnotherapy is still employed. Therapy following learning theory is now advised for some patients.

Medications are also used in treatment. Patients with neurotic disorders are now likely to be of more concern to nurses in community work and in private practice.

In DSM III, the neuroses are no longer in a class to themselves; they are subsumed under other headings (see Appendix C).

SOMATOFORM DISORDERS: CONVERSION DISORDERS

The conversion disorder[25] differs from psychosomatic reactions in that the anxiety is alleviated by the symptom, the symptom is expressed symbolically, and there are usually no structural changes within the body that threaten life. In a sophisticated society, conversion reactions are generally rare in psychiatric practice, although it must be recognized that these individuals often go to faith healers and others and therefore do not appear for professional assistance. However, conversion reactions still do appear in individuals. The first patient I saw with hysterical paralysis could not move her right leg. The chief of psychiatry inserted a spinal needle into the muscle, and the patient sat as if she had not been touched at all. This dramatic demonstration convinced skeptical students of the impact and importance of the unconscious life of the individual.

Another patient was admitted to the psychiatric unit from the general hospital with paralysis of his legs. He was thirty-four years old and had had eleven operations in the past five years. The patient exhibited *la belle indifférence* (complacency in the presence of his disability). Now, he was confined to his wheelchair, and the *secondary gain* involved was thought to be related to (1) the money (compensation) received from his disability (which took place after a back injury) and (2) the fact that the patient could focus all of his previous symptoms upon the disability and therefore not worry about them.

A conversion disorder is differentiated from malingering, which is a conscious simulation of disability. For example, the patient who makes up her own eye medicine and applies it to keep the pupils dilated and

[25] In the conversion type, the special senses are affected, causing symptoms of blindness, deafness, anosmia, anesthesias, and paralyses.

achieve a status of blindness does not have the same problem as the individual whose wife is killed in an accident and who becomes blind on the spot.

Conversion disorders are more likely to occur during catastrophes. In a highly technological society such as ours, their occurrence does not assume the importance they had in other centuries. During the time of Florence Nightingale, for instance, they were fashionable and socially acceptable.

Groups sometimes exhibit mass conversion disorder, *i.e.,* among some political, religious, and erotic group activities. In a stressful group situation, rumors are fabricated, exaggerated, and circulated. Conversion disorder and organic changes may occur together. Sometimes physical changes are primary and conversion is superimposed. At other times, the conversion disorder precedes the organic changes. Conversion disorder has to be differentiated from organic nerve disease. It is very difficult for some nurses to accept the fact, for example, that the pathogenesis of convulsive seizures can be a conversion disorder. The nurse's observations are very important in assisting the team to achieve better understanding of the underlying psychodynamics and to formulate a treatment plan.

Since one of the most anxiety-producing situations for a person is severance of communication, the nurse can help the patient by maintaining a nonjudgmental attitude toward him and keeping communication channels open. The nurse can visit in the home and, by example, influence family members to do likewise. Reassurance that function will be restored can be helpful.

In the dissociative disorders, alterations in the patient's state of consciousness appear. Attempts to deal with anxiety can result in a walling off of some parts of consciousness from others. Amnesia is one result; fugue states, and multiple personality are others. *The Three Faces of Eve* (Thigpen and Cleckley, 1957) exemplifies the problems of a patient with a multiple personality. The *primary gain* provided by these states is the defense against anxiety supplied by the symptoms.

The amnesia patient may be discovered miles away from home and loved ones without any idea as to how he got there. The amnesia may be circumscribed (for a certain period of time), anterograde (from the traumatic situation forward), or retrograde (for all events prior to the trauma).

ANXIETY DISORDERS: PATIENTS WITH OBSESSIVE-COMPULSIVE DISORDERS

Unwelcome and unwanted thoughts, urges, and actions characterize the person with an obsessive-compulsive disorder. They are repetitive, and the patient views them as nonsensical; however, he is unable to stop them. These individuals separate an idea from its associated affect, which is repressed and expressed later as an obsession. The ritual of the compulsion negates an unacceptable urge.

The libido theory of Freud explains obsessive-compulsive behavior in terms of fixation at and of regression to an anal–sadistic level of organization without solving the oedipal conflict. Rado's (1974) theory of obsessive-compulsive disorder cites the conflicts of the child in relation to his defiant anger and fear toward parents who are trying to socialize him, as central to its genesis. From the standpoint of learning theory, obsessive-compulsive behavior derives from a conditioned stimulus to anxiety. The person learns that a certain action reduces anxiety and thereby continues the behavior. Because the action reduces the pain of anxiety, it becomes fixed into a learned pattern and behavior.

Obsessive-compulsive patients have periods of self-doubt and vacillate back and forth before making decisions. They may rush back into the house to see if the gas is turned off, or if the garage door is locked. An unwanted tune may enter the mind and remain there. Patients may wash their hands and bodies excessively as if they have been contaminated with some virulent microorganism. Lady Macbeth's compulsive hand washing was an attempt to symbolically cleanse herself of murder, thus exhibiting the defense mechanism of *undoing.* Other patients count the number of people in a room, touch all objects while walking down a hall, or step on all the cracks in the sidewalk. They may also have a terrible fear of impending disaster associated with harm to self or others. Severe obsessive-compulsive behavior is difficult to treat. Psychoanalysis or psychoanalytically oriented psychotherapy is preferred. A patient with this disorder may appear for psychiatric treatment only after losing a job, alienating family members, and spending all the family money. I once had a patient who had a compulsion to sit on the toilet all day and another who could never wear the same set of clothes twice without their being cleaned between wearings. Another patient collected all her stools in a drawer in her room and became severely anxious every time they were removed.

Mr. W., a thirty-five-year-old butcher with a wife and three children, gradually, over a period of a few years felt that everything was contaminated except his bedroom. Because the business was owned by the extended family, his disorder affected all the other family members in that he finally could no longer work or support his family. He and his family had spent thousands on various "cures" before coming to the psychiatric unit. He also went into a panic when he saw a dog. Mr. W. checked out of the hospital against advice before completing treatment.

These are examples of severe disability; patients with less severe obsessive-compulsive disorders are usually treated on an outpatient basis.

Nursing Care

The nurse should assess levels of anxiety that the patient feels and intervene before the patient becomes panicky or has to go through the rituals. In institutional settings, the nurse can note the compulsions and take required action to preserve life. For example, if the patient spends most of the day washing his hands, his nutritional state will suffer, and his skin will become excoriated. If his compulsion is interfered with, his anxiety level heightens; thus, it is up to the nurse to find a way to help the obsessive-compulsive patient meet his basic needs. A warm, permissive nurse who does not feel threatened by the patient's rituals will usually be able to help him meet his basic needs. It is best to make individual schedules together with the obsessive-compulsive pa-

tient, so that plenty of time is given for the patient's rituals. The patient is expected to adhere to the schedule. Limits have to be set within the realm of social reality. If the patient makes all the other patients wait for leaving on a planned outing, he will probably be ostracized from the group. If the patient is in a general medical–surgical unit, nurses should avoid a collision of "nursing rituals" with the rituals of the patient.

In the one-to-one nurse–patient relationship, informal contacts, in addition to those formally contracted, should be made to allay anxiety and increase the patient's security. As for any patient, anticipation of needs conveys to the patient that he is an individual instead of "just a carcass" as one patient put it. Encourage cathartic expression of rage and fear and teach the patient ways to relax. Listen carefully to verbalizations and focus on current problems. Because the patient's waking hours may be totally occupied with obsessions and compulsions, diversion is important. The nurse should determine the interests of the patient, plan diversion in the patient's schedule, and participate with him.

It is important to avoid adopting a perceptual set about the patient and acting as if every day is the same. The nurse who has broad interests—*e.g.,* in music, literature, theater, art, sports, and current events—will help the patient find enjoyment.

A lot of repair work may be called for to help the patient restore his position within his family. The nurse's attitude toward the patient influences the family members, and discussing his limitations with them can help them to better understand the behavior.

ANXIETY DISORDERS: PATIENTS WITH PHOBIAS

In the case of phobias, there is an intense, persistent, irrational fear of objects or situations such as dogs or high places. At the same time, the person who is phobic is capable of reality testing and conscious of the fact that these objects or situations are not harmful to him. The original source of his fear is repressed, and anxiety is symbolically displaced to the object or situation from the original object or situation of which the individual is unconscious. For example, a man with an unresolved oedipal conflict gets a job where the boss is similar to his father. This situation triggers a reenactment of the childhood conflict, and by the unconscious use of the mental mechanism of displacement, the man develops a phobia of dogs. Manifestations of phobias range from a mild faintness to panic. The more common phobias include fear of animals (zoophobia), fear of open spaces (agoraphobia), fear of closed spaces (claustrophobia), fear of dirt and germs (mysophobia), and fear of heights (acrophobia). Other phobias encountered less frequently are aerophobia (fear of air), nyctophobia (fear of night), phonophobia (fear of sounds), carcinomatophobia, ylophobia (fear of forests), thanatophobia, hydrophobia, zelophobia (fear of jealousy), xenophobia (fear of strangers), and syphilophobia. There are many others. Childhood is fraught with phobias of many kinds.

To understand the meaning of phobias, one has to reconstruct earlier events in the life of individuals and to study the structure of the symbolic content. The phobia itself is the manifest content of the neurotic disorder; the underlying content is veiled by the phobia. Phobias also represent some regression in that the individual has some restriction of activity not caused by objective reality. *Identification* with the feared object can also occur, for example, with an animal. Counterphobic behavior may appear in the phobic individual in which he voluntarily seeks out dangerous situations. For example, a man who has a phobia of snakes consistently goes hunting where there are copperheads and cottonmouths and spends hours reviewing the process of action if bitten by these snakes. Many persons with phobias simply avoid the object or situation where they might encounter the experience. This adaptation is sufficient for individuals who do not have a phobic reaction to the *mental image of the object or situation.*

Ms. P., a twenty-one-year-old university student, has had a snake phobia since childhood. Needless to say, she does not go swimming in lakes and rivers, does not hike, camp out, or garden. She enters treatment where hierarchies of phobic threat are presented: first, merely talking about

snakes, next, pictures of snakes, and so on. At the last hierarchy—exhibition of a real snake—she dropped out of treatment.

Several different therapies are now used in the treatment of patients with phobias of which some are discussed in the following. The *psychoanalytic approach,* based on the analysis of inner conflicts, may, with these individuals, include some educational and supportive measures as well as systematic psychoanalytic treatment and active intervention. *Behavioral therapy,* based on the view that phobias are nothing more than maladaptive habits, is now used in the treatment of phobias. Systematic desensitization, developed by Wolpe and Lazarus (1966), is the technique used, together with relaxation procedures. Hierarchies of phobic threat are established by the patient and the therapist to which the patient is subsequently desensitized. *Implosive therapy* includes some psychoanalytic concepts such as the difference between the manifest and repressed objects of anxiety. This therapy floods the phobic patient to the phobic object or situation or to the fear that the object or situation represents (Stampfl and Levis, 1967). Short-term therapies may relieve the symptom but insight-oriented therapy is needed where there is a deep disturbance.

NURSING CARE

Collection of data relevant to the total life situation and personality of the patient is of great importance in treatment. The phobic patient needs to feel protected and have dependency needs met. Close collaboration of all members of the psychiatric team can aid in understanding the psychodynamics and to establish treatment goals.

In the one-to-one nurse-patient relationship, the nurse encourages the phobic patient to ventilate, stays with the patient if he has a phobic encounter to allay anxiety, and makes every effort to be reassuring.

CATASTROPHIC STRESS

Catastrophic stress refers to situations and events where entire groups or communities are affected. In a catastrophe, the individuals have been subjected to overpowering experiences such as a natural disaster as in a flood, epidemic, tornado, earthquake, or a social disaster as in a concentration camp or war. The whole group of individuals is subjected to similar astounding disruptions. A disaster is usually thought of as being acute, *i.e.,* occurring very suddenly, unexpected, and doing a lot of damage.

An acute disaster is usually an intensely emotional experience in which the individual experiences: (1) psychological shock, (2) disbelief, (3) realization, and (4) adaptation or maladaptation. Mental imagery of the events are sharp and clear.

For the acute disaster itself, there may be a *threat phase* in which planning can be done. Hurricanes and tornadoes are predicted, change courses rapidly, and come and go. For earthquakes, the threat phase is prolonged. The *warning phase* may be a matter of seconds as in a plane crash or hours as in some floods. Other disasters come without warning. The *impact phase* can be for a few seconds as in a plane crash and earthquake or for days as in being taken hostage or trapped in a mine explosion. During this period the convergence phenomenon occurs where crowds gather, watch, and wait. In the *inventory phase* people observe and figure out what happened. In the last phase, the *remedy phase,* rescue begins. Some people recover from their psychological numbness, depersonalization, their perceptions of reality are sharp and clear, and they begin to help. People sometimes work unceasingly until all possible people are rescued, then rehabilitation occurs. Many people adapt quickly, take stock of what happened, clean up after a flood, sort out their things, start to rebuild their homes in the same place, and recover.

The first thing for the nurse to do in a disaster is to control her own anxiety. Removal of the person in catastrophic stress from the anxiety-provoking situation to a protective environment is desirable. Assessment of level of anxiety provides the data for nursing action. Because anxiety is communicated interpersonally, separate the anxious individual from others, if possible. To alleviate the acute emotional reaction, show interest, concern, get a short review of the precipitating factors by asking what happened and listen. Often, the severely anxious person pinpoints the last critical event as being the one that upset him. Even a few minutes of talking about what happened may relieve the anxiety. Speak directly and clearly in short, uninvolved sentences: "Come with me," "What happened?" "Sit down," "Drink this," "Let's walk." It is a relief to the person that someone else takes over and makes decisions. For comforting the person, touch helps: Put an arm around him, hold his hand, stroke his head. Touch and togetherness help; stimulation of the person to the immediate sheltered environment connects him with it instead of the hazardous event he has just experienced.

Tolerance for stress varies with the individual; therefore, many people are able to assist others undergoing catastrophic stress. Put them to work doing something; others may need a place to lie down, a hot drink, and a blanket. The provision of a protective environment and a supporting attitude help. The military method is: removal from front lines, food, bath, sleep, catharsis, and company. Most people feel relieved when they receive friendly, noncoercive attention in a protective environment.

Post-traumatic Stress Disorder. Post-traumatic stress disorders are associated with traumatic events that are outside of the range of the usual human experience, for example, concentration-camp victims and victims of war. They can be acute, chronic, or delayed (American Psychiatric Association, 1980).

Characteristics of this condition are: "psychic numbing," or diminished responsiveness to the external world, re-experiencing the traumatic event in a variety of ways such as nightmares or actual behavioral reliving of the traumatic events (especially among veterans of war). The person may complain that ability to feel emotions has decreased and that he feels detached from others. Some persons become excessively alert, insomniac, and have overactive startle responses. When the person comes into contact with a stimulus that reminds him of the original trauma, he may suddenly feel or act as if the event were occurring. Anxiety, depression, irritability, difficulty in concentration, impulsive behavior, and drug dependence are characteristics associated with post-traumatic stress disorder. The person may feel guilty that he is alive when others have died and may have memory loss for some events.

A disaster can also be chronic in that a series of events can lead to, for example, poverty, where large groups of individuals remain stuck at poverty level and for various reasons are unable to change it (Erikson, 1976).

When individuals are faced with the usual stresses of life, the stimulus barrier protects the ego but when the stress is overwhelming, the mental processes become disturbed. However, not every person manifests the same degree of disruption, time of onset, or duration of disruption, and this establishes that "every person has a breaking point."

The people of Buffalo Creek, West Virginia, as a result of a devastating flood on 26 February 1972, experienced *collective trauma,* a loss of communality (Erikson, 1976). The whole network of human relationships that made up their daily lives was disrupted. Survivors had increased concerns with illnesses and compensation, lost interest in keeping their households, and no longer felt they were in control of their own lives. Reestablishment of communality is very difficult, where a whole community has been destroyed.

For veterans of war, rap groups have been set up in various places for sharing of experiences among people who are willing to listen. A new counseling program was established in late 1979 away from established VA Centers (which many veterans of the Vietnam War tend to avoid). Encouraging the veteran to talk about his experiences helps. Listening and being nonjudgmental are important.

Eating Disorder: Anorexia Nervosa

Anorexia nervosa is now being seen more often; not only in the United States but in other countries as well. The reasons for its increase are unknown. It is now recognized as having the characteristics of a fear of fatness and a *relentless pursuit of thinness,* often following mild obesity. Bulimia followed by induced vomiting are common.

Bruch (1973, 1974, 1978) reports work with patients who have psychogenic malnutrition and warns against assigning the same problem to patients simply because they have a similar emaciated appearance. Bruch describes the person with the *primary syndrome* and the *atypical* group. In the primary syndrome of anorexia nervosa, the characteristic features are as follows: preoccupation with food, hyperactivity, striving for perfection, delusional denial of being thin, and pursuit of thinness in the struggle for an independent identity.

Three outstanding disturbed psychological functions are present in the patient with anorexia nervosa: (1) There is a delusion about the body image in which the true anorexic displays an absence of concern. (2) Accurate perception or cognitive interpretation of body stimuli is disturbed, i.e., the patient is unable to recognize hunger and the whole eating pattern is disorganized. Patients are hyperactive, deny fatigue, and have (3) a sense of ineffectiveness in everything they do, indicating a deficit in initiative and autonomy. Unable to control other things, they begin to control their bodies. The patient may be preoccupied with food, collect cookbooks, spend a lot of time grocery shopping and teaching others about nutrition. The patient may refuse treatment, adopt various subterfuges about eating, and hide her cadaverous appearance in stylish loose clothing. Her energy seems boundless but she complains of exhaustion; good grades in school are usually the result of long hours of study. Despite the skeleton-like appearance, the patient misperceives her size although saying she knows she is thin.

Bruch (1978) describes anorexics as being stuck in the stage of childhood thinking called concrete operations by Piaget (see Chap. 1) and having the moral judgment of childhood. Bruch views the anorectic as not having separated–individuated from parents. Thomä (1967, 1977) described anorectics as having very diverse psychopathological pictures. Freud equated anorexia nervosa with melancholia and related it to undeveloped sexuality. He also advised that psychoanalysis should not be attempted in a case of hysterical anorexia (Freud, 1957, p. 264).

In the atypical group, the concern is with the eating function itself and weight loss is incidental. Atypical patients do not follow a pattern. The distinguishing signs of anorexia from other conditions of cachexia and weight loss are (1) it occurs mostly in teenage females although it also occurs in males; (2) the reduction in dietary intake is psychically determined; (3) vomiting occurs and is sometimes self-induced; and (4) amenorrhea, constipation, and hyperactivity are present (Thomä, 1967). The condition can lead to death.

A slow pulse (56 to 60) and respiration (12), and a subnormal temperature (one half to one degree below normal) occur. Although the patient remains active and energetic, there is a significant weight loss. This is so marked that the skin is drawn tightly over the bones, the body is covered with lanugo, and the sufferer presents a cadaverous appearance.

Patients with anorexia nervosa are usually first treated medically and referred to psychiatry only after medical treatment has failed. If they are taking laxatives, enemas, or diuretics, they may be in electrolyte imbalance in addition to their state of starvation and require emergency treatment.

The aim of treatment is to restore normal nutrition and to resolve the psychological conflicts. The goal of psychotherapy is to help the patient uncover her own resources and abilities. If the patient is to recover she must perceive her body image correctly. In addition to individual psychotherapy, work with families is necessary. A variety of medications have been used in treatment as well as the biological therapies of psychiatry and psychotherapy. Thomä reports that there is no doubt that those patients under his care who receive psychotherapy have the best prospect for recovery (1967, p. 62). Bruch (1978, p. 108) cites behavior-modification therapy as *adding* to the inner turmoil and helplessness of these patients.

NURSING CARE

The person with anorexia nervosa has a better chance for recovery the earlier it is discovered and treatment is started. Nurses have a responsibility for recognizing it in patients *and in their own families* and helping people get early treatment. The school nurse, through educational programs, can assist teachers, parents, and others in the recognition of this disorder. One of the principal nursing problems centers around dietary intake. Forced feeding does not solve the problem although it may have to be done as a life-saving measure. Hyperalimentation may be instituted. Self-induced vomiting can reduce temporary effects of tube feedings. High protein-high caloric liquids are tolerated by some patients instead of solid foods. The nurse must take a firm attitude that eating is required. Sitting with the patient at mealtime may help, or spoon feeding if the patient will not feed herself; if it is possible, get her food that she will eat. Several small feedings throughout the day may be best to start with instead of three large meals. Care must be taken that contacts with the patient are frequent, that the patient is sought out at various times other than at meals, and that the nurse conveys warmth, empathy, and a sense of caring for the patient. The nurse must be ready to expect deceptive and manipulative behavior. The patient should be weighed daily at the same time and before eating. Care must be taken that the patient has not concealed something heavy on her body to keep her weight up, for example.

The loneliness of the anorectic patient is acute; she may use all sorts of subterfuges to keep from participating in occupational and recreational activities but must not be forgotten. In the one-to-one nurse–patient relationship, it is important to establish rapport and trust. The nurse should help the anorectic patient become aware of her own thoughts, feelings, and actions through listening and providing new experiences. Expectations should be set that the patient express her own needs; the nurse should question the patient about them and not go ahead and plan for needs without the patient's participation. Listening to the patient and verbalizing to her what strengths you see may help her discover her strengths, feel more effective, and begin to review herself as autonomous. The patient needs to be made aware of how her behavior affects others; the nurse should verbalize her own reactions to the patient in a nonthreatening manner and assess the patient's reaction. Focusing on the patient's current symptoms and discussing them openly as they occur can aid the patient in learning new ways to interact with others.

Vivian Meehan, R.N., is founder and president of a national organization called Anorexia Nervosa and Associated Disorders. This organization offers many services (all free) including information and referral, counseling, self-help groups, a listing of therapists, hospitals, and clinics treating anorectics, and educational programs. The organization also sponsors a program for early detection and the value of early treatment and encourages research on the disorder. The address is: Anorexia and Associated Disorders, Suite 2020, 550 Frontage Road, Northfield, Ill., 60093.

For this pioneering work, Vivian Meehan received the first American Nurses' Association Creative Nursing Award (1979).

Summary

This chapter on patients under stress focuses on psychic trauma, conflict, tension, and anxiety with emphasis on identifying the defenses against and forms of anxiety. The therapeutic tasks of the nurse are outlined. Stresses of sensory deprivation and overload upon the individual are presented, effects described, and the concepts of confinement, immobilization, and social isolation emphasized.

Some background discussion of the stimulus barrier and of the development of the body image is included in this chapter. Stigma resulting from multiple causes is presented. Impaired body image is discussed with some concentration on the phantom experience. Changes of body image due to cancer of the breast, obesity, and pregnancy are discussed with reference to therapeutic and preventive nursing action.

Some psychosomatic reactions of patients are included in this section, which concludes with discussion of the main neurotic disorders and anorexia nervosa.

References

AMERICAN CANCER SOCIETY: *Cancer Facts and Figures*. New York: 1979.

AMERICAN PSYCHIATRIC ASSOCIATION: *Diagnostic and Statistical Manual: Mental Disorders*. Washington, D.C.: American Psychiatric Association, 1952.

————: *Diagnostic and Statistical Manual of Mental Disorders,* II. Washington, D.C.: American Psychiatric Association, 1968.

————: *A Psychiatric Glossary.* Washington, D.C.: American Psychiatric Association, 1980.

————: *Diagnostic and Statistical Manual of Mental Disorders,* III. Washington, D.C.: American Psychiatric Association, 1980.

AYD, FRANK J.: *Recognizing the Depressed Patient.* New York: Grune & Stratton, Inc., 1961.

BEEBE, CHRISTINE: "Psychiatry for the Student Nurse," *American Journal of Nursing,* **XXI**:7:450–54, April 1921.

BENJAMIN, JOHN D.: "Developmental Biology and Psychoanalysis," in Greenfield, Norman S., and Lewis, William C.: *Psychoanalysis and Current Biological Thought.* Madison: University of Wisconsin, 1965, pp. 57–80.

BOBAK, IRENE: "Self-image: A Universal Concern of Women Becoming Mothers," *Bulletin of the San Francisco County Nurses' Association,* 20:2, 1969.

BRUCH, HILDE: *Eating Disorders: Obesity, Anorexia Nervosa, and the Person Within.* New York: Basic Books, Inc., 1973.

————: "Eating Disturbances in Adolescence," in Arieti, Silvano, ed.: *American Handbook of Psychiatry,* Vol. II New York: Basic Books, Inc., 1974, pp. 275–93.

————: *The Golden Cage: The Enigma of Anorexia Nervosa.* New York: Vintage Books, 1978.

BUHLER, CHARLOTTE: *Values in Psychotherapy.* New York: The Free Press of Glencoe, 1962.

CANNON, WALTER: *The Widsom of the Body.* New York: W. W. Norton Co., 1932.

CAPLAN, GERALD: *Principles of Preventive Psychiatry.* New York: Basic Books, Inc., 1964.

CASTELNUOVO-TEDESCO, PIETRO, ed.: *Psychiatric Aspects of Organ Transplantation.* New York: Grune and Stratton, 1971.

DERRICK, H. FRED: "How Open Heart Surgery Feels," *American Journal of Nursing,* 79:2:276–285, February 1979.

DUFFY, E.: *Activation and Behavior.* New York: John Wiley & Sons, 1962.

DURKHEIM, EMILE: *Suicide.* New York: Free Press, 1951.

EISENDRATH, ROBERT M.: "The Role of Grief and Fear in the Death of Kidney Transplant Patients," *American Journal of Psychiatry,* 123:3:381–87, 1969.

ELLIS, ROSEMARY, JACKSON, C. WESLEY, RICH,

ROSEMARY, HUGHEY, GEORGE ANN, and SCHLOTFELDT, ROZELLA M.: "Suggestions for the Care of Eye Surgery Patients Who Experience Reduced Sensory Input," *ANA Regional Clinical Conferences.* New York: Appleton-Century-Crofts, 1967, pp. 131–38.

ENGEL, GEORGE L.: *Psychological Development in Health and Disease.* Philadelphia: W. B. Saunders Co., 1962.

———: "Psychological Aspects of Gastrointestinal Disorders," in Arieti, Silvano, ed.: *American Handbook of Psychiatry.* Vol. 4. New York: Basic Books, Inc., 1975, pp. 653–692.

ERIKSON, KAI T.: *Everything in Its Path: Destruction of Community in the Buffalo Creek Flood.* New York: Simon and Schuster, 1976.

EVANS, F. M. C.: "Visiting Older People: A Learning Experience," *Nursing Outlook,* 17:3:20–23, March 1969.

FRANK, LAWRENCE K.: "Tactile Communication," *ETC,* 16:31–79, 1958.

FRANKL, VIKTOR E.: *Man's Search for Meaning.* Boston: Beacon Press, 1959, pp. 106–107.

FRENCH, T. N., and ALEXANDER, F.: *Psychogenic Factors in Bronchial Asthma.* Psychosomatic Medicine. Monograph 4. Washington, D.C.: National Research Council, 1941.

FREUD, SIGMUND: "Beyond the Pleasure Principle (1920)," in *Standard Edition of the Complete Psychological Works of Freud,* Vol. XVIII. London: The Hogarth Press, 1955, pp. 7–65.

———: *Standard Edition of the Complete Psychological Works of Freud,* Vol. VII. London: The Hogarth Press, 1957.

GEDIMAN, HELEN K.: "The Concept of Stimulus Barrier: Its Review and Reformulation as an Adaptive Ego Function," *International Journal of Psychoanalysis,* 52:243–57, 1971.

GLUCKSMAN, MYRON L., and HIRSCH, JULES: "The Response of Obese Patients to Weight Reduction," *Psychosomatic Medicine,* 31:1:1–7, January–February 1969.

GORMAN, WARREN: *Body Image and the Image of the Brain.* St. Louis: Warren H. Green, Inc., 1969.

Grand Illusion, Film, by Jean Renoir, 1938.

GRINKER, R. R., SR., and SPIEGEL, J. P.: *Men Under Stress.* Philadelphia: Blakiston, 1945.

GROSSNIKLAUS, DAURICE MCCULLAUGH: "Nursing Interventions in Anorexia Nervosa," *Perspectives in Psychiatric Care,* 18:1:11–16, Jan/Feb. 1980.

GUYTON, ARTHUR C.: *Function of the Human Body.* Philadelphia: W. B. Saunders Co., 1969, pp. 349–54.

HATHAWAY, K. B.: *The Little Locksmith.* New York: Coward-McCann, 1943, p. 41.

HAWTHORNE, NATHANIEL: *The Scarlet Letter.* Boston: Houghton Mifflin, 1883.

HIGHLEY, BETTY: "Antepartal Nursing Intervention," *Nursing Forum,* II:63–80, 1963.

HOFFER, WILLIE: "Development of the Body Ego," *Psychoanalytic Study of the Child,* Vol. 5, New York: International Universities Press, 1950, p. 19.

HORNEY, KAREN: "Culture and Neurosis," in Millon, Theodore, ed.: *Theories of Psychopathology and Personality.* Philadelphia: W. B. Saunders Co., 1973. pp. 157–62. *American Sociological Review,* 1:221–30, 1936.

———: *The Neurotic Personality of Our Time.* New York: W. W. Norton and Company, 1937.

JAMISON, KAY R., WELLISCH, DAVID K., and PASNAN, ROBERT O.: "Psychosocial Aspects of Mastectomy: I. The Woman's Perspective," *American Journal of Psychiatry,* 135:4:432–436, April 1978.

KANE, FRANCIS J., and SIMES, LEE: "Phantom Urinary Phenomena in Hemodialysis Patients," *Psychosomatics,* 18:5:13–22, December 1977.

KELLERMAN, JONATHAN, RIGLER, DAVID, and SIEGAL, STUART E.: "Psychological Effects of Isolation in Protected Environments," *American Journal of Psychiatry,* 134:5:563–565, May 1977.

KEMPH, JOHN P.: "Psychotherapy with Donors and Recipients," in Castelnuova-Tedesco, Pietro: *Psychiatric Aspects of Organ Transplantation.* New York: Grune and Stratton, pp. 145–158, 1971.

KENNERLY, SADIE L.: "Breast Cancer: Confronting One's Changed Image," *American Journal of Nursing,* 77:9:1430–1432, September 1977.

King Rat, Film, Columbia, 1965.

KNAPP, PETER H.: "Psychosomatic Aspects of Bronchial Asthma," in Arieti, Silvano: *American Handbook of Psychiatry.* Vol. IV. New York: Basic Books, Inc., 1975, pp. 693–708.

KUBIE, LAWRENCE S.: "The Nature of the Neurotic Process," in Arieti, Silvano, ed.: *American Handbook of Psychiatry,* Vol. III. New York: Basic Books, Inc., 1974, pp. 3–16.

A Late Inmate of the Glasgow Royal Asylum for Lunatics at Gartnavel, 1947. (No other publication data available.)

LOWENTHAL, MARJORIE F.: "Social Isolation and Mental Illness in Old Age," in Neugarten, Bernice L., *Middle Age and Aging.* Chicago: University of Chicago Press, 1968.

LUCHTERHAND, ELMER: "Prisoner Behavior and Social System in the Nazi Concentration Camps," *International Journal of Social Psychiatry,* 13:4:245–64, 1967.

MAIN, T. F.: "A Fragment on Mothering," in Barnes, Elizabeth, ed.: *Psychosocial Nursing.* London: Tavistock Publications, 1968.

MANN, THOMAS: *The Magic Mountain.* New York: Knopf, 1946.

MEERLOO, JOOST A. M.: *Illness and Cure.* New York: Grune & Stratton, Inc., 1964.

MENNINGER, KARL: *The Vital Balance.* New York: The Viking Press, 1963.

MURRAY, CECIL D.: "Psychogenic Factors in the Etiology of Ulcerative Colitis and Bloody Diarrhea," *American Journal of the Medical Sciences,* 239:248, 1930.

NEMIAH, JOHN C.: "Anxiety: Signal, Symptom, and Syndrome," in Arieti, Silvano, ed.: *American Handbook of Psychiatry,* Vol. III. New York: Basic Books, Inc., 1974, pp. 91–109.

NOBLE, MARY ANN: "Communication in the ICU: Therapeutic or Disturbing?" *Nursing Outlook,* 27:3:195–198, March 1979.

RADO, SANDOR: "Obsessive Behavior," in Arieti, Silvano, ed.: *American Handbook of Psychiatry,* Vol. III. New York: Basic Books, Inc., 1974, pp. 195–208.

RANGELL, LEO, in Furst, Sidney S.: *Psychic Trauma.* New York: Basic Books, Inc., 1967, pp. 50–80.

RUFF, G. E., and LEVY, E. Z.: "Psychiatric Research in Space Medicine," *American Journal of Psychiatry,* 115:793–97. 1959.

_____ and THALER, V. H.: "Studies of Isolation and Confinement," *Aerospace Medicine,* 30:599, 1959.

San Francisco Chronicle, 31 August 1979.

SARTRE, JEAN PAUL: *No Exit and Three Other Plays.* New York: Vintage Books, 1956.

SCHILDER, PAUL: *The Image and Appearance of the Human Body.* New York: International Universities Press, 1950.

SCHULMAN, CAROL A., RICHLIN, MILTON, and WEINSTEIN, SIDNEY: "Hallucinations and Disturbances of Affect, Cognition, and Physical State as a Function of Sensory Deprivation," *Perceptual and Motor Skills,* 25:1001–24, 1967.

SCHULZ, DUANE P.: *Sensory Restriction.* New York: Academic Press, Inc., 1965.

SEEMAN, MELVIN: "On the Meaning of Alienation," *American Sociological Review,* 24:783–91, 1959.

SELYE, HANS: *The Stress of Life.* New York: McGraw-Hill Book Co., Inc., 1956.

_____: "The Evolution of the Stress Concept," *American Scientist,* 61:692–99, 1973.

SMITH, ELAINE C., LIVISKIE, SHARON L., NELSON, KATHERINE A., and McNEMAR, ANN: "Reestablishing a Child's Body Image," *American Journal of Nursing,* 77:445–447, March 1977.

STAMPFL, T. G., and LEVIS, D. J.: "Essentials of Implosive Therapy: A Learning Theory Based Psychodynamic Behavioral Therapy," *Journal of Abnormal and Social Psychology,* 72:496–503, 1967.

STEVENSON, ROBERT LOUIS: *A Child's Garden of Verses.* New York: Charles Scribner's Sons, 1901, p. 5 and p. 21.

_____: *Dr. Jekyll and Mr. Hyde.* New York: Charles Scribner's Sons, 1897.

SUSSKIND, DORTHY, and FRANKS, CYRIL M.: Notes taken from lecture and demonstration of behavioral therapy. Kujbischeff Sanitorium, Yalta, U.S.S.R., July 30, 1968.

THIGPEN, H., and CLECKLEY, H. M.: *The Three Faces of Eve.* New York: McGraw-Hill, 1957.

THOMÀ, HELMUT: *Anorexia Nervosa.* New York: International Universities Press, 1967.

_____: "On the Psychotherapy of Patients with Anorexia Nervosa, *Bulletin of the Menninger Clinic,* 41:5:437–452, September 1977.

TILLICH, PAUL: *The Courage to Be.* New Haven, Conn.: Yale University Press, 1952.

TITCHENER, JAMES L. et al.: "Acute or Chronic Stress as Determinants of Behavior, Character, and Neurosis," in Arieti, Silvano, ed.: *American Handbook of Psychiatry,* Vol. III. New York: Basic Books, Inc., 1974, pp. 39–60.

TUKE, DANIEL HACK (M.D.): *Insanity in Ancient and Modern Life, with Chapters on Its Prevention.* London: Macmillan & Co., 1878.

WELLISCH, DAVID K., JAMISON, KAY R., and PASNAN, ROBERT O.: "Psychosocial Aspects of Mastectomy: II. The Man's Perspective," *American Journal of Psychiatry,* 135:5:543–546, May 1978.

WEYBREW, BENJAMIN B.: "Patterns of Psychophysiological Response to Military Stress," in *Conference on Psychological Stress.* New York: Appleton-Century-Crofts, 1967, pp. 324–62.

WILDE, OSCAR: "The Ballad of Reading Goal," in Maine, G. F., ed.: *The Works of Oscar Wilde.* London: Collins, 1948, p. 822.

WISSER, SUSAN HISCOE: "When the Walls Listened," *American Journal of Nursing,* 78:6:1016–1017, June 1978.

WITTKOWER, ERIC D., and WHITE, KERR L.: "Psychophysiologic Aspects of Respiratory Disorders," in Arieti, Silvano, ed.: *American Handbook of Psychiatry,* Vol. 1. New York: Basic Books, Inc., 1959, pp. 690–707.

WOLPE, JOSEPH, and LAZARUS, ARNOLD A.: *Behavioral Therapy Techniques.* Oxford: Pergamon Press, 1966, pp. 54–101.

Suggested Readings

ALVAREZ, WÂLTER C.: *The Neuroses.* Philadelphia: W. B. Saunders Co., 1951.

BARCAI, AVNER: "Family Therapy in the Treatment of Anorexia Nervosa," *American Journal of Psychiatry,* 128:3:286–90, September 1971.

BELL, JANICE M.: "Stressful Life Events and Coping Methods in Mental-Illness and Wellness Behaviors." *Nursing Research* 26:2:126–140, March/April 1977.

BIBRING, GRETE L., DWYER, THOMAS F., HUNTINGTON, DOROTHY, S., and VALENSTEIN, ARTHUR F.: "A Study of the Psychological Processes in Pregnancy and of the Earliest Mother–Child Relationship," *Psychoanalytic Study of the Child.* New York: International Universities Press, 1961, Vol. XVI, pp. 9–72.

BLEESTONE, HARVEY, and McGOHER, CARL L.: "Reaction to Extreme Stress: Impending Death by Execution," *American Journal of Psychiatry,* 119:5:393–96, November 1962.

BOVE, ALFRED: "The Cardiovascular Response to Stress," *Psychosomatics,* 18:4:13–17, October 1977.

BRAY, G. A.: *The Obese Patient.* Philadelphia: W. B. Saunders, 1976.

CHRISTOPHERSON, LOIS: "Cardiac Transplantation; Need for patient counselling," *Nursing Mirror,* 149:1:34–39, July 5, 1979.

BRUCH, HILDA: "The Insignificant Difference; Discordant Incidence of Anorexia Nervosa in Monozygotic Twins," *American Journal of Psychiatry,* 119:5:393–96, November 1962.

———: "Perils of Behavior Modification," *Journal American Medical Association,* 230:1409–1422, 1974.

———: "Obesity and Anorexia Nervosa," *Psychosomatics,* 19:4:208–212, April 1978.

CAMERON, DYNTHIS F. et al.: "When Sensory Deprivation Occurs," *The Canadian Nurse,* 68:32–34, November 1972.

CASPER, REGINA C., and DAVIS, JOHN M.: "On the Course of Anorexia Nervosa," *American Journal of Psychiatry,* 134:9:974–978, September 1977.

CLEAVER, ELDRIDGE: *Soul on Ice.* New York: Dell Publishing Co., Inc., 1968.

CLEVELAND, S. E.: "Personality Characteristics, Body Image, and Social Attitudes of Organ Transplant Donors versus Nondonors," *Psychosomatic Medicine,* 37:313–319, August 1975.

DLIN, BARNEY M., PERIMAN, ABRAHAM, and RINGOLD, EVELYN: Psychosexual Response to Ileostomy and Colostomy," *American Journal of Psychiatry,* 123:3:374–81, September 1969.

DUBOVSKY, STEVEN L., GETTO, CARL J., GROSS, SUSAN ADAMS, and PALEY, JUDY A.: "Impact on Nursing Care and Mortality: Psychiatrists on the Coronary Care Unit," *Psychosomatics,* 18:3:18–27, August 1977.

DUMAS, RHETAUGH G., and LEONARD, R. C.: "The Effect of Nursing on the Incidence of Postoperative Vomiting," *Nursing Research,* 12:12–15, 1963.

ENGEL, G. L., and SCHMALE, A. H.: "Psychoanalytic Theory of Somatic Disorder: Conversion, Specificity and the Disease Onset Situation," *Journal of the American Psychoanalytic Association,* 15:334–65, 1967.

FENICHEL, OTTO: *The Psychoanalytic Theory of Neurosis.* New York: W. W. Norton & Co., Inc., 1945.

FRASER, T. M.: "The Effects of Confinement as a Factor in Manned Space Flight," National Aeronautics and Space Administration, Washington, D.C., 1966 (NASA CR-511).

GOFFMAN, ERVING: *Stigma.* Englewood Cliffs, N.J.: Prentice-Hall, Inc., 1965.

GORNEY, RODERICK: "Interpersonal Intensity, Competition and Synergy: Determinants of Achievement, Aggression and Mental Illness," *American Journal of Psychiatry,* 128:4:43–45, October 1971.

GOTTSCHALK, LOUIS A., HAER, JOHN L., and BATES, DANIEL E.: "Effects of Sensory Overload on Psychological State," *Archives of General Psychiatry,* 27:451–57, October 1972.

GREENACRE, PHYLLIS: "Certain Relationships Between Fetishism and the Faulty Development of the Body Image," *The Psychoanalytic Study of the Child,* Vol. 8. New York: International Universities Press, 1953, pp. 879–98.

GREENWOOD, ALLEN: "Mental Disturbances Following Operation for Cataract," *Journal of the American Medical Association,* 91:1713–15, December 1, 1928.

GRINKER, ROY R.: "The Psychosomatic Aspects of Anxiety," in Spielberger, Charles D., ed.: *Anxiety and Behavior.* New York: Academic Press, Inc., 1966, pp. 129–42.

HARLOW, HARRY F., and WOOLSEY, CLINTON N.: *Biological and Biochemical Bases of Behavior.* Madison: University of Wisconsin Press, 1958.

HAVEKAMP, KATHARINE: *The Empty Face.* New York: Richard Marek, Publisher, 1978.

IZARD, CARROLL E., and TOMKINS, SILVARS: "Anxiety Is a Negative Affect," in Spielberger, Charles D., ed.: *Anxiety and Behavior.* New York: Academic Press, Inc., 1966.

JANIS, IRVING L.: *Psychological Stress.* New York: John Wiley & Sons, Inc., 1958.

KARUSH, AARON, DANIELS, GEORGE E., O'CONNOR, JOHN F., and STERN, LENORE: "The Response to Psychotherapy in Chronic Ulcerative Colitis," *Psychosomatic Medicine,* 31:3:201–26, May–June 1969.

KLEINMAN, CAROL S.: "Psychological Processes During Pregnancy," *Perspectives in Psychiatric Care,* **XV**:4:175–180, Oct.-Nov.-Dec., 1977.

KOBRZYCKI, PAULA: "Renal Transplant Complications," *American Journal of Nursing,* 77:4:641–643, April 1977.

LAUFER, MOSES: "The Body Image, the Function of Masturbation and Adolescence," *The Psychoanalytic Study of the Child,* Vol. 23. New York: International Universities Press, 1968.

LAVIE, PERETZ, HEFEZ, ALBERT, HALPERIN, GILA, and ENOCK, DANIEL: "Long-Term Effects of Traumatic War-Related Events on Sleep," *American Journal of Psychiatry,* **136**: 2:175–178, February 1979.

LEVENKRON, STEVEN: *The Best Little Girl in the World.* Chicago: Contemporary Books, Inc., 1978.

LIFTON, ROBERT J., and OLSON, ERIC: "The Human Meaning of Total Disaster," *Psychiatry,* 39:1–18, February 1976.

LINN, L. et al.: "Patterns of Behavior Disturbance Following Cataract Extraction," *American Journal of Psychiatry,* 110:281–89, 1953.

LOWENTHAL, M. F., and ROBINSON, B.: "Social Networks and Isolation," in Binstock, R. H., and Shanas, Ethel, eds.: *Handbook of Aging and the Social Sciences.* New York: Van Nostrand Reinhold, 1967, pp. 432–456.

MAHLER, M. S.: "Thoughts about Development and Individuation," *The Psychoanalytic Study of the Child,* Vol. 18. New York: International Universities Press, 1963.

MINTER, RICHARD E., and KIMBALL, CHASE PATTERSON: "Life Events and Illness Onset: A Review," *Psychosomatics,* 19:6:334–339, June 1978.

MINUCHIN, SALVADOR, ROSSMAN, BERNICE L., and BAKER, LESTER: *Psychosomatic Families.* Cambridge: Harvard University Press, 1978.

NORRIS, CATHERINE M.: "Body Image: Its Relevance to Professional Nursing," in Carlson, Carolyn E., ed.: *Behavioral Concepts in Nursing Intervention.* Philadelphia: J. B. Lippincott Co., 1978, pp. 5–36.

OKURA, K. PATRICK: "Mobilizing in Response to a Major Disaster," *Community Mental Health Journal,* 11:2:136–144, 1975.

ORBACH, SUSIE: *Fat is a Feminist Issue.* New York: Paddington Press, 1977.

PALAZOLLI, MARA: *Self-Starvation.* New York: Jason Aronson, 1978.

RUBIN, REVA: "Body Image and Self-Esteem," *Nursing Outlook,* 16:6:20–23, June 1968.

RUESCH, JURGEN, and PRESTWOOD, A. RODNEY: "Anxiety—Its Imitation, Communication and Interpersonal Management,"

Archives of Neurology and Psychiatry, 62:527–50, November 1949.

SAINT-EXUPERY, ANTOINE DE: *Night Flight.* New York: Signet Classics, 1942.

SAYERS, SHEILA: "Puerperal Psychosis," *Nursing Times,* 72 (20):774–776, 1976.

SCHMITT, FLORENCE E., and POWHATAN, J.: "Psychological Preparation of Surgical Patients," *Nursing Research,* 22:2:108–17, March–April 1973.

SHONTZ, FRANKLIN C.: *The Psychological Aspects of Physical Illness and Disability.* New York: Macmillan Publishing Co., Inc., 1975.

SLONIM, A. R.: "Effects of Minimal Personal Hygiene and Related Procedures During Prolonged Confinement," Aerospace Medical Research Laboratories, Springfield, Va.: U.S. Department of Commerce, 1967.

SOLOMON, PHILIP, KUBZANSKY, PHILIP E., LEIDERMAN, P., HERBERT, MENDELSON, JACK H., TRUMBULL, RICHARD, and WEXLER, DONALD: *Sensory Deprivation.* Cambridge, Mass.: Harvard University Press, 1965.

SPITZ, RENE A.: "Hospitalism: An Inquiry Into the Genesis of Psychiatric Conditions in Early Childhood," *The Psychoanalytic Study of the Child,* 1:53–74, 1945.

STONE, CHARLES B.: "Psychiatric Screening for Transsexual Surgery," *Psychosomatics,* **XVIII:** 1:25–27, Jan.-Feb.-March 1977.

STUNKARD, ALBERT J., and MENDELSON, MYER: "Obesity and the Body Image I. Characteristics of Disturbances in the Body Image of Some Obese Persons," *American Journal of Psychiatry,* 123:11:1297–1300, April 1967.

——— and BURT, VICTOR: "Obesity and the Body Image II. Age at Onset of Disturbances in the Body Image," *American Journal of Psychiatry,* 123:11:1443–47, May 1967.

THOMPSON, SUE: "Anorexia Nervosa: Hungry for Knowledge—but not for Food," *Nursing Mirror,* 149:2:29–32, July 12, 1979.

TIERNEY, ELIZABETH ANN: "Accepting Disfigurement When Death is the Alternative," *American Journal of Nursing,* 75:12:2149–2150, December 1975.

VERNON, CHARLES R.: "Psychiatric View of Cardiac Rehabilitation," *Journal of Rehabilitation,* 24:6:18–19, November–December 1958.

VIGERSKY, ROBERT, ed.: *Anorexia Nervosa.* New York: Raven Press, 1977.

VOLICER, BEVERLY J.: "Patients' Perceptions of Stressful Events Associated with Hospitalization," *Nursing Research,* 23:3:236–238, May–June 1974.

WALTERS, CATHRYN, SHURLEY, JAY T., and

PARSONS, OSCAR A.: "Differences in Male and Female Responses to Underwater Sensory Deprivation; An Exploratory Study," *The Journal of Nervous and Mental Disease,* 135:4:302–309, October 1962.

WEINSTEIN, SIDNEY, RICHLIN, MILTON, WEISINGER, MARVIN, and FISHER, LARRY: "Adaptation to Visual and Nonvisual Rearrangement," Washington, D.C.: National Aeronautics and Space Administration, January 1967 (NASA CR-663).

WEISMANN, A. D., and HACKETT, T. P.: "Psychosis After Eye Surgery, Establishment of a Specific Doctor—Patient Relation in the Prevention and Treatment of 'Black Patch' Delirium" *New England Journal of Medicine,* 258:2:1284–89, 1958.

WINKLER, WIN ANN: "Choosing the Prosthesis and Clothing," *American Journal of Nursing,* 77:9:1433–1436, September 1977.

WOLF, STEWART G., and WOLFF, HAROLD G.: *Human Gastric Function.* London: Oxford University Press, 1943.

WOLFF, HAROLD, G.: "Stressors as a Cause of Disease in Man," in *Stress and Psychiatric Disorder.* Mental Health Research Fund Proceedings. Oxford: Blackwell Scientific Publications, 1961, pp. 17–31.

WOLPE, JOSEPH, BRADY, JOHN PAUL, SERBER, MICHAEL, AGREES, W. STEWART, and LIBERMAN, ROBERT PAUL: "The Current Status of Systematic Desensitization," *American Journal of Psychiatry,* 130:9:961–65, September 1973.

_____: "The Behavior Therapy Approach," in Arieti, Silvano, ed.: *American Handbook of Psychiatry,* Vol. I. New York: Basic Books, Inc., 1974, pp. 941–57.

World Health Organization: "Neurophysiology and Behavior Science in Psychiatry," *WHO Chronicle,* 22:5:204–207, May 1968.

_____: "Controlling Hypertension: Community Care and Mutual Aid Through Neighborhood Clubs," *WHO Chronicle,* 32:11:448–450, November 1978.

ZUBEK, JOHN P.: "Counteracting Effects of Physical Exercises Performed During Prolonged Perceptual Deprivation," *Science,* 142:3591:504–506, October 25, 1963.

_____: *Sensory Deprivation: Fifteen Years of Research.* New York: Appleton-Century-Crofts, 1969.

6

The Problem of Loss[1]

LEARNING OBJECTIVES / Persons studying this chapter should be able to:

1. Define depression
2. Describe the characteristics of depression in infancy, childhood, adolescence, and adulthood
3. Describe the onset and characteristics of a major depressive episode
4. Define pseudoanhedonia, nihilism, introjection, and object loss
5. List five guidelines for the nurse in recognition of depression
6. List ten guidelines important in the nursing care of a patient in a depressive episode
7. Define hypomania, and bipolar affective disorder
8. List ten guidelines important in the nursing care of a patient in a manic episode
9. Define: grief, mourning, catharsis, denial, isolation, and anticipatory grief
10. List four phases of grief and mourning
11. Describe the characteristics of grief
12. Discuss current burial customs and contrast them with earlier periods
13. List five ways to assist bereaved adults
14. Discuss ways to help children view death
15. Describe five stages of the process of dying
16. List ten guidelines important in the nursing care of the dying patient

Sadness and grief for the loved and lost are perhaps the most powerful emotions affecting humans. Inability to cope with these feelings has tragic consequences that can shatter a person's life. Sorrow, one of the most painful affects, needs to receive more attention in nursing practice. The problem of loss is a primary focus in caring for the mental patient who is encouraged to bring his feelings into the open and discuss them with helping persons. Depression[2] in relation to loss and its painful affects is emphasized in this book because of the prevalence of depression not only in psychiatric patients but in severely physically ill patients where loss is in the forefront and which, for the most part, goes unrecognized and therefore untreated. In general nursing, the feeling of loss that a patient endures because of conditions inherent in his illness and hospitalization has not been dealt with adequately.

Although young nursing students, for the

[1] Loss refers to the lack of external and internal supplies required by the individual to satisfy his basic needs.

[2] There are strong theoretical positions based on loss being a primary basis of depression. This psychological position, presented here, does not negate additional points of view, for example, that depression may emerge from many factors: sociocultural, genetic, the amine hypothesis (see Chap. 16 for discussion), disturbances in endocrine function, and others.

most part, have not experienced great and intense losses at the time they enter the profession, they must prepare themselves to help patients and their families through crises of development, life, and illness and through the ultimate crisis of life—death. They can do so only by understanding and watching for the many ways in which feelings arise and are expressed, both verbally and nonverbally.

This chapter deals with the ways in which people handle their feelings of loss of body parts, function, capacity, or accustomed environment.

Depression and Normal States

Many people say they are depressed when their usual feeling of well-being is lessened. A lowering of mood resulting from internal or external factors may influence others to comment that they are "feeling blue" or "having the blues." "Blue Monday" is a common colloquialism referring to the day following the weekend traditional time of rest and relaxation when unfinished work and responsibilities must be resumed, distasteful as they may be, and joys and pleasures be put aside. Sadness, dejection, and despondency are synonyms for "blue" feelings. Premenstrual and postpartum "blues" are well known but not fully understood. They are thought to be connected with changes in endocrine patterns. "Feeling blue" may also be a mood related to loneliness, grief, and mourning, and feeling sorrow for one's self and condition. Other adjectives that describe this lowering of mood are gloomy, hopeless, discouraged, pessimistic, unhappy, downhearted, and low. They all describe an affect that is a normal response. It is emotional pain that can be thought of as analogous to physical pain. Just as physical pain is not illness per se, so emotional pain is not mental disorder. A deep intensity of this affect, however, is usually labeled depression.

These low spirits may be observed in the older person who has just given up hope of maintaining his independence. In persons of all ages, it is a familiar mood caused by feeling trapped in a situation from which there is no apparent escape. Broken love affairs and failure to meet goals long sought may result in an unhappy state. It may arise in students who receive a lower grade in an examination or on a term paper than they had expected. Patients admitted to the hospital for diagnostic tests or for long-term illness may become discouraged about the results or their lack of progress.

Certain people develop depression in response to stress and loss; others may, for example, develop changes in physical health and still others make healthy adaptations.

Depression is used essentially in three different ways. One refers to the affect of sadness and feelings of disappointment that are experienced by everyone. A second use of the term "depression" refers to depression as a mood disorder, in which changes in mood constitute the major symptom. Young people between the ages of eighteen and twenty-nine have a higher incidence of mood depression than any other age group (Secunda, 1973). The depressive mood disorder is thought to be one of the bases for drug dependence. The third use of the term refers to a *major depressive episode;* it is more than one affective change; it carries with it a complexity of body symptoms, changes in motivation, and behavior. Whereas in all depressive states, the affect of sadness may be equally painful, the difference between them relates to the fact that self-depreciation and helplessness are greater in clinical depression. Therefore, the differentiating factors between the states relate to behavior. A continuum between the low mood of the normal person and the person with a major clinical depressive episode is accepted by most clinicians. A prolonged state of depressive affects may deepen into a major depressive episode that has a greater number of symptoms and is more difficult to reverse.

Depressive neurosis as a diagnostic entity now appears as "dysthymic disorder" under the heading of affective disorders in the new *Diagnostic and Statistical Manual of Mental Disorders III* (1980).

Depression

". . . nothing has been discovered which directly and specifically removes the mental pain of the melancholic, and yet, broadly speaking, the recovery rate is high."[3]

Depression, in this culture one of the most common reactions to loss, is probably experienced by all to some degree during the life span. The degrees of depression are discussed at conferences of psychiatrists, psychiatric nurses, and other professionals. Depression is one of the oldest mental disorders. It is known from antiquity and is described in Job's lament.

"Perish the day I was born
and the night which said,
  'A man is conceived,'
May that day be darkness.

Why did I not die at birth
Come forth from the womb and expire?"[4]

People who become clinically depressed often have had difficulty in the past with their feelings of helplessness and hopelessness.

Depression is a "state of feeling sad; psychoneurotic or psychotic disorder marked by sadness, inactivity, difficulty in thinking and concentration, and feelings of dejection; a reduction in activity, amount, quality of force; a lowering of vitality or functional activity."[5] Depression may be a symptom of any illness or it may constitute its principal component.

In depression there is a failure to perform usual daily tasks; work may mount up as the depressed person feels overwhelmed by the things he has not accomplished. The depressed person may fail to do household chores, expect other family members to do them instead, but still be able to go to work. As the depression deepens the person will not be able to go to work and eventually becomes psychologically immobilized.

Pseudoanhedonia[6] is prominent, and the person worries about everything. Often preoccupation with suicide and feelings of guilt occurs. Cognitive disturbances may include a paucity of thinking, inability to concentrate, indecisiveness, and continuous worrying, often about events long past. Preoccupation with sin, feelings of unworthiness, and concern about death may predominate. Pain and suffering is reflected in the facial expression of the depressed person. Beck (1974) emphasizes a cognitive theory of depression and describes a "cognitive triad" as follows: (1) The depressed person considers himself as worthless; (2) the depressed person sees all that he has done in his life a failure; and (3) the depressed person views the future as filled with difficulties. Beck attributes many of the symptoms of depression as arising from these cognitive changes; i.e., if the person thinks he is no good, then he will behave as though he is of no value.

BODY SYMPTOMS

Preoccupation with the body is a common symptom, especially preoccupation with the body organs. A feeling of malfunction or other disorder of the organs will often bring the patient to the doctor or outpatient clinic for the first time. In this connection, it is worth noting that high body concern is socially acceptable, whereas "losing one's mind" is still something of a stigma in this country. Actual *physical* changes may be present; therefore, the examiner must be alert to this possibility. Other symptoms are loss of interest in one's usual pursuits—a kind of withdrawal from social contacts, family members, neighbors, and fellow employees, impotence and lack of interest in sex, weight loss, constipation, amenorrhea, insomnia, hypersomnia, anorexia, fatigue, heightened tension, inability to concentrate, and increased restlessness. The mood is one of great sorrow, and crying spells may come without warning. A feeling of tightness in

---

[3] *One Hundred and Fourteenth Report of the Retreat, York, A Registered Hospital for the Treatment of Mental Diseases, 1914, p. 11.*
[4] The Book of Job, 3:3–12.
[5] *Webster's New Collegiate Dictionary.* Springfield, Mass.: G. and C. Merriam Co., Publishers, 1977.

[6] Pseudoanhedonia refers to the loss of interest or pleasure in things formerly pleasurable.

the head as though wearing a closely fitting cap is often expressed by the suffering patient.

Patients may display a diurnal mood; i.e., they will feel very low early in the morning hours and cheer up later in the day.

Depressed persons fail to maintain their personal appearance. They do not bathe, they neglect personal hygiene, and their hair and skin may appear oily. If they are menstruating, they may forget to use napkins or tampons. In severe stages, people pace up and down, wring their hands, and say they are worthless and deserve to be shot. They may ask for electroconvulsive treatment or say they deserve no treatment but death. Suicidal thoughts may occupy the waking hours of the depressed person, who may attempt, often successfully, to kill himself. The highest risk for suicide occurs when the patient is going into a depression or coming out of it. Agitation may be marked, with pacing, sighing, wringing of the hands, pulling the hair, scratching the skin. Psychomotor retardation may appear as very slow speech, slowness to respond to others, a low tone of voice, and very slow movements. Paranoid ideation may be present with ideas of reference and delusions. Nihilistic[7] delusions may occur as well as delusions of guilt, of having committed an unpardonable sin, poverty, or self-depreciation.

Features associated with depression in prepubertal children are clinging, refusal to go to school, and fear of death. In boys, antisocial behavior may be present.

In adolescents, features associated with depression are aggression, acting out, running away, restlessness, pouting, irritability, withdrawal, increased appetite and weight gain, slovenliness, and a feeling of being misunderstood.

OCCURRENCE OF DEPRESSION

Loss is one of the major causes of depression. The loss may be real, symbolic, or fancied; it may stem from childhood or from the immediate past. Depression may come

from loss of love or the feeling of being important to others, two of the basic needs essential to positive mental health.

OBJECT LOSS

The love of objects is based upon the love of the child for the mother or mother substitute. The first response to threatened object relationships is anxiety and a subsequent reaction to object loss may be depression. The ego establishes object relationships, evaluates threats to these relationships, and attempts to protect them. When the ego meets overwhelming loss, depression may result. Object loss, be it a body part, death of a loved one, receiving bad news (which may threaten object loss), or being fired, may trigger the dread of abandonment and activate the feeling of "No one will want me because I have no legs," or "Who will love me now that I am nobody's child?" Object loss is felt intrapsychically, the highly valued aspects of life are gone, and ego-object relationships are broken. Grief is the specific subjective reaction to object loss, and if it is resolved, depression is avoided.

Depression has its origins in unconscious guilt deriving from relationships with the lost object. The superego punishes the ego, and unconscious ambivalence and hostility toward the lost object are redirected toward the self. When the beloved object is lost, the support of the object to the ego is gone, anxiety arises as a reaction specific to the danger that the loss entails, the libido (id) becomes detached from the object, and the result is psychological and physical immobility. When the relationship with the lost object has been ambivalent, the superego is especially punitive and harsh. A depressed person with an overpunitive superego internalizes hostility through the process of identification with the lost object by introjection[8] and incorporation and hurts himself. If externalization or projection occurs, the person hurts someone else, sym-

---

[7] *Nihilistic* refers to the delusion that the self, or part of the self or some other object does not exist.

[8] Introjection is a defense mechanism whereby loved or hated external objects are symbolically absorbed within oneself. It is related to a more primitive defense mechanism, incorporation, in which the symbolic person or parts of a person are figuratively ingested, e.g., the mother's breast (American Psychiatric Association, 1980).

bolically, in actuality, or both simultaneously. The threatened loss of an object relationship may trigger a similar response.

ANACLITIC DEPRESSION

Anaclitic depression is a syndrome of a depressive nature shown by infants who lose a love object during the latter half of the first year of life, namely, the mother or mother substitute (Spitz and Wolf, 1946). It is the infant prototype of the adult clinical depression and is manifested by three phases: (1) *protest,* in which crying, apprehension, and struggling occur; (2) *despair,* a quiet stage in which the infant may refuse to eat and fall into a state of marasmus; and (3) *detachment,* in which the infant withdraws (Bowlby, 1969). The term "anaclitic" refers to the infant's depending on the mother for his love and security. Children with anaclitic depression exhibit a dejected expression and posture. They appear vague and helpless and seem to have a distaste for motility.

OTHER TYPES OF DEPRESSION

Individuals who become depressed are likely to be shy, oversensitive, and inclined to worry too much. Delicately balanced emotionally, they are very self-conscious. The unconscious mechanisms involved in depression are regression, oral sadism, anal traits, a primitive return to a hedonistic level of existence, a desire to return to the womb, and a sense of being wronged.

There are also elements of sadomasochism, self-depreciation, and perfectionism in the depressed person. The patient may feel a loss of prestige, both in and out of the family, a loss of sexual love and function, and a sense of abandonment by his loved ones.

Depression involves rage intended for someone else turned back onto the self. Menninger (1938) wrote that with every suicide there is one of three complaints: (1) the wish to kill, (2) the wish to be killed, or (3) the wish to die. If the helping person is too nice, the depressed patient may feel unworthy and may kill himself; on the other hand, if the helping person is too harsh, the depression may deepen. The therapist,

therefore, must be very sensitive to the balance between supporting the overly punitive superego and encouraging the ego functions in communication with the depressed person. For example, assets of the patient can be deservedly complimented and shortcomings realistically pointed out at the same time, with psychological support readily available from the therapist.

Perfectionistic, high-performance, and maximum-performance people who are constantly going at high rates of speed are particularly susceptible to depression when their work has been interrupted. Depressive states also occur frequently in older people who have experienced a sudden change for the worse in their lives. Enforced retirement, death of a loved one, loss of a limb, and removal to a nursing home are serious problems to the aged. An unexpected change in health status brought on by a stroke or accident, particularly one that requires long periods of hospitalization with no prospect of return to former levels of functioning or to one's own home, may understandably precipitate depression. Very often, the patient's apathy, following upon such a personal catastrophe, is attributed to senile processes, although the cause may in fact be a reversible depression. Nurses sensitive to their patients' feelings and needs can do much to uncover the roots of the symptomatology and help in the recovery process.

Research shows that the first months of institutionalization constitute a difficult period for the aging, one in which some of the most adverse psychological effects occur (Lieberman, 1968). In addition, effects that have previously been attributed to confinement in an institution are now considered aspects of the waiting period, in which crises about separation and loss are being experienced. The fantasies and symbolic meanings of institutionalization that occupy the patient's mind during this period may be related more to his psychological changes than to the institutionalization itself. Both concepts are of great relevance to the nurse's preventive role in dealing with feelings of separation, loss, and despair in patients.

Depression can occur with any abrupt change in body image, during any of life's crises, and at other stress points in the life cycle. They are evident in all age groups. Childhood depression, the "old soldier syndrome," and the "empty nest syndrome" all occur. Depression in older groups may be characterized by loneliness and a preoccupation with physical illnesses (Schwab et al., 1968). Other physical disabilities that give rise to depressive episodes are hysterectomies, rapid weight gain, amputations, mastectomies, pregnancy, colostomies, and strokes. *Anniversary depressions* are a special category; a specific date recalls to the patient the extent of a previous loss. One patient, Mrs. P., became depressed every year at the beginning of the deer season when her husband left her to go hunting. Severe scars on young people and mutilating operations on old people may evoke particularly strong depressive reactions. With other conditions, such as arthritis and metastatic cancer, there may be chronic depression.

The characteristics and symptoms of depression as described above may not all occur in one person at any one time, but any of them is indicative of its existence. In all cases, however, differentiation must be made between the clinical definition of depression and its lay meaning of sadness of a transitory nature that is causally related to an immediately preceding event.

The person with a dysthmic disorder (depressive neurosis) falls into the clinical definition. This disorder is characterized by an intensity of depression due to an internal conflict or to a known event such as the loss of a love object as explained by the following patient:

Franklin A., aged thirty-one, was admitted to the psychiatric unit after jumping from the fourth floor of a downtown hotel where he worked. Estranged from his parents, and married at eighteen, he shortly afterward joined the Navy. Bored with the Navy, he transferred to the Army. Working with top secret papers and tapes, he was accused of giving out information. Before his court martial, he went AWOL and got a job in a hotel. At this time, his only brother was killed in action in the Navy. He began drinking alcohol, gave himself up, and spent five months in an Army prison. Afterward, he returned home to his wife and two children. Although able to employ himself in a valued job, he felt bored, drank heavily, and stopped meeting his obliga-

tions as a husband and father. His wife divorced him three years ago, at which time he transferred within the hotel system to another city, worked for three years, and finally was fired because of drinking. The loss of the job was the recent event precipitating the suicidal gesture.

Franklin's depression was thought to have been triggered by the loss of his brother; he tried to handle it by drinking. In turn, he lost his wife and children and later his job. Although he was in a good position at work he felt guilty in it and expressed the thought that he had stepped on and cheated others on the way up. He tried to overcome anxiety, guilt, and tension by alcohol and finally suicide seemed the way out.

In the hospital, he slept poorly, was uninterested in maintaining his personal hygiene although he said, "I'm a handsome dude when I'm cleaned up," and sat around in hospital clothes preoccupied and silent unless approached. In group meetings he was attentive but silent until the feeling of failure was expressed by others and when asked what he thought, he replied that he felt the same way. In one-to-one encounters, the nursing student established rapport, helped him talk about his feelings, showed him some card tricks that sparked his interest, ate lunch with him, went for walks with him, and helped him get interested in macrame.

In addition, Franklin was treated with imipramine, psychotherapy, and milieu therapy. Within three weeks his depression lifted and he made plans to go to an alcoholic rehabilitation unit for further treatment.

The following patient was diagnosed as having a depressive episode:

The patient, Jack A., sixty-four years old, was admitted to the psychiatric hospital following a suicidal attempt one day after his wife died of a long illness. He suffered from profound depression, with psychomotor retardation, insomnia, anorexia, and neglected personal hygiene. He blamed himself for the death of his wife and this was about the only verbalization he made.

The treatment for this patient was milieu therapy, psychotherapy, and antidepressants. After two months of this treatment he was not any better. Therefore, electroconvulsive therapy was administered, the depression lifted, and he was discharged home.

THE NURSE'S ROLE IN RECOGNITION OF DEPRESSION

Recognition of depression in others is of major importance in nursing. Because they spend more time with patients and families than other professionals, nurses are in a particularly important position with regard to recognizing depression. A depressed patient may not present a clear-cut, easily recognized pattern. Changes in usual behavior, such as refusing to eat, bathe, or apply the other body care, wearing dark colors, and slowing down in usual activities, may be taken as cues. A family member may say that the person does not do the things he used to do, does not seem to like to be with people, is irritable, and easily bursts into tears. One of my patients with chronic depression literally spent months building a white garden to help herself overcome her melancholia. The depressed person may have had many absences in his work record before finally reaching the point where he is unable to make the effort to get out of bed. The distressed family may ascribe such behavior to laziness or other factors. Nurses learn to consider behavioral changes as events to be probed because of their significance in regard to the patient's underlying motivation.

Constant reference to melancholy or morbid subjects may precede depression. A patient may also firmly assert, "I want to die; why don't you leave me alone?" When asked by the nurse how he is feeling, he may respond sadly, "I am no good to anybody," and begin weeping. Some patients who are depressed as a consequence of multisurgery become surgical invalids; others are repeatedly admitted to general hospitals for series of diagnostic tests. Still others become iatrogenically dependent on drugs.

Professionals often mistake depression in older persons for organic mental disorder. Irritability in the aged, a common sign of depression, is also often confused with organic mental disorder. I am reminded of many older patients, severely depressed, whose mood lifted dramatically after treatment for the depression. Patients and families are thereby relieved of their chronic suffering by early recognition and treatment of depressive conditions. The constellation of losses suffered by older persons makes them particularly vulnerable to depression; the constant loss of love objects, changes in body image, and other losses add to their loss complex. Many problems of older persons relate to the problem of loss.

Nurses have the responsibility of becoming cognizant of the mental state of their patients and of conveying their observations and clinical inferences to the attending physicians. Suggestions for psychiatric referral of patients are often welcomed by physicians who are frustrated and puzzled by the persistence of symptoms in the presence of negative diagnostic tests. The patient, too, is helped by the nurse in accepting psychiatric treatment because of the nurse's role as a sympathetic and knowledgeable person whose interest is in his recovery.

The importance of listening has previously been discussed: listening carefully to the words that your patient speaks, the inflection, pitch of voice, and expression. For example, when the patients says, "Yeah, I'm really finished," with a sort of finality when you ask if he has finished his bath, he may be saying something extremely significant about himself. He may, for instance, be telling you that he did not pass his Ph.D. orals, that he is a failure as a father and husband, or that he has used up his life span. Tone of voice, inflection, and emphasis on certain words communicate feelings. Pick up verbal cues from your patient and analyze them. You may be saving a life.

Preoccupation with body functions, neglect of personal appearance, masked facies, and refusal to see loved ones may all be indications of depression. A spurt of angry words from a previously calm patient may furnish a clue as to how he has been feeling all along. Actions directed against self are also important, such as refusing to take medications or prescribed treatment and refusing to eat. Tears or the traces of tears and sniffling as you enter the room or home may evidence depressed feelings. A patient who has lost his sense of humor is definitely depressed. A depressed person may injure himself; accidents should therefore be fully investigated.

The depressed patient may feel a chronic

fatigue and discouragement because simple tasks become Sisyphus-like in nature. A hospitalized depressed patient stated that he felt like he had the whole world on his shoulders. A patient may feel overburdened by his work load and be unable to take on any new responsibilities that demand a change in interaction. Depressive affects can easily be overlooked by physician and nurse, especially when they appear in a patient some time after treatment has begun. Nurses prepared to anticipate symptoms and to look regularly at the inner lives of their patients can perform primary preventive service in the interest of the mental health of patients and families.

Because of the prevalence of depression in the United States, nurses in all areas of practice should help persons work through their feelings where losses occur. School nurses and community nurses need to be more aware of the emotional needs of children. Nurses in university health services help students deal with situations where self-esteem is lost and depression could result.

Because of the high incidence of depression in middle-aged women, particular attention should be given to helping individuals prepare for this phase of life by developing life-long interests that build self-esteem. The changing role of women and the women's movement have helped many middle-aged women to perceive new ways of self-fulfillment.

Beginning students may look for just one etiological event to explain the onset of depression. In developing multifactoral concepts of human behavior, however, one must consider the totality of the patient's experiences in assessing his response to change. How the individual adapts to conditions at any developmental stage in his life is largely predicated on his total life pattern, his hopes, desires, and fears, and the successes and failures of past performances.

THERAPEUTIC TASKS

For the infant who has lost his mother, provision of a mother substitute serves as the balm. In the depressed patient, self-esteem must be regained; feelings that have turned inward must be turned outward. The therapeutic task is to free the ego so the libido can seek a new love object. The first task of the nurse is to get acquainted and to learn the facts of a case. The next step has three aspects: getting the patient to talk, exploring the source of pain, and encouraging catharsis. It may sometimes be necessary to use nonverbal communication as a starting point. Helping the patient to express his internalized anger is a central part of nursing action. With verbalization, the patient brings his feelings to the surface where he and the nurse can exmine them, discuss them, and mitigate them through interaction.

Interest and concern alone are sometimes all that is needed. Emotional support is necessary, the support given through understanding, patience, and love. Love is the main thing—being with the patient and communicating to him that you are on his side; staying with him on a gradually diminishing basis, each day expecting more and more of him; calling on the telephone between visits if the patient is at home. You can do a lot in a five-to-ten-minute phone call to help lift his spirits.

To be aware from the first of the individual's needs and his likes and dislikes is essential. The depressed person is immobilized; therefore, needs have to be anticipated. Patients often lie or sit and wait to see if others are interested enough to make the overture to ascertain their needs. Keenly aware of the interactions of others, they easily feel slighted. They are crying for attention without knowing how to ask for it.

Relief from the punitive superego must be achieved when the severely depressed person accepts his fate and requests that you hasten his death. Provision for atonement needs to be made. Some patients feel that hospitalization is atonement enough; others feel that electroconvulsive treatment is appropriate punishment and that they will rapidly come out of their depression after its administration. It is important for the nurse to make a sharp assessment of each patient in regard to task assignment. For the depressed individual whose self-concept may be so poor that he thinks he is good for nothing, fulfillment of a daily responsibility may renew his sense of purposefulness. The provision for atonement will be different for various individuals. Menial chores may help some patients wash away theoretical sins symbolically. Such jobs could include scrubbing kitchens and floors, washing windows and walls or dishes and clothes, cleaning cupboards and drawers. Polishing and waxing cars, painting walls, and cleaning sidewalks are suitable menial chores. Polishing shoes is also a good menial task in a hospital or a home setting. Other kinds of jobs that regularly have to be done such as desk work may be suitable for other patients.

Depressed patients are accident-prone and should not drive a car or any other motorized vehicle. They can get along for quite a while without eating, but they must have fluids. The depressed person may have lost a lot of weight; therefore, a high-caloric diet may be prescribed by the physician. Between-meal feedings may also help the patient's nutritional state. If at home, the nurse may need to teach the family member responsible for meal preparation to help the depressed patient meet his nutritional needs. The amounts of fluid intake and output require close attention; the patient's temperature should be taken regularly, and all staff should be alert for infections or other manifest body changes.

The depressed person should be observed closely for sleep. Without sleep, exhaustion may occur and the mental state of the individual may become more severe. Personal hygiene may require assistance from the nurse—bathing, shaving, grooming, applying makeup, keeping clothes in order, and changing clothes. Setting a schedule for bathing, feeding, and other personal hygiene can help get the depressed person mobilized. *The nurse's presence also helps allay anxiety.* Depressed patients should be weighed weekly; an increase in weight will, in most cases, reflect the lifting of the depression.

Close observation of the patient and his environment is required for his safety. The dangerous time for the depressed person as far as suicide is concerned is when he is going into or coming out of a depression. It is important, however, to place responsibility on the patient for his own actions. Nurses have been known to go to pieces after a patient has killed himself, even though there was nothing they could have done to prevent it.

Depressed patients may prefer to eat by themselves rather than in the dining room at the regular dining hour. Sometimes they have to be spoon-fed. To avoid constipation, they should be offered food that aids elimination, fluids between meals, and regular exercise. The release of internalized aggression in a socially acceptable manner through exercise and sports is therapeutic to the depressed person. Nurse and patient walking together and throwing a medicine ball back and forth may lead to longer walks and group sports such as volleyball.

Patients who are depressed should not be pushed into making decisions. At first all decisions may have to be made for them, with the nurse assessing and timing them each day until the patient can *very soon* assume responsibility. As the depression lifts, the nurse should watch for the turning point at which the patient can make decisions about his own care. Signs of this turning point may be the first good night's sleep in a long while, a relaxed, mobile facies, assisting another patient, or performing for himself some aspect of personal hygiene. Regaining appetite and gaining weight may be cues for the lifting of the depressive mood and the patient's ability to make more decisions for himself.

As early as possible, the depressed person should participate in group activity. Singing simple familiar songs is a beginning. Often the nurse will have to take the patient by the hand and sing with him the first time he is part of a group. Being with others in group singing or even just sitting evokes the herd instinct, described by one person as the "warm body" theory. It can be very comforting to the depressed person.

Individuals who are depressed frequently have no hobbies and have not participated in recreational activities since they were in grade school or high school. The nurse is the person who can best assess the appropriate time and activity for the patient in this area. At the beginning making simple things, easily finished in one session (the familiar pot holder, for example), is recommended. There is nothing quite so therapeutic as the sense of accomplishment, of creation, no matter how elementary the project.

Depressed patients receiving medication must be observed closely for therapeutic effects and other changes. They should be questioned about their symptoms and possible side effects, since they may not volunteer the information. Medication may be given to induce sleep, but with extra caution to guard against hoarding, since attempted suicide is a possibility. It is also necessary for the nurse to keep the menses record of the depressed female patient and to make sure she uses napkins or tampons during menstruation. Handing such items to the patient may be the beginning of her caring for herself.

If the patient is spoon-fed, he should be offered the cup and the fork at each feeding to encourage self-help. Verbalizing to the patient that you know it is a difficult time for him acknowledges his pain and his depressed state, but it also connotes that the difficulty is time-bound and will not last forever.

There are no universals in the care of the depressed patient. You have to feel with each patient what he is like, what is most painful to him, and what can be done about his condition.

In summary, the level of depression is best measured by the ability of the person to function in his usual setting. The mildly depressed person is quiet, inhibited, and has an unhappy expression. His thoughts may be pessimistic and self-derogatory. Self-depreciating remarks are truly meant for the lost love object. He feels inadequate, discouraged, and hopeless, is unable to make decisions, and has difficulty with his usual intellectual activities. He is too concerned with personal problems and may complain a great deal.

The moderately depressed person has a feeling of unpleasantness, is tense, and feels pain. He is absorbed in a few topics of a very melancholy nature such as death and pseudoanhedonia.

The person who becomes more severely depressed is dejected, feels rejected and unloved, and is anxious and perplexed. He is preoccupied; concentration, attention, and memory are impaired; he may have feelings of unreality and be unable to think.

It is at this stage that the vegetative systems become most affected, resulting in anorexia, constipation, loss of weight, and other symptoms. Delusions are likely to be self-accusatory or expressive of guilt and unworthiness. Suicidal thoughts tend to be present. The patient may be monosyllabic, have psychomotor retardation, and show a neglected appearance and a dejected facies. The severely depressed person should be informed repeatedly that if he follows instructions he will gradually improve (Ayd, 1961). Reiteration of support, reassurance, and dissuasion from taking on anything difficult are also recommended. All instructions should be explicit and repeated frequently; rest and relaxation should be provided. If a patient cannot perform his job, his self-concept will receive a blow if he attempts to continue working. Taking a temporary leave of absence or reducing the work load may be advisable.

Depression may occur in proximity to a known event such as bereavement in which grief work is incomplete, business failure, broken love affairs, and other adversities. Following bereavement those who become disturbed tend to have prolonged grief or to have a delayed reaction to bereavement (Parkes, 1972). When not associated with a known event, depression may be the result of conflict between instinctual wishes and drives in which guilt, ambivalence (particularly love and hate feelings), and hostile impulses toward others are turned inward toward the self. The person who is wounded and hurt and feels unwanted, neglected, and disappointed is prevented by a punitive superego from expressing his feelings outwardly. He is therefore compelled to direct his hostility to his own ego. Some features of melancholia, according to Freud (1917), are borrowed from grief; others have resulted from the process of regression from narcissistic object choice to narcissism.

Manic Episode

Manic episodes usually appear before the age of thirty, whereas depressive episodes may appear at any age, including childhood.

Depressive disorders are much more prevalent than manic episodes. Depression is more common in females whereas manic episodes are about equally divided between men and women. The principal characteristics of a manic episode are a change in mood to one of heightened euphoria, expansiveness, or irritability. The mood may be unusually cheerful, the expansiveness a continuous overenthusiasm for everything in the environment, and the irritability expressed when the person is thwarted. Hyperactivity occurs and social interactions become intrusive. The mood is labile, shifting within moments, hours, or days from anger to depression. Delusions may be present, usually in response to some grandiose scheme or to a person.

Other persons with major affective disorders may exhibit a bipolar disorder in which there are severe mood swings of elation and depression with recurrent manic and depressed states and remissions. A mild bipolar disorder is a cyclothymic disorder.

There are many theories with regard to the development of bipolar disorders. Their occurrence in the same family suggests a hereditory factor. Studies of monozygotic and dizygotic twins support the genetic point of view (Kallman, 1953). Other biological correlates have been described, such as, the pyknic[9] body build and the mesomorphic[10] somatotype.

Recently it has been hypothesized that elation is accompanied by an increase in brain catecholamines.

From the psychoanalytic side, mania is a flight into reality in which some regression occurs in both the ego and the superego. Mania is considered a defense against depression. An understanding of the psychodynamics of the depressive affect is therefore fundamental to comprehension of the elated joy of the manic patient.

BEHAVIOR

Manic patients are breezy, capricious, and extroverted. They may accomplish a great deal and may be well liked by their associates. They stand out in a crowd, seem to have limitless energy, and may be the life of the party. This stage is referred to as *hypomania,* and during this phase behavior is purposeful, much work is accomplished, and others wonder just how the person manages to be so vigorous.

In his spiraling *mood of elation,* the patient becomes expansive. He may consider himself increasingly powerful and wealthy and will spend money wildly on luxuries at the merest whim. Bold schemes are devised that may easily fall apart. Irritability occurs, and hasty separations may ensue within families. Very little introspection seems possible for the elated patient; insight also varies with the degree of the mania.

The manic patient's witty comments have an infectious quality, and there is a saying in the profession that "everybody loves a manic." Immediately thwarting demands of the manic patient may, however, incur swift, uninhibited action from the patient. Professionals and others may become the focus of verbal attacks peppered with obscene expressions. The manic patient is very suggestible and distractible, flitting from subject to subject and from activity to activity. His attention span is short. The hypomanic patient writes copiously. Reams of letters may be forthcoming, which may create some turbulence. He can be absorbed with creating, even with a collection of rags that he may tear into bits and use as decorations for himself. His handwriting is large and bold, with words printed and underlined, and he often writes standing up. Constructing rhymes may occupy his attention, or making some elaborate drawing for a new invention. Clifford Beers wrote on wrapping paper (Deutsch, 1937).

All scraps of paper are, of course, precious to the patient and should be carefully saved for him. One patient in a manic state came to the hospital with rough drawings of a self-watering planter. He had great ideas of setting up an industrial plant near the hospital so that all the patients could be employed in it and make the planters for international distribution. He had planned that all proceeds would go to the hospital. Another patient designed a wheeled vehicle with a sail to travel over

[9] "One with broad head, thick shoulders, large chest, short neck, and stocky body" (Thomas, 1973).

[10] The predominance of the structures of the body developed from the mesodermal layer of the embryo (Hinsie and Campbell, 1960; Patten, 1968).

the western prairies. Clifford Beers, hospitalized after a suicide attempt in 1900, while passing from a state of profound depression to one of extreme exaltation and approaching recovery, shaped in his mind a worldwide movement for the protection of mental patients. Later, *A Mind That Found Itself* (1908) resulted from the notes he made on wrapping paper while he was hospitalized. It is still widely read. Beers founded the National Committee on Mental Hygiene in 1909 (Deutsch, 1937).

Manic episodes may be recurrent; thus, someone within the family constellation and the patient himself may quickly perceive the hypomanic affect and seek treatment. The use of medications may eliminate the necessity for hospitalization. One patient I know gets so angry in her beginning manic phase that she tears up the linoleum at home. This is the signal to the family for taking her to the psychiatrist for medication.

As the hypomanic patient goes into an acute state of mania, if he is not furiously writing he will be talking continuously. He will have a constant and speeded-up stream of speech in which he makes puns and rhymes; speech and laughter will be very loud. His ideas come so fast that, even though he is highly loquacious, he simply does not have time to express them in complete sentences. This results in a flight of ideas. The ideas will most likely be connected (one idea leading to another) although the first idea is only partially expressed. Ideas may be expressed that border on delusions of grandeur. Clang associations may occur in acute states in which the patient expresses himself with words that have similar sounds but different meanings. The nurse who is a careful listener will be able to capture some of this material, which is somewhat like free association. If the nurse is able to understand it, she will better understand the patient and be better able to assist in treatment.

The psychomotor activity is accelerated in speech, and the muscular activity of the patient is also greatly increased. The manic patient is constantly on the go and in the hospital will soon learn a great deal about the other patients and the staff. He does not appear to feel fatigue. According to Morozov and Romasenko (Moscow, no date), this lack of fatigue is due to the increase of sugar in the blood and the utilization of more sugar. The level of lactic acid is low because it is rapidly eliminated from the blood. This explains why patients do not tire easily in the manic state if their carbohydrate intake is sufficient. Manic patients may decorate themselves with cosmetics until they have a garish appearance and wear brightly colored clothes in rather unusual arrangements. Numerous tinkling, jangling objects may be part of their costume. Some patients may remove their clothing and make erotic overtures to those around them.

THERAPEUTIC TASKS

If the manic patient is first observed by the nurse in his home, an early referral may be made and hospitalization avoided. Environmental manipulation may be of therapeutic value to the hypomanic patient who is chronically unable to express his anger at being taken advantage of by family members. Treatment by the psychiatrist is most likely to be a combination of lithium carbonate, antipsychotics, and psychotherapy. Hospitalization may be required in acute states. Psychotherapy will not be of the uncovering type because discussion of conflict material may increase the overactivity. In these instances, psychotherapy will be rather direct reassurance. In the past, electroconvulsive therapy, narcosis therapy, hydrotherapy, and other types of treatment were used for manic patients. These methods are still used by some psychiatrists here and in other countries. Hydrotherapy is a major part of treatment in the Soviet Union.

Therapy advised by the physician or psychiatrist may be reinforced by the nurse. Nurses are usually nonthreatening and can often help a family member take responsibility for seeing that the hypomanic patient takes his medications and gets needed rest. In the nursing care of manic patients in the acute phase, the principal aim is to prevent exhaustion. Directing the patient, distracting him, setting limits, and administering his medications to provide relief from overactivity are main points in nursing care. The patient must be protected from himself. His sensorium is clear except in very severe mania, his memory is good, and his judgment is somewhat impaired.

The nurse must also assess the potentials of the patient and enlist his aid in his care. Examination of his body for neglected cuts and bruises or other traumata is important, as are observation and communication to him of the signs of his physical and mental state in a concerned and noncritical manner. For example, "You are really keyed up around these people. Here is your coat. We are going for a walk."

Manic patients can be hypercritical of others, and the nurse should be prepared for criticism of dress, makeup, coiffure, and perfume. If something about your appearance does not suit the patient, he will let you know about it. If the nurses are men, other criticisms may be made. Few are exempt. Amorous overtures to particular psychiatrists and/or nurses may be made by the manic patient. When they are absent, he may compose long amorous letters and poems to these individuals and fill their mailboxes.

The following patient is an example of someone who did not wait to be asked questions.

The patient, Tom G., is a forty-eight-year-old edentulous man who was admitted to the psychiatric unit after he visited the local newspaper office and made plans to start his own paper. His girl friend had just been arrested for disturbing the peace and the patient did not have thirty-five dollars to bail her out. He telephoned his father and threatened to kill him or himself if the father did not give him the thirty-five dollars; so the father telephoned the police. The patient has had several previous admissions. On admission, he states that he is a professional poker player and that he bet seventeen thousand dollars on one card and lost. He is euphoric, irritable, has a short attention span, pressure of speech, and increased motor activity. He has been unable to sleep for three or four nights. As the nursing student approaches him at the door to the nurses' station, the patient initiates the conversation:

Patient: You want to talk with me, don't you?
Student: Yes, my name is Nancy C. Let's sit down.
Patient: I need a cigarette first. Get me a cigarette and you can ask me all the questions you like. (Student gets a cigarette from the office for him and returns.)

Patient: O.K., ask me anything you like.
Student: Why are you here?
Patient: Them damn police brought me here because of my father. I knew it was him. I came early this morning. I've been here five or six times. This ain't the only place I been either. I like it here. I know all the staff. The people are very warm and human. Excuse me for a minute (gets up and gives his cigarette to another patient). (Sits down and scratches his ear, rubs his eyes and face. Gets up again and asks for a cigarette from another patient walking by, is in constant motion.)
Student: What medication are you on at home?
Patient: Lithium. I'm supposed to take it five times a day but I'm *very* busy. I do a lot of running around. I'm a street man and I don't like carrying pills around with me (opens a stick of chewing gum and pops it into his mouth). I'm chewing gum to satisfy my oral gratification, sucking, chewing, biting, eating, sex, and drinking. You know I'm excited and depressed at the same time (gets up and gives the rest of his cigarette to another patient).

The role of the student during this contact was to assess the mental status of the patient and help him to think about his future plans. The patient continued to speak freely of his condition and his life. At the meeting of the psychiatric team, the student presented her findings, the patient was placed back on lithium, 300 mg five times daily, discharged, and referred to the outpatient team for follow-up.

ENVIRONMENT

The protected *environment* of the hospital itself aids the patient, who is relieved of the demands of job or housekeeping and family duties and surrounded by helping persons. The acutely manic patient is easily stimulated by bright colors, loud sounds, and other people. The nurse may use soothing, restful music as an aid. Maintaining the same nurses and providing a private room without bright lights and colors can help. Acutely excited patients may require the constant attention of at least one nurse because they tend to be impulsive and easily distracted. Visitors are inadvisable. After the acute phase is over, manic patients may then be eased into group activities.

NUTRITION AND ELIMINATION

The manic patient is overactive and therefore too busy to eat. A high-vitamin, high-caloric diet will help prevent exhaustion and weight loss. In acute manic states, patients should be weighed daily. Frequent small meals will be taken by the overactive patient who is too busy to sit down and eat. He should be given finger food such as sandwiches, apples, celery, carrot sticks, and raisins or other dried fruit that can be taken and eaten *en passant.* Offering milk shakes and other fluids and holding the glass to prevent the patient from trying to throw it is one way to get him to take nutrients. Constipation is a problem but can be prevented by attention to intake of nutrients and fluids.

PERSONAL HYGIENE

The manic patient needs assistance with personal hygiene. Clothing should be durable and easily put on and removed. The excited patient has no time for tedious fasteners and other complex arrangements, although he may festoon himself with available baubles. It is important to help the patient to control the use of cosmetics and jewelry. A male patient may take a quick shave upon suggestion. Since he is likely to hit only the high spots, someone else may have to complete the job. Bathing may present a problem with the busy, overactive patient. Assist him to gather needed articles for bathing; otherwise he may come from the bathroom *au naturel* looking for something like the soap! Attention should be given to the coiffure, nails, and oral hygiene of the manic patient, as well as to the maintenance of his wardrobe. The nurse should be alert to the fact that foreign objects may be stuffed into body orifices. During the bath a nurse can ascertain whether the patient has received any injuries during the day that might have gone unobserved.

Items from other patients may have been purloined. This may come to light only when the patient is getting his clothes ready for the laundry and emptying his pockets. Discreet return of such items to their rightful owners may avoid numerous headaches. Manic patients often change clothes several times a day and they may enter the rooms of others for their clothing. Preventive measures such as asking other patients to keep their belongings inside cupboards and drawers can be instituted, as well as discussing this behavior at community meetings.

SOMATIC COMPLAINTS

Because these patients are so keyed up, they only inadvertently inform you about something that should receive attention, such as chest pain or bleeding from some body orifice. If the patient has flight of ideas, he will include any symptoms in his flight of ideas. The alert nurse will *regard every complaint* with seriousness, explore it, record it, and bring it to the attention of the physician. Although the patient's primary diagnosis may be of psychogenic origin, he may develop other problems during the course of his disorder. Be careful to avoid the trap of considering only people's psychological needs when you are in a psychiatric facility.

SETTING LIMITS

Manic patients are into everybody else's business, and occupy themselves by arranging and rearranging things. Limits must be set upon their behavior within their ability to respond in order to aid them in their group relationships and to prevent exhaustion.

MEDICATIONS

Administration of medications may pose a nursing problem. A refusal at one moment may be acceptance at the next. Make use of the suggestibility and distractibility of the manic patient, diverting his attention when required and directing it to the task at hand. You might talk about something else, have the medications in one hand and a paper cup of water in the other, and say firmly and directly, "Mr. Z., here are your medications, open your mouth," as you hold the medicine cup to his lips. Medications may have to be given by parenteral routes if the patient will not take them orally. All efforts should be made to administer medications with the least amount of exertion on the part of the patient. Usually at least one nurse on duty will be able to give the patient his medications orally. I have seen patients who would take medications only from other patients but would take them faithfully in this manner. A manic patient may hoard lithium and other medications for patients who are "worse off than I am" or for "more difficult times." Some patients with recurrent episodes may persuade a new psychiatrist to give them larger doses than they really need for the purpose of hoarding.

SLEEP AND REST

Although most people need their daily rest, manic patients may not feel the need for sleep. Removing exciting stimuli from the patient's environment in the early evening will help prepare him for sleep. Playing a quiet game of cards or chess, or quiet conversation, a hot bath, warm milk, and a back massage will encourage sleep. These patients may go off to bed at their regular hour and awaken two hours later fully refreshed; adequate doses of medication may be required to ensure a full night's sleep. It is up to the patient and the nurse to make these judgments and request needed medication from the attending psychiatrist. Often orders for medication for excited patients are written *pro re nata*. As the mania subsides, patients sleep without so much medication; they also begin to gain weight. It is the nurse's responsibility to be aware of the amount of sleep a manic patient gets and to suggest tapering off the sleeping medication as soon as this is feasible. Enforcing daily rest periods can also help prevent exhaustion.

DIRECTING ACTIVITY

The excess energy of the manic patient should be directed into constructive channels. Exercise requiring the large-muscle groups is appropriate if it is done in moderation. The excited patient cannot concentrate on precise work. In the hospital unit, making beds and exercising are suitable. If the patient can safely perform his part of the chores in the milieu of the hospital unit, it will help his group relationships, which may have suffered as a result of his impulsive behavior. These chores may sometimes be done after most of the other patients have gone out, in order to avoid overstimulation. Running, gymnastics, splashing in the swimming pool, walking, and building something are all appropriate activities.

Patients with bipolar affective disorders will most likely have recurrences. Preventive techniques can be used to avoid extreme mania. An example is discussing with the patient how he feels when he is approaching a manic state and advising him how to get help. One patient I know regularly signs herself into the hospital when she becomes aware of symptoms; previously she was taken to the hospital by the police.

Patients may now also be treated by their family physicians before they spiral into the dangerous delirious manic state. The overactive patient may also fall into the schizoaffective diagnostic category. The aim of nursing care in this group will also be toward pevention of exhaustion in addition to employing the techniques necessary for working with schizophrenic patients (see Chap. 9). Patients with delirious mania may have developed it gradually, going through the two previously described states of hypomania and acute mania. However, in some instances, a full-blown delirious mania may develop suddenly. The patient is incoherent, and his sensorium is clouded in all three spheres. He is highly overactive for no seeming purpose. Hallucinations and delusions are likely to be present. Exhaustion may be quickly reached, and signs of dehydration appear (e.g., dry mouth and lips, flushed face, fast pulse, and fever) unless preventive measures are initiated quickly.

From a psychotherapeutic standpoint, a goal is to aid the patient to progress to where he can consciously regard loneliness and separation without overactivity.

Care of the overactive patient is demanding for the nurse, who must be keenly aware of the "contagiousness" of his overactivity. As patients recover and spend weekends and other times at home before discharge, the nurse also aids them in dealing with lonely feelings by being an available and interested listener and reflecting feelings.

Following are descriptions of two manic patients:

The patient, Helen R., is a thirty-three-year-old

rotund woman admitted to the psychiatric unit in a very hyperactive state. Her husband states that she has slept very little for three days. Dancing and singing, she now exhibits increased psychomotor activity, pressure of speech, and flight of ideas. She is wearing a shocking pink pantsuit and a dramatic hairdo with her jet-black hair in a tall pouf and flowing down her back with a red rose on the side. She wears another red rose laid just inside her blouse—"just like the one I put in my mother-in-law's coffin," she informed the nurse. (The death of her mother-in-law was thought to have precipitated her admission.) She wore rings on all her fingers, heavy makeup, and three necklaces. She approached every newcomer with the prospect of selling vitamins and collected names and addresses in a notebook on which she had inscribed in bold, block letters HELEN OF TROY. She also carried around several newspaper clippings about diets, which she wanted everyone to read. On the ward, at other times, she was constantly cleaning; she made all the beds in the women's dorms for one week. To the men around her, she made erotic gestures and remarks and took it upon herself to watch over a dependent, depressed patient. She also promised everybody a job at a prominent downtown hotel, a diamond ring, or some other luxury selected just for that person.

The treatment of the patient included milieu therapy, individual psychotherapy, and lithium carbonate. After about a week, she became calmer and in about three weeks was back to her normal mood.

This episode began when the following patient's thesis was due:

Larry R., twenty-six years old, is a graduate student at a local university. He is elated, in constant motion, has pressure of speech, flight of ideas, is dehydrated and exhausted. He characterizes himself as "one Chinaman against the world." He has not shaved for several days and his clothing is soiled. Larry's parents state that he has not slept in a week but, instead of sleeping, has remained up all night, cooking, arranging and rearranging all of his books, writing, rewriting, and throwing away notes for his thesis. In the hospital, he is placed on lithium therapy and in the locked unit.

What nursing measures would you institute for this patient and why? Stop now and think through the situation. Discuss your ideas with someone else.

The Process of Grief and Mourning

Grief is a sequence of subjective states that follow loss and accompany mourning. Mourning indicates a broad range of reactions to loss and also refers to symbols of loss such as widows' veils and black armbands. It is not a morbid condition; on the contrary, for the bereaved, absence of mourning is abnormal. Mourning comprises the set of psychological processes aroused by the loss of a love object. In a broad range of reactions to loss, these processes are linked together and result in healthy or unhealthy adaptation to reality. Loss is a crisis to which the helping person can aid the sufferer achieve a healthy adaptation. Mourning is analogous to inflammation in physiology; several signs and symptoms may be included.

In grief, the loss of a loved person makes the world seem poor and empty. Other serious deprivations, such as loss of freedom in institutionalization, loss of country, and loss of neighborhood, will also produce grief. In the grieving person who suffers from object loss there is no significant fall in self-esteem, but there is some self-accusation. In contrast with melancholia in which the object loss may be trivial and the causative factors largely internal, the emotional loss in grief is attributed to an object that has been strongly desired, wanted, or loved and has become part of the person's ego by a process of assimilation, incorporation, or introjection. A feeling of loss originates within the ego of the person; his hurt and disappointment generate hostile, angry feelings. The superego turns these feelings against the incorporated object and the ego, and the patient experiences the pain of depression.

PHASES OF GRIEF AND MOURNING

Bowlby (1968) describes four phases of grief and mourning. The first is the phase of numbing, the initial shock phase; the second phase has outbursts of anger or other distress signs; the third is yearning for the lost figure, a searching in the mind for the lost figure; and the fourth is healing and reorganization.

Consider the experiences of loss that you observe in patients under your care: those who lose body parts (organ or limb); those whose body images change for other reasons; those who lose their homes because of a disaster, moving, or relocation (as in urban renewal); those who are dying; those who are bereaved; and those who lose pet animals. For a picture of the loss complex, add to these loss of money, job status, hearing, vision, sexual drive, and the ability to move about. The wish to remain whole and intact is fundamental to the human being. Since the first part of the ego to develop is the body image, changes in it arouse the most emotional resistance (Rochlin, 1965). What Spitz and Wolf (1946) called anaclitic depression is now included in the loss complex (Levin, 1965, p. 209). Everyone at some time experiences grief and mourning. Persons rebuffed or rejected, as in divorce and broken love affairs, may also experience the process.

There is a basic overall pattern of grief and mourning in adults, amounting to a definite syndrome in acute grief. Intense emotional pain is felt: a feeling of loneliness accompanied by tightness in the throat, choking, sighing, crying, and an empty feeling in the abdomen. Others may vomit, lack muscular power, or feel another intense subjective distress described as tension or anguish. A feeling of emptiness prevails, and the mourner tends to avoid people, preferring to be left alone. Images of association with the deceased constantly occupy the individual's waking life. The mourner reviews all aspects of his life with the deceased; the fact that the love object no longer exists requires that the life energy be withdrawn from the lost love object (Freud, 1917). There is a struggle between reality and what used to be, with reality gaining ascendancy as the natural outcome.

The amount of time required for accomplishing grief work is an individual matter, but time is an important factor in giving needed help. The helping person must be at the patient's side right from the start.

Waiting until the mourning period is over is useless, because by this time resolution will have been achieved, possibly in an unhealthy manner. For a healthy resolution, preventive techniques must be initiated early. In one community, quiet visitors from the mental-health center keep the mourner company, wash the dishes, and help with other chores. In other communities such concern is shown by neighbors and church members.

During the time of grief and mourning, the bereaved is overwhelmed by a sense of helplessness and a concern that perhaps he could have done something to prevent the death. Tears and sobbing come without warning when memories of the deceased occur, when friends visit, and when sympathy is offered. The mourner lacks energy and feels as if he bears the burdens of the world. In the first phase of numbness, a definite sense of unreality prevails, as if all the happenings of the death were a bad dream. The voice of the deceased may be heard, as one hears voices or has mental images just before sleep, yet the mourner recognizes that it is unreal.

The mourner may evidence a loss of concern and warmth for others and show irritability and anger. He may wonder, "Why did this have to happen to me?" or, when reminded of the happy decades he spent with his love object, retort, "Well, I could have had a lot more!" The individual is overwhelmed with yearning for the lost object, and much of his mental life may be occupied with fantasies of its return.

The dream life of the mourner may be filled with nightmares, especially when there has been an accidental death of a loved one. Dreams of earlier relationships with the deceased may be frequent.

When the grief work is done, there is emancipation from bondage to the deceased; readjustments are made to the environment, and new relationships are formed. The lost object takes a different place in the individual's memory, and behavior is reorganized toward a new object.

A dramatic example of unresolved grief and mourning for a spouse is exemplified by Queen Victoria, who kept Albert's suite of rooms in the castle exactly as they were when he was alive. In addition, the queen commanded that fresh clothing be laid on his bed and water set in the basin every evening for nearly forty years.[11] Moreover, after his death *every bed* in which she slept had attached to it on the right-hand side, at the back above the pillow, a photograph of Albert as he lay dead.

In some cultures, such as the Anglo-American, thoughts and feelings with regard to loss are suppressed and deemphasized. In others, loss may be dramatized. Patients should be viewed within the context of their cultures. The bereaved plead for sympathy and support, express anger, and seek understanding. In our culture these aspects of grief are not easily expressed. If grief work is unaccomplished, the thoughts and behavior of the mourner are still directed toward the lost object, hostility may be displayed, unreasonable appeals for help may be made, and the presence of the deceased will be felt in the home. The household may be maintained as before, with clothes and other belongings of the deceased kept in their places. Insomnia may become a problem, accompanied by preoccupation with body functions. Persons close to the deceased may feel that they are getting the disease or condition that caused the death of their loved one. When this happens, family members finally agree or are self-impelled to seek out their physician. For each family member it is a time of reassessment of family roles and rearrangement of family tasks. Hostility may be directed to others, especially the physician, and some recrimination may be expressed for his ineffectiveness in preventing the death of the loved one.

Adults have difficulty with grieving in a family in which attachment behavior[12] is regarded without sympathy, for example, where crying is discouraged because it is "babyish" and "bad." When a person who has grown up in such a family suffers loss, he may be inclined to stifle his grief; members of his family are the least likely to be able to help. A girl whose family advocated courage and civilized behavior at all times especially in the face of adversity, lost her mother at the age of twelve years. She did not shed a tear. Six months later, when her horse died, she wept uncontrollably.

During national tragedies (as, for example, when John F. Kennedy, Martin Luther King, and Robert Kennedy were assassinated), oceans of tears are shed by people who bottled up their feelings when disaster struck closer to home. For the first time in history, mass worldwide grief and mourning have become possible. The therapeutic effects on many people throughout the world of simultaneous mourning for a lost leader has been neither noted nor measured, but the possibility merits consideration.

Death, Dying, and Bereavement

One of the ways to learn about death is to recall your first experience with it. Attitudes toward death are strongly conditioned by the strength of the ties that integrate the individual with the social organization. The problem for each of us is how not to die alone. The first contact with death has important implications for lifelong attitudes toward it. Stop now and think of the first death you recall. Share your thoughts with another person. My first memory is of my grandmother wrapped in a shroud and lying on a red couch. For years I carried this image until I checked it out with someone who had also attended her funeral. In actuality, my grandmother had been lying in a white casket, not on a red couch. What I had done in converting the image was associate the color of blood (red) with death.

In nursing and medicine, there is now an intellectual social awakening to the needs of dying patients. This movement was spearheaded by Glaser and Strauss (1965) and Jeanne C. Quint (1967), who worked together at the University of California at San Francisco in a six-year research project that

---

[11] Strachey, Lytton: *Queen Victoria.* New York: Blue Ribbon Books, 1921, pp. 402–404.

[12] Attachment behavior refers to instinctive behavior in animals. The function of attachment behavior is protection from predators.

gathered data from five schools of nursing in the Bay Area.[13]

People prepare for their own deaths through experiencing those of pets, friends, classmates, and acquaintances as well as the deaths of family members and other loved ones. In out culture, only the aged are likely to refer to death in open conversation. Children and other young people may never have seen anyone die (except via the mass media) or been in the presence of a dying person. Death is denied in many ways, and various avoidance techniques are common in our culture, as shown by the many euphemisms relating to death.

In the hospital, reference to the dying person as the "terminally ill" or "the patient with a negative prognosis" and, in some cases, the furtive removal of the body to the morgue testify to these avoidance techniques. Funeral directors advertise the installment buying of funerals as "sunrise plans" and advise buyers of the services to purchase the watertight vault. In the funeral home, the corpse (man or woman) is often made up to look "lifelike," even if the person never wore makeup. The euphemisms describing death and the attempts of morticians to preserve bodies act as defenses for our helplessness in the face of death. The corpse is viewed in a "slumber room," and the deceased is referred to as the "dear departed."

At one time in America, the corpse was washed by close friends, wrapped in a shroud, and buried in a pine box.

CULTURAL BELIEFS ABOUT THE DYING

The belief in an afterlife is pancultural. For the Buddhist, it is nirvana; for the Scandinavians, Valhalla; for the pre-Christian Greeks, Elysium; for the Persians, the Abode of Song; and for the Western world, heaven. Nirvana may be achieved at death, but it may also be achieved in life, when the spiritual struggle over karma has

[13] For her pioneer work on the nurse and the dying patient, Jeanne Quint Benoliel was recognized by her profession at the American Nurses' Association Convention, Atlantic City, 1976.

brought to an end the series of deaths and rebirths, and the long-sought state of extinguishedness ends the need of another rebirth.

A primitive view regarding death was that provision for the physical needs of the deceased helped him to a longer life after death. Archeologists have been able to describe previous cultures after studying their grave sites. The glorious treasures of the burial chambers of Tutankhamen show us, more than three thousand years after his death, the power of the belief in an afterlife. Fear of touching a corpse derives from the idea of death as something that comes and gets you.

Among the Romans, the attitude toward a corpse was mystical and supernatural; contact with one was alarming. However, the Romans did not manifest so much a fearful attitude toward spirits as they did an interest and desire through ritual to effect communion of the upper and lower worlds. The *dies parentales* held in February were holidays for performance of appeasement rites to the dead. The *lemuria* in May allowed the Romans to rid themselves of anxiety by spitting out black beans and saying, "With these I redeem me and mine," thereby banishing the spirits (Bendann, 1930). Holbein's series of engravings show Death as a dancing skeleton with clinging pieces of putrefied flesh, gathering people to him as he sees fit. The artist Rowlandson's *Dance of Death* deals with a similar theme.

The motif of the death dance is found in French literature and folk songs from the thirteenth century through the high point of its popularity, the middle of the sixteenth century. In the theme of the three dead and three living men (Huizinga, 1924; de Caumont, 1886), three young noblemen meet three hideous dead men who tell them of their past grandeur and warn the noblemen of their imminent end. One can see this theme in the frescoes of the Campo Santo at Pisa, the oldest pictorial form of the death dance. The Church of the Innocents at Paris, which has been destroyed, had carvings on the same theme. A "dance of the dead" was actually performed in fifteenth-century France.

Since the thirteenth century, the mendicant orders had admonished the populace about death to such an extent that there were public outcries against the practice. By the fifteenth century the engraver and the carver made the dance of death graphic as well. The theme was widely dispersed throughout central and western Europe, possibly due to the revival of trade and commerce and the renewal and growth of city life. In addition to poetry, folksongs, sculptures, woodcuts, manuscripts, performances, miniatures, and tapestries portrayed the dance of death. It represented or reflected the feeling of the populace toward the warnings made by the Church, but it also showed that death was the great equalizer in that it took away pope, cardinal, bishop, friar, and priest. Wars and plagues made death a common acquaintance.

BURIAL CUSTOMS

The burial customs of the Middle Ages were a constant reminder of death. Cemeteries were the preferred places of burial, and rich and poor were buried without distinction. Because of the belief that the human body decomposed in nine days, bodies were quickly disinterred to make room for others; skulls and bones were heaped up along the cloisters and left for all to see. During the plagues, corpses were collected in the streets and piled in the charnel houses for mass burials. The rulers and potentates were put to rest in the cathedrals, frequently in coffins carrying life-sized representations of the decedents on their lids. The urge to be buried in home soil led English soldiers abroad to cut up dead warriors (as was done with Henry V), boil the remains, and return them to the homeland.

In the daily life of the medieval person, death was preached from the pulpit, bones of skeletons were stacked for all to see, and the power of death was omnipresent. On the way home from wars or from tilling the soil, the medieval person probably thought of heaven, and of angels, devils, and death. Appearances of the latter were familiar from cathedral sculptures, chapel frescoes, descriptions by priests, and the visible skeletons serving as daily reminders that Death could strike at any time. The

dance of death glorified death; the realism of death helped popularize the idea. Without warning and without acceptance of bribes, Death dragged human beings of all stations and ages into the dance and rejoiced.

PRESENT CUSTOMS

The contrast afforded by today's customs is marked, for the starkness of death is hidden away discreetly in hospitals, funeral homes, and distant cemeteries. People are usually taken to a hospital to die, and their care is turned over to the hospital personnel. When death does come, the body is removed immediately, impersonally, and even furtively. At one sanitarium situated high on a hill, corpses were sent to the bottom of the hill on a trolley running through a specially constructed tunnel, like soiled laundry down the chute. Although this measure was conceived to protect the patients from the sight of the corpse, all of them knew exactly when the trolley began its descent.

National mourning for great persons has become familiar to all of us; flags are at half-mast, schools close, work stops, and the funeral is televised for all to watch in the privacy of their own homes.

Following deaths in America, black and purple wreaths are sometimes placed on the front doors of houses; men occasionally wear black armbands, and women dress in black and sometimes wear mourning veils. The hearse is black and, in military funerals, the caisson and horses are black.

A cross-cultural study made of 127 elderly San Franciscans showed that death was the most frequently reported stress (Anderson, 1964). The loss of a spouse represented death's most serious threat to native Americans. Some Europeans, however, gave the loss of mother as the greatest of life's stresses. Persons with religious affiliations reported the death of loved ones as stressful more often than did persons without expressed religious affiliations. Women mentioned death more often than men, but men elaborated more upon the circumstances of death, the process of dying and the ordeal of death itself. Men also showed greater empathy in that they expressed suffering for the afflicted, whereas the women in their death recalls did not give empathy as the primary feeling. They were more likely to speak of the effect of the consequences of loss upon themselves, e.g., the misery of managing alone. In this study it was determined that loss of spouse was most stressful to the poor.

THERAPEUTIC TASKS

Ambivalence is common in mourning and is perhaps the cause of the intense pain of bereavement. Freud said in *Mourning and Melancholia* (1917) that no one gives up a love object, that there is a fixation of the memory of the lost object.

The work of mourning, the grief work, can be centered around a pool of shared images. Talking about the deceased with a friend or therapist will help create these. Some widows form groups that meet regularly for years and share remembrances of happier times and experiences with their spouses. The therapeutic potential of interpersonal relationships is mobilized and put to use in widow-to-widow programs organized in community mental-health programs. One such program noted that lending a friendly ear and a shoulder to cry on and helping other family members to be considerate were all of benefit to the bereaved widow (Silverman, 1969). People participating in these programs will remind a newly bereaved widow that the deceased husband would have liked her to do things in a certain way that will restore her equilibrium. The pain of bereavement is gradually neutralized by discussing the deceased in great detail. When the work of mourning is done, an unpainful picture of the loved one emerges, to be stored in the memory and recalled without suffering. The following is an example of unfinished grief work completed years later.

The patient, a young boy now sixteen years old, son of a prostitute, was placed in an institution by his mother at the age of two years. Later on he lived in foster homes. He was followed up by his psychiatrist several times a year in an effort to maintain continuity of the relationship (Bowlby, 1968). The boy made a plan to find his mother and then go to America to find his father, who he thought was an American serviceman. He discussed the plan with the psychiatrist, who listened but did not criticize it, although he thought it was quite impracticable. Eventually the boy told the therapist that he believed the plan was difficult to accomplish and that even if he succeeded in it, he might not be welcomed by his parents.

The boy finally came to accept this own reality: If he found his lost parents, they would be strangers. Maybe they would not be so glad to see him. He had a picture in which the lost person was present and one in which the person was gone. Someone's listening to him and showing care and sympathy helped him work through his conflicting images.

Immortality may be discussed and ideas about it reviewed. It is a very personal subject and may be expressed in terms of belief in an afterlife. Identification with the deceased may occur, not in the sense of one's becoming more like the dead person, but by retaining the image of the loved one painlessly through accepting certain thoughts and feelings.

CATHARSIS

One of the principal therapeutic tasks should be aimed toward securing catharsis, which can be defined as an effective discharge of feelings with resultant relief. It is the healthful release of thoughts and feelings through "talking it out" and experiencing the appropriate emotional reactions. If anger is expressed openly, the person gets over it. One newly bereaved widow beat up the physician; other people may get angry at the nurses. The climate can be set by the nurse for expression of angry feelings. Take the initiative to become acquainted with the family.

Nurses can take family members aside and help them to express their feelings about the dying patient. If the family knows that anger toward the physician and others may occur, it may help to advise them to engage in physical exercise for release of aggressive feelings. A long walk can be immensely helpful. Older family members who have experienced loss before and who understand the feelings may be enlisted to aid the younger ones during the crisis. An example of how a nursing student helped one family follows:

A student, during a visit to Mr. and Mrs. J., learned that a grandson's divorced mother and father had just died within a few weeks of each other. Besides helping Mr. and Mrs. J. with their own grief and mourning about the loss of their son and former daughter-in-law, the student felt that they needed assistance in helping their grandson in this crisis. Since the new stepmother seemed unable to help Tommy, the student talked with Mrs. J. (the stronger one of the retired couple) about helping Tommy to express his feelings, informing his teachers about the loss of his parents, and getting the school counselor to talk with Tommy, all of which were carried out.

The manner in which grief is expressed is determined by the previous relationship with one's mother or mother substitute. If the person feels self-reproach or guilt, he needs someone who will listen to him. Thoughts that appear real to him may seem unreal to the therapist. The nurse can help the bereaved review their relationship with the deceased. A mourner who feels self-reproach or guilt needs to perceive the positive aspects of his relationship to the deceased and may require reassurances from the nurse that he did all he could to help the deceased get well or die without pain.

The unresolved grief of Doctor Zhivago resulted in his thinking that he saw his loved one on the street after the revolution. Pursuing this image, he met his death (Pasternak, 1958). The therapist's work is to determine the feeling that is to be expressed and to help the mourner express it. If the person tries to turn back time he may become involved in a painful struggle with the past. If encouraged, however, to return to the time of bereavement and to review it in detail with a friend, relative, or therapist, a much better chance of relieving sorrow is possible. To give words to sorrow is important. The mourner's helper or therapist serves as a companion who gives emotional support and who has time to discuss hopes, desires, plans for the future, regrets, reproaches, and disappointments.

We help our patients decide their own reality, as in the following example:

Mrs. P, a patient who developed metastatic cancer, was greatly worried about her aged mother, who lived across the country. The old woman lived alone and held firmly to independence without accepting needed aid from physicians and acquaintances. The patient, preparing for her own death, was greatly relieved when she received news of her mother's death.

If the patient has not had time to grieve and mourn, as during a disaster or war, time and place should be set aside to complete the grief work. The treatment during World War II of grief-stricken Royal Air Force officers by T. F. Main (1968) is an example. The officers were removed from active duty with a diagnosis of combat fatigue. They had lost all their buddies and sat and stared, neither eating nor moving. Main hypothesized that they needed time and a place for grieving. Each was then given a dark room for a few days with no interruptions, except for meals, in order to accomplish his grief work. Often this treatment was sufficient.

People need privacy to give vent to their feelings in our culture; many cannot cry in the presence of others. The nurse can ask others to leave the bereaved alone or may ask the grieving patient to go to a secluded place. The climate is thereby set for the expression of sorrow, and the patient is encouraged to assume his role obligation of discussing feelings of loss, guilt, rage, and hostility if they are present.

Nurses should also help the patient who has lost a roommate or neighbor by death to express his feelings about the event. In a psychiatric unit, death is quite rare, but when it happens, it should be handled in a matter-of-fact manner and announced to the patients. Enough staff should be present at that time to help the patients express their thoughts and feelings within a group. Time must be found to accomplish this task.

HELPING CHILDREN VIEW DEATH

The age and level of development of the individual determine his manner of expression of grief. We need to know more about how children and adolescents express their feelings about death. One of the best films about how children view death is *Forbidden*

Games. Some family members may consider it strange that children and adolescents do not cry but instead continue playing baseball or their other usual activities. If the young people cannot verbalize, these exercises may be their catharsis; in fact, the young mourner may display fierce competition. Retiring into seclusion to listen to music or a particular achievement at school may be other forms of catharsis. The child's behavior at a time of death is a dramatic example of the need to look beyond manifest behavior for understanding people and being able to help them. "Manifest behavior with analysis of its corresponding conflicts is a notoriously unreliable index to an understanding of psychology on a level that is beyond behaviorism."[14]

Parents who are experiencing loss, as of a spouse, need assistance in expressing their thoughts and feelings. They can be helped not to deny their feelings while in the presence of their children, but to express them. On the other hand, they can be advised to avoid becoming hysterical around the children. One child whose mother had died and whose father explained that she was dead and would be buried in the ground the next day asked him, "How will she breathe and who will feed her?" (Barnes, 1964). Children may feel that the death of a mother is contagious and avoid a friend whose mother has just died. If children see death only as sleep, which is one of the more common ways that parents explain death to a very young child, they may fear sleep themselves and be unable to take naps and go to sleep at night. Clearly stating to a child that a dead person does not breathe, eat, or sleep may help him to better understand death.

A bereaved child may blame the surviving parent for his loss. Many children cannot cry at the death of parents because they are angry at being left alone. The surviving parent may be so absorbed in his own grief that he forgets about the child.

A six-year-old girl lost her younger sister and her mother's attention and denied and repressed her hostility at that time (Lampl-deGroot, 1976). Reconstruction of the

event in psychoanalysis at the age of twenty revealed that the affect and mode of mourning were similar to that of the adult and thus this early experience contributed to the patient's tendency to be depressed.

The life-style of the family will affect their capacity for tension management and emotional support at the loss of one of its members. If you consider the death of Senator Robert Kennedy, and the help given to the children at the time of their loss, you have an example of children's involvement in the reality of the situation of death. It is of importance to note that the life-style of the Kennedy family includes much support for its children. On the night that Robert Kennedy was shot, family friends checked the bedrooms of the children; thirteen-year-old David was found to have watched the tragedy of his father's death on television. The family friend held David in his own arms, giving him body contact comfort, and stayed in the room to share his grief (Caplan, 1968). The older children with the stronger egos were brought to their father's hospital room. The involvement of the children in the funeral—for example, standing guard at the casket; one was a pallbearer—kept them within the family circle during this tragedy.

The child can easily and immediately transfer affectional ties to a mother substitute. (The adult analog would be the widow who quickly remarries following the death of her husband.) The mourning period gives the adult mourner time for detaching emotional energy from the lost object. Only after a longer period of time does the adult mourner make the transfer. Denial is very strong in children. One child said, "If my mother were dead, then I would be all alone" (Wolfenstein, 1966). Here the child's concept of death is one of abandonment. He cannot conceive of his mother leaving him; therefore, he cannot conceive of her death.

With children, there may also be magical thinking for the mother to return; it serves to bring back the lost parent. Children in a group may avoid talking of death if one of their members has lost a parent. Regression is common, often characterized by a return to thumbsucking and clinging to dolls. Games of playing dead enable chil-

---

[14] Rochlin, Gregory: *Griefs and Discontents: The Forces of Change.* Boston: Little, Brown & Co., 1965, p. 59.

dren to act out their feeling about death. Displacement onto animals may also occur; their concern about the animals may actually represent concern for the dead parent. An active child may suddenly become quite passive or a naughty child unusually well behaved.

There is a difference of opinion about the age at which mourning can occur. Bowlby says it may occur at six months of age. Anna Wolf (1957–1958) writes that between the ages of five and nine children may grasp the finality of death but not until ten or eleven can they have something approaching adult comprehension of death. On the other hand, a child may intellectually understand death but the emotional impact will be too much for him. According to Furman (1964), mourning is dependent upon the ability to have a concept of death. The age that this ability occurs may certainly vary in different children.

ADOLESCENCE AND MOURNING

Adolescence can be considered the initiation into mourning; it must be experienced before the individual can perform grief work in reaction to future losses. Some view adolescence as a trial mourning itself, the breaking off of childhood ties and the detachment from parental figures. Adolescence then may be thought of as a necessary prerequisite for the mourning process. It is important not to confuse normal adolescent behavior and conflicts with the work of mourning. The renunciation of childhood may be accompanied by much pain unrelated to death.

In the adolescent mourner, particularly boys, crying may be considered a sign of weakness and will not be evident. The glorified and idealized parent of childhood is returned to in fantasy life. Mourning at a distance may occur, as in the previously cited example of the twelve-year-old whose mother died and who remained stoical but cried profusely when her horse died. Mastery may be returned to as in childhood, where a very detailed verbal account of the death is given to another.

DYING, BUT NOT ALONE

Apart from this lying, or in consequence of it, the most wretched thing of all for Ivan Ilyich was that nobody pitied him as he yearned to be pitied. At certain moments, after a prolonged bout of suffering, he craved more than anything—ashamed as he would have been to own—for someone to feel sorry for him just as if he were a sick child. He longed to be petted, kissed, and wept over, as children are petted and comforted. He knew that he was an important functionary, that he had a beard turning grey, and that therefore what he longed for was impossible; but nevertheless he longed for it. And in Gerassim's attitude toward him there was something akin to what he yearned for, and so Gerassim was a comfort to him. Ivan Ilyich feels like weeping and having someone to pet him and cry over him, but in comes his colleague Shebek and instead of weeping and being petted Ivan Ilyich puts on a grave, stern, profound air, and by force of habit expresses his opinion on a decision of the Court of Appeal, and obstinately insists on it. The falsity around him and within him did more than anything else to poison Ivan Ilyich's last days."[15]

The process of dying can only be experienced by the dying person himself. However, it is thought that the dying person goes through a process of grief and mourning for his own death. The last phase of life brings with it what was previously thought to be detachment from objects, but which now is viewed as an introspective involvement in holding one's self together. An extreme fear of death may be due to primitive fears of abandonment stemming from childhood. Kubler-Ross's study of over two hundred dying patients resulted in a description of five stages of the process of dying: (1) denial and isolation, (2) anger, (3) bargaining, (4) depression, and (5) acceptance (Kubler-Ross, 1969). These stages are similar to the phases of grief and mourning described by Spitz (1945) and Bowlby (1968). In the assessment process the nurse must be sensitive to and aware of what the dying patient is experiencing. People are different; everybody does not experience dying in the same way.

Phase 1: Denial and Isolation. Denial is a

[15] Tolstoy, Leo: *The Death of Ivan Ilyich* (1886). Baltimore: Penguin Books, 1960, pp. 143–44.

defense mechanism that protects the ego. With the dying patient it is not interfered with and usually gives way later in the dying process. *Isolation* is a defense mechanism in which an intolerable act, idea, or impulse is separated out from the emotion connected with it. Isolation allows the dying patient to speak of death and life together. In this phase the dying person's response is "It cannot have happened to me."

Students often wish to hasten the process of verbalization of feelings with regard to death and fail to understand (in their own hastened learning process) that defense mechanisms actually function to protect the ego. A patient's fear of breaking down completely in front of the nurse or his family must be respected.

Phase 2: Anger: In this phase, dying patients may tend to blame others for their condition, complain of their care, and ring their call bell frequently. Patients should be able to vent their anger without nurses reacting personally to it.

To determine how much the patient knows about his condition, ask the physician what information he has given the patient, his chances of survival, and how much time he has left. Awareness of oblique ways in which some patients may express their feelings must be uppermost in your thoughts as you care for the patient. Probing for feelings is not the answer.

Phase 3: Bargaining: The bargaining state is characterized by attempts to negotiate with the helping persons for more time to live or for a few days without pain. It has three qualities: postponement of death, a reward for the patient who does the best that he can, and a self-determined deadline. Mr. L., who had Hodgkin's disease, "bargained" with the hospital staff to "go home once more for my son's birthday." Pulling himself together for this event, he did go and returned to the hospital only to die a few days later.

Phase 4: Depression: The feeling of loss occurs in this phase. The patient becomes depressed, and prepares himself for his own death.

Phase 5: Acceptance: In this phase the work of mourning for his own death has occurred and the person accepts the inevitable.

PERCEPTION OF DEATH

Patients come to their own realization of death at their own pace. They can see expectation of it in our eyes, our manner, and our faces. Dying patients pick up clues from their relatives with regard to their deaths. When dying is prolonged, the patient can feel changes within his own body and come to his own conclusions. The patient perceives a decline in energy level. He is aware of losing or gaining weight and, often, of increasing infirmity. He knows he must depend on others to assist him because he can no longer get up to go to the bathroom and bathe himself, for example. He feels other changes in his body, e.g., increased or decreased pulse and respiration. Answering a simple question such as "How sick are you?" may help your patient tell you what he knows about his condition. A dying patient may greet you with the announcement, "Nurse, I won't be here much longer." If the nurse is calm about her own feelings about death she will be able to sit with the patient, listen to what he has to say, help him express his sorrow, and repeat her visits. Nonverbal communication can be most meaningful to the patient in conveying that you care when words themselves may fail to do so.

Ask the family of the dying patient how the patient has reacted to a previous loss and about his philosophy of life. Relatives welcome the opportunity to talk about their loved ones. If there are no relatives or significant others, the nurse can get this information from the patient himself. Talking about what people live by is one approach. Another is to discuss the best and the most difficult things in life. Information about how previous losses have been met may be of help or they may not. New crises call for new adaptive mechanisms. It is no longer claimed that the same defenses hold forth throughout the life span. In hospitals where there is staff transiency and turnover, it is imperative that information be passed on to nurses on different shifts so that each nurse who enters a dying patient's room does not expect catharsis. Usually, in a hospital with many staff members, patients will feel closer to one or two nurses. Know about and consider these nurse–patient ties in making patient assignments. Similarly, if the human relationship has become important to the patient, the nurse will not break it off but will remain with the patient throughout his last days. Nurses may have guilt feelings about their dying patients, especially those on clinical assignments where death is frequent. Discuss these feelings with others as they occur.

Everybody needs a confidant. Find out if the patient has anyone who shows care and concern about what is happening to him and make it possible for that person to stay with the patient during his last hours. Be in tune with what your patient is experiencing. Students tend to look for formulas of behavior for themselves in relation to their dying patients. They sometimes blame the physician for not telling the patient what is happening to him. In discussing this matter in class one day, one student reported a change in her attitude when a young physician told her about a patient of his who committed suicide after he told her she was going to die.

THE NURSE'S ACCEPTANCE OF DEATH

Inasmuch as dying patients will discuss their own deaths with their nurses, if with anybody, it is essential that nurses examine their own thoughts and feelings about death as they care for patients. Fear of death is probably common to everyone.

Reviewing your earliest memories of death can aid in understanding feelings; sharing them with other students is also helpful. Many young people may never have experienced the death of a person, but almost everyone can recall the death and burial of a pet. Review what you did and what you felt the first time you had experience of death. Share your experiences with your peers. Although I had experienced death in my life several times before I went to nursing school, I still remember the first two dying patients I had, both of whom suffered from bacterial endocarditis. One was a twelve-year-old boy, the same age as one of my brothers. He was the youngest patient on the unit, a large men's medical

unit in a teaching hospital. The concern of the other patients in the sixty-bed unit was touching. I was the only night nurse, and I was assisted by one orderly. This dying boy's needs were anticipated by the other patients, who were very sick themselves.

In the uninitiated, feelings of despair and frustration may be evoked by the dying patient. Guilt may also be felt because of one's failure to help the dying person. To overcome these feelings, nurses and other helping persons often feel impelled to make frantic efforts to save patients—suggesting, for example, surgery, parenteral feedings, or oxygen. Nurses who witness multiple deaths in a short space of time, as in an intensive-care unit, or who otherwise take care of terminal patients need a defined place and time to discuss their feelings about dying and death. Such an arrangement is practiced in a cancer-research unit in a large medical center. The hospital chaplain attends weekly staff conferences; after the nurses ventilate their feelings about death, they proceed with the usual discussion of nursing problems. Weekly conferences for nursing staff in some intensive-care units are now held to assist nursing staff with their feelings about death.

STYLE OF DEATH

Everyone has a right to a dignified death. Nurses have a responsibility to the individual to assist him to die in the style that he chooses. Keep the patient as comfortable as possible. Instruct the family and all the staff that the sense of hearing is the last to leave the body. Admonish them to take care with what is said within the patient's presence even though he may appear totally insensitive to the world around him.

One of a person's greatest fears is that of dying alone. If no friend or relative is attending the patient in the last hours, stay with the patient yourself. Patients who are being treated in large medical centers often come from long distances and may therefore not have the comfort of their families when they are dying. Older people may not have surviving friends or relatives to be with them. Reassure your patients that you will be with them to the end.

Family members who are visiting the dying patient may feel quite lonely, and they too will need the nurse's assurance and assistance. They may feel they are not doing enough, or they may wish unconsciously to hasten the death. Guilt may also be present because of old, unresolved conflicts with the dying person.

ANTICIPATORY GRIEF[16]

It is thought that individuals who are assisted to work through anticipatory grief will also have been assisted in bereavement. To increase understanding of anticipatory grief, Hampe (1975) identified needs of twenty-seven persons with chronically ill terminal spouses: (1) *those related to the dying person:* to be with the dying spouse, to participate in the care of the dying spouse, to be assured of comfort of the dying spouse, and to be informed of the spouse's condition; (2) *those related to the mate:* to be informed of the impending death, to express own emotions, to be accepted, supported, and comforted by staff, and to have comfort and support from family members.

HOSPICE

The *hospice* movement is now providing a better way for terminally ill patients to die. Hospice service includes: attention to biopsychosocial needs, an interdisciplinary team (including volunteers), the family, structured staff support, and coordination of inpatient and outpatient care. Home, day, night, inpatient care, and bereavement counseling constitute complete hospice service. A hospice focuses on caring, a friendly, cheerful social environment, psychological and spiritual support, physical comfort, and control of pain and symptoms. The hospice movement is a humanistic approach to nursing care. Dr. Cicely Saunders opened St. Christopher's Hospice (London) in 1967. Two hundred groups in the United States are now planning or have opened a hospice (Brown, 1978). One hopes that this humanistic movement spreads to nursing homes and hospitals.

[16] Anticipatory grief is an awareness of an impending death/loss; it follows a pattern similar to bereavement.

PHYSICAL COMFORT

There are many books that deal with the physical needs of the dying patient. Following are suggestions of some things nurses can do to make the last days more pleasant for those who are dying. All things that we do for ourselves should be anticipated by the nurse and carried out without the patient's having to ask for them: oral hygiene for mouth breathing, care of the skin, repositioning, care of the hair and nails, helping the patient's intake by getting suitable foods, and observing the output. Assisting the patient with the body arts, such as shaving, shampooing, and applying makeup, will help the patient and the family by minimizing to some extent the ravages wrought by the disease in the patient's appearance. Personal care of this nature is invaluable to the patient, who is made to feel that someone cares for him and who gets the basic comfort of being touched. *It is important that these procedures be carried out until the end; they convey to the patient that someone still cares about him.*

ATTITUDES TOWARD DEATH

The nurse has a responsibility to help patients use their last moments to the fullest. The following is an excellent example of a caring staff:

Mr. C. had leukemia. He was in his late twenties, and had a wife and a three-year-old son. He was told by his physician that he had probably three months to a year to live and that he would be helped during his illness. The nursing staff and the physician helped him to plan his time so that he could be with his family as much as possible. He spent much of his time at home, returning to the hospital when he had an infection. Eight months later he went into terminal coma while in the hospital.

It should be noted that many people approach death with a minimum of fear. The following is an example of the serenity of an older person approaching ninety years of age. Her husband had predeceased her and three of her six children had died, one only two weeks earlier. She lived alone in the old house where she had spent most of her life. She told her visiting nursing student:

I don't really have a great fear of dying. In fact, sometimes when I get lonely, I almost pray that God will take me. I guess He just isn't quite ready for me yet.

The fear of dying can be present in any patient. The following situation is an example of a patient who verbalized his fear of death.

The patient is an old Italian man, Mr. B., who raised vegetables on the outskirts of the city when he was younger and now lives in the same house surrounded by subdivisions. He has a deeply lined face, a thin body, and an unsmiling demeanor. Now in his second week postsurgery in which he had a prostatectomy, he complains bitterly to all who will listen that his bed has been wet all night, that no one came to check him but the little Chinese girl, and that he is afraid that he is ready for Colma.[17] It was difficult to get across to the night staff that Mr. B. was very shy and could not bring himself to allow a young girl to change his dressings and his bed. As a result, he did not ask for help and no one took the initiative to check his bed. Mr. B. became more and more anxious and began to complain about the meals, the small bathroom, and being ready for Colma. The nursing staff became more and more irritated, held a conference, and decided to set limits on his behavior. They felt very pleased with themselves when Mr. B. stopped complaining. At this point they learned that he had developed a fistula and would require a colostomy as an interim measure. Then guilt arose in some of the nurses and they became very solicitous of the patient.

What are the nursing problems involved in the case described above? What actions would you have taken and why? Discuss them with others.

SPIRITUAL NEEDS

Nurses who are sensitive to the needs of the dying will give priority to these needs. Reading part of the patient's Bible to him may be a help; comfort may also be received from the presence of a minister or priest. Some dying patients who have

[17] The location of the burial grounds for citizens of San Francisco.

broken their ties with the Church may not think of asking for religious consolation until the nurse suggests that the chaplain come in and talk with them. The following situation is an example of how a nursing student helped a patient to establish contact with the minister of his church:

Mr. A. was diagnosed as having lung cancer and was told by his physician that he has perhaps two to three months to live. He is in a ward with three other men who have minor surgical problems. The student learned that the patient lives alone. He is divorced and his children live across the continent and do not write to him. The student, thinking of spiritual needs, asked the patient if he would like to see his minister. When the patient refused, the student pursued the matter until he told her that he had not gone to church for twenty or thirty years, that his old church was far across the country, and that he did not know any ministers. The student dropped the subject and went on to something else. Later, she found out the days the Episcopal minister regularly visited the hospital and arranged a meeting at which she told him about her patient, mentioning that he had a fatal disease, that he had not been to church for a long time, had no family in the area, and needed a friend. The minister agreed to visit the patient who, when he was subsequently informed of the fact, seemed pleased and relieved.

At the time of death even unbelievers may become believers or agnostics.

MEDICATIONS

Nurses sometimes require assistance in making decisions about whether to give p.r.n. (at their own discretion) medications to the dying person; they may feel that the patient himself should be consulted and his wishes honored during his final days. Judgment about pain medication requires a thorough knowledge of many factors: the patient's pain tolerance, severity of pain, and whether or not the patient himself wishes to remain aware of what is happening to him. A frank discussion with the patient may elicit his own thoughts and feelings about his style of dying. Some people wish to be fully conscious even when they are suffering. Incorporate the wishes of such patients and their families into your nursing-care plan and team conferences. Others prefer to be "knocked out" or "unaware." Time is also a factor in this type of decision. Many things need to be done: letters written, a will drawn up, farewells made to family and friends. These matters should not be delayed too long, because dying patients are no longer interested in what they are leaving behind and may not be capable of handling their affairs.

THE SILENCE OF DEATH

Two months before my father died I went with him to his physician for treatment of the lymphoma that had suddenly enveloped his body. In spite of his increasing fatigue, he went about his work as usual. Finally becoming bedridden, he read his Bible, made his peace with God, and one morning called all of us individually to his bedside to say good-by. "Be a good girl and don't forget me" were his last words to me. He went quietly into coma that afternoon and died two hours later. Because his face was disfigured, his body was prepared by the mortician and placed in a pine box in the same room where he died. Friends and neighbors called and sat with the corpse until it was time for the funeral, which was held in the local church. Burial was in the adjacent graveyard among the wild flowers of the earth that he loved.

I have given this example as a contrast to the more common style of dying, most likely to occur in hospitals with nurses in attendance.

After all of the pertinent knowledge of medical science has been exhausted in treating the dying person, the family and nurses wait. Family members may be torn between the wish to prolong the contact and the desire to get it over with. Help the family members to decide among themselves that at least one person will take the responsibility for staying with the dying relative. Sitting, caring, touching, and showing concern become all that is left for the nurse to do. The nurse who sits at the side of a dying person and holds his hand until the last breath feels a oneness with the experience and suffering of humanity and realizes the evanescence of life. When life finally leaves the body, the stillness and silence of death can leave the living with the feeling of hope that someone will do the same things for them when their time comes.

Summary

In this chapter, some aspects of the problem of loss have been discussed. Depression, as a frequent outcome of feelings of loss, is differentiated from normal states. The prevalence of depression is described and ways for the nurse to recognize depressive affects outlined. Nursing care of patients with affective disorders is presented. In a section on grief and mourning, the central aim of the nurse to help the bereaved complete their grief work is stressed. Some aspects of the social and intellectual movements in nursing designed to make possible better understanding of the dying patient and the bereaved family are discussed, with a focus on the nurse's therapeutic tasks.

References

AMERICAN PSYCHIATRIC ASSOCIATION: *A Psychiatric Glossary.* Washington, D.C.: 1980.
_____: *Diagnostic and Statistical Manual of Mental Disorder,* III. Washington, D.C.: 1980.
ANDERSON, BARBARA GALLATIN: "Death as a Subject of Cross-Cultural Inquiry." Presented at the International Congress of Social Psychiatry, London, 1964.
AYD, FRANK: *Recognizing the Depressed Patient.* New York: Grune & Stratton, Inc., 1961, pp. 118–25.
BARNES, MARION J.: "Reactions to the Death of a Mother," *The Psychoanalytic Study of the Child,* Vol. 19. New York: International Universities Press, 1964, pp. 334–57.
BECK, AARON T.: "Depressive Neurosis," in Arieti, Silvano, ed.: *American Handbook of Psychiatry,* Vol. III. New York: Basic Books, Inc., 1974, pp. 61–90.
BEERS, CLIFFORD WHITTINGHAM: *A Mind That Found Itself* (1908). Garden City, N.Y.: Doubleday, Doran & Co., Inc., 1921.
BENDANN, E.: *Death Customs, an Analytical Study of Burial Rites.* New York: Alfred A. Knopf, Inc., 1930.
BOWLBY, JOHN: Notes from Symposium on "Separation and Loss." San Francisco Psychoanalytic Institute, San Francisco, 1968.

———: *Attachment and Loss: Attachment,* Vol. 1. New York: Basic Books, Inc., 1969.

BROWN, ESTHER LUCILE: "Nursing, What Direction. The Humanizing of Patient Care." Paper delivered in conjunction with the LA County-University of Southern California Medical Center Centennial, 16 September 1978.

CAPLAN, GERALD: "Lessons in Bravery." *McCall's,* pp. 85ff., September 1968.

CAUMONT, M. A. DE: *Abecedaire en Rudiment d'Archeologie.* Caen: F. Le Blanc-Hardel, 1886.

DEUTSCH, ALBERT: *The Mentally Ill in America.* Garden City, N.Y.: Doubleday, Doran & Co., Inc., 1937.

DRACUP, KATHLEEN A., BREU, CHRISTINE S.: "Using Nursing Research Findings to Meet the Needs of Grieving Spouses." *Nursing Research,* 27:4:212–216, July–August 1978.

Forbidden Games (Jeux Interdits), Film, Robert Dorfman, 1952.

FREUD, SIGMUND: "Mourning and Melancholia" (1917), *The Collected Papers,* Vol. IV. London: The Hogarth Press, 1949, pp. 152–70.

FURMAN, ROBERT A.: "Death and the Young Child," *The Psychoanalytic Study of the Child,* Vol. 19. New York: International Universities Press, 1964, pp. 321–33.

GLASER, BARNEY, and STRAUSS, ANSELM: *Awareness of Dying.* Chicago: Aldine Publishing Co., 1965.

HAMPE, SANDRA OLIVER: "Needs of the Grieving Spouse in a Hospital Setting," *Nursing Research,* 24:2:113–120, March–April 1975.

HINSIE, LELAND E., and CAMPBELL, ROBERT JEAN: *Psychiatric Dictionary.* New York: Oxford University Press, 1960.

HOLBEIN, H.: *The Dance of Death.* London: Hamilton, Adams and Company, 1887.

HUIZINGA, JOHAN: *The Waning of the Middle Ages.* New York: Anchor Books, 1954. (First published in 1924.)

KALLMAN, F. J.: *Heredity in Health and Mental Disorders.* New York: W. W. Norton, 1953.

KUBLER-ROSS, ELIZABETH: *On Death and Dying.* New York: Macmillan Publishing Co., Inc., 1969.

LAMPL-DE GROOT, JEANNE: "Mourning in a 6-Year-Old Girl," in Eissler, Ruth S., ed.: *The Psychoanalytic Study of the Child.* Vol. 31 New Haven: Yale University Press, 1976, pp. 273–281.

LEVIN, SIDNEY: "Depression in the Aged," in Berezin, Martin A., and Cath, Stanley H., eds.: *Geriatric Psychiatry: Grief, Loss and Emotional Disorders in the Aging Process.* New York: International Universities Press, Inc., 1965.

LIEBERMAN, MORTON A., PROCK, V. N., and

TOBIN, S. S.: "The Psychological Effects of Institutionalization," *Journal of Gerontology,* 23:3:343–53, July 1968.

MAIN, T. F.: "The Hospital as a Therapeutic Institution," in Barnes, Elizabeth, ed.: *Psychosocial Nursing.* London: Tavistock Publications, Inc. (Barnes and Noble, Inc., in U.S.), 1968.

MENNINGER, KARL: *Man Against Himself.* New York: Harcourt, Brace & Co., 1938.

MOROZOV, G., and ROMASENKO, V.: *Neuropathology and Psychiatry.* Moscow: Moscow Peace Publishers (no date).

MOTTO, JEROME: Notes taken from lecture at symposium on "Psychiatric Problems of Aging," Mendocino, Calif. 1968.

One Hundred and Fourteenth Report of the Retreat, York, A. Registered Hospital for the Treatment of Mental Diseases, 1914, p. 11.

PARKES, COLIN MURRAY: *Bereavement: Studies of Grief in Adult Life.* New York: International Universities Press, Inc., 1972.

PASTERNAK, BORIS LEONIDOVICH: *Doctor Zhivago.* New York: Pantheon, 1958.

PATTEN, BRADLEY M.: *Human Embryology.* New York: The Blakiston Division, McGraw-Hill, 1968.

PIRENNE, HENRI: *Economic and Social History of Medieval Europe.* New York: Harcourt, Brace & Co., 1936.

QUINT, JEANNE C.: *The Nurse and the Dying Patient.* New York: Macmillan Publishing Co., Inc., 1967.

ROCHLIN, GREGORY: *Grief and Discontents: The Forces of Change.* Boston: Little, Brown and Co., 1965.

SCHWAB, JOHN H., BROWN, JUDITH M., HOLZER, CHARLES E., and SOKOLOF, MARILYN: "Current Concepts of Depression: The Sociocultural," *The International Journal of Social Psychiatry,* 14:3:226–34, 1968.

SECUNDA, STEVEN K.: *The Depressive Disorders: Special Report: 1973.* Department of Health, Education and Welfare Publication No. (HSM) 73–9157. Washington, D.C.: U.S. Government Printing Office, 1973.

SILVERMAN, PHYLLIS ROLFE: "The Widow-to-Widow Program," *Mental Hygiene,* 53:3:333–37, July 1969.

SPITZ, RENE A.: "Hospitalism. An Inquiry into the Genesis of Psychiatric Conditions in Early Childhood," in Freud, Anna, ed.: *The Psychoanalytic Study of the Child,* 1:53–74, 1945.

SPITZ, RENE, and WOLF, KATHERINE M.: "Anaclitic Depression," *The Psychoanalytic Study of the Child,* 2:313–43, 1946.

STRACHEY, LYTTON: *Queen Victoria.* New York: Blue Ribbon Books, 1921, pp. 402–404.

THOMAS, CLAYTON L., ed.: *Taber's Cyclopedic Medical Dictionary*, 12th ed. Philadelphia: F. A. Davis, 1973.

TOLSTOY, LEO: *The Death of Ivan Ilyich* (1886). Baltimore: Penguin Books, 1960.

Webster's New Collegiate Dictionary, Springfield, Mass.: G. and C. Merriam Co., Publishers, 1977.

WOLF, ANNA: "Helping Your Child to Understand Death," *Child Study*, 35:36ff., Winter 1957–58.

WOLFENSTEIN, MARTHA: "How is Mourning Possible?" *The Psychoanalytic Study of the Child*, Vol. 21. New York: International Universities Press, 1966, pp. 93–123.

Suggested Readings

ALBERT, AUGUSTA: "A Brief Communication on Children's Reactions to the Assassination of the President," *The Psychoanalytic Study of the Child*, Vol. 19. New York: International Universities Press, 1964, pp. 313–24.

ARIETI, SILVANO: "Affective Disorders: Manic-Depressive Psychosis and Psychotic Depression," in Arieti, Silvano, ed.: *American Handbook of Psychiatry*, Vol. III. New York: Basic Books, Inc., 1974, pp. 449–90.

BECKER, ERNEST: *The Denial of Death*. New York: The Free Press, 1973.

BEREZIN, MARTIN A., and CATH, STANLEY H., eds.: *Geriatric Psychiatry: Grief, Loss and Emotional Disorders in the Aging Process*. New York: International Universities Press, Inc., 1965.

BROWN, NORMAN O.: *Life Against Death*. Middletown, Conn.: Wesleyan University Press, 1959.

BOWLBY, JOHN: *Attachment and Loss: Separation, Anxiety and Anger*, Vol. II. New York: Basic Books, Inc., 1973.

CLAYTON, PAULA J.: "The Effect of Living Alone on Bereavement Symptoms," *American Journal of Psychiatry*, 132:2:133–137, Feb. 1975.

CRAVEN, JOAN, and WALD, FLORENCE S.: "Hospice Care for Dying Patients," *American Journal of Nursing*, 75:10:1816–22, October 1975.

DAVIS, JOHN M.: "Overview: Maintenance Therapy in Psychiatry: II. Affective Disorders," *American Journal of Psychiatry*, 133:1:1–13, January 1976.

FREIHOFER, PATRICIA, and FELTON, GERALDENE: "Nursing Behaviors in Bereavement: An Exploratory Study." *Nursing Research*, 25:5:332–337, Sept.–Oct. 1976.

FREEDMAN, ALFRED M., KAPLAN, HAROLD I., and SADOCK, BENJAMIN J., eds.: *Comprehensive Textbook of Psychiatry*-II. Baltimore: Williams and Wilkins Co., 1975.

GORNEY, ROBERT J., and HORTON, FREDERICH T.: "Pathological Grief Following Spontaneous Abortion," *American Journal of Psychiatry*, 131:7:825–27, July 1974.

ILFELD, FREDERIC W.: "Current Social Stressors and Symptoms of Depression," *American Journal of Psychiatry*, 134:2:161–166, Feb. 1977.

INGLES, THELMA: "St. Christopher's Hospice," *Nursing Outlook*, 22:12:753–763, December 1974.

KALKMAN, MARION E.: "Recognizing Emotional Problems," *American Journal of Nursing*, 68:536–39, March 1968.

———— and DAVIS, ANNE J., eds: *New Dimensions in Mental Health—Psychiatric Nursing*. New York: McGraw-Hill, 1980.

KOLB, LAWRENCE C.: *Modern Clinical Psychiatry*. Philadelphia: W. B. Saunders Co., 1977, pp. 439–480.

LAUFER, MOSES: "Object Loss and Mourning During Adolescence," *The Psychoanalytic Study of the Child*, Vol. 21. New York: International Universities Press, 1966, pp. 269–93.

LINDEMANN, ERICH: "Symptomatology and Management of Acute Grief," *American Journal of Psychiatry*, 101:141–48, 1944.

MENDELS, J.: "Biological Aspects of Affective Illness," in Arieti, Silvano, ed.: *American Handbook of Psychiatry*, Vol. III. New York: Basic Books, Inc., 1974, pp. 491–523.

MOGUL, KATHLEEN M.: Women in Midlife: Decisions, Rewards, and Conflicts Related to Work and Careers," *American Journal of Psychiatry*, 136:9:1139–1143, September 1979.

OSTERWEIS, MARIAN, and CHAMPAGNE, DAPHNE SZMUSZKOVICZ: "The U.S. Hospice Movement: Issues in Development." *American Journal of Public Health*, 69:5:492–496, May 1979.

PADILLA, GERALDINE V., BAKER, VERONICA E., and DOLAN, VIKKI A.: *Interacting with Dying Patients: An Inter-hospital Nursing Research and Nursing Education Project*. Duarte, Calif.: City of Hope National Medical Center, 1975.

PAIGE, ROBERTA LYDER, and LOONEY, JANE FINKBEIN: "Hospice Care for the Advanced Cancer Patient," *American Journal of Nursing*, 77:11:1812–1815, November 1977.

PATTISON, E. MANSELL: "Help in the Dying Process," *American Handbook of Psychiatry*, Vol. I. New York: Basic Books, Inc., 1974, pp. 685–702.

QUINT, JEANNE C., and STRAUSS, ANSELM L.: "Nursing Students, Assignments and Dying

Patients," *Nursing Outlook,* 12:24–27, January 1964.

_____: "The Threat of Death: Some Consequences for Patients and Nurses," *Nursing Forum,* 8:2:286–300, 1969.

ROCHLIN, GREGORY: "Loss and Restitution," *The Psychoanalytic Study of the Child,* Vol. 8. New York: International Universities Press, 1953, pp. 288–309.

_____: "The Dread of Abandonment," *The Psychoanalytic Study of the Child,* Vol. 16. New York: International Universities Press, 1961, pp. 451–70.

ROSS, CHARLES W.: "Nurses' Personal Death Concerns and Responses to Dying-Patient Statements," *Nursing Research,* 27:1:64–48, January–February 1978.

STODDARD, SANDOL: *The Hospice Movement: A Better Way of Caring for the Dying.* New York: Vintage Books, 1978.

STOLL, RUTH I.: "Guidelines for Spiritual Assessment," *American Journal of Nursing,* 79:9:1574–1577, September 1979.

UJHELY, GERTRUD: "Preventive and Therapeutic Nursing Care," *Nursing Forum,* 5:2:23–35, 1966.

_____: "What is Realistic Emotional Support? *American Journal of Nursing,* 68:758, 1968.

WALD, FLORENCE S., and HENDERSON, VIRGINIA: "Death and Dying," in Henderson, Virginia, and Nite, Gladys: *Principles and Practice of Nursing.* New York: Macmillan Publishing Co., Inc., 1978, pp. 1929–2007.

WARD, BARBARA J.: "Hospice Home Care Program," *Nursing Outlook,* 26:10:646–649, October 1978.

WAUGH, EVELYN: *The Loved One.* New York: Random House, 1948.

WOLFENSTEIN, MARTHA: "Loss, Rage and Repetition," *The Psychoanalytic Study of the Child,* Vol. 24. New York: International Universities Press, 1969, pp. 432–60.

7

Aggression

Patriotism is not enough;
I must have no hatred or bitterness for anyone.
　　　　　　　　　　　　　　　EDITH CAVELL

DEFINITION AND ORIGINS

Freud (1920) postulated that aggression[1] derives from and is part of one of the two major instincts of the person, the instinct for death (Thanatos).[2] (The other is Eros,

---

[1] "*Aggression* is a forceful, physical, verbal, or symbolic action. It may be appropriate and self-protective, including healthful self-assertiveness, or inappropriate. It also may be directed outward toward the environment, as in explosive personality, or inward toward the self as in depression." (From *A Psychiatric Glossary*, copyright 1980, American Psychiatric Association.)

[2] In Greek mythology Thanatos was the personification of death, the son of Nyx (night) and brother of Hypnos (sleep).

the instinct for life.) Aggression covers the spectrum of intrusive attacking behaviors.

Today, the primitive drives or the instinctual aspect of the personality are conceptualized as the id. As the ego develops, the *pleasure–pain principle,* which is dominant with instinctual drives, is modified and adapted to become the *reality principle.* The *pleasure–pain principle* tries to deal with pain in a manner that brings the individual the most pleasure; it represents the libido. It is a mechanism of mental life aimed toward the reduction of tension due to undischarged drives. The *reality principle* refers to the inclusion of the influences of the outer world within the personality. According to Freud, instinctual drives are energies invested in various body areas; they enhance specific biological and psychological functions with pleasure; behavior is toward pleasure, and to avoid unpleasure, there is a compulsion to repeat behavior and we strive to repeat what is pleasant. As the child

211

develops, the pathways of discharge of aggression change; for example, between early childhood and latency, words take the place of muscular actions. It is in this phase that swear words are relished by the child, serving as a defense against aggression taking the form of muscular action; it is also here that the child is taught to count to ten before acting. Aggression in psychotic children may occur for many reasons, one of them being a healthful discharge of aggressive impulses. Other aggressive acts may be for the purpose of defending the ego, for example, when defenses are weakening, as a defense against anxiety, as a reaction of the superego against id impulses, and also as an expression of a sort of powerless rage. Bender (1969) states that hostile or destructive aggression in children is the result of developmental pathology in the context of a disturbing situation that has disorganized the normal drives of the developing child. She further states that murderous, hostile aggression is not a normal pattern for children. Freud (1957) thought that aggressive behavior rests on different physiological aspects of the body.

According to Anna Freud (1972), the child's pleasure in constructive activity is libidinal, whereas his pleasure in destruction is aggressive; they exist together and each is the derivative of a primary id tendency. Furthermore, the observation of early aggression in toddlers shows that attack derives expressly from the aggressive drive. Toddlers are extremely aggressive toward each other; they bite, kick, pull hair, and hit but, initially, the victim of the attack dissolves into tears instead of defending himself. Only later does the toddler learn self-defense. The conclusion is therefore drawn that *aggression in service of defense is learned and mediated by the ego.*

Mahler and associates (1973) describe a period of growth and development in the child in which the euphoric aspects require assistance from others, namely, the mother figure; if these aspects are submerged, the aggressive drive becomes uppermost and is projected onto others. As a result, the world may be divided into good and bad and consequently the child divides himself into good and bad. Mahler and associates think these mechanisms may provide the beginnings of paranoid features; behaviorally, the child clings and is moody and coercive.

The frustration–aggression hypothesis of Dollard and associates (1939) purports that frustration increases with rank and territory of the person. Berkowitz (1962) views aggression as not automatically accompanying frustration or threat; instead, he sees it as relative to the degree and amount of frustration, the power of the individual to react against the aggressive act, and one's values against aggression. In past centuries aggressive acts might lead, for example, to a duel, a type of confrontation unlikely today. Dueling served as a sanctioned outlet for individuals or groups in conflict. After the duel, amicable relations were expected to be resumed.

In modern times, in the highly ritualized sport of fencing one may symbolically "pick off" one's adversary by winning a bout; afterward both parties remove their protective masks, approach each other, smile, shake hands, and thank each other. Competitive sports are ritualized forms of aggressive behavior.

Although some groups are more aggressive than others, all cultures experience aggression to some degree. The evocation of aggressive behavior depends on a number of antecedent conditions, e.g., the arbitrariness of the frustration, the power to retaliate against the aggression, and the presence of values against aggression.

Aggression has been described by an ethologist as the fighting instinct[3] in beast and humans directed against members of the same species (Lorenz, 1963).

Gorney (1971) proposes that in societies where we see the most intense interpersonal relationships, we see also the highest level of cultural achievement and intrapsychic conflict. He poses the thought that aggression and mental disorder might be diminished by reducing the intensity of interpersonal relationships.

Aggression is usually easily perceived, and the concept of constructive aggression

[3] "*Instinct* is generally understood to be a specific response pattern—invariant in its development, maturation, and expression—that occurs to some quite specific cluster of stimuli from the environment" (Holloway, 1967, p. 40). (Copyright, 1967, The American Museum of Natural History.)

is well known. The child who uses magical thinking to release aggression may also experience guilt when, for example, he wishes that his father would die and the parent does die. A guilt reaction to unexpressed aggression is probably normal for the adolescent. In the ten-to-fifteen-year-old, depression is linked to unexpressed aggression. Sadism and murder are extreme forms of outward aggression; masochism and suicide are examples of extreme inward aggression. A classical example of hatred poses the question of the origins of aggression. For example, Medea, cast off by Jason for a young wife, killed her rival, Glauce, and her own three sons by Jason, all of whom she loved. A more recent example was Hitler's annihilation of the Jews under his autocratic rule of Germany. It must be remembered that homicide, rape, spouse abuse, child abuse, parent abuse, and incest occur in families. A study by Silver and associates (1969) covering three generations of families of abused children supports the view that violence breeds violence and that a child who experiences violence has the potential of becoming a violent member of society as he grows older.

DISPLACEMENT

Aggression may be aroused by frustration, threats, or annoyances. Displaced aggression directs hostile feelings toward a person or an object other than the one that causes the frustration. The person who has a hard day at work and comes home and yells at his spouse or kicks the dog is one example of displacement. Another example is provided by a psychotic child in a residential treatment center who, when frustrated in his relationships with peers, bites the nursing staff.

The need for expression of aggression arising from intrapsychic tensions and the need for resolving an external conflict are dissimilar. Intrapsychic tensions may be released toward one of several different people, whereas external conflicts between persons or groups may be resolved by arbitration or negotiation.

NEED FOR RELEASE OF AGGRESSION

Release of aggression as in play, hunting, work, and other physical activities may be greatly altered when patients are hospitalized, at times of other stresses, and when the usual outlets for aggression are not available. For example, a blind person may verbally attack an agency, reject it, or make excessive demands on it. His family may also join in the attack. Nursing students are familiar with the many biting remarks that some patients make about the institutions serving them, and about the professionals caring for them. The intimacy, sustained close contact, and heightened interaction that nurses experience with patients provide fertile ground for arousal of hostility and tension as well as the more positive affects of rapport (Coser, 1956). The rivalry—e.g., the traditional dislike of the French for the Germans and vice versa—between nations also serves as a channel for release of aggressive feelings. The competitiveness between nations symbolized in the Olympic Games can now be vicariously experienced throughout the world through the medium of television.

INAPPROPRIATE AGGRESSION: SUSPICION AND HOSTILITY

Suspicion is the imagination of the existence of some fault, defect, guilt, or falsity when there may be slight evidence for its existence or none. It precedes hostility. The suspicious person tends to question motives of others over minute matters, mull over the consequences, and later confront individuals with long and involved analyses of their motives. Hostility refers to an unfriendly, antagonistic manner, to resentment, grudges, and resentful acts. All humans experience hostility. It is common for everyone to feel aggressive when frustration is encountered and handle it by adjusting, adapting, changing one's perceptions, or leaving. In a nonhuman primate society, there is no alternative to bluffing; if the bluff is called, fighting occurs. Humans, however, have language; they can explain, reason, and negotiate (Washburn, 1969). Hostility usually emerges after much rumination over an imagined slight. Buss (1961) makes the point that a hostile remark such as "I hate you" voiced by a person who is alone is not aggressive until there is someone to hear it. Hostility is one way that patients who are threatened react to the threat. If the threat can be removed, the hostility is not needed.

The following terms describe behavior of hostile persons; picky, resentful, argumentative, antagonistic, uncooperative, aggressive, irritable, caustic, sarcastic, rude, critical, resistant, begrudging, ignoring, demanding, litigious, complaining, scapegoating, gossiping, blocking, derogating, threatening, and rejecting (verbally and nonverbally). Inflicting physical injury, making barbed remarks, and joking at someone else's expense are all examples of hostility.

NURSING INTERVENTION

Aggressiveness in patients may stir up anxiety in the nurse. The patient who is sarcastic, irritable, and resentful and who constantly complains about the hospital, the physician, and the other staff may put you in a defensive position without your actually knowing whether his complaints are justifiable. Try to discover if there is indeed a basis in fact for the sarcasm. If there is none, perhaps your patient is releasing aggression because his normal manner of handling it is unavailable. The nurse can help by listening, offering alternative solutions to problems, and helping the patient to be secure enough so that aggressive behavior is no longer necessary. One nurse's approach to a patient whom most of the nurses described as "demanding" was to simply explain to the patient what she was going to do and

how she would do it before she started anything. The patient responded in a receptive way, and the student was satisfied with her discovery. Taking the initiative, after explanation to the patient—what Ruesch (1961) calls unaggressive directness—indicating that the patient is expected to carry through his therapeutic regime, may really communicate to him. One student reports a situation as follows:

The patient was referred to as "demanding" by the nursing staff who volunteered the information that she always had her light on for something. The previous evening the patient had rung the supervisor to get someone to answer her light, which she said had been on for twenty minutes. When I tried to get her to help change the colostomy bag, I could see that she was frightened and I suspected that she also was scared that the surgeon may not have been able to remove all of the cancer. So I explained everything I was doing, step by step, and that I would help her the next time and be with her this evening. I tried to anticipate her needs and help her meet them. I asked her about her feelings, what happened yesterday, and then I listened. The patient poured out her pent-up thoughts and feelings about the colostomy and how she feared rejection by her husband. I also explained how the unit was staffed during the evening and the kinds of problems the other patients on the unit were experiencing. Later, the patient changed her colostomy bag with my support and thanked me for helping her.

The student had noted the insecurity and apprehension of the patient, made herself available, and used her professional authority for leverage only after assessing the individual needs of this "demanding" patient.

Patients with more severe problems who cannot express anger and hostility may be aided by the therapist to do so. The patient immediately past his psychotherapeutic hour often is upset and may require a release of aggressive feelings. The individual who does not receive gratification from his usual modes of expressing aggression should be assisted to develop new ways to decrease tension.

The hostile patient expects the nurse to be hostile in return. If the nurse rises to the challenge, it is likely to increase the patient's tension and result in a fight. Other ways of responding may disarm the hostile patient. Turning a verbal attack into something that can be laughed about can drain off tension (Ruesch, 1961, p. 150). Humor is one of the popular coping mechanisms; having a good laugh makes almost anything seem less formidable.

Running away from the hospital is sometimes attempted by patients, and efforts by staff to thwart such attempts will probably be met by aggression. The nurse should be aware of the usual habits of patients. A sudden decision to join a group of patients for an outing that has previously been consistently refused or a frantic accumulation of possessions when visitors are about to leave is a nonverbal cue to what the patient may have on his mind.

Hostility from patients is probably one of the most difficult things to deal with in nursing. Some people are more sensitive to hostility than others. When hostility is encountered for the first time in a patient, you may have a tendency to flee the situation or to make a counterattack, both of which are quite natural but neither one of which benefits the patient. Help him identify what is threatening, frightening, or annoying to him and accept the patient as he is. Accepting him as he is implies that you will not pass moral judgment on him. It does not mean abandoning the patient in his psychological state but implies that you perceive the strengths within the individual and can therefore help him to move on to greater potentials. Setting limits on behavior and disapproval of behavior communicate to the patient that you care about him but not particularly about some of his behavior. *Avoid reacting to hostility as if it were personally directed toward you.* It is important to accept the feelings of the hostile patient and to give him the opportunity to clarify them with you. The following is an example of what one nurse did.

A teenage patient, Valerie, became belligerent, rude, and verbally abusive to a nurse who took it personally and retaliated by becoming verbally abusive to the patient. The nurse thereby lost control of the situation and the patient's abusiveness spiraled. Another nurse, observing the event, went over quietly to Valerie, took her by the hand, walked to a corner with her, sat with her until she calmed down, and then interested her in something else.

The action of the second nurse let the patient know that she was accepted for herself. The nurse's presence and calm manner acted as comfort to the patient. Since anxiety itself communicates rapidly to others, the nurse, to be helpful to the patient, must learn to control her own anxiety. The serene, authoritative manner of the nurse communicates to the hostile patient whose whole personality is *not* oriented toward hostility. Retaliation or the use of the talionic principle is discarded in therapeutic work. A word of caution is included here: Students should not mistakenly use these therapeutic techniques in life situations where their own self-preservation may be at stake.

Signs of mounting tension can be noted by the nurse, who can prevent the patient from hurting others, destroying objects, and injuring himself. Increased motor activity, angry facial expressions, stereotyped movements, and tremulousness may be some of the cues. Doing some habitual thing in a different manner than usual may be another sign of mounting tension.

The nurse can help by providing support to the patient who is learning to express anger and by not denying her own anger. Make clear to the patient that destructive aggression is not acceptable. The use of suggestion can direct the patient to socially acceptable outlets such as pounding. Fear of losing self-control may accompany release of pent-up hostility; the patient may ask you to help him not to lose complete control. Remove the patient from the group to his room or similar privacy, remain with him, touch him, hold him, and talk with him. If possible, the same person assigned to help him meet his needs should be available to him through periods of aggression.

Breaking all the windows may temporarily release tension, but the destruction remains as a reminder of the guilt involved. The nurse sets limits here in that property and people are not to be physically attacked and helps the patient verbalize hostility or work it out in other ways. Talking through events that lead to expressions of hostility can help the patient learn new ways of handling aggression. Assist the patient immediately when he is able to talk about it, not tomorrow or next week.

SECLUSION AND RESTRAINT

Seclusion and restraint are measures undertaken as a last resort.

A seclusion room should have shielded lights, shielded electrical outlets, unbreakable windows (if any), a window for observation, and be lockable. It should also contain a bed bolted to the floor so that the patient can be restrained. Seclusion is used mostly for (1) safety (of patient and others) and (2) decrease of sensory stimulation. Patients sometimes choose to put themselves in open seclusion for impulse control referred to as "cooling off."

During the past decade, hospital violence seems to have increased and more attention is now being given to assaultive behavior. Assaultive–aggressive behavior may be impulsive, occur as a reaction, premeditated, or self-inflicted.

Countertransference reactions of anger and fear in therapists have been cited as interfering with the management of violent patients (Lion et al., 1973). Violence can erupt in a therapeutic milieu if staff are unclear about setting limits. Patients may misinterpret the actions of others and lash out due to various reasons. One study of violence among psychiatric patients reports that most violence came from patients who were diagnosed as schizoaffective (Applebaum, 1975). Not enough attention is given to the effects of assaultive patients on nursing staff. One study reported that one in every four qualified nurses over the age of fifty has a visible physical defect from aggressive acts by patients (Ernst, 1975). Not enough attention is given to the destructiveness of furnishings by aggressive psychiatric patients in hospital units. Budget makers need to take this into consideration in maintenance of an aesthetically pleasing environment.

Recently on an acute inpatient unit, a patient set two fires in the dayroom (a wastebasket and the telephone book) to distract the staff from his attempt to break the window with a chair to jump from the seventh floor. After that didn't work he removed the ceiling in the bathroom, climbed into the space for wires and vents, and tried to get out. The patient was secluded, restrained, and given medication.

Threatening gestures such as raising the fist, hitting the wall, verbal threats, and throwing objects are cues to assaultiveness.

A calm, self-confident, decisive attitude of the nurse (and other staff) is essential in managing assaultive behavior.

Limitations on aggression for the patient who fears losing control can be very meaningful to him. Verbal controls should be used first and the patient expected to control himself.

Try to ally yourself with the hostile, aggressive patient for something instead of against something and thereby assist the patient toward constructive use of aggressive feelings. Medication may be given to help. If this fails, then the patient needs to know that the staff will prevent harmful acts by physical restraint. Do not try to seclude or restrain the patient without sufficient resources to carry it out. Teamwork is necessary for the physical restraint itself and should be practiced together so each knows what to do when a patient needs seclusion and restraint. The patient may be put into a seclusion room only, but leather restraints may also be applied to wrists, ankles, and body if the patient is hurting himself. All harmful objects must be removed from the patient when he is secluded. While the seclusion and restraint are being carried out, some staff should remain with the other patients. A special form is then made out with the reason for restraint, the time, the type of restraint, and behavior of the patient at fifteen-minute intervals. After the patient calms down and can control himself, he is removed from restraints and seclusion. All involved in restraining the patient should then meet together to discuss what happened and to check themselves for injury. The patient should also have the opportunity to verbalize thoughts and feelings. An emergency community meeting may be called for full discussion.

TRUST

Suspicious and hostile patients watch every move you make, every nuance and inflection of your voice, and mull them over. Take the initiative and make the overture to your patient, even if you anticipate a hostile encounter. This bolsters the self-esteem of the patient. Trust is not likely to be established right away, but persistent interest communicates to the patient.

If you are on a home visit, the way you react to other members of the family—or, if in hospital, to other patients—communicates to the suspicious, hostile patient. An impersonal, hasty manner of one staff member may also communicate to the hostile patient that he may expect the same treatment from all the members of your profession and therefore further eliminate possibilities for the development of trust. Empathize with the patient and assess his particular situation so that you can be more aware of his expectations of you. Patients who are suspicious and hostile are keenly aware of actions of staff and patients that are different from the particular culture of that psychiatric unit, e.g., staff members who give their attention to each other instead of the patients. If the whole ward is going on a picnic, the suspicious patient will wait to see if the nurse has remembered his special needs, for example, his medications, and ponder possible motivations if these have been overlooked. A promise for the smallest item should not be forgotten.

The therapeutic task of the nurse is to help the hostile patient regain and perceive self-esteem. Removing his working defenses is opening a psychic wound and should be avoided. Belittling others (derogation) is a defense; as the patient belittles others, they become less threatening to him. Hostile individuals, beneath their thorny and bristly exteriors, are really insecure; their aggression may be a facade covering their insecurity. Belittling the nurse may result when the nurse has not gained the patient's trust and supported his ego.

ACTIVITIES FOR THE RELEASE OF AGGRESSION

Activities that involve pounding, running, hitting, and cutting release aggression. For immobilized patients, a set of exercises requiring muscles that are not immobilized can be run through regularly. Vicariously "participating" in a much-loved television game may afford an effective outlet. Watch-

ing boxing and wrestling matches where someone else does the "clobbering" perhaps enables the vicarious releases of aggression. Being able to discuss a favorite competitive game and how effective one is in it can also release aggression. The identification with a particular ball team, jockey, or driver of a racing car and watching, hearing about, or discussing their competitive actions help release aggression. For example, one older patient in his nineties now almost blind, home-bound, living alone, with all relatives dead, loved horse racing. The nursing student enlisted the aid of her boyfriend to learn something about racing so she could discuss it with the patient. The animation on his face was the reward for her. For some, a punching bag, ping-pong, hammering, tennis, running, or a fast fencing bout provides release of aggression.

In a hospital unit, pounding metal as in copper work or metal sculpture and the pounding and kneading necessary to prepare clay for the potter's wheel are outlets. The classic example given for the sublimation of aggression is the surgeon who instead of expressing his aggression just by cutting people up does it by performing a precise operation. Typing and piano playing and various tasks carried on each day in a hospital can be made available to the patient. Nurses may use other methods for helping patients release aggression such as the use of boffers and psychodrama.

THE NURSE'S HOSTILE FEELINGS

Any feeling of hostility in the nurse toward a patient must receive careful attention and self-examination through introspection and discussion with others. The continuous giving to others may drain the nurse emotionally, and hostile behavior may ensue. In at least one large medical center where many organ transplants are done, the nurses who care for these patients have psychiatric nursing consultation available to them and also regular group sessions with a psychiatrist. One student reported her work in an intensive-care unit where a patient thought he was being done away with, got up, and walked despite his condition and all the tubes. Instead of working on establishing trust the nurses became angry at the patient.

The Paranoid Person

The paranoid person misperceives ordinary events within his environment and feels that everything relates to himself. He has excessive suspicion, hostility, and rigidity, and reality testing is impaired. Possibly throughout his life he has been unable to trust anyone. The paranoid person may not be able to get along with anyone and therefore lives alone, or at odds with those with whom he does live. He has a basic insecurity, is full of pride, and has been unable to develop satisfactory social skills. He is rigid and self-centered in his personality organization. He is sensitive to situations that make him feel inferior and most likely had a childhood in which his parents made demands of him that he could not meet. As a child he was sensitive and narcissistic. He uses overcompensation for feelings of inferiority, and his compensatory mechanisms involve status and prestige. He tends to deal with problems by brooding and introspection, and there may be delusions and ideas of self-reference and influence.

The differentiation of paranoid disorders from paranoid personality disorder and paranoid schizophrenia is unclear (*Diagnostic and Statistical Manual of Mental Disorders,* III, 1980).

Paranoia, in the form of self-reference, delusions, hallucinations, negativism, and disturbances of associations and affect, does not usually occur until after adolescence and is most frequent after the age of thirty. It often appears after or during a *real* crisis situation for the patient. Therefore, it must be remembered that the delusions of the paranoid person may have some basis in fact. Delusions of jealousy, persecutory delusions, and grandiose delusions are commonly present. The disorder begins with an uncertainty of identity, a misidentification of others, a feeling of self-disorganization, rage, projection, and unstable and changing ego boundaries; depersonalization

and nihilism may appear, anxiety increases, repression no longer works, regression occurs, and feelings of being controlled by an influencing machine may be present. In addition, a pseudocommunity labeled "they"—the watchers, listeners, and persecutors—may develop. This pseudocommunity is thought to represent introjected parental figures, now projected, usually toward the parent of the same sex, or toward others who may represent parental figures. Strong rage and strong love feelings are thought to be fixated at infantile levels, and this ambivalence toward love objects, then, is carried on into adulthood. The paranoid person fails to establish stable heterosexual object relations and fights against intensive homosexual feelings. The paranoid schizophrenic person's preoccupation with ideas of homosexuality, thought by Freud (1911) to be the basis of paranoid delusions, may derive from the parents' confused gender identities and failure to have maintained their gender-linked roles (Lidz, 1973). According to Cameron (1974), the paranoid person who develops delusions of grandeur is attempting to recapture lost object relationships.

As an adult, the person who is developing paranoia may sustain an injury to the ego and feel frustration and hate; ambivalence reappears and energy is withdrawn from the libido toward the hostile energy and projected as delusions of persecution. Unable to tolerate the anxiety aroused by the ambivalence, in the unconscious, "I hate him" is transferred to projection to "He hates me." These persecutions may represent superego figures. The paranoid person, underneath the facade of *hauteur* and the paranoid stare,[4] feels inferior and may develop delusions of power and influence as compensatory mechanisms. He is ready to fight anything that threatens his security; the paranoid grandiosity enhances his self-esteem.

Denial and projection become major mechanisms in the paranoid person. Denial

---

[4] The paranoid stare makes most people feel uncomfortable and thus succeeds in isolating the individual even further, thus giving grist for the mill of suspicion.

is thought to play a role in psychoses similar to that of repression in neurotic disorders. Patients who are paranoid have often suffered much in early childhood from parental figures.

Delusions of persecution become prominent; auditory hallucinations are usually of a threatening nature or accusatory. The person may feel that he is being pursued, becomes desperate, and turns to aggression and assaultiveness in a self-defensive effort to protect himself, or he may take flight, attempt to withdraw, flee, hide himself, injure himself, or commit suicide.

One patient, a twenty-seven-year-old man, had seen the film *The Exorcist* two times in one week. Subsequently, he ingested cleaning powder and poured soap and cleaning powder into his eyes to "exorcise the devil in himself."

J. D., age twenty-one, was picked up by the police in an expensive, downtown hotel where he had checked in under the pseudonym of a French duke. He had also written a letter to the FBI as follows:

Agent W
US Secret Service
Washington, D.C.
I tried to reach you but to no avail. I'm still sick in my own way. I want still to kill the president and end this farcical government. I'm tired of hospitals that do no good. At _____ they really helped me, and I may try to get back there but I don't think I'll make it. I bought a gun and we'll head to LA where I'll meet comrades in arms. Agent A. knows nothing of this—he noticed I was nervous but only because I had my gun on me. From here I'll try to phone to Washington, if you don't try to stop me first. Please don't cause I don't want to cause anyone unnecessary problems or hurt anyone. Neither of my parents know of my intentions; only Mrs. H. knows or might know. You were good to me. You really helped.

The letter was not signed but was written clearly and the return address simply gave the name of a French duke. On admission it was found that the patient had visions and heard voices—"They tell me to destroy." He also stated, "I am one of the French dukes . . . I'm among the aristocrats. I use titles; if Nixon took the title of king I'd support him completely." In addition, he was tense, anxious, suicidal, homicidal,

and depressed. It was also found that, in the past, he had poured rat poison in the family milk supply.

Some paranoid individuals may get along quite well in the community with some support and with only occasional periods of exacerbations as does the following person:

Elsa D., age fifty-two, is admitted to the inpatient service by the home visiting team after a telephone call from the manager of the hotel where she lives. He reported that she had been a model tenant for two years but had recently stopped eating, began talking to herself, standing on the street corner counting her money, and tossing her hands to the sky. She seemed to be fighting imaginary people, no longer spoke with friends, was two months behind in paying her rent, and had stopped responding to her name.

On admission, she is angry, loud, suspicious, hostile, and states that her husband has been poisoning her. "He has been giving me liver poison especially since I am not Jewish," she says. She accuses the nurse of trying to poison her and says to the psychiatrist, "No thank you, Dr. Aesop, I've had enough of your fables and all that poison the nurse is giving me." She misidentifies the staff and says to the nurse, "I knew you when you were a little girl. I will sue you for a million dollars." Despite her belligerence and unwillingness to talk about herself, she cooperated with the treatment plan.

Later, it was learned that she was under the care of a psychiatrist, was taking phenothiazines, but that every two years or so she stopped taking her medications and would have to be admitted.

The following is a person with an acute paranoid break for the first time:

The patient, Mr. N., is a twenty-six-year-old male who is employed at a local department store. He comes to the psychiatric emergency services at 1:00 A.M. with his girl friend and parents. He is delusional, agitated, and disoriented to time, place, and person. He says, "I was kidnapped. I've been arrested three times tonight and I don't know why. I've been locked up three days without bread and water. I haven't slept for three days due to the police. I'm a pro-baseball player from Cincinnati. I'm worth one hundred thousand dollars. My stomach and back hurt. People from Texas are coming to kill me. I don't want to die."

The patient made threats to kill unspecified people "before they kill me." The patient has lived with his girl friend (and with parents) for six years. He is agitated and crying and does not recognize his parents. His parents and girl friend say there have been no problems or disagreements. His mother states, "He's a good boy; he never got into trouble."

This patient was admitted to the locked inpatient psychiatric unit and placed on moderate suicide precautions. Haldol 5 mg. IM *prn* for agitation was ordered by the physician. After a few weeks of milieu therapy, and psychotherapy, he was discharged to his home and referred to a private psychiatrist.

Politics, religion, and sex are common themes in the content of the paranoid patient's verbalizations as follows:

"I was president of North Vietnam, they want to kill me—they're (family) all Nazis. They are multimillionaires and they are letting me starve to death. My uncle is applying for prime minister of the U.S.

The Communists are taking over Washington, they need to kill the Jews. Want to hear a Jewish joke? Hitler is alive! He is taking over Washington. I saw him in a hospital there. I think all the Nazis are dead—I hope Hitler is dead.

I like to masturbate and fantasize about masturbating women. I was Indian chief of the Apaches. They appointed me because they loved me."

The behavior of the following paranoid person exemplifies the feeling of being ready to flee from persecution:

When asked why he was at the hospital, the patient replied, "They chained my wrists and ankles and dragged me through the streets. I've never been treated so badly. I was packing—I couldn't pack any faster. I have a Steinway piano and Hemway organ. I'm a musician. I love music. I had my two-hundred-dollar drapes folded. I'm going to sell my things, buy a station wagon, and go to Mexico. I won't be a citizen anymore."

NURSING CARE

In order to help the paranoid person, trust is essential to develop and to be retained. Through trust and confiding in a neutral person who does not take sides, reality can become more apparent than the pseudocommunity and anxiety is therefore lessened. The patient needs to express his fear and anger to a kind, helpful, but somewhat detached person (if the therapist gets too close, it will be too threatening to the patient). The nurse does not agree with the delusions of the patient or argue with the patient about them. Instead, communication should be directed to the real world.

The paranoid individual is very sensitive to restrictions of liberty; therefore, posted rules in inpatient units and explanations of any deviations from them are necessary in order to help the patient understand that he is not being singled out and to avoid increasing suspicion and hostility. Manners often keep aggression in hand, and paranoid persons may appear overly courteous and often relate easier to nurses who are themselves polite and courteous.

TREATMENT

The work of Otto Allen Will, Jr. (1961), with a paranoid schizophrenic patient demonstrates the use of psychoanalytic concepts in a therapeutic procedure, which emphasized, (1) dependable, clear, and secure interpersonal relationships, (2) identifications with the therapist and others who were acceptable, comprehensive, and could be an enduring, reliable part of the self-concept, and (3) a relationship where anxiety felt as a threat of loss was diminished. Psychotropic drugs are widely used in the treatment of paranoid persons.

Since counteraggression reinforces the patient's delusions, in the nurse–patient relationship a lack of counteraggression is necessary; intellectual challenges may be encountered with the patient, and relationships explored matter-of-factly. It must be remembered that there is some truth in the delusions of the paranoid person. Truthfulness and promises must be rigidly adhered to by the nurse. A promise made, however small, is remembered by these patients, and if unfulfilled, is taken as rejection and becomes further food for insecurity. The nurse does not agree with the patient's delusions, but instead helps him use other defenses in adaptation. The account of the therapist who entered into the delusion of his patient is dramatically presented in the "Jet-Propelled Couch" (Lindner, 1955).

Summary

This chapter presents aggression from the social, ethological, and psychiatric points of view. The need for release of aggression is discussed as being common to everyone. Suspicious, hostile, and paranoid behavior is described and implications for nursing presented.

REFERENCES

AMERICAN PSYCHIATRIC ASSOCIATION: *Diagnostic and Statistical Manual of Mental Disorders.* III. Washington, D.C.: 1980.
_____: *A Psychiatric Glossary.* Washington, D.C.: 1980.
APPLEBAUM, PAUL S.: "Patterns of Violence Among Psychiatric Inpatients," in American Psychiatric Association: *Scientific Proceedings in Summary Form,* Washington, D.C.: American Psychiatric Association, 1975, pp. 141–142.
ARIETI, SILVANO: *American Handbook of Psychiatry,* Vol. III. New York: Basic Books, Inc., 1974, pp. 641–43.
BENDER, LAURETTA: "Hostile Aggression in Children," in Garattini, S. et al, eds.: *Aggressive Behavior.* New York: John R. Wiley & Sons, Inc., 1969, p. 322.
BERKOWITZ, LEONARD: *Aggression: A Social Psychological Analysis.* New York: McGraw-Hill Book Co., 1962.
BUSS, ARNOLD H.: *The Psychology of Aggression.* New York: John Wiley & Sons, Inc., 1961.
CAMERON, NORMAN A.: "Paranoid Conditions and Paranoia," in Arieti, Silvano, ed.: *American Handbook of Psychiatry,* Vol. III. New York: Basic Books, Inc., 1974, pp. 676–93.
COSER, LEWIS A.: *The Functions of Social Conflict.* New York: The Free Press of Glencoe, 1956, p. 62.
DOLLARD, J., DOBB, L. W., MILLER, N. E., MOWRER, O. H., and SEARS, R. F.: *Frustration and Aggression.* New Haven, Conn.: Yale University Press, 1939.
ERNST, K.: "Aggressive Acts by Psychiatric Patients as Reported by Staff. A Retrospective Reconstruction," *Psychiatria Clinica* (Basel), 8:4:189–200, 1975.

FREUD, ANNA: "Comments on Aggression," *International Journal of Psychoanalysis,* 53:163–69, 1972.
FREUD, SIGMUND: "Three Essays on the Theory of Sexuality," *Standard Edition of the Complete Psychological Works of Sigmund Freud.* London: The Hogarth Press, 1953, pp. 135–243.
_____: "Beyond the Pleasure Principle" (1920). *Standard Edition of the Complete Psychological Works of Sigmund Freud,* Vol. XVIII. London: The Hogarth Press, 1955, pp. 44–61.
_____: "Psycho-analytical Notes on an Autobiographical Account of a Case of Paranoia (Dementia Paranoides)" (1911). *Standard Edition of the Complete Psychological Works of Sigmund Freud,* (The Case of Schreber), Vol. XII. London: Hogarth Press, 1958, pp. 3–82.
_____: "On Narcissism: An Introduction," *Standard Edition of the Complete Psychological Works of Sigmund Freud,* Vol. XIV. London: Hogarth Press, 1957, pp. 73–102.
_____: "Instincts and Their Vicissitudes," (1915). *Standard Edition of the Complete Psychological Works of Sigmund Freud,* Vol. XIV. London: Hogarth Press, 1957, pp. 117–40.
GORNEY, RODERIC: "Interpersonal Intensity, Competition and Synergy: Determinants of Achievement, Aggression, and Mental Illness," *American Journal of Psychiatry,* 128:4:436–45, October 1971.
HOLLOWAY, R. L.: "Human Aggression: The Need for a Species Specific Framework," *Natural History,* 76:10:40–43, December 1967.
LIDZ, THEODORE: *The Origin and Treatment of Schizophrenic Disorders.* New York: Basic Books, Inc., 1973, p. 14.
LINDNER, ROBERT M.: *The Fifty Minute Hour.* New York: Rinehart, 1955.
LION, JOHN R., and PASTERNAK, STEFAN A.: "Countertransference Reactions to Violent Patients," *American Journal of Psychiatry,* 130:2:207–210, 1973.
LORENZ, KONRAD: *On Aggression.* New York: Harcourt, Brace & World, Inc., 1963.
MAHLER, MARGARET S., BERMAN, ANNI, PINE, FRED: "Danger Signals in the Separation–Individuation Process," unpublished paper, 1973.
RUESCH, JURGEN: *Therapeutic Communication.* New York: W. W. Norton & Co., Inc., 1961.
SILVER, LARRY B., DUBLIN, CHRISTINA C., and LAURIE, REGINALD: "Does Violence Breed Violence? Contribution from a Study of Child Abuse Syndrome," *American Journal of Psychiatry,* 126:3:404–407, September 1969.
WASHBURN, SHERWOOD L.: "The Origins of Aggressive Behavior," *Mental Health Program Reports-3.* Washington, D.C.: U.S. Department

of Health, Education and Welfare, 1969, pp. 255–72.

WILL, JR., OTTO ALLEN: "Paranoid Development and the Concept of Self," in *Chestnut Lodge Symposium: Papers Presented on the Fiftieth Anniversary, 1910–1960.* Washington, D.C.: William Alanson White Psychiatric Foundation, 1961.

Suggested Readings

ANDERS, ROBERT: "When a Patient Becomes Violent," *American Journal of Nursing,* 77:7:1144–1149, July 1977.

ARIETI, SILVANO: "Schizophrenia: Symptomatology and Mechanisms," *American Handbook of Psychiatry,* Vol. I. New York: Basic Books, Inc., 1969, pp. 475–84.

_____: "Schizophrenia: The Psychodynamic Mechanisms and the Psychostructural Forms," *American Handbook of Psychiatry,* Vol. III. New York: Basic Books, Inc., 1974, pp. 551–87.

BERES, DAVID: "Clinical Notes on Aggression in Children," in Eissler, Ruth, ed.: *The Psychoanalytic Study of the Child.* New York: International Universities Press, Inc., 1952, pp. 241–63.

BERKOWITZ, LEONARD, ed.: *Roots of Aggression.* New York: The Atherton Press, 1969.

BLUMENTHAL, MONICA D.: "Resentment and Suspicion Among American Men," *American Journal of Psychiatry,* 130:8:876–80, August 1973.

BRENNER, CHARLES: "The Psychoanalytic Concept of Aggression," *International Journal of Psychoanalysis,* 52:137–43, 1971.

BROOKS, BEATRICE R.: "Aggression," *American Journal of Nursing,* 67:12:2519–22, December 1967.

CHRISTIE, L. S.: "Conflicting Needs and Concepts in Psychiatric Hospitals," *Nursing Times,* 71:51:2036–2037, 1975.

CLACK, JANICE: "Nursing Intervention into the Aggressive Behavior of Patients," in Burd, Shirley F., and Marshall, Margaret A., eds.: *Some Clinical Approaches to Psychiatric Nursing.* New York: MacMillan Publishing Co., Inc., 1963.

COFFMAN, JUDITH ANN: "Anger: Its Significance for Nurses Who Work with Emotionally Disturbed Children," *Perspectives in Psychiatric Care,* VII:3:104–11, 1969.

FLYNN, GERTRUDE E.: "Hostility in a Mad, Mad World," *Perspectives in Psychiatric Care,* VII:4:152–58, 1969.

FREUD, SIGMUND: *Civilization and Its Discontents.* London: Hogarth Press, 1953. (First published 1930)

GRIER, WILLIAM H., and COBBS, PRICE M.: *Black Rage.* New York: Basic Books, Inc., 1968.

GUTHEIL, THOMAS G.: "Observations on the Theoretical Basis for Seclusion of the Psychiatric Inpatient," *American Journal of Psychiatry,* 135:3:325–328, March 1978.

HODGE, IAN LODGE: "Treatment or Punishment? A Nineteenth-Century Scandal," *Psychological Medicine,* 6:1:143–149, 1976.

JAHODA, MARIE: *Race Relations and Mental Health.* Place de Fontenoy, Paris: United Nations Educational, Scientific and Cultural Organization, 1960.

JAMES, DAVID J.: "Practical Care of the Aggressive Patient," *Nursing Times,* 68:1352–53, October 1972.

KIENING, SISTER MARY MARTHA: "Hostility," in Carlson Carolyn E., ed.: *Behavioral Concepts and Nursing Intervention.* Philadelphia: J. B. Lippincott Co., 1978, pp. 128–140.

KNEISL, CAROL R., and KELLY, HOLLY S.: "Introduction to the Conference on Hostility in the Nurse–Patient Interaction," *Perspectives in Psychiatric Care,* 7:4:153–58, July–August 1969.

LATHROP, VALLORY G.: "Aggression as a Response," *Perspectives in Psychiatric Care,* XVI:5–6:203–205, September–December 1978.

LEBON, GUSTAVE: *The Crowd.* London: Ernest Benn Limited, 1952.

LION, JOHN R.: "Conceptual Issues in the Use of Drugs for the Treatment of Aggression in Man," *Journal of Nervous and Mental Disease,* 160:2:76–82, 1975.

LION, JOHN R., MADDEN, DENIS, and CHRISTOPHER, RUSSELL: "A Violence Clinic: Three Years Experience," in American Psychiatric Association: *Scientific Proceedings in Summary Form.* Washington, D.C.: American Psychiatric Association, 1975.

LIPP, MARTIN R.: *Respectful Treatment: The Human Side of Medical Care.* Hagerstown, Md.: Harper & Row, Publishers, 1977, pp. 112–114.

PENALVER, MEG: "Helping the Child Handle His Aggression," *American Journal of Nursing,* 73:9:1554–55, 1973.

P. O. REPRINTS: "Understanding Hostility," *American Journal of Nursing,* 67:10:2131–50, October 1967.

RESTAK, RICHARD M.: *The Brain: The Last Frontier.* New York: Doubleday and Co., Inc., 1979.

STASTNY, JOY P.: "Helping a Patient Learn to Trust," *Perspectives in Psychiatric Care,* 3:7:16–28, 1965.

STEWART, ALLEN T.: "Handling the Aggressive Patient," *Perspectives in Psychiatric Care,* XVI:

5–6:228–234, September–December 1978.

STRINGER, MARGE: "Therapeutic Nursing Intervention Following Derogation of the Nurse by the Patient," *Perspectives in Psychiatric Care,* 3:4:36–38, 1965.

WAELDER, ROBERT: *Basic Theory of Psychoanalysis.* New York: International Universities Press, 1960.

THOMAS, MARY DURAND: "Trust," in Carlson, Carolyn, ed.: *Behavioral Concepts and Nursing Intervention.* Philadelphia: J. B. Lippincott Co., 1978.

VOINESKOS, G.: "Locked Wards in Canadian Mental Hospitals: The Return to Custodialism," *Canadian Medical Journal,* 114:8:689–694, 1976.

WHITAKER, CARL A.: "Psychotherapy of the Absurd: With A Special Emphasis on the Psychotherapy of Aggression," *Family Process,* 14:1:1–16, 1975.

8

The Suicidal Crisis

LEARNING OBJECTIVES / Persons studying this chapter should be able to:

1. Define suicidology, psychological autopsy, suicide equivalents, lethality assessment
2. Discuss the epidemology of suicide in the United States and the implications for nursing
3. Discuss determinants of suicide
4. List eight fables about suicide
5. Describe the affects associated with the suicidal person
6. List the components of a lethality rating
7. List guidelines for nursing care of a suicidal person at high risk (a) in a psychiatric unit (b) in a general hospital
8. Describe the effect of suicide upon the victim–survivors

There is but one truly serious philosophical problem, and that is suicide.
ALBERT CAMUS, "An Absurd Reasoning," *The Myth of Sisyphus*

Operatic suicides are very dramatic and the affects are diverse. They range from the fear of *Peter Grimes* to the jealousy of *Wozzeck* and the despair of *Tosca.* The theme of romantic love and the unwillingness of one to live without the other is exemplified in the tragedy of *Romeo and Juliet.* Suicide prevention in antiquity probably began with Plutarch, A.D. 46–119 (Choron, 1968).

The National Save-a-Life League, which is located in New York City, is the oldest suicide-prevention organization in this country. It was founded by Rev. Harry Marsh Warren in 1906. Besides offering counseling and emergency help, it maintains a twenty-four-hour telephone service. In England the Salvation Army established an antisuicide department as early as 1906 (Stengel, 1964, p. 118). The Samaritans, founded in 1953, comprise a group of ministers and lay people with physician consultants. Similar organizations exist in many towns and in other countries. The Samaritans help others by offering friendship, care, concern, and love and have become international (Varah, 1965).

The incorporation of suicide-prevention centers within public-health services at both federal and local levels gives a new emphasis to this problem. More research into suicide has therefore been made possible. The National Institute of Mental Health Center for Studies of Suicide Prevention was established in October 1966. It was dissolved and converted to a section on Crisis Intervention, Suicide, and Mental Health Emergencies in 1972. Founded in 1967, the American Association of Suicidology is the first nationwide organization to be dedicated to the scientific study of suicide prevention. The association stimulates research, education, and training in suicidology,[1] disseminates knowledge through programs and publications, and encourages the application of research to the understanding and reduction of self-destruction in the person. The first Annual National Conference on Suicidology was held in Chicago in 1968. Subsequently the International Association for the Prevention of Suicide has been formed and is involved in much-needed research.

A new school of suicidology open on the interdisciplinary levels gives impetus to better understanding that may lead to more effective preventive techniques. The *Bulletin of Suicidology,* published from 1967 through 1971, aided in communication of findings and knowledge of organizational structures; the Journal *Suicide and Life-Threatening Behavior* is the official publication of the American Association of Suicidology.

The study of suicidology is aimed at reducing the self-destruction of persons. The purpose of the National Institute of Mental Health Center for Studies of Suicide Prevention was to assist, encourage, support, and catalyze research, in addition to training, supporting, and demonstration activities related to suicide theory and suicide prevention throughout the country. It was designed to further basic knowledge of the problem of suicide and to develop techniques for aiding the suicidal individual.

In the study of suicide, the psychological autopsy has given further understanding that may lead to more effective preventive efforts. The psychological autopsy focuses on the intention of the deceased in relation to his own death. It represents an attempt by a team of professionals to clarify cases in which the motivation for suicide is unclear. Information is secured from a number of persons and a reconstruction is made of the life-style of the deceased and the last few days of his life. After the information is discussed by the team, a confidential written report is given to the medical examiner (Curphey, 1968). Family members and others involved have remarked on the benefits

of talking with the team performing the psychological autopsy. The team therefore performs a double function: research into the conditions surrounding the suicide and the therapeutic function of aiding the survivor–victims.

Epidemiology

The suicide rate for the United States is usually reported as between ten and twelve per one hundred thousand. Reported suicides per year now exceed twenty-five thousand, although it is generally believed that a more accurate figure would be two to three times greater. Suicide has ranked among the twelve leading causes of death in the nation at large for several years. Stigma is attached to suicide, and attempts to cover it up are made by physicians and families. Over four thousand of the twenty-five thousand suicides are in the fifteen to twenty-four age group; many cases go unreported. For the age group fifteen to twenty-four, the suicide rate was 4.0 in 1957 and 12.2 in 1975 (U.S. Division of Vital Statistics, 1976).

For 1977, the overall suicide rate per one hundred thousand people in the United States was 12.5 (see Fig. 9).

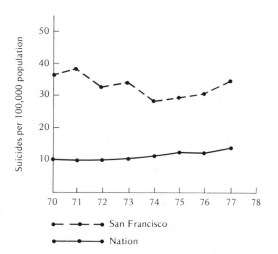

FIGURE 9. Comparison of Suicide Rates of San Francisco with the Overall Rates of the United States.

---

[1] Suicidology is the study of suicide and suicide prevention as well as related phenomena of self-destruction.

In Hendin's (1975) study of fifty college students over a six-year period, it was found that high proportions of suicidal students had lost a parent or felt the bond of emotional death.

A recent study of suicide in Cuyahoga County, Ohio (1959–1974), shows a marked increase in suicide among teenagers and young adults and among nonwhite males; older white males had the highest rate of suicide, reflecting the national picture (Ford et al., 1979). Alcohol was present in the blood of one fourth of those dead on arrival and at levels of intoxication of 20 per cent of the DOA's. Disrupted affectional relationships figure prominently in the suicides of person who suffer from alcoholism.

Hart and Keidel (1979) emphasize the importance of suicide prevention by the school nurse. Detection of those at high risk, counseling, educating school personnel, parents and students, and referral are important aspects of the school nurse's role. Because of the vulnerable age group, schools and college campuses should have access to suicide prevention. A geriatric hot line is also an integral part of the Suicide Prevention Center of San Francisco.

Suicide is shown to be a significant factor in mania, depression, and schizophrenia (Winokur and Tsnang, 1975). As alternatives to hospitalization are developed and deinstitutionalization has occurred, large numbers of people with mental disorders now live in the community instead of the more protective environment of the mental hospital. Nurses in community settings (and others) now have more responsibility for risk detection and assisting those individuals in suicidal crisis.

There is also evidence that suicide is more prevalent in those who have incurable diseases and those in war, although the incidence of suicide in the population at large decreases during wartime. Suicide through self-neglect may be more widespread than documented, especially among those experiencing the crises of aging, poverty, loneliness, and desolation. Suicide is linked to alcoholism and homicide. Suicide in accidents, especially automobile accidents, may go unrecorded as suicide. Studies of the psychodynamics of death have resulted in changes in the concept of the modes of death, e.g., the NASH classification: natural, accident, suicide, and homicide (Shneidman, 1969).

Suicide is higher among the single, widowed, separated, and divorced; males outnumber females. In the United States, it is more prevalent among whites than nonwhites. Migrants to a district, the foreignborn, native-born American youth, the aged, and those living alone have distinctly higher suicide rates. In most areas of the world, physical and mental illness, social isolation, death of a loved one, and loss of status (particularly upon retirement), together with the sudden lowering of income, are associated with suicide in the aging (World Health Organization, 1968). In San Francisco, which has been called the suicide capital, a study by Seiden (1967) shows that only 5 percent of suicides are from the Golden Gate Bridge. The fact that San Francisco's alcoholism rate is very high influences its suicide rate. San Francisco is a relatively small city, but there is a large area in the central city where suicide rates are high. San Francisco's median age is eight years higher and the single population 35 percent greater than in the country as a whole. All these factors contribute to the high suicide rate.

Etiology

TYPES OF SUICIDE

The motivation for suicide was considered by Freud to be directed against the introjected love object, a kind of murder of the self. It has been a generally accepted view that suicide is internalized aggression. Durkheim (1951) categorized suicide into three types: *egoistic,* where the person no longer finds life palatable and therefore kills himself; *altruistic,* that is, required by society; and *anomic,* in which society is lacking in its support to the individual. Added as a footnote to these three types of suicide was another, which has received little attention: *fatalistic* suicide.

. . . the suicide deriving from excessive regulation, that of persons with futures pitilessly blocked and passions violently choked by oppressive disciplines . . . the suicide of very young husbands, of the married woman who is childless . . . But it has so little contemporary importance and examples are so hard to find . . . Do not the suicide of slaves . . . belong to this type, or all the suicides attributed to excessive physical or moral despotism? To bring out the ineluctible and inflexible nature of a rule against which there is no appeal, and in contrast with the expression "anomy" which has just been used, we might call it *fatalistic suicide.*[2]

No more than half a century has elapsed since the time of Durkheim; therefore, such cases of fatalistic suicide are now perhaps more evident. The all-too-familiar example of the person who kills himself when his fraudulent activities are discovered or who is jailed for minor violations of authority may fall into this category. In a study of forty-two Black men who killed themselves in New Orleans, the critical factor of fear and impotence in dealing with the police and other authorities was seen as relevant to suicide (Breed, 1969).

In De Vos's (1973) psychocultural concept of suicide, he adds to the traditional ones of Durkheim a new category: *egocentric* suicide. It is differentiated from the egoistic suicide in that there is greater emphasis on frustration and aggression in egocentric suicide as contrasted with the loss and despair of egoistic suicide.

DETERMINANTS OF SUICIDE

Freud considered the instinct for life (Eros) and the instinct for death (Thanatos) to be present in everyone and in conflict. At times of stress, the destructive part of the suicidal person gains ascendancy.

Based on Freud's view that, unconsciously, persons identify with introjected love objects and that both feelings of love and hate occur with introjection, the suicidal person attempts unconsciously to want the internalized love object dead.

[2] Durkheim, Emile: *Suicide.* New York: The Free Press, 1951, p. 276.

Menninger (1938) described three components of every suicide: the wish to kill, the wish to be killed, and the wish to die. He also pointed out that self-mutilation is a "compromise form of suicide" constituting a victory of the life instinct over the death instinct (Menninger, 1938, p. 285). Meerloo (1962, p. 25) notes that "there is also the secret belief in mystical rescue and revival; an urge to make a magic offering to the gods; and many other motivations contributing to the act."

Because children are so dependent on love objects for gratification and since identification and other levels of growth have not been completed, destruction of introjected love objects is too painful. Therefore, children rarely commit suicide (Schechter, 1957, p. 131). However, in the suicidal child, the hostility toward the parent is turned inward and desperate attempts are made to regain contact with the parent. Feelings of rage, helplessness, and worthlessness are developed. Although there are many motivations for suicide in children, the primary one is real or threatened loss of a love object (Schechter, 1957, p. 141). The treatment of the suicidal child is to reestablish gratifying object relationships.

If the target of aggression is another person rather than oneself, the homicide rate increases, as in the legitimized act of war (Henry, and Short, 1954, p. 102). Aggression, instead of being directed against the self as in suicide, is directed outwardly in war.

Disruptions of social relations have also been postulated as etiological factors in suicide. For example, broken homes and parental loss in childhood predispose to depression and suicide in later life (Dorpat et al., 1968). Since children are the age group likely to have the most status integration on a wide scale, this may account for their low suicide rate (Gibbs and Martin, 1964).

Suicides below the age of ten years are not reported nationally, although hospitals are currently receiving more latency-age children who have made suicidal attempts.

Cultural determinants of suicide must be studied in every case. The influence of society in the determination of the particular kind of human being under consideration requires emphasis. In the Black culture, abandonment by husband or boyfriend, guilt about pregnancies, and rejection of their children are factors in the suicide of women (Hendin, 1969). Also, a history of childhood rejection in Black men and women may add to the higher urban suicide rate among young Black adults than that of their white counterparts (Hendin, 1969, p. 106). A connection between conscious overt violence, including homicide, and self-destructive behavior, including suicide, is made by Hendin, who describes the experience of being Black in our culture as generating violence. The Black man is thus faced with the problem of controlling it (p. 48).

In adolescence, the reawakening of the oedipal conflicts, the emergence of heightened emotional stresses, and sexual urges that may be strongly tabooed are etiological factors. The Icarus complex has been noted as a factor in suicide, especially in Japan and the Soviet Union, where failure in exams denotes loss of status and wounded ambition (Meerloo, 1962).

A study of family determinants of suicide potential by Richman (1971) on one hundred families cites characteristics of a majority of over one hundred families with suicidal problems as follows: (1) intolerance for separation, (2) symbiosis without empathy, (3) fixations upon childhood patterns and social roles, (4) closed family system, (5) a characteristic pattern of dealing with aggression, (6) scapegoating, (7) sadomasochistic relationships, (8) doublebind and other communication disturbances, (9) acting out the negative side of the family, (10) family fragility, (11) family depression, and (12) intolerance of crises.

Suicidal equivalents are alternate expressions of self-destruction. Accidental injuries, antisocial acts, engagement in dangerous activities, and cigarette smoking are familiar examples.

The suicidal person feels love and hate together; ambivalence is marked. He also feels the urge for life and the urge for death. The suicidal person slashes his wrist and cries for help at the same time. The first person who survived the suicidal leap from the Golden Gate Bridge decided between the time she jumped off and before she hit the water that she wanted to live and, despite broken bones, swam to safety.

On the other hand, there is more to suicide than hostility (Shneidman, 1966). Shneidman refers to dependency as a factor with critical affects of helplessness and hopelessness. "I can't survive in this world" and "I'm too far gone for anyone to help me" are expressions of these affects.

Patients who are depressed may be particularly suicidal, although not all suicidal patients are depressed. The most vulnerable times for the depressed patient are when he is going into or coming out of a depression. Seventy to 80 per cent of completed or attempted suicides are due to depressive disorders (Kiev, 1979).

The following facts and fables about suicides are pertinent to the practice of all helping persons.

Facts and Fables About Suicide

1. *Fable:* People who talk about suicide don't commit suicide.
   Fact: Of any ten people who kill themselves, eight have given definite warnings of their suicidal intentions.
2. *Fable:* Suicide happens without warning.
   Fact: Studies reveal that the suicidal person gives many clues and warnings regarding his suicidal intentions.
3. *Fable:* Suicidal people are fully intent on dying.
   Fact: Most suicidal people are undecided about living or dying, and they "gamble with death," leaving it to others to save them. Almost no one commits suicide without letting others know how he is feeling.
4. *Fable:* Once a person is suicidal, he is suicidal forever.
   Fact: Individuals who wish to kill themselves are "suicidal" only for a limited period of time.
5. *Fable:* Improvement following a suicidal crisis means that the suicidal risk is over.
   Fact: Most suicides occur within about three months following the beginning of "improvement," when the individual has the energy to put his morbid thoughts and feelings into effect.
6. *Fable:* Suicide strikes much more often among the rich or, conversely, it occurs more frequently among the poor.
   Fact: Suicide is neither the rich man's dis-

ease nor the poor man's curse. Suicide is represented proportionately among all levels of society.

7. *Fable:* Suicide is inherited or "runs in the family."

Fact: It follows individual patterns.

8. *Fable:* All suicidal individuals are mentally ill, and suicide always is the act of a psychotic person.

Fact: Studies of hundreds of genuine suicide notes indicate that although the suicidal person is extremely unhappy, he is not necessarily mentally ill.[3]

RITUAL SUICIDES

In Japan, *hara-kiri* may be carried out when there is a change of status of the individual. The *kamikaze* pilots of World War II achieved a form of *hara-kiri* that accorded them great honor. The rite of *suttee* in which the Hindu wife throws herself on her husband's funeral pyre and is cremated with his body is still illegally practiced in India (Carstairs, 1958, p. 74). The ritualized self-disembowelment by the famous Japanese novelist Yukio Mishima, at age forty-five, is described by Iga and Yamamoto (1973) as the "sword" (aggression) aspect of the cultural traditions of Japan, whereas the suicide of Yasunari Kawabata, at the age of seventy-two, by gas, emphasizes the "chrysanthemum" (resignation and despair) aspects. The recent (1978) and apparently rehearsed suicides of the People's Temple members in Guyana is an example of mass suicide in its most extreme form. Public immolations and suicide viewed on television signify the intensity of feelings involved for the act itself and the martyristic nature of the suicides.

ALIENATION

There is a resurgence of loneliness in our society; it is not physical loneliness, but the loneliness of the crowd or loneliness of self. Loneliness refers to being without company,

destitute of friendly companionship. Being lonely refers to self. That there is more loneliness today is symbolic of the fact that institutions do not offer a sense of belonging. Being human is inseparable from being social; yet loneliness can be experienced in relation to others and to oneself. It can therefore occur when one is physically close to others. Alienation in modern society is real. The power and attraction of groups that invite the individual to examine his mirror-image self and the mirror of his social image through the group experience is a possible indication of the alienation in contemporary society. Even families involve themselves in these group experiences for better understanding of individual members and the unit as a whole. The technological modern society seems to have discarded the church social, the annual family reunion, and other kinds of small gatherings where people could observe the yearly differences, take in new members, note the members missing either by death or for other reasons, and thereby feel an identity of self and with the group. Can institutions in the mass society provide a sense of belonging?

In our society, although we may sympathize with others, it is culturally forbidden to feel sorry for ourselves. It is important to distinguish between social isolation and loneliness. The former is an objective condition such as the situation of a hermit. It refers to having few contacts with family, neighbors, or significant others. Loneliness is subjective; it is a feeling and may be unrelated to social isolation (Townsend, 1963).

We as a people are dissatisfied with self and are generally striving for some kind of improvement of self. It is not uncommon to see students in their seventies. People with higher degrees attend evening classes and take trips to foreign countries to "sit in on classes there." Students with perfectly respectable grades of "C" and "B" often say disappointedly, "I *could* have gotten an A." People in our society are not taught to be alone; there is push for conformity, to be with others, to be beset with decibels and other stimulants. Children are not taught the value of solitude or how to deal with it and derive benefit from it. For the most part, the solitary experiences of moun-

[3] Shneidman, Edwin S., and Farberow, Norman L.: "Some Facts About Suicide." Washington, D.C.: Superintendent of Documents, Public Health Service Publication No. 852, 1965, pp. 3–5.

taintop, prairie, desert, taking an ocean voyage, or being snowbound have disappeared; ways of finding solitude are seldom sought in the crowded city. Perhaps the alienation results from the daily physical closeness and encounters with hundreds of people in an urban environment. Alienation may be a defense since interacting to any personal degree with all the individuals one meets in an urban environment would quickly deplete one's energy sources.

Fromm (1962) points out that in our society, a society of consumers, we are surrounded by innumerable *things* in whose creation we have not participated directly—we know only how to use or to consume them—and that this alienates us from ourselves. The recent interest in handmade items and country living may help overcome alienation.

The love of solitude and time for contemplation as a method of self-renewal has been virtually lost in our society where a person who is not at work feels he must be constantly entertained. Stimulus flooding may leave us with a psychological numbness (Keniston, 1967). Toynbee (1968) states that one of the features of human nature that makes us human is the faculty of spiritual contemplation.

Flight from feeling, detachment, fragmentation of feeling, and lack of belief in each other were prevalent in college students studied by Hendin (1975). He makes a plea for saving our emotional environment to make life worth living.

The dynamic interaction of self-worth, degree of ego strength, and number and availability of alternatives offered by our culture determines the amount of alienation for each one of us.

The era of transitory relationships may require alienation as a method of survival. On the other hand, however, nursing students are asked to overcome alienation. In nursing, there is an intimacy between the nurse and the patient that calls for involvement. The student's wish to be needed is met by the helpless, dependent, horizontal patient who depends on the nurse for his sustenance and comfort. When someone is needed, he is not likely to be lonely. Understanding oneself and one's relation to the society in which he lives is a prerequisite to being an effective nurse. It is not all learned at once and in fact all throughout life there are continuous glimmers of further understanding, if one seeks it. It in part prepares the nurse to better help patients who are lonely, fear death, are helpless, have financial problems, are paralyzed unexpectedly, and can never resume the level of wellness formerly experienced.

The intensive study of suicide during the sixties reveals it as a method of communication. Causes for suicide are likely to be multiple, and one traumatic event may be the precipitating factor after a series of preceding ones. To save a life, all professionals need to learn to be sensitive to the nuances of those individuals under their care. The profound loneliness of the suicidal patient with the subsequent cry for help needs to be understood, heard, and acted upon.

Nursing Intervention

With the suicidal patient the only significant intervention is prevention. The principal preventive technique is for a concerned person to show to the suicidal person that he really cares for him in a very deep way, that he will be there and that he will not desert him. Nurses are with patients and families throughout many stresses and can readily encourage this attachment behavior. Attention to their needs during these emotional crises may prevent suicide. Suicide-prevention centers have now been established in the nation for receiving telephone calls from the distressed potential suicidal person; others send out teams for home visits. Suicide-prevention services are an integral part of comprehensive crisis intervention.

Suicide is now viewed as communication: when, how, and where it takes place; to whom it is directed; and what is the content of the message. Nursing has previously been mostly concerned with patients who were hospitalized; now in the era of community mental health, nursing is concerned with preventive efforts in an anticipatory way. When the suicidal attempt comes, it may be too late. The challenge is to find populations at risk and to assist these individuals and families to meet their basic needs and crisis situations.

RECOGNITION OF THE SUICIDAL CRISIS

Aggression directed inward toward the self may result in suicide or the contemplation of suicide. Most suicidal patients give a warning. It is up to you to hear it and to respond. Cues may be verbal or nonverbal. The stresses of life and the process of passage through the usual developmental phases of life are all danger points. Changing jobs, leaving home for school, loss of job, marriage, inability to keep up grade point averages, divorce, death, and rejection are phases of the life arc in which anticipatory work is needed for prevention. A child who requests a blue casket and a blanket of flowers if he dies is telling you something serious. There are at least two dynamics found in lethal attempts: hostility and anxiety; therefore, these two facets of human behavior are critical phases and it is up to the helping person to note behavior and to do something about the suicidal person. Those people who want to kill themselves are ambivalent; they want to live and they want to die at the same time. Eros is stronger than Thanatos for most people; therefore, suicide prevention is possible.

Asking how to leave one's body to a medical school may be a hint of suicide, and saying, "I'm going to shoot myself" is a direct announcement. A fellow student who says that he cannot concentrate or who declares, "I'm all washed up," or who keeps saying over and over, "I'm no good," "It's my fault—I'm responsible," is asking for help. A sudden change in a person from being happy-go-lucky and cheerful to irritability, solemnity, and anger may be an indication of suicidal thoughts. Giving things away, making a will, and checking on insurance are indirect cues, although these behaviors may be normal preparation for death in older persons. In over one half of suicidal deaths, the person who kills himself indicates that he will do so to others. There seems to be a three-month interval following the suicidal crisis in which the patient is dangerous to himself (Shneidman and Farberow, 1959). School problems, family problems, and drug abuse are some of the precursors of suicide. Early secondary prevention at this stage can be effective.

Preventive efforts include observation and assessment of developmental tasks and helping patients to attain those tasks they have not accomplished. The helping person uses growth-promoting, problem-solving approaches.

Suicidal children are often those who do not take part in school activities and who do not have any close friends. In the adolescent, if the drive toward independence from parents is interfered with by cultural problems and a low opinion of himself, there is increased alienation, which may make him more vulnerable to suicide. Hot lines and rap lines are usually non-Establishment, nonpsychiatric, and nonprofessional and are often used by young people for assistance.

With a distressed person, emergency evaluation is required to assess his self-destructive potentiality. Psychiatric first aid may be administered via the telephone interview where a relationship must be established and maintained and trust secured if one is to provide the needed help. Taking a history from the distressed individual reminds him of his identity; it also provides information about the strengths of the patient. Emergency evaluation may also involve a home visit or a visit to another institution such as a school or hospital. For a potentially suicidal person, the emergency evaluation requires that the therapist get information, assess the lethality, and decide on action very quickly. The suicidal crisis calls for help on the spot.

For persons who telephone, at least five steps are designated in the treatment process: "(1) Establishment of a relationship—maintain contact and obtain information; (2) identification of and focus on the central problem; (3) evaluation of suicidal potential; (4) assessment of strength and resources; (5) information and initiation of therapeutic plans" (Farberow, 1967).

ASSESSMENT OF LETHALITY

Lethality is the probability of suicidal risk for a person. Agencies usually develop forms for recording data about the individual using the service, *i.e.,* name, age, sex, race, address, telephone number, and so on, although some telephone crisis services do not take the name of the caller.

In the establishment of a relationship, clear identification of both individuals should be made. The goal is to evaluate lethality. Direct, specific questions are asked about suicide. In the identification and clarification of the central problem, it is important to help the patient recognize central and secondary problems. Evaluation of the suicidal potential is made from the following criteria, which have been empirically derived by the Los Angeles Suicide Prevention Center. By use of these criteria, judgment is made about the lethality of the suicidal person and designated high, medium, or low.

1. *Age and sex:* The suicide rate increases with age, and men are more likely to kill themselves than women.
2. *Suicide plan:* This is probably the most important of the criteria. How well laid out is the plan? Are the means to carry it out available? Possession of a gun and making a plan for jumping or hanging constitute high risks. People who are psychotic and have bizarre plans are also high risks. A detailed plan and means available to carry it out are maximal lethality.
3. *Stress:* Stress must be evaluated from the patient's viewpoint. If stress and symptoms are severe, the situation calls for immediate assistance. "Why are you feeling suicidal now?" is the direct question to ask. Typical stresses are: loss of loved one, job, or health, threat of prosecution, and so forth. Suicide attempts are often made following the loss of or separation from a love object, at anniversaries of the loss, and at subsequent times when other losses occur such as that of a valued pet.
4. *Symptoms:* It is important to assess the symptoms. What is the person thinking and feeling? Is he in control of his behav-

ior? If his behavior is out of control, he is a high risk for suicide. Suicidal thoughts and feelings occur in many psychological states; the most common are depression, agitation, and psychotic states with delusions and hallucinations. Depressed patients are at very high lethality, at the onset and the decline of the depression.

5. *Resources:* Internal and external resources of the person, and resources of the community are all considered in the evaluation of lethality. Who is available for aid? Family? Friends? Neighbors? Clergy? Is the person already in contact with a therapist? Is there a history of ambivalent relationships with others? Does the person have a place to stay, something to eat, and money to live on? All efforts should be made to get as many others concerned about the person as are available. The less resources available, the higher the danger.
6. *Life-Style:* Is the person stable or unstable and is the suicidal behavior acute or chronic? It is important to differentiate between the extremely acute lethal person and one who is chronically dependent. When people whose lives are stable, and who are in acute stress, seek help, it is a significant contact. These people need immediate help. People whose lives are chronically disturbed, who have prior suicidal behavior, and are now in a downhill course constitute a high-risk group. Caution should be taken with the chronic suicide attempter to be certain he has not exhausted his resources.
7. *Communication:* The most important aspect of communication is whether or not the person is still in contact with other people, or is he telling you that his will is made and that he means to end it all? When the content of communication is directed toward others, the reaction of these individuals is important in the evaluation.
8. *Reaction of significant others:* The significant others are evaluated in terms of being helpful or not helpful. If the significant other sees the need for help and attempts to help get assistance, this is a positive communication to the suicidal person.
9. *Medical status:* People over sixty-five tend

to kill themselves because of physical illness and loneliness. If a person is over sixty-five, lives alone, has lost a spouse, has made a previous suicidal attempt, and is physically ill, he is a high risk. Physical body changes may be the signal of increasing hopelessness and helplessness.

At high risk are older persons, the alcoholic, the person who has previously attempted suicide, and those with severe mental disorders. Suicide risk is also increased by catastrophic stress, availability of lethal weapons, and contact with others who have made suicide attempts (Shneidman, 1976, p. 45).

Evaluation of homicidal intent should also be made according to history of assault, threats, plans, and possession of weapons.

If the person can accept help and respond, this is hopeful. The therapeutic plan is made on the basis of evaluation of the suicidal status and the information obtained about him. All available resources should be tapped for help, including nonprofessional and professional. The universal factors in suicide are thought to be isolation, separateness, and aloneness. The task of the therapist is to indicate awareness of his presence to the patient and to acknowledge that things are hurting. Suicidal patients are ambivalent, and the patient can be reassured that suicidal feelings are time-limited. Those who cannot ask for help are considered by some to be the most lethal. They are often seen in community mental-health centers and psychiatric hospitals. It is important for the nurse to *be on the side of Eros and thereby support life.*

The person who receives the telephone call for help assesses the lethality of the caller and the kind of problem that led to the crisis. Face-to-face contact teams are necessary for response to some requests for help; therefore, some community mental-health centers have developed outreach teams (McGee, 1974). It is definitely easier to assess the more obvious aspects of the potentially suicidal patient such as age, sex, job, a place to live, and availability of emotional support of others. However, the critical factors of strength are much more difficult to determine, for example, the ability to cope, to bear up under physical pain and

mental anguish, to relate to other people, and to accept help (Beck, 1974). Whether the suicidal person is at the other end of the telephone or face to face, the same principles of assessment and assistance apply. The mobile go-and-see team may be able to do a more thorough assessment in a home visit than by telephone. Intervening may sometimes therefore take the form of "breaking and entering" if the patient is unconscious, or it may also take the form of removing firearms, pills, and alcohol. For a person who is suicidal, it is very important in crisis intervention to elicit plans for the next few hours or days. This involves him with the events of life and with the support systems, for example, if it is the weekend, until his appointment or until he goes to work on Monday. Continuity of care and follow-up are crucial aspects of crisis service to suicidal persons.

Hendin (1964) evaluated suicidal patients on a scale of one to three with regard to their suicidal intent: the patient with (1) minimal intent, (2) moderate intent, and (3) maximal intent. Patients with maximal intent to die may accidentally survive and will continue in the maximal-intent group unless atonement has been reached by the intended act. Those with minimal intent may also accidentally die, as in the rejected lover's simulating taking poison that actually *is* poison. The patients in the moderate-intent group are indecisive. They may be the ones who jump from bridges and decide during the fall and before they hit the water to swim to safety.

In a recent study of nursing personnel (twelve R.N.'s, three licensed practical nurses, and fourteen paraprofessionals) of three psychiatric inpatient units of general hospitals in western New York, sixty-nine percent were not familiar with the term, "lethality assessment" (Barbee, 1978). If this reflects current knowledge elsewhere, an enormous nursing-education job needs to be done.

If the person is not hospitalized, the nurse first encountering the suicidal patient has the responsibility to assist the person and his family or friends to get help. Knowledge of the particular community facilities is therefore very necessary, in addition to the ability to assess the situation and to give psychiatric first aid. The book *Doctor Zhivago* portrays all too well the hushing up of the suicidal attempt in former times, which is still all too prevalent in the twentieth century (Pasternak, 1958). The frantic pleas to the physician, the anguish, the pain, and the hushed-up episode—all speak eloquently of society's attitude toward the person who tries to kill himself. It is time now that we are approaching the twenty-first century to abolish the hidden suicide attempt and to do all that we can to assist those who cry for help. They may be our dearest friends, family members, professors, roommates, colleagues, or complete strangers. The message is the same.

PREVENTION OF SUICIDE

Detention may propel the depressed person into a suidical attempt. Careful attention must be given to the psychodynamics of each individual. The traditional nursing safeguards such as twenty-four-hour observation and removal of harmful objects from the environment are not used in some psychiatric units. The responsibility put upon the patient is considered to be of value in prevention of suicide. Where the nursing staff uses the traditional safeguards, the ego of the depressed patient may be lowered further. Even with the most vigilant observations and removal of harmful objects from the environment, patients manage to attempt to kill or do kill themselves. Before entry to a hospital, one patient hid a razor blade in the innersole of her shoe and carefully reglued the inner sole back into place. Another had hidden a large box of phenobarbital tablets in a facial-tissue box that she brought with her to the hospital and took all of them the night she was admitted. Still another patient had thirty Nembutal capsules in the bottom half of a pack of cigarettes, having cut the cigarettes in half, put the capsules back in the package, and replaced the halved cigarettes. Another patient in bed under the watchful eyes of nurses managed to turn over and slice his veins with a piece of glass that was previously hidden in the pocket of his pajamas. One patient who succeeded in his suicidal attempt had taken phenobarbital and iodine

and slashed his throat from ear to ear as well as his wrists and his antecubital veins. Due to his poor conditions, physicians were unable to suture his throat, although they did succeed in lavaging his stomach with starch. The patient was conscious until death and wanted to live. I still remember the suffering in his eyes.

Suicide reflects hopelessness, helplessness, and fearfulness within individuals. It can be recognized and help can be given to prevent it. It is important to be open and level with the suicide patient, to discuss it with him fully. Suicide-prevention centers and others have the working philosophy that one must convey to the suicidal person that someone cares deeply. However, if one's own philosophy and affect is one of hopelessness, this may itself push the potential suicide over the brink. People live up to expectations, and how the nurse feels deeply affects the patient and his family. Hope must be sought by the nurse; all thoughts and actions (behavior) pyramid toward this point. The following is an interaction between a nursing student and her suicidal patient, a teenage girl:

The patient, Diane, feigned illness, avoided group therapy, and finally, after being questioned, said that she wanted to get sick so she would not be sent home. She stated that she had already caused her parents too much sorrow.

Nurse: Why?
   Patient: I've saved my medications since I've been here. I've intended to kill myself ever since I've been here. [She sat forward in her chair with her head hanging down and looking at the floor.]
   Nurse: Do you still feel like taking your own life?
   Patient: I don't know.

The student and the patient proceeded to talk about love and friendship and the patient related how her best friend closed the door in her face when she went to visit with her the last time she had been home on leave. The interaction ended with the student's saying forcefully and earnestly to the patient.

Nurse: Diane, I feel very strongly that you can get well and gain a desire to live. It's some-

thing each one of us has to discover. Life in some ways is very good and in other ways is very bad. Now, we can talk about this for a long time but ultimately the decision is yours. Let me help you. We can find some of the things that make life worthwhile.
Patient: O.K.

The student acknowledged the feelings of Diane, especially the feeling of rejection. She also immediately and openly asked about her suicidal thoughts. She expressed directly her belief in Diane as a person and quite pointedly put some responsibility on Diane's shoulders. After working with this patient for four and one half months the student terminated, as required by the curriculum. The student received the following note:

Dear Miss H.,
I call you this because it really takes a lady to do what you did. I haven't even opened the gift yet, but I feel I should write and let you know how thrilled I am. I'm writing this in pencil because tears blot ink, and I do want you to be able to read this.

I'm also writing this to thank you for all you have done for me. I would probably be doing all my foolish things if it hadn't been for you yet. Believe me I am very grateful, and always will be. I was afraid the hospital wouldn't be able to help me, but now that I see they can and already have, I'm going to do my best to get well.

Thanks again for everything. With all my love,
D.

P.S. Please write.

There were many other examples of emotional support to this patient by the student and others in the mental hospital. The foregoing interaction represents part of an interaction at a time when Diane was quite suicidal.

The following is a note written by a distraught, extremely suicidal nineteen-year-old to his dead fiancée before admission to the psychiatric ward. The patient was in a searching phase; he found some people in the telephone book with the same name as the finacée, telephoned, and wanted to see them.

I have been dreaming about the month of May (six months ago when the financée died). I was walking to school through the orchard and could hear your footsteps as you always ran to meet me. I don't know what to do with myself. I'm in a daze. I want to run or jump off a huge cliff or through a window on a high building or something to release the tensions inside me. I dream about it and pretend that you are really with me inside. You know I tried to kill myself twice before I ever met you. I'm so scared I'm gonna die soon. I need you to protect me from myself. I have it all planned.

With psychiatric treatment, this patient's depression lifted and he was discharged after three weeks.

Hospitalized patients may take the time of weekend leaves to commit suicide. Often it is the psychiatric nurse who knows the moods of the patient as part of the psychiatric team playing a most vital role in the determination of the appropriate timing of weekend leaves in the course of the patient's mental disorder. The circumstances of leaves should be known and include what the family and patient plan to do, where they will be, and what help can be secured if the suicidal feelings emerge.

Within the psychiatric unit itself, the change of shifts and mealtime are times that patients use to commit suicide. One young man hung himself on the door to his room with a coat hanger during the morning hours at the change of shifts after report was given and patients were being awakened to prepare for breakfast. Known by the nursing staff to be suicidal, he was carefully observed by them. It was determined that only ten minutes had elapsed between the time he was observed by nursing staff and when he was found hanging. Mouth-to-mouth resuscitation and heart massage elicited no responses. Other times when staff and other patients are occupied may be sought. Weekends and holidays where the policy is to provide only a "skeletal" staff and where the patient may feel very keenly alone may be the times chosen.

Visiting hours when the depressed person receives no visitors is another crucial time. The importance of doing special things appropriate to the season for patients who stay in the hospital on weekends and holidays is of significance in prevention. Verbal acknowledgment that it is difficult to be in the hospital at these special times may be of benefit to the patient, who may express anger or other emotions related to his conditions. The thoughtfulness of the dietary department in providing traditional foods, using decorations made by the patients for the dining room, and initiating group discussion of former holidays and family traditions may be especially helpful. Celebration of birthdays provides recognition of the patient as a person.

Initiation of discussion of various traditions may be a catalyst for prevention, especially if the patients are of different cultural backgrounds. Here is where knowledge of anthropology is useful to the nurse. If the nurse has not already learned something about the cultural background of the patient, then it is imperative to read, inquire, and find out. Knowledge of the great religions of the world, their holidays, and religious practices is of considerable import in acknowledging individual identity.

It is important to be aware of whether or not your suicidal patient is sleeping at night. With this person, who probably suffers insomnia, the dark, sleepless night may culminate in a particularly difficult time during the early morning hours. It may be at these times that the patient needs the nurse the most. Depression often lifts after a suicidal attempt as though atonement has been achieved. When patients confide in you their fantasies in which death is a means of gratification, suicide is a very great danger. Depressed patients who find the early morning hours black and melancholy may rush into activity in efforts to ward off suicide. The tension of some depressed patients can be easily felt, *i.e.,* a very tense, determined gait, vigorous scrubbing of the face, bathing, and splashing water. A depressed patient who had killed her best friend was subsequently in psychiatric treatment. Some months after her release, she suggested a suicide pact for the entire family, while on a trip. Rehospitalized, she persuaded the intern on duty one Sunday afternoon to give her permission to go out with her family to visit friends where she jumped to her death from their high-rise apartment.

Patients may watch and wait for such a time to talk the inexperienced person into giving him permission to go out with relatives and, in turn, persuade the relatives to take them to places where suicide is possible. Absences of helping persons involved with the suicidal person must be prepared for very carefully.[4]

It is important to be aware that the patient who suddenly becomes better or who suddenly begins making decisions or whose depression has lifted is at a vulnerable point and requires particular forcefulness of help and hope at this period. The person who is feeling better may have the psychic energy to do away with himself, whereas he did not have this energy when he was severely depressed.

A clinical nurse specialist worked with suicidal patients and the staff in one large (1,000-bed) mental hospital (Summer and Gwozdz, 1976). As a result of their work serious suicidal behaviors were reduced.

Important in the admission to a psychiatric unit of a suicidal patient is securing a contract with the patient that he will tell staff when he is feeling suicidal.

Suicidal precautions in one locked general-hospital psychiatric unit involve three levels of risk from zero to high risk. Suicidal risk is evaluated by the admitting physician and an order written on the patient's chart. Nursing staff assess lethality and make recommendations to the physician.

Nursing staff, however, can put patients on suicidal precautions at any time deemed necessary by them. Patients with no risk follow usual procedures. Patients who are at moderate risk are assigned to a staff member for a one-to-one relationship and observation and are continuously assessed for suicidal ideation. They may use sharps but return them to the nurse after use. Accompanied passes are possible. Patients who are at high risk use sharps *only* under supervision. For patients with high risk, the staff member is expected to be at elbow distance from the patient and for a patient with slightly less acuity but still at high risk, the staff member may be within observation distance of the patient.

The patient at high risk is also assigned

[4] Some suicide-prevention centers advise their staff to be available for some of their patients on a twenty-four-hour basis, due to the rapport established between the two people.

to a room observable to nursing staff and leaves the door open at all times. One practice is for the suicidal patient to sleep on a cot in the day room at night or to pull his bed out into the hall and sleep there. A staff member searches the patient and his possessions. Drugs can be concealed in the patient's hair and body orifices or taped to the body in various places. Suicidal risk is assessed continuously and precautions removed only after documentation of behavioral changes in the patient's chart and by a physician's order.

In some psychiatric inpatient units, suicidal patients are not admitted unless they contract to tell the staff if they are feeling suicidal. Instead, they are referred to a locked inpatient unit.

In a general hospital, if you find that your patient is suicidal, get someone to stay with him, an experienced nurse who does not leave the room unless relieved by another experienced nurse. For patients who take sleeping pills, slash their throats, and fill themselves with poisons, the general hospital is the most likely place they will be taken. The emergency room of a general hospital is usually equipped with antidote charts, drugs necessary in treatment, lavage equipment, and other aids to assist in overcoming suicidal attempts. Nurses who first encounter patients who have attempted suicide should be able to elicit from the patient exactly what he has done without adding to the guilt that is usually already present over the attempt of the person to take his own life. This very first encounter is the chance to instill hope in the patient. The nurse may also be able to assist families and friends who accompany the patient in this crisis. If hospitalization occurs, the patient and his family will most likely be under the care of a physician and psychiatric consultation provided. Nurses have a responsibility to see that the patient gets the help he needs. Many patients have an idea of how to help themselves, and the nurse can use the resources within the patient himself. A person who has temporarily been without hope sees no hope for the future. Therefore, follow-up is crucial. Patients who have survived suicidal attempts also often have suggestions about how to help others.

Although some professionals advocate stripping the environment of the hospitalized suicidal patient of all suggestions and methods of suicide, I have found common sense to be of help here.

It is good judgment to have the patient in the general hospital on the ground floor, if possible, close to the nurse's station, and in a private room. The watchful eyes of the nurse on the suicidal patient can be likened to those of the nurse in a surgical recovery room who watches the patients recovering from the effects of anesthesia. This idea of caring, simultaneously with observation, can have a therapeutic effect.

The nurse caring for patients who have suffered a debilitating disease or who have been diagnosed as having cancer should be especially aware of the effects upon the patient, who may choose to have his own style of death, that of suicide. One patient who had a stroke and after recovery participated in a class for students advised the students to never leave a razor around as a temptation to their patients who had just suffered a stroke. Patients with chronic disease may give up and subsequently die as a result.

There is a tendency in general nursing to heal the physical body without much attention to the mental life of the patient. Some general hospitals now employ psychiatric nurses to canvass the wards, find those who need help, and provide it themselves.

EFFECT OF SUICIDE UPON THE NURSE

In caring for patients who have attempted suicide, the nurse's anxiety level may rise. Repressed self-destructive urges are aroused in others by the suicidal act. The suicides and suicidal attempts of others bring to our own consciousness aspects of death and consideration of our own death. The nurse has the responsibility for management of anxiety within self and avoiding communication of it to others. In addition, the nurse has the responsibility for helping other nursing personnel on the pyschiatric team handle their anxiety by role modeling to them and helping them express their feelings.

EFFECT OF SUICIDE UPON THE VICTIM–SURVIVORS

The two-sidedness of death is a fundamental feature of death—not only of the premature death of the spirit, but of death at any age and in any form. There are always two parties to a death; the person who dies and the survivors who are bereaved (Toynbee, 1968).

Suicide has a stigmatizing effect upon the survivors, the "psychological skeleton in the closet," with the resultant search for the motive for the death (Shneidman, 1976). All family members and/or significant others need help to come to terms with their feelings about the suicide. Provision of emotional support at these times is important to the mental health of the survivors in the bereavement crisis. Being available, being undemanding, and assisting in practical ways all help. Emotional support from the nurse may be the decisive factor between successful adaptation and maladaptation.

Summary

In this chapter, attention is given to the study, epidemiology, and prevention of suicide. Some populations at risk are named and etiology of suicide is discussed. Responsibilities of the nurse in the recognition of the suicidal crisis and assessment of lethality are presented and intervention outlined.

References

BARBEE, EVELYN L.: "Lethality Assessment: Whose Role?" *Issues in Mental Health Nursing,* 1:67–84, 1978.

BECK, AARON T., RESNIK, HARVEY L. P., and LETTIERI, DAN J.: *The Prediction of Suicide.* Bowie, Md.: The Charles Press Publishers, Inc., 1974.

BREED, WARREN, in Hendin, Herbert, ed.: *Black Suicide.* New York: Basic Books, Inc., 1969, p. 135.

CAMUS, ALBERT: *The Myth of Sisyphus.* New York: Vintage Books, 1960.

CARSTAIRS, G. MORRIS: *The Twice-Born.* Bloomington: Indiana University Press, 1958, p. 74.

CHORON, JACQUES: "Notes on Suicide Prevention in Antiquity," *Bulletin of Suicidology,* pp. 46–48, July 1968.

CURPHEY, THEODORE J.: "The Psychological Autopsy," *Bulletin of Suicidology,* p. 41, July 1968.

DE VOS, GEORGE A.: *Socialization of Achivement: Essays on the Cultural Psychology of the Japanese.* Berkeley: University of California Press, 1973, p. 453.

DORPAT, THEODORE L., JACKSON, JOAN K., and RIPLEY, HERBERT S.: "Broken Homes and Attempted and Completed Suicide," in Gibbs, Jack P., ed.: *Suicide.* New York: Harper & Row, 1968.

DURKHEIM, EMILE: *Suicide.* New York: The Free Press, 1951 (first published 1897).

EVANS, FRANCES MONET CARTER: "Suicidal Patients in General Hospitals," *Bulletin of the San Francisco Nurses Association,* 22:1, January–February 1971.

FARBEROW, NORMAN L.: "Crisis, Disaster and Suicide: Theory and Therapy," in Shneidman, Edwin S., ed.: *Essays in Self-Destruction.* New York: Science House, Inc., 1967, p. 388.

FORD, AMASA B., RUSHFORTH, NORMAN B., RUSHFORTH, NANCY, HIRSCH, CHARLES S., and ADELSON, LESTER: "Violent Death in a Metropolitan County: II. Changing Patterns in Suicides (1959–1974)." *American Journal of Public Health,* 69:5:459–464, May 1979.

FREUD, SIGMUND: *Collected Papers,* Vol. 5. London: The Hogarth Press, 1950, p. 135 (first published 1922).

———: *Standard Edition of the Complete Psychological Works of Freud.* Vol. XVII. London: The Hogarth Press, 1955, pp. 7–64.

FROMM, ERICH: "Alienation Under Capitalism," in Josephson, Eric, and Josephson, Mary: *Man Alone: Alienation in Modern Society.* New York: Dell Publishing Co., 1962, pp. 56–73.

GIBBS, JACK P., and MARTIN, WALTER T.: *Status Integration and Suicide.* Eugene, Ore.: University of Oregon, 1964.

——— ed.: *Suicide.* New York: Harper & Row, 1968.

HART, NANCY A., and KEIDEL, GLADYS C.: "The Suicidal Adolescent," *American Journal of Nursing,* 79:1:80–84, January 1979.

HENDIN, HERBERT: *Suicide and Scandinavia.* New York: Grune & Stratton, Inc., 1964, p. 14.

———: *Black Suicide.* New York: Basic Books, Inc., 1969

———: *The Age of Sensation.* New York: W. W. Norton, 1975.

HENRY, ANDREW F., and SHORT, JAMES F.:

Suicide and Homicide. New York: The Free Press of Glencoe, 1954, p. 102.

IGA, MAMORU, and YAMAMOTO, JOE: "The Chrysanthemum versus the Sword in Suicide: Yasunari Kawabata and Yukio Mishima," *Life-Threatening Behavior,* 3:3:198–213, Fall 1973.

KENISTON, KENNETH: "Drug Use and Student Values," in Hollander, Charles: *Background Papers on Student Drug Involvement.* Washington, D. C.: United States National Student Association, 1967, pp. 121–30.

KIEV, ARI: *The Courage to Live.* New York: Thomas Y. Crowell, 1979.

MCGEE, RICHARD K.: *Crisis Intervention in the Community.* Baltimore: University Park Press, 1974.

MEERLOO, JOOST A. M.: *Suicide and Mass Suicide.* New York: Grune & Stratton, Inc., 1962, p. 25.

MENNINGER, KARL: *Man Against Himself.* New York: Harcourt, Brace and Co., 1938.

PASTERNAK, BORIS LEONIDOVICH: *Doctor Zhivago.* New York: Pantheon, 1958.

RICHMAN, JOSEPH: "Family Determinants of Suicide Potential," in Anderson, Dorothy B., and McLean, Lenora J.: *Identifying Suicide Potential.* New York: Behavioral Publications, Inc., 1971.

ROSS, MATHEW: "Suicide Among College Students," *American Journal of Psychiatry,* 126:2:220–25, August 1969.

SAN FRANCISCO DEPARTMENT of PUBLIC HEALTH, 1980.

SCHECTER, MARSHALL D.: "The Recognition and Treatment of Suicide in Children," in Shneidman, Edwin S., and Farberow, Norman L., eds.: *Clues to Suicide.* New York: McGraw-Hill Book Co., 1957.

SEIDEN, RICHARD H.: "Suicide Capital? A Study of the San Francisco Suicide Rate," *Bulletin of Suicidology,* pp. 1–10, December 1967.

SHNEIDMAN, EDWIN S., and FARBEROW, N. L.: "Suicide and Death," in Feifel, Herman: *The Meaning of Death.* New York: McGraw-Hill Co., 1959.

——— and FARBEROW, N. L.: *Some Facts About Suicide.* Washington, D. C.: Superintendent of Documents, Public Health Service Publication No. 852. 1965.

———: "Preventive Suicide," *American Journal of Nursing,* 65:5:111–16, May 1965.

———: Notes taken from lecture on "Depression," Napa State Hospital, Imola. Calif., 1966.

——— ed.: *Essays in Self-Destruction.* New York: Science House, Inc., 1967.

——— ed.: *On the Nature of Suicide.* San Francisco: Jossey-Bass, Inc., 1969.

SHNEIDMAN, EDWIN S., ed.: Suicidology: *Con-temporary Developments.* New York: Grune and Stratton, 1967.

STENGEL, ERWIN: *Suicide and Attempted Suicide.* Baltimore: Penguin Books, 1964.

SUMNER, FRANCES C., and GWOZDZ, THERESA A.: "A Nurse for Suicidal Patients," *American Journal of Nursing,* 76:11:1792–96, November 1976.

TOWNSEND, PETER: *The Family Life of Old People.* Baltimore: Penguine Books, 1963.

TOYNBEE, ARNOLD: *Man's Concern with Death.* London: Hodder and Stoughton, 1968.

UNITED STATES DIVISION OF VITAL STATISTICS: *Vital Statistics Report,* Vol. No. 13. Washington, D.C.: U.S. Government Printing Office, 1976.

VARAH, CHAD, ed.: *The Samaritans.* New York: MacMillan Publishing Co., Inc., 1965.

WINOKUR, GEORGE, and TSNANG, MING: "The Iowa 500: Suicide in Mania, Depression, and Schizophrenia," *American Journal of Psychiatry.* 132:6:650–651, June 1975.

WORLD HEALTH ORGANIZATION: *Prevention of Suicide.* Public Health Papers No. 35. Geneva: 1968.

ZILBOORG, GREGORY: "Considerations on Suicide, with Particular Reference to That of the Young," *American Journal of Orthopsychiatry,* VII:15–32, January 1937.

Suggested Readings

BAKAN, DAVID: *Disease, Pain and Sacrifice.* Chicago: University of Chicago Press, 1968.

BATCHELOR, I. R. C.: "Suicide in Old Age," in Shneidman, Edwin, and Farberow, Normal L., eds.: *Clues to Suicide.* New York: McGraw-Hill Book Co., 1957, pp. 143–51.

BEALL, LYNNETTE: "The Psychopathology of Suicide in Japan," *The International Journal of Social Psychiatry,* 14:3:213–26, Summer 1968.

BELL, KAREN KLOES: "The Nurse's Role in Suicide Prevention," *Bulletin of Suicidology,* 6:60–65, Spring 1970.

BENEDICT, RUTH: *The Chrysanthemum and the Sword.* Boston: Houghton, Mifflin Co., 1946.

BRONFENBRENNER, URIE: "The Origins of Alienation," *Scientific American,* 231:2:53–61, August 1974.

BOURNE, PETER G.: "Suicide Among Chinese in San Francisco," *American Journal of Public Health,* 63:8:744–50, August 1973.

CHORON, JACQUES: "Concerning Suicide in Soviet Russia," *Bulletin of Suicidology.* pp. 31–36, December 1968.

DILLER, JULIE: "The Psychological Autopsy in Equivocal Deaths," *Perspectives in Psychiatric Care,* **XVII**:4:156–161, July–August 1979.

DUBLIN, LOUIS I., and BUNZEL, BESSIE: *To Be or Not To Be: A Study of Suicide.* New York: Harrison, Smith and Robert Maas, 1933.

———Suicide: *A Sociological and Statistical Study.* New York: Ronald Press Co., 1963.

FLINN, DONE E., SLAWSON, PAUL F., and SCHWARTZ, DONALD: "Staff Response to Suicide of Hospitalized Psychiatric Patients," *Hospital and Community Psychiatry,* 29:2:122–127, February 1978.

HATTON, CORRINE HATTON, VALENTE, SHARON MCBRIDE, and RINK, ALICE: *Suicide: Assessment and Intervention.* New York: Appleton-Century-Crofts, 1977.

MCKEGNEY, F. PATRICK, and LANGE, PAUL: "The Decision to No Longer Live on Chronic Hemodialysis," *American Journal of Psychiatry,* 128:3:267–47, September 1971.

MOORE, GORDON L., and WESTERVELT, JR., FREDERIC B.: "Suicidal Behavior in Chronic Dialysis Patients," *American Journal of Psychiatry,* 127:9:1199–1203, March 1971.

NEWTON, J.: "Suicide by Fire," *Medicine, Science, and the Law,* 16:3:177–179, 1976.

SHNEIDMAN, EDWIN S., FARBEROW, NORMAN L., and LITMAN, ROBERT E.: *The Psychology of Suicide.* New York: Science House, 1970.

———ED.: *Death and the College Student.* New York: Behavioral Publications, 1972.

WORLD HEALTH ORGANIZATION: "Suicide and the Young," *WHO Chronicle,* 29:5:193–98, May 1975.

9

Relating to Withdrawn and Autistic Patients

LEARNING OBJECTIVES / Persons studying this chapter should be able to:

1. Describe the onset of withdrawal as seen in patients with schizophrenia
2. Discuss at least three theories of the determinants of schizophrenia
3. Define: withdrawal, autism, depersonalization, hallucination, illusion, delusion, regression, social-breakdown syndrome, recidivism.
4. List ten guidelines important in the nursing care of the withdrawn, autistic patient

5. Describe the process of development of the social-breakdown syndrome.
6. Name four psychiatric services that serve as alternatives to hospitalization
7. Name six needs of schizophrenic patients in aftercare
8. Describe: transitional services, day treatment, halfway house, therapeutic social club, foster-family home, residential-care home, and the colony of Gheel

Patients in different age groups and with numerous diagnostic categories may evidence withdrawal and autistic[1] behavior. The psychosis in which these behaviors is most dramatically presented is schizophrenia. In the *Diagnostic and Statistical Manual of Mental Disorders, III,* there are five diagnostic categories under the heading of schizophrenic disorders (see Appendix C).

Bleuler described schizophrenia in terms of four primary symptoms: ambivalence,[2] inappropriate affect, autism, and loose associations. Inappropriate affect refers either

to lack of emotional response (apathy) or an emotional response that is the opposite of a normal response. Loose associations refer to a disturbance in thinking evidenced by verbalizations that are not connected; the thought content is bizarre and incomprehensible, and the accessory symptoms of delusions, illusions, and hallucinations may also be present.

The main disturbances in people with schizophrenic disorders can be grouped as follows: (1) disturbed thinking, i.e., loose associations, delusions, (2) disturbed feeling—apathy and inappropriate affect, (3) disturbed perception, i.e., illusions and hallucinations, (4) disturbed volition—autism and withdrawal, and (5) disturbed behavior, i.e., bizarre behavior (Mitchell, 1974).

Disturbed language and communication are also present as well as a disturbed relationship to the external world, disorganiza-

---

[1] Autism is a form of thinking characterized by extreme self-absorption and egocentric ideas in which ideas are distorted and the person is preoccupied with inner thoughts.

[2] Ambivalence refers to the presence of opposite emotions, ideas, attitudes, or wishes toward a situation or object.

tion of a previous level of functioning, and disturbed identity referred to as a loss of ego boundaries. Consider the following patient and pick out the main disturbances:

A twenty-four-year-old man admitted to the crisis unit had recently broken off with his girl friend. Subsequently, she moved back to the South. Now, he states, "I'm wired up to her and to robots; I hear robot voices and human voices." The patient also states that he is bothered by the voices and that "I will be very relieved when they are gone." He says that he wants "to get unwired" and to "break the telephoto communication and cybernetic frequency" with the lady in Georgia. He also says that he hears voices of Louis Armstrong and from Deuteronomy.

Recognition of Withdrawal[3]

With the new focus on preventive intervention, nurses in all areas of practice aid in the early recognition of withdrawn and autistic behavior so that something can be done about it in its early stages. The withdrawn person will not ask for things for himself. He is often alone. He may be described by his family as being a very good, quiet baby "who never cried much," and by his teacher as being a "model child," "bright," and "never in any trouble." He may regard himself as unpopular and unliked; he avoids people, stays in his room at home, sleeps a lot, and more and more drops out from daily associations and activities. Withdrawal is not to be confused with solitude, which is necessary to think things through, reflect upon previous actions, and plan new ways of doing things. The temporary bizarre habits and patterns of life occurring during adolescence are not to be mistaken for autism and withdrawal. The withdrawn person's fantasy world more and more occupies his thoughts and he behaves according to the pleasure–pain principle instead of the reality principle. Withdrawal strikes at the ego, and the activities of daily living no longer seem important. The pa-

[3] Withdrawal refers to the retreat from the world of reality.

tient may stop bathing, shaving, and eating and spend his days and nights in bed. Bizarre gestures, mannerisms, activities, and use of body arts may be the first cues in the recognition of withdrawal and autistic behavior.

Many older people are now being seen in psychiatric practice who are diagnosed schizophrenic for the first time who present in the form of withdrawal and paranoid ideation. Since the prodromal signs and symptoms may pass unnoticed by family members, the condition may be under way long before it comes to the attention of professionals. In our technological urban society, it will probably first come to the attention of people where the person works, goest to school, or buys his groceries. Community-health nurses, industrial nurses, and others may be able to institute secondary preventive measures, as well as self-help groups for the elderly.

Determinants

Although no specific determinant of schizophrenia has been found, there are broad indicators of risk: (1) genetic predisposition, (2) psychogenic factors—for example, familial disorganizaton, schizophrenogenic mother hypothesis, double-bind, pseudomutuality, marital schism and skew, transmission of irrationality, symbiosis, defective object relations, and (3) sociocultural factors in which a pathogenic environment associated with migration, poverty, deprivation, and neglect are prominent. From the biological point of view, it has been suggested that there is a disturbance of amine metabolism in schizophrenia.

From a developmental point of view, Lidz (1978) merges Piagetian and psychoanalytic theory. He describes the belief of the schizophrenic patient that what others are saying and doing centers on him as being similar to Piaget's egocentrism. He maintains that the schizophrenic patient's family of origin is always disturbed. Theories about the etiology of schizophrenia follow nature versus nurture.

How the Patient Feels About Himself

The withdrawn, autistic patient may imagine that he "smells funny" or "looks peculiar." He may feel that people look at him in a condescending manner and are out to get him. He may assume grotesque body positions. The patient may appear to be preoccupied with a dream world but he is acutely aware of everything said and done within his presence. His posture and stance may indicate a turning inward. He may not be able to look at anyone fact to face because, as one patient expressed it, "Everyone knows more than I do." Plans for the future are vague and unrealistic. The patient suffers from a feeling of rejection and lack of self-esteem. The way he protects himself is by withdrawal from emotional involvement with people. He does not trust or confide in anyone and others may view him as indifferent. He seldom shows emotion about his likes and dislikes and does not feel much enthusiasm for anything.

Loss of reality contact is very frightening to a person, who may stand in one place and stare continuously at you in an attempt to focus on a real person.

Depersonalization

Depersonalization refers to feelings of unreality or strangeness concerning either the environment, the self, or both. In the patient with autistic behavior, there is a loss of ego boundaries; the ego cannot differentiate between the real world and the inner world. One patient, upon admission, stated, "I don't want to kill you. I think you're a part of me." For patients with indistinct ego boundaries, it is important for the nurse to maintain physical distance to avoid increasing the patient's anxiety. Interest and affect, formerly directed toward conscious aspects of existence, become attached to the unconscious, and withdrawal results. The behavior of the patient seems mechanical. The patient feels himself changed—he seems unable to identify his own personality; it seems indistinct. In attempts to rationalize these feelings the patient may develop nihilistic ideas that parts of himself are strange and do not belong to him. He may develop further nihilistic ideas that he is dead. Feelings that one side of his body is different from the other, that fluids are backing up into the blood, that he is turning into the opposite sex, that he is being charged with electricity, that he has no stomach, that he is drowning or dying may preoccupy the patient.

The following is an example of a patient who verbalized his nihilistic ideas:

The patient, a twenty-one-year old man, thought that he had no penis; food represented male organs and homosexuality to him and therefore he would not eat.

Many autistic patients, however, will not verbalize their feelings and fantasies. Withdrawn patients are hypersensitive to nuances of feeling, ordinary communication is dropped, and attention is shifted to absorption with the self.

Fantasy Life

The autistic patient's fantasy life defends the ego. In his dereistic world, hallucinations, delusions, and illusions may act as defenses. When the therapist enters the world of the patient in such a manner that the patient no longer needs these defenses, he gives them up for more healthy ones.

"In June, upon the little table
Between the beds, he saw a dish
Of strawberries. As they lay
there, so ripe, ruddy, delicious
For an hour he played with his delay
then in delight
Put out two fingers towards the wished-for,
Ate for the first time."[4]

[4] Clarke, Austin: "Mnemosyne Lay in the Dust," from *The Collected Poems of Austin Clarke* (The Dolmen Press and Oxford University Press, 1974) p. 343, is a long poem recording a mental breakdown and recovery. By permission.

HALLUCINATIONS

A hallucination is a false sensory perception without an actual external stimulus. The visual hallucinations immediately preceding sleep and other somnolent states are known to almost everyone. The hallucinations resulting from fatigue, dehydration, and exposure are epitomized in the mirage of the desert traveler. As sleep loss progresses, there is an increased unevenness of mental functioning (Williams et al., 1962). Sensory deprivation produces hallucinations, mostly visual, but some kinesthetic. Those individuals who have had anesthetics preceding surgery have probably had the experience of both visual and auditory hallucinations. Hallucinations induced by hallucinogenic drugs are now well known. The environment of the patient in a general hospital in which he is isolated from loved ones and rather powerless may contribute to altered mental states and resultant hallucinations.

One autistic patient who was talking to herself, when asked to whom she was speaking, stated that sometimes her thoughts became so intense that she could hear her mother and father saying threatening things to her. She said she knew that her father and mother were not present but that the thoughts persisted and she answered them out loud. People who live alone or who may be doing very concentrated work often talk to themselves in response to their own thoughts. In these instances, the hold onto reality is kept, however. Hallucinations may involve any of the senses; auditory hallucinations are most prominent in patients with autistic behavior. Their presence, if not verbalized, may be inferred from behavior. The listening posture and demeanor of your patient may indicate that he hears voices. Impulsive and aggressive actions on the part of the patient may be in response to inner voices as well as the inactivity and dream world of withdrawal. Threatening, unfriendly, inner voices may issue commands or caustic appraisals. They tend to occur during periods of mounting anxiety and to represent voices of "significant others" in the life of the patient: parents, spouses, children, and grandparents. The voices may be helpful to the patient in that they accompany him through various activities. One patient reported voices that were active in achievement of orgasm (Modell, 1962).

Patients may also verbalize their hallucinations very directly.

ILLUSIONS

Illusions are misinterpreted sensory perceptions. An illusion can affect any of the senses. For example, a patient who heard airplanes flying over the hospital said that their sound was the voice of her estranged husband.

DELUSIONS

A delusion is a false belief out of proportion to culture. It is to be differentiated from illusions and hallucinations in that it involves thought, not sensory perceptions.

A patient, age twenty-five admitted two weeks after an abortion, described her auditory hallucinations as "guilty voices after me from death." She had been found walking nude in the park covered with mud and explained her delusion: "I am God so I took a mud bath in the park to cleanse myself." She was preoccupied and spent time setting up maneuvers between the Japanese and Americans at Midway and made rockets from the milk cartons.

Another patient on admission heard voices from "my sister and brother-in-law. They will contact me in an emergency through the system to get me a message from Jesus Christ—to test my Christianity. I have to choose between God and the devil. I am in a secret job. 6–3–8–1–7. Don't mind me; I'm crazy."

Therapeutic Tasks

The principal aim of the therapist is to relieve the anxiety of the patient, the difficulty he has in communication, and the feeling he has of being unrelated to others. Psychotropic drugs are now widely used in treatment.

PROTECTED ENVIRONMENT

A protected environment may relieve the withdrawn and autistic patient of some of his fears, or it may bring on still others. One teenage patient, when hospitalized, thought that the round windows on the doors of the hospital rooms were portholes and that he was therefore in a ship, not only a ship but a sinking ship and that he was drowning. His facial expression and actions expressed terror at this time. However, he was also mute upon admission and it was only much later, as he recovered, that he related this fear to me. Unverbalized fear can be felt by the nurse who is sensitive to the needs of her patients. Being with the individual who is afraid, in a nonthreatening manner, aids the patient to perceive your support. Stating and restating to the fearful patient the reality of time, place, and person will help.

A warning note must be made here about a protected environment for withdrawn patients. The open-door policy of hospitals may give the patient freedom to further withdraw. It becomes rather easy for the patient to spend his entire day on solitary walks, sleeping, or wound up in other activities by himself. In a large mental-hospital setting, it is quite common to observe autistic patients sidling up to the hollows of trees so as to be inconspicuous or standing under covered areas talking and gesturing to themselves. On the hospital unit you may find an autistic patient in a remote area of a room or sitting under a table with his jacket pulled over his head unraveling bits of cloth or tearing paper into little pieces.

DEVELOPING RAPPORT

For the withdrawn and autistic patient, it may take a long time before he can display affect toward you. Attempts to pull away the veil of the dereistic world and bring in reality require that you convey persistent interest in the patient, that you show consistency in amount and time of communication with him, and that contacts with the patient allow enough time to do this.

The autistic patient fears closeness because of the hurt that he has received. Being close entails being able to feel and to express feelings with the other person. Autistic patients may not be able to do this. Feelings may be discussed but the autistic patient will often discuss them in terms of someone else's feelings, *not his own.* Since parents were perceived as being too cold or too threatening or too close and rejecting, he does not feel that anyone can love him for what he is and is ambivalent about what he should be like. In fantasy, he may have developed his own identity in a "community" such as the "Yeeries" of Deborah in *I Never Promised You a Rose Garden* (Green, 1964) and feel reluctant to give up this fantasied identity. His wishes for love and to be loved are confused with feelings about formerly painful relationships. The first task of the nurse is to assure the patient of his identity and worth as a person by conveying to him that you are interested and care about him.

Identifying the specific needs of the patient conveys the idea that you care for him. Since anxiety influences and interferes with communication, all communication should be simple and easily related to the real world. Patients should be in a milieu in which they can exert some control and in which simple social relationships are possible. Powerlessness, isolation, and purposelessness merely add to hallucinations. As a therapeutic relationship is established, the patient feels more secure and the need for hallucinations as defenses against anxiety disappears. On the other hand, the hallucinations met in long-term autistic patients are likely to be rather stereotyped and long-lasting.

Anxiety is hypothesized to be the antecedent of hallucinations, illusions, and delusions. These symptoms are reflections of hopes, wishes, and fears of the patient; they are defenses against anxiety. They are indicators of the unconscious life of the patient and require careful attention to be understood. The work of the nurse is focused toward helping the patient to relieve his anxiety where these defenses are no longer required.

There are periods in which patients seem free of hallucinations; it is important for the nurse to be cognizant of these times and to show interest and concern for the patient and to convey interest in him as a person and not just in his hallucinations.

If the patient's behavior indicates to you that he may be hearing voices, ask him about them. Say, for example, "Tell me about the voices you say you hear. . . . Whose voices are they? Are they friendly to you? Are they unfriendly to you? When do you hear them? Have you heard them at similar times before?" If the voices or other hallucinations frighten the patient, the nurse should be ready to provide a safe environment for him. Stating to the frightened patient where he is and who you are and that it is a safe place may provide the needed comfort.

The work of the nurse is centered around helping the patient to establish what is real and what is unreal. The patient may, for example, believe that you are a spy. Establishing contact with the patient, gaining trust, and being with him in an ego-supportive role can help him to perceive the real world. Establishment of ego boundaries aids in anxiety reduction. If the hallucinations, delusions, and illusions are defenses against anxiety, they will not occur when the patient's fractured ego is once more whole. Assisting the autistic patient to relate to other patients may help him to give up his world of unreality. The nurse and other members of the therapeutic team do not agree with the delusions, hallucinations, and illusions of patients. Neither do they argue about them. A simple, forcefully put response such as "I don't hear any voices" or "You might be mistaken" helps the patient to distinguish between the real and the unreal world. Verbatim recording should be done, which gives a lead to the inner life of the patient and may be of central importance in his care. There is a need for more research and knowledge about hallucinations as well as other behavior of autistic patients.

All these interventions cannot be done at once. It may take a long time for the autistic patient to trust you enough to confide in you what is on his mind.

MOTHERING CARE

In the establishing phase of the nurse–patient relationship, most of your time may be taken up with helping the autistic patient to meet his mothering needs, that is, bathing, feeding, personal hygiene, dressing, and grooming. Patients may perform some of these things for themselves; others will require assistance in most all of them. Still others will only partially attend to their needs. For example, it is quite common for the autistic patient not to tie his shoelaces. A simple act such as tying the patient's shoelaces for him may be the key to establishment of rapport. Your body language communicates clearly to the patient how you feel about him. No two people, for example, bathe a patient exactly alike. Gertrud Schwing (1954), assuming that autistic patients were primarily orally deprived, used physical ministrations, including feeding and caressing to relate to her patients. Rosen (1953) forcefully confronted the patient with interpretations of unconscious motivation and a mystique of personality. With the aid of attendants he assumed total care of the patients, often adding them to his household. Sechehaye (1951) used what she called symbolic realization to contact withdrawn patients through a symbolic return to mother. Bettelheim's work (1955, 1968) with autistic children documents the influence of the human relationships. Fromm-Reichman's (1950) technique of intensive psychotherapy with autistic patients was shaped on the empathic response. Sullivan (1953) focused on the interaction between the therapist and the patient at the moment that it occurred. The "here and now" received emphasis in his approach. Bateson and Jackson (1956), using the "double-bind" theory, treated the entire family. The social psychiatric approach used in treatment by Main (1946), Jones (1953, 1968), Wilmer (1958), Bierer (1948), and others added a new dimension to the intensive psychotherapeutic approach.

Awareness that mutual withdrawal can occur is a spur for the nurse to pursue the establishment of rapport. Verbalize to the patient how you think he feels and ask him whether or not you are correct. Indicate that you think he is capable of recovery and tell him that he has to make the decision to want to be helped. Restate your expectations so that the patient still knows that you have them. It is here with the autistic patient that your conversations and other efforts may be one-sided for a long time, before the patient develops trust and is otherwise responsive to you. The work of Ward (1969) with a silent patient records one verbal sound, a grunt, during her entire contact with him. One-sided relationships are at first difficult. You learn to be alert for small changes in your patient that indicate movement toward trust; for example, when your patient first looks at you, gets up when you present yourself, or takes your hand.

When nurse–patient relationships are one-sided and there is little movement toward progress, there may be a tendency to depreciate one's own efforts since no effects are discernible. Nurses may fall back on one facet of interpersonal relationships, i.e., "to accept people as they are," and steadfastly defend their position. Part of this position is to stoutly declare that they have no right to delve into the lives of their patients and that they furthermore do not have the skills to help mental patients or the time to spare to do so if they could. If you should find yourself approaching this position, try to look at the fact that if you understand something about human motivation and also accept people as they are, you are much better equipped to help those who cannot help themselves. If understanding the "why's" of behavior is necessary for the health of our patients, why not help search for it in order to help each person realize his greatest potential—whatever that may be for him?

REGRESSION

Regression with symptoms of dependence occurs in almost every illness. It may be temporary or, as in patients with autistic behavior, prolonged. Regression implies a return to a former level of development. A healthy person can regress as in play, and then return to his developmental level quite readily. This has been called regression in service of the ego (Kris, 1952). In schizophrenia, *teleologic regression* refers to a return to lower levels of functioning for the purpose of relieving anxiety. However, it is progressive in the sense that it fails to relieve anxiety and tends to repeat itself (Arieti, 1974). Regression may also occur

in crisis situations such as the birth of a new sibling, childbirth, hospitalization, or with the debilitating diseases and conditions in which there are disturbances of body image. It is a human tendency to regress under stress.

The nurse may be repulsed by the severely regressed patient. Anger is commonly felt, and the thought may occur that the patient really could do something himself about his regressed state. On the other hand, the regressed patient may progress rapidly forward only to regress back to his former state. You may find yourself discouraged or lose interest in the patient who seems unable to recover. You may also feel that you have personally failed. The problem of withdrawal, autistic behavior, and regression may cause you to be perplexed and bewildered. It may be difficult to comprehend the meaning of such behavior, especially in adults. Some scientific people seem to be able to work more comfortably in situations where causes of phenomena are quickly and easily identified. Since there are no exact formulas to follow in interpersonal relationships, you will need to develop and to follow your own way in working with people. An assessment of ego strengths of the patient is one way to begin. Determine where the patient is and work from that point. This knowledge will help you to set more realistic goals. Severely regressed patients in great numbers are no longer seen on the back wards of some mental hospitals as they were in the past where great efforts in "habit training"[5] were made by the nursing staff. But regression still occurs. The degree of regression can also be assessed and a picture put together of what the patient was like before the regression. Avoid attempting to get the regressed patient to achieve a level of wellness unknown to him or impossible for him to achieve. Knowing what kind of person you are dealing with—his assets and liabilities—will help you to make a more realistic nursing-care plan and therefore better aid the patient to achieve the highest potential of

---

[5] Habit training refers to the retraining of severely regressed patients to use the toilet themselves and to otherwise meet their own needs in personal hygiene and to feed themselves.

which he is capable. In order to do this, you will need to know the following:

His patterns of coping
How the patient views himself
How the patient has adapted himself
How the patient has coped with the crises in his life cycle
The nature of his relationships with others

Pooling the information about the patient and his situation by the therapeutic team gives each person involved the opportunity to give and to take information and to formulate a better plan of care. If you get to know something about your patient's goals in life, his educational background, how his life has been spent, i.e., jobs held and jobs aspired to, his hobbies and his other interests, you will have the beginnings of assessment of his strengths.

When you develop a fundamental cognitive understanding of the patient's problem, you may feel discouraged because you have the problem of the patient in the forefront of your mind instead of the patient as a person. You may also feel angry because you are doing all the work in the relationship and the patient is making no effort whatsoever. Hope for recovery of your patient may then disappear. If you perceive that the patient himself appears not to want to get well, you may feel further hopelessness. It is well known from the studies of Stanton and Schwartz (1949), Caudill et al. (1952 and 1958), Greenblatt et al. (1957), Tudor (1952), and others that how the staff feels readily communicates to the patient. Adverse feelings influence behavior of the patient; therefore, the nurse's feelings of frustration, hopelessness, and discouragement have to be dealt with. Frustration may be high on your list because you have tried everything that you know how to use. You may feel worthless and inadequate and wonder whether or not you will ever be able to help the patient or anyone else. You may feel angry at the patient because of the way he has made you feel.

Students who have developed countertransference to their patients, for example, as a sibling, often become angry at the psychiatrist and psychologist who diagnose the patient as schizophrenic or some other clas-

sification and adamantly champion the patient's cause. Once a patient who had been a member of my social club and a student at the same university had a psychotic break while playing the role of Ophelia in her drama group on campus. She was admitted to the mental hospital, and I found her on the unit where I was assistant head nurse. Later she was presented at grand rounds as a possible candidate for prefrontal lobotomy. I persuaded and encouraged her as well as I could to present the part of herself that I knew as a contrast with her state of mutism. I felt angry at her psychiatrist who had not been able to achieve rapport with her and was therefore recommending that the answer to her problem was a prefrontal lobotomy. I felt a kind of sibling loyalty to her and a strong urge to protect her from the neurosurgeons. As it turned out, at grand rounds, she was quite open and responded readily to the questions of the interviewer, the chief of psychiatry. Despite her accessibility at that event, the staff recommended that she have a lobotomy, which was refused by her mother.

There is no substitute for experience with regressed patients. Talk it over with someone with more contact with regressed patients than yourself. Try to understand the limitations of other professionals as well as your own. Remind yourself that the condition of the patient did not occur overnight and that predicting an end point to regression is a tricky endeavor for the most experienced professional. Hope for recovery of your patient can reemerge as you develop self-insight and a better understanding of the motivation underlying the regression.

As you get to know your patient better, you will be able to observe his healthy behavior and, in the development of your short-term and long-term goals in nursing care, get a better idea of what can be accomplished and the next steps in that direction. Looking for the strengths of your regressed patient and nurturing these like a delicate plant helps him to blossom into full flower and gives the impetus for recovery.

It is the consistency of daily goals and daily expectations that conveys to the patient that you care about him. Weekly or monthly goals may also be set in collaboration with the therapeutic team. Patients may have periods of great forward spurts toward recovery and then go backward. The nurse can be ready for these reverses and starts and not get too excited about them but calmly set about expecting the patient to move forward again. In the case of acute physical illnesses in individuals, regression may be lifesaving and therefore encouraged. However, in mental disorder, regression is a fundamental issue. A psychiatric milieu that fosters powerlessness, regression, and conformity and provides no ways for patients to perform purposeful activity and to take responsibility will probably not enable the regressed patient to make much progress.

During regression, magical thinking may particularly emerge. Try to be aware of what your patient is expecting by the process of magical thinking and point out social reality to him.

In psychoanalytic theory, ambivalence derives from the oral stage of development and subsequent phases. Your patient who has regressed to an earlier phase of development will show other characteristics of that period of development. If your patient is regressed to the oral stage of development, ambivalence is therefore activated. There is an element of indecisiveness in the patient's behavior. The ambivalent patient may agree to play ping-pong with you and stop right in the middle of the game. Another example is the patient who expresses love on one hand and hate on the other. For instance, the patient who hugs you delightedly and, at the same time, unconsciously wants to kill you. Another example is the patient who alternately reaches out toward people and subsequently withdraws from them. The nurse can support behaviors that move toward reality testing and assist the patient to be more cognizant of social reality, as below:

Patient: What would you do if I pushed you off a five-story building? What would you do?
Nurse: I would probably be dead and you would lose a friend. Then how would you feel?

Another patient, in his twenties, who lives at home and tells you that he does not trust his mother—that he would like to be on his own but at the same time cannot accept different living arrangements—is expressing ambivalence. Extremes of ambivalence coupled with negativism accompanying regression may result in marked indecision. The nurse makes decisions for the patient where necessary and helps the patient move toward his own decisions.

TERMINATING WITH AUTISTIC PATIENTS

The anger felt by the patient toward the nurse who is leaving him may help the patient to achieve independence. If he can feel anger, tolerate it, and express it in an adult manner, without feeling that he is disintegrating, a definite advance has been made (see Fig. 10). Anger may be expressed obliquely as, for example, the patient who does not keep his appointment with you. Or, he may "forget" his appointment with you because he fears that he may be unable to control his anger. The nurse begins discussion of termination upon first contact with the patient and again long before the last contact with him. If you have talked about loss and expressed feelings about it during the nurse–patient relationship, termination will be better understood. Former losses are reactivated and it is the work of the nurse to help the patient express his feelings about these losses. One patient, Mr. C., now forty-seven years old, at termination spoke of the girl that he dated in high school. Others speak of death, perhaps not their own, but the death of other patients. Nearing termination, Mr. C. noted the hearse at the hospital morgue and commented that "someone must have died— sometimes two die within a day on the wards where the old people are. Most of these people do not have anyone to think about them." Although Mr. C. could not express directly his feelings about termination, through the death of someone else, he made an appeal to the student to be remembered and perhaps be mourned for when he died (Doane, 1963). (The reader is referred to the section on grief and mourning in Chap. 6 for review.) The patient mourns for the nurse with whom he has developed a meaningful relationship and with whom he has been able to be him-

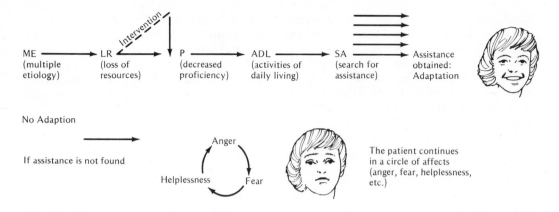

ME ──────▶ LR ◀─────▶ ▼ P ──────▶ ADL ──────▶ SA ──────▶ Assistance
(multiple   (loss of   (decreased   (activities of   (search for   obtained:
etiology)   resources)   proficiency)   daily living)   assistance)   Adaptation

No Adaption

──────▶

If assistance is not found

Anger

Helplessness   Fear

The patient continues
in a circle of affects
(anger, fear, helplessness,
etc.)

Therapeutic intervention occurs at LR where loss can become an experience in
which there is growth instead of a painful intrapsychic wound.

FIGURE 10. Adaptation. In the Process of Nurse-Patient Interaction, both the Nurse and the Patient May Grow, and After Termination, Each Takes a Place in the Memory of the Other.

self. Autistic patients need a great deal of help to express feelings. Saying directly that "it is all right to cry when you say good-by" may be the cue. Another may be to state your own feelings, as, "I feel sad that we have to say good-by," or "leaving is like leaving high school." Emotional termination may occur before the last meeting. Help the patient to review the time that you have spent together by reviewing it before the last meeting and mentioning the date that you began and the events of the relationship. In the terminating phase, patients may suddenly open up with a rush of feelings. In the reluctance to terminate, they may express loneliness, self-depreciation, and guilt. The nurse can counteract the reluctance to terminate by discussion of the patient's growth and maturation and by encouragement (Fromm-Reichman, 1950). Although one student and patient had spent many hours together during the semester, it was only during the last five minutes of the relationship that the patient herself could "reach out." She did this by grabbing the student's hand, squeezing it, and exclaiming, "Oh, Margaret, please don't forget me. . . ." The student held the patient's hand with both of hers and said, "I won't forget you."

Patients may tell you about their former physical ailments or newly developing ones as if in an effort to keep you with them.

They may also praise others on the team and say that these people helped them more than you did. In this, the patient is disdaining any transference that implies that you are important to him in any way. One patient at the time of termination got a job and informed the nurse, "I'm leaving you."

Nursing students often use a cultural ritual to assuage termination pangs of their patients and of their own by holding farewell teas, coffee hours, picnics, and other outings. Sometimes the patients themselves plan these events for the students. If such an event is planned, the other work of termination should have already been accomplished. Teenage patients in particular often manage to get cake and coffee for their departing students.

The factor of time is very important; last appointments should be made so that you can be with your patient longer than usual if he requires it. Much work of the relationship is often accomplished during the last few nurse–patient contacts. If your interaction has centered around an activity such as going for a walk or card playing, then you may wish to continue this during the last visit. Sometimes another patient may join you, which can also be a catalyst for expression that this is the last time you and your patient are meeting and also may provide a basis for therapeutic patient–patient interaction after you leave. Other staff may also be of assistance at termination. One staff member said to the student who was with her patient, "It was good to have you here. How long have you been here?" The patient, usually taciturn, proceeded to answer, "Four months," and went on to tell of all the things he and the student had done together.

Students and their patients sometimes plan group outings, and during the terminating phase these can be used to help the patient perceive that others are terminating at the same time and to talk about loss in a group. If the student and patient are also known to other staff and patients, when the nurse leaves, the patient has someone with whom he can communicate a pool of shared images. Helping your patient plan to fill up the appointment time that you have had with him is an important facet of termination. Other patients are often sensitive to this need and their help can be enlisted. If the patient is being reassigned to another nurse, inform the patient and inform the nurse of your work with the patient. A summary should be made and added to the patient's record.

SEPARATION OR "LITTLE TERMINATIONS"

Autistic patients seem to find separation difficult and may regress during the absence of the nurse unless careful attention is given to holidays, vacations, intersessions, and illnesses of the nurse. Nurses can prepare their patients for their absences by informing them of the time and occasion for them. If the absence is lengthy, during the interim write a note to your patient reaffirming your next appointment. The use of professional calling cards with dates for the next appointment can also be something for the patient to refer to and consider. Reminding the patient that other staff are available in case of need and informing the other staff yourself that you will be gone can indicate to the patient that you are concerned about him. Concentration on the patient's feelings of loss during these separations can act as a focal point for understanding his feelings of loss. Holidays alone can be periods of life in which loss is most acutely felt. The nurse can aid the patient to discuss former

holidays and his feelings about them. Nursing students often send their patients a commemorative card at these times. Some psychiatrists on vacation send cards to their patients to indicate that they are remembered.

NURSE'S NEEDS

Termination with autistic patients may be particularly anxiety-provoking for the nurse. If there is no one to continue the nurse–patient relationship, the student may wish to continue as before. The student needs guidance to consider the reality of the situation as well as support for her own feelings. The student may also feel pushed to get the patient "well" before leaving, not recognizing that the patient's recovery cannot be so easily tied to a schedule. If the nurse can perceive the efficacy of preventive techniques at the time of termination, the patient will derive more benefit from the nurse–patient relationship than a hurried push for recovery that is not in tune with the timetable of the patient. How the patient himself reacts to termination will clearly affect the nurse's needs. The nurse directs all possible attention to prevention in the terminating phase. Therapeutic termination or prevention of desolation becomes your aim—not to get the patient 100 per cent well the day that you leave.

Recording

Written nurse–patient interactions help the nurse to analyze and interpret communication with the patient. Evaluation, introspection, and reflection upon the events between you and your patient can lead to insights filled with affect and poignancy. In learning to work with patients, one of the major educational aims is to become conscious of one's own communicative behavior.

Written work aids introspection and objectivity and can be put aside after its initial use for future reference. Since almost all professionals who work in a similar intensive manner with patients have supervision and/or consultation by a more experienced professional or, in the case of the experienced worker, a colleague, both written records and verbal accounts are helpful to both participants. As a student, your instructor will usually require either written nurse–patient interactions, tape recordings, or videotapes for your perusal and analysis, and also as an initial basis for discussion in individual conferences with you.

Nursing Care of Two Patients

The patient, A. T., age sixty-five, following a thoracotomy-lobectomy for cancer became progressively anxious and out of touch with reality and was admitted to the inpatient psychiatric service. Now ambulatory and capable of self-care, her constant appeal to the nursing staff was "Will you help me?" which exemplifies what Arieti (1974) calls *teleologic regression.* Her request for help was repeated over and over again and many times the help was requested for different things. She referred to a picture of a man on the wall in the dayroom who was speaking to her and expressed the belief that the doctor was going to slit her throat and that "they" were talking about her, especially the nursing staff. Two years after retirement, A. T. had developed cancer. Three weeks postoperative she developed feelings of despair and inadequacy and had some recognition that she could not cope. In the hospital, these vague feelings became perceptible to her as the conviction that "they" were unfriendly to her. The perception of the indefinite abstract feelings in the concrete is referred to by Arieti (1974, pp. 217–23) as *the process of active concretization* and they became hallucinations. For example, A. T. began to smell an awful odor coming from her body and to ask whether or not anyone else smelled it. She also constantly asked whether or not she looked all right in an effort to maintain ego boundaries. She also visualized the head of her bed as jumping up at her and preventing her from breathing.

A most important part of her nursing care was to help her to test reality, i.e., to state that the bed was not moving, that there was no one speaking to her from the wall, and to orient her toward reality as exemplified in the following interaction:[6]

Student: Hello, A., how are your feelings today?
Patient: I'm fine, dear. Are you a social worker?
Student: No, I'm a nursing student. We talked yesterday, remember?
Patient: [Nods head in assent.] You know he told me to get the food ready. I'm so worried about doing that.
Student: Who told you to get the food ready?
Patient: The man over there on the wall. I heard his voice.
Student: Tell me about this man you say you hear.
Patient: He told me to give the food out.
Student: I don't see a man. Where is this man you say you see?
Patient: He's right there on the wall [indicating the movie screen].
Student: A., that's a movie screen. It is a blank screen. The movies are shown on that during the afternoons. There is no man on it. There is a television in the other corner.
Patient: Television in that corner [thoughtfully, and looking toward the corner where the television is]. Oh, that's a screen [as she reexamines the movie screen and sounds as though she is beginning to perceive it for what it is].

Subsequently this patient was encouraged to talk about her work before retirement (she had cooked in a local cafeteria for thirty years), to discuss the news she had just heard on television, to remember her friends, where they lived, what they do, and to relate the events of her day in an attempt to assist her to reestablish ego boundaries and to try to accept the fact that she was in friendly surroundings.

Reorganization of the self therefore was encouraged and made possible by the nurse who had already established a trusting relationship and who shared the immediacy of the environment and experiences in a clear-cut, dependable way, which was readily evaluated and characterized by a congruence of communication both verbal and nonverbal.

Although the nurse–patient relationship is telescoped below within this one paragraph, it is intended that the reader perceive some of the nursing care of this patient before the use of ataraxics and without the use of any of the therapies such as electro-

---

[6] Courtesy of Maggie McKenna, Student, University of San Francisco, School of Nursing, 1974.

convulsive treatment. It is intended to portray the influence of one person on another.

Another patient, Opal S., was mute, withdrawn, autistic, and restless. She did not stay in her room or sit alone but paced up and down the hospital unit a great deal. Most of the early contacts with Opal centered around mothering care such as feeding, grooming, elimination, and medications. In Opal's dereistic world, verbal messages were ignored. For example, suggestions that she take a shower and get ready for bed went unheeded. But getting her clean clothes and other personal effects ready, taking her by the hand, and stating simply, "Opal, it's time for your shower. Come on, your things are ready," and giving her a tug gave her the aid that was needed. At times, her negativism was so strong that she refused all approaches by pulling away. In these instances, compromises were made, such as agreeing that she did not have to shower today if she did not feel like it but had to wash her face and hands, brush her teeth, and change her clothes, and take one the next day. At times, Opal became very angry, shadow-boxed, and was assaultive to the nurses. Signs of mounting tension were clearly observable in her increased pacing, rapidity of smoking, angry facial expression, and tremulousness. Removing her from the group, sitting down with her, holding her, lighting her cigarette, and talking with her about how she felt were calming actions. If her tension went unnoticed, it spiraled rapidly into attacking someone or some object in the environment. If the nurse assigned to Opal to help her meet her needs was available, it seemed that calming her was accomplished somewhat more easily. Since Opal was mute, her needs were anticipated by nonverbal cues, her facial expression, especially her eyes, and her body language. Displeasure, pain, pleasure, ambivalence, and determination were evidenced by this type of communication and were very useful to the nurse in ascertaining the patient's needs. It was also important to convey to her that she could tolerate anger and not be consumed by it. The firm touch and voice of the nurse through these aggressive periods were intended to convey to the patient that the "bad me" had not eliminated the caring person from her dereistic world.

In the case of Opal, ataraxic drugs were administered after two and one-half to three months of the condition described above. She was also seen in psychotherapy by her psychiatrist all during her hospitalization and was discharged when she became able to handle her own affairs under his continued care.

The patient's preference for one nurse may create jealousy among staff members. Discussion of all patients at nursing-care conference helps to clarify that all patients and all nurses do not relate in the same way to each other. It is important, however, that all patients have at least one person on the nursing staff with whom they feel comfortable and in whom they feel free to confide. One of the advantages of the availability of a diverse staff in a psychiatric setting is that the chances are increased that the patient will be able to relate to at least one staff member. I have rarely observed patients in a treatment setting who did not have some member of the staff they related to quite positively.

Other Therapies

In addition to the human relationship, various other therapeutic endeavors have been attempted and many are still being used in some parts of the world for these patients. Since the etiology of schizophrenia is unknown, various therapies are prescribed. Psychiatrists who are oriented to the biological school tend to use biological therapies. Those oriented to the psychological school tend to treat their patients with the human relationship or a combination of psychotherapy and biological treatments. Psychosocial therapies are in a new ascendance. The effect of the human relationship pervades all the therapies, and some psychiatrists, learning of new therapies for autistic patients, advise less experienced colleagues to hurry and try the new treatment "while it is still effective." Since there is considerable attention given to all patients who are receiving new therapies, the effect of a new treatment may be due to the human relationship instead of the particular treatment being administered.

Regardless of the ailment of the patient, the nature of human beings remains the same. When old problems are faced and conquered, new ones arise. As you contact and work with autistic patients you will develop your own theories about the etiology of their problem.

The Social-Breakdown Syndrome and Long-Term Illness

The social-breakdown syndrome is thought to be sociogenic, and the pioneering effort to remove it began in England during the forties and fifties where more humane care in some large institutions began, the open-door policy was initiated, restraints were less in evidence, emphasis on voluntary admissions was made, and more services were made available in the patient's own community. Continuity of care was emphasized with attention given by the same person following the patient throughout his disorder. During the late fifties the American Public Health Association gave mental health priority, and the Program Area Committee on Mental Health named the social-breakdown syndrome (American Public Health Association, 1962). The Dutchess County Experiment at Hudson River State Hospital led the way to a new reorganization of services to attack the disability of chronicity, which in turn showed a decrease of social-breakdown syndrome with *no additional services added except precare* (Hunt et al., 1961). In the meantime, federal funds have assisted in the development of community-based programs on a nationwide scale.

Geographical rearrangements were made in large institutions to facilitate the process; for example, one ward would be set aside for inpatient care of individuals from a designated catchment area. Aggression, soiling, regression, and muteness in patients became rare. Under the auspices of the World Health Organization I studied the delivery systems of mental-health services in the United Kingdom, Holland, Denmark, and Sweden during 1961–1962, and some aspects of the role of the nurse in these services is described in *The Role of the Nurse in Community Mental Health* (Evans, 1968). Excellent well-organized services with nurses prominent in the delivery systems in these communities preceded the development of decentralized services in the United States. The importance of continuity of care and coordination of services was emphasized in a study by Evans et al. (1965).

Patients who have been institutionalized for many years now living in residential-care facilities in communities exhibit the social-breakdown syndrome in addition to their mental disorder. Often fearful of going out of the house alone, they remain inside waiting for directions from the caretakers, the cook, or someone from the local community mental-health services to visit or take them someplace. Since some are unable to manage their own medications, these are passed out to them by the caretaker or some other designated person in the home. After long years of hospitalization, ties with families and with significant others have long been severed. Resocialization programs established in the community are most likely to be made with other people in a similar situation. Receiving welfare[7] may further add to the "patient role."

The social-breakdown syndrome is described as disability associated with psychosis but not necessarily a component of any specific psychosis (Gruenberg, 1967, 1970, 1974). It is the name given to the deterioration of psychiatric patients and is seen very frequently in patients who are schizophrenic. The social-breakdown syndrome has as its beginnings a decrease of recreational activities, an absence of initiative in being with people or an unenthusiastic social participation, neglect of self, and nuisance or dangerous behavior (Gruenberg, 1967). When the person comes to the attention of the care-giving system, he may be termed "gravely disabled" or "a danger to self or others."

Several steps are identified in the process: (1) For a variety of reasons the person cannot meet the demands made on him. (2) There is an increased suggestibility. (3) The patient, family, neighbors, or significant others see that something is wrong and seek assistance. (4) The person is hospitalized. (5) The person is introduced to the hospital routine and rules and begins to feel comfortable there. (6) The person is unable to carry out his usual (although diminishing) social exchanges; for example, visitors may be limited. (7) The person begins to identify with the staff and tries to be a "good patient" or he takes the role of the "bad patient"

---

[7] H.R.1 made possible the direct grant to the mentally disabled as of January 1, 1974.

(Gruenberg, 1967). Thus, the stage is set for chronicity. Since the patient has broken off from the usual activities of life and has the added stigma of being a mental patient, the psychiatric services become a way of life. Often, family and friends visit less and less, and the person who does not recover in a specified period of time is then discharged to residential services.

The decentralized services now work with the philosophy of providing assistance to disturbed individuals very early in the process to avoid the social-breakdown syndrome. If, for example, the individual cannot meet the demands made upon him, assistance at this point helps him through the immediate crisis and frees him to work on underlying problems. Alternatives to hospitalization have been developed and short-term hospitalization determined to be sufficient in many cases. The problems of linking precare with aftercare, provision of continuity of care for the patient, monitoring quality of care, and follow-up are far from being solved. Sheltered workshops and resocialization programs are helping but are slow in developing. Acceptance of community mental-health services within the community itself continues to be a problem.

Although the social-breakdown syndrome occurs in many people with schizophrenia, it is not limited to that diagnostic group. The central cities now have a large population of both young and old who are more or less lost to the community mental-health services who live in dilapidated hotels, in the parks, in vacant houses, or under freeway approaches and who come into the delivery system when they become upset and a nuisance to others.

Community Treatment for the Chronic Patient

Community treatment now includes alternatives to hospitalization and aftercare. Hospitalization for the most part does not prepare patients for living in the community. When large numbers of mental patients were discharged from hospitals, community treatment programs had to be established for them. Community care facilities are now dealing with patients who were hospitalized for many years in the state public mental hospitals as well as patients newly diagnosed. The majority of these individuals are schizophrenic and require assistance with the activities of daily living, are especially vulnerable to stress, are dependent, have difficulty in getting jobs and in forming interpersonal relationships.

ALTERNATIVES TO HOSPITALIZATION

Facilities are being developed to treat patients in the community instead of inpatient hospital services. The goals are: to maintain the patient's ability to cope with the activities of daily living or to teach these skills, to avoid dependency, and to provide treatment in the least restrictive setting.

Psychiatric emergency services may use crisis intervention where they keep a patient for several hours until he is stabilized and can return to his living situation.

Residential settings especially designed as alternatives to hospitalization are now being developed for patients thought to be able to be sustained by this short-term care. Soteria House is a residential treatment center for young schizophrenics with their first break. It provides a permissive, unstructured milieu by paraprofessionals to help patients through their psychosis, usually without medications (Mosher and Menn, 1978).

Instead of being admitted to the hospital, some patients can be treated at home where families are willing to keep the patient and to participate in treatment.

Some patients have been admitted to "crisis homes" instead of the hospital. Private homes provide shelter and support with outreach from the mental-health services (Polak and Kirby, 1976).

Aftercare

Although aftercare services affect all mental patients, they are discussed under this heading because schizophrenic patients make up a large portion of patients in mental hospitals who subsequently need prolonged aftercare services and who are high on the readmission rate.

Many patients are discharged to their own homes, and continue in outpatient treatment without the need for additional care.

In 1966 the Center for Studies of Schizophrenia was organized in the National Institute of Mental Health. A major goal of the Center was to coordinate the efforts of research, training, and services throughout the country. Attention was also given to the treatment of patients in new types of facilities so as to provide for individualization of care and to avoid the chronicity of "warehousing" the patient.

It is now established that aftercare reduces recidivism. In addition to providing supportive services and interpersonal therapy, aftercare probably serves to keep the patients on medications, thus preventing exacerbations (Test and Stein, 1978). Current studies do not separate out the types of aftercare services that are most effective in the community treatment of the chronic patient (Merrill, 1969). The effect on the family of the presence of the patient can also be determined and the help of relatives elicited and acknowledged.

One of the most important factors in aftercare of patients is that they be accepted. The hospital patient on a weekend leave to his home who finds that his room is now used for storage readily gets the idea of what his family thinks of his return. The patient who has been in a mental hospital and adjusted to the institutional life is all too often thrown out into the community and into the hectic affairs of everyday life without the ability to keep up. Unless he and his family receive the assistance they need, the patient will probably very quickly be readmitted. There is no substitute for the home visit to assess the family ecology and interaction. For example, a patient now in his early twenties who has been severely mentally disordered since the age of twelve has a mother who now refuses to talk about her son. In a home visit, the nurse was confronted by the mother who immediately stated, "To be perfectly honest with you, I don't want a thing to do with you and what you are doing with Tom." She became

rather upset that the nurse was "delving into the past" of Tom and felt that it was too painful for him. She also stated that "it wouldn't do any good for you to try and find out about Tom's past life; we've been over it many times and it will never do any good." This mother based her criteria for her son's improvement on the time when he would make more friends and socialize more, which was precisely what Tom had not been able to do since he was twelve years old. It is doubtful whether this home will ever be a place to foster the mental health of this patient unless the attitude of the mother changes.

Upon leaving the hospital, schizophrenic patients may require aftercare. Help may be given to them in the form of (1) finding a job and a place to live, (2) follow-up and psychological support, (3) assisting the patient and his family through crisis periods, (4) general health supervision, (5) supervision of medications, and (6) socialization.

The mental patient returning to the community needs someone to attach himself to. Families also need this kind of person to help them with their special problems. The nurse can be the person to appear when needed and to follow the patient and his family until the need is dissipated.

In the Cassel Hospital, United Kingdom, where whole families are admitted, nurses begin their aftercare *before* the prospective family is admitted (Webster, 1968, p. 176). The work of the nurses in precare can add a new dimension to the treatment plan and also to plans for aftercare. They visit the home beforehand to accomplish at least the following:

To assess adjustment, pressures, and interrelationships around the "sick" member
To find a way to help the family overcome resistances to care
To begin the nurse–family relationship
To offer the family an opportunity to clarify any questions about hospital admission

In preadmission visits, the nurse also determines whether or not it is advisable to separate the patient from the family. Seeing the patient as a part of his particular sociocultural milieu aids the nurse to assess needs accordingly.

TRANSITIONAL SERVICES

Transitional services refer to those facilities and services established for psychiatric patients to aid in moving them from hospitalization to independent living.

DAY TREATMENT

The day hospital and the day-treatment center are nonresidential modalities used as alternatives to the mental hospital. Day treatment was originally designed for patients who were not in an acute stage of mental disorder. More recently the concept of an acute day-treatment center has emerged. In one of San Francisco's catchment areas patients who are hospitalized in the inpatient services are taken to the acute day-treatment center daily. In this model, inpatients are known to the staff who will be working with the patient upon discharge. Patients may also be referred to day treatment for a limited period upon discharge from the inpatient service.

Included with the concept of the acute day-treatment program was a community-based workshop project for the chronic mentally disabled patients with an outreach to the patients in board and care homes. The goals of the treatment program were resocialization and independent living. Group therapy, arts, crafts, cooking groups, outings, and yoga were offered in this program. Patients could sell their crafts. A nutritious and inexpensive lunch was prepared for one day. The following is an example of a day-treatment schedule:

Mondays 9:15–3
    Community Introduction
    Teams A and B
    Relaxation Group
    Activity Planning Meeting
    Lunch
    Housing
    Small Group
    OT
Tuesdays 9:15–3
    Community Introduction
    Teams A and B
    Ladies' Club
    Lunch
    Women's Group

    Community Survival Group
    Folk Dancing
Wednesdays 9:15–4
    Community Introductions
    Teams A and B
    Art Lab
    Lunch
    Small Group
    Music Group
    Staff Meeting
Thursdays 9:15–4
    Community Introductions
    Teams A and B
    Outing
Fridays 9:15–4
    Community Introductions
    Teams A and B
    OT
    Lunch
    Small Group
    Swimming

Day treatment has an increasingly important role to play in the treatment of schizophrenic patients (and others) nationwide.

HALFWAY HOUSES

Halfway houses provide a sheltered living arrangement for discharged patients. Halfway houses are residences in the community designed to assist the expatient to participate in community life with the goal of progressing to independent living. A halfway house is usually designed to accept persons who are considered by clinicians to be able—after a designated period of stay—to be independent. Emphasis is upon self-care, school or work, and socialization. Patients are expected to participate in structured activities and the treatment program. Halfway houses are a kind of dormitory living in the community and accommodate several patients. Patients either have a single room or share a room. Bathrooms and cooking facilities are usually shared and patients expected to maintain their own rooms and laundry. Patients pay rent, plan their own meals, and share the kitchen work. They come and go as they wish. A committee made up of residents and the director plans special events and hears complaints of the residents. Most halfway houses serve only patients with mental disorder, men or women, and get referrals from an agency. Also, most patients who are referred to halfway houses have a potential to adjust to society and to get a job. Most require little supervision and are willing to work toward an early discharge from the house. Halfway houses share certain common functions: (1) residence, (2) transition, (3) socialization and resocialization, (4) vocational assistance, and (5) other ancillary treatment services (Landy and Gleenblatt, 1965).

OTHER TRANSITIONAL SERVICES

Transitional services usually provide accessible counseling and socialization. Socially isolated patients have been found to have higher readmission rates than those with some form of social contacts (Dudgeon, 1964). Aiding the discharged patient to socialize is therefore high on the list of priorities in aftercare. The patient who has adjusted himself to institutionalization with staff-planned and staff-directed social activities needs a great deal of help in deciding and planning what to do when discharged. Therapeutic social clubs for discharged patients can be used.

The first therapeutic social club was originated by Joshua Bierer in the United Kingdom after his arrival there from Vienna in 1938. The first club of this kind in the United States, Fountain House, originated in 1948. Although there are many psychiatric social clubs now throughout the United States, each one is different. The principal aim of the clubs is rehabilitation. They emerged from the therapeutic community concepts initiated by Main (1946), Jones et al. (1953), and Bierer (1948 and 1962), in England.

These clubs are for the benefit of individuals who have suffered mental disorder and who have been hospitalized. They are for those who have fragile egos and who are more vulnerable to the stresses and rejections of daily life than most other people and for those who suffer from long-term disturbances. Individuals who use the clubs have few relationships with others. Where relationships occur, closeness is lacking and social isolation is severe. They need to be accepted by others in a milieu in which few

demands are placed upon them. Common elements of social clubs are that they are (1) community based, (2) noninstitutional, (3) intrinsically social, (4) offer democratic emphasis, (5) have preference for horizontal merging of staff and volunteer roles, and (6) group activity (Grob, 1968).

The primary aim of the psychiatric social club is to help the discharged mental patient to return to community life and work. The social club is a social–vocational model in that it emphasizes job counseling, personal adjustment counseling, group therapy, and housing services. Mabel Palmer (1966) has written a guide for development of a therapeutic social club.[8]

Senior centers within the community can also be used. Knowledge of the existing community facilities will help you to assist your discharged patient to make use of them. All large cities have many recreational facilities accessible to all age groups. Self Help for the Elderly in San Francisco is credited with decreasing the suicidal rate among Chinese men.

Patients may also go to foster-family homes, homes inspected and approved by professionals where patients live with designated families who are paid for their care. After finding a job, the patient may then move to other accommodations. Availability of industry and other types of housing is a necessary inducement to independent living. Foster-family homes have often been located in rural areas where jobs and other types of housing were not easily found. This care is also used for patients who do not require hospitalization but who need some continuous supervision in activities of daily living.

Departments of vocational rehabilitation may assist the patient in getting a job. Counselors attached to community mental-health centers are now doing this. A sheltered workshop may be the best place for those patients who require supervision. We do not have enough sheltered workshops in our psychiatric services.

---

[8] The reader is referred to F. M. C. Evans: *The Role of the Nurse in Community Mental Health.* New York: Macmillan Publishing Co., Inc., 1968; for further discussion of transitional services.

RESIDENTIAL CARE HOMES

As community mental-health facilities developed, residential care homes have emerged in some states and counties. These homes in my own community house both patients from the back wards of mental hospitals and those newly admitted to community mental-health centers who cannot care for themselves in individual living arrangements. These homes are referred to as board and care homes. Having been socially isolated in remote state mental hospitals, patients often continue to be isolated in these homes. Institutional control of visitors, food, time, sleep, recreation, work, sex, and money has added to the helplessness and dependency. These individuals need help to deal with the activities of daily living and to participate in decision making and problem solving. Assistance is needed in bathing, nutrition, medications, sexual counseling, and management of time and finances. Medical, dental, and psychiatric care of these individuals needs improvement (see Chap. 3).

The residential care homes provide room and board for patients. Sometimes the operator lives on the premises; often he does not. The cook and the maids then become the people most often seen by the residents. The resident may have his own room or may share a room with others. The house itself tends to be Victorian and located in the poorer areas of the city. Once-elegant stairways, chandeliers, and stained-glass windows attest to past eras of gracious living. A former master bedroom may now be subdivided into four.

The following is a description of a patient in one of these homes:

The patient, R. F., is now twenty-nine years old. He has been hospitalized for nine years at a local state hospital with a diagnosis of chronic, undifferentiated schizophrenia. R. F. wears thick-lensed spectacles, a fragment of a beard, and clothes that give the appearance of being hastily assembled but carefully chosen for color. His skin is pale and he is very thin. He is taking ataractic drugs on prescription and often complains of insomnia. He decorates his room with pieces of cloth and paper of special significance to himself. Periodically the caretaker requires housecleaning because of the fire hazard. When the aftercare services staff come to the home weekly for activity groups, R. F. selects which groups he will participate in and usually goes along if there is a trip to an art museum or if one of the staff is going with whom he can discuss art, music, and poetry. He is seen once a month by the medical doctor who visits all the patients in the home at one time and this visit is paid for by Medi-Cal. If necessary, two psychiatric treatment visits per month are available and are paid for by Medi-Cal.

The following patient went directly to a residential care home from the inpatient unit of the community health center:

K. B., a former ballet dancer, is now fifty-two years old. There are no known relatives or friends. Twice during the previous three years she was hospitalized with a diagnosis of catatonic schizophrenia with paranoid features and treated with psychotherapy and ataractic drugs. Her delusion is that Black people are out to get her; therefore, she remains in her apartment in the center of the city with her pet parakeet and does not go out to buy food. The outreach team from the local mental health center take her food to her. A nursing student in a follow-up home visit was almost bodily ejected from the apartment. Two days later the patient was found by the newspaper boy during the early morning hours in the apartment house elevator stuck between floors. On readmission, she is mute, and lies in bed in the fetal position without eating. Refusing oral medications and food, she is given ataractic drugs intramuscularly and is tube-fed. A conservatorship is obtained and the patient sent to a residential care home housed in a community mental-health center complex in the central city where staff are available in the complex twenty-four hours a day.

Relegated to the back wards of the state hospitals and long accepting the "patient role," rehabilitation of these individuals is difficult. Although in a humanistic sense the quality of life is better in the community than in the dehumanizing environment of large state institutions, the basic problems of the patient with chronic schizophrenia remain unchanged. Although these patients are considered "burned out" and "hopeless" by many institutional staff, the professionals of community mental-health facilities are now picking up the challenge.

Some houses are oriented to work as on a farm or ranch. Others may be called a lodge, for example, where patients live together with little supervision and run their own business, or work at various jobs.

Satellite housing is now developing where a group of residents (two to four) who have lived together in a halfway house move to an apartment (Kresky et al., 1976).

Hostels are also now being developed as permanent homes (Carpenter, 1978).

Two towns (New Haven and Troy, Missouri) now receive expatients into community life (Keskiner and Zalcman, 1974).

Thousands of patients formerly housed in state public mental hospitals now live in the community; many of these individuals are schizophrenic and some have been institutionalized as long as thirty to forty years. Due to this change the state hospital has become a facility used as a last resort (Rachlin et al., 1979). This change in locus of care has resulted in the need for new methods of treatment. Aftercare services that provide supportive group psychotherapy, socialization therapy, interdisciplinary therapists and follow-up were found by Donlon and Rada (1976) to be effective and economic treatment.

Evidence for the efficacy of maintenance antipsychotic drugs to prevent relapse of the schizophrenic patient was found by Davis et al. (1976) in their summary of twenty-five studies. However, for patients who are on maintenance medication all should be examined periodically to determine whether they need it (Davis, 1975).

Because of the high rate of schizophrenia at the lowest social class of urban areas, Kohn (1976) suggests that experiences of this social class foster a limited view of social reality and that, in turn, impairs the ability to cope. For example, simple jobs, low educational level. constricted freedom of action, and a belief that Fate cannot be controlled are constricting factors.

The relocation of patients from state public mental hospitals that were structured and controlled to a nonstructured community environment creates new adjustment problems. A study of the social organization of former patients diagnosed as schizophrenic who live in SRO (single room only) hotels found that they had significantly fewer social networks[9] and that social networks can function in a preventive and therapeutic role in a community (Sokolovsky et al., 1978). In this study, rehospitalization was found to be dependent upon two factors; psychopathology and social network size (Cohen and Sokolovsky, 1979). The importance of persisting linkage of social contacts needs to receive more attention by care-giving personnel. Social isolation, alienation, and anomie of patients in urban areas are problems to be faced. Halfway houses, landlord-supervised cooperative apartments, board and care homes, and single-room-only hotels comprise a large component of current community facilities for schizophrenic patients.

GHEEL

One situation in which mental patients have been accepted and cared for since the fifteenth century is the colony of Gheel in Belgium. It was originally one of the many shrines dedicated to different saints whose cures were famous in the medieval period. The shrine at Gheel was dedicated to St. Dymphna, and mental patients were brought there in large numbers to be cured. From the time of "miracle cures" until now, mental patients have come to Gheel for family treatment. At Gheel the mental patient is accepted. The medical center of the colony of twenty-seven thousand inhabitants is a mental hospital for three hundred fifty patients with its own staff. Over two thousand patients live in Gheel. The colony is Gheel itself and is split into sections, each with its own psychiatrist and two to three qualified male nurses. The nurses visit patients in their foster homes, talk with the patients and the foster family, see if and how the patients work, look after the bedrooms, clothing, and food, and give instructions to foster parents. They are responsible for the psychiatric part of the treatment. Each morning there is a conference of all staff involved. Gheel is agricultural and two thirds of the patients live on farms. It is

[9] Social network refers to interpersonal relationships linking individuals with other individuals.

the philosophy of the colony that farm work offers a great variety of activities and that a job can be found for everyone.

Summary

This chapter concerns itself with withdrawal and autistic behavior. Emphasis is placed upon recognition of withdrawal and ways that nurses may be of aid in case finding, direct care, and referral. Due to the incidence of schizophrenia and the social-breakdown syndrome, attention is focused in this chapter on needs of and ways to aid these individuals.

References

AMERICAN PSYCHIATRIC ASSOCIATION: *Diagnostic and Statistical Manual of Mental Disorders,* III Washington, D.C.: American Psychiatric Association, 1980.

AMERICAN PUBLIC HEALTH ASSOCIATION: Program Area Committee on Mental Health. *Mental Disorders: A Guide to Control Methods.* New York: American Public Health Association, 1962.

ARIETI, SILVANO: *Interpretation of Schizophrenia.* New York: Basic Books, Inc., 1974, pp. 217–23.

BATESON, GREGORY, and JACKSON, DONALD D.: "Toward a Theory of Schizophrenia," *Behavioral Science,* 1:4:251–64, 1956.

BETTELHEIM, BRUNO: *Love Is Not Enough.* New York: The Free Press, 1955.

_____: *Truants from Life.* New York; The Free Press, 1955.

_____: *The Empty Fortress.* New York: The Free Press, 1968, pp. 233–342.

BIERER, JOSHUA, ed.: *Therapeutic Social Clubs.* London: H. K. Lewis, 1948.

_____: "Great Britain's Therapeutic Social Clubs," *The Journal of Hospital and Community Psychiatry,* 13:203f f., April 1962.

CARPENTER, MARY: "Residential Placement for the Chronic Psychiatric Patient: A Review and Evaluation of the Literature," *Schizophrenia Bulletin,* 4:3:384–398, 1978.

CAUDILL, WILLIAM, et al.: "Social Structure and Interactive Processes on a Psychiatric Ward," *American Journal of Orthopsychiatry,* 22:314–33, April 1952.

_____: *The Psychiatric Hospital as a Small Society.* Cambridge, Mass.: Harvard University Press, 1958.

CLARKE, AUSTIN: "Mnemosyne Lay in the Dust" from *The Collected Poems of Austin Clarke* (The Dolmen Press and Oxford University Press, 1974), p. 343.

COHEN, CARL, and SOKOLOVSKY, JAY: "Schizophrenia and Social Networks: Ex-patients in the Inner City," *Schizophrenia Bulletin,* 4:4:546–560, 1978.

DAVIS, JOHN M.: "Overview Maintenance Therapy in Psychiatry: I. Schizophrenia." *American Journal of Psychiatry,* 132:12:1237–1245, December 1975.

DAVIS, J. M., GOSENFELD, L., and TSAI, C. C.: "Maintenance Antipsychotic Drugs Do Prevent Relapse: A Reply to Tobias and MacDonald," *Psychological Bulletin,* 83:3:431–447, 1976.

DOANE, LEONA: *The Therapeutic Termination of Interpersonal Relationships.* Unpublished master's field study, Boston University, 1963.

DONLON, PATRICK T., and RADA, RICHARD T.: "Issues in Developing Quality Aftercare Clinics for the Chronic Mentally Ill," *Community Mental Health Journal,* 12:1:29–36, Spring 1976.

DUDGEON, YVONNE M.: "The Social Needs of the Discharged Mental Hospital Patient," *The International Journal of Social Psychiatry.* 10:1:45–54, Winter 1964.

EVANS, F. M. C.: *The Role of the Nurse in Community Mental Health.* New York: Macmillan Publishing Co., Inc., 1968.

_____ and ESQUIVEL, PIEDAD: "A Family Study Project: Coordination of Psychiatric and Public Health Nursing for Basic Baccalaureate Students," in *Nursing in Community Mental Health and Retardation Programs.* New York: National League for Nursing, 1965.

FROMM-REICHMANN, FRIEDA: *Principles of Intensive Psychotherapy.* Chicago: The University of Chicago Press, 1950, pp. 188–94.

GREEN, HANNAH: *I Never Promised You a Rose Garden.* New York: The New American Library, 1964.

GREENBLATT, MILTON, LEVINSON, DANIEL J., and WILLIAMS, RICHARD H.: *The Patient and Mental Hospital.* New York: The Free Press, 1957.

GROB, SAMUEL: "Psychiatric Social Clubs Come of Age," Hartford, Conn.: The Connecticut Association for Mental Health, 1968.

GRUENBERG, ERNEST M.: "The Social Breakdown Syndrome—Some Origins," *American Journal of Psychiatry,* 123:12:1481–89, June 1967.

_____: "The Social Breakdown Syndrome and

Its Prevention," in Arieti, Silvano, ed.: *American Handbook of Psychiatry*, Vol. II. New York: Basic Books, Inc., 1974, pp. 697–711.

———: "The Epidemiology of Schizophrenia," in Arieti, Silvano, ed.: *American Handbook of Psychiatry*, Vol. II. New York: Basic Books, Inc., 1974, pp. 448–63.

——— and HUXLEY, JUDITY: "Mental Health Services Can Be Organized to Prevent Chronic Disability," *Community Mental Health Journal*, 6:6:431–36, December 1970.

H. R. 1: *Social Security Amendments of 1972*. Washington, D.C.: U.S. Government Printing Office, 1972.

HUNT, R. C., GRUENBERG, E. M., HACKEN, E., and HUXLEY, M.: "A Comprehensive Hospital-Community Service in a State Hospital," *American Journal of Psychiatry*, 117:817–21, 1961.

JONES, MAXWELL, BAKER, A., FREEMAN, THOMAS, MERRY, JULIUS, POMRYN, B. A., SANDLER, JOSEPH, and TUXFORD, JOY: *The Therapeutic Community*. New York: Basic Books, Inc., 1953.

———: *Beyond the Therapeutic Community*. New Haven, Conn.: Yale University Press, 1968.

KESKINER, A., and ZALCMAN, M: "Returning to Community Life: The Foster Community Model." *Diseases of the Nervous System*, 35:419–426, 1974.

KOHN, M. L.: "Social Class and Schizophrenia: A Critical Review and a Reformulation," *Schizophrenia Bulletin*, 1(Experimental Issue No. 7):60–79, 1973.

KRESKY, M., MAEDA, E. M., and ROTHWELL, N. D.: "The Apartment Living Program: A Community-Living Option for Halfway House Residents." *Hospital and Community Psychiatry*, 27:153–154, 1976.

KRIS, ERNST: *Psychoanalytic Explorations in Art*. New York: International Universities Press, Inc., 1952, p. 177.

LANDY, DAVID, and GREENBLATT, MILTON: *Half-Way House*. Washington, D.C.: U.S. Department of Health, Education, and Welfare, 1965.

LIDZ, THEODORE: "A Developmental Theory," in Shershow, John C., ed.: *Schizophrenia: Science and Practice*. Cambridge: Harvard University Press, 1978, pp. 69–95.

MAIN, T. F.: "The Hospital as a Therapeutic Institution," *Bulletin of the Menninger Clinic*, 10:3:66–70, May 1946.

MERRILL, GEORGIA: "How Fathers Manage When Wives Are Hospitalized for Schizophrenia," *Social Psychiatry*, 4:1:26–32, 1969.

MITCHELL, ROSS: "Advances in Psychiatry—7: Schizophrenia," *Nursing Times*, 70:32:1234–36, Aug. 8, 1974.

MODELL, ARNOLD H.: "Hallucinations in Schizophrenia Patients and Their Relation to Psychic Structure," in West, Louis Jolyon, ed.: *Hallucinations*. New York: Grune & Stratton, Inc., 1962.

MOSHER, L. R., and MENN, A. Z.: "Lowered Barriers in the Community: The Soteria Model." In Stein, Leonard D., and Test, Mary A. eds.: *Alternatives in Mental Hospital Treatment*. New York: Plenum Press, 1978, pp. 75–113.

PALMER, MABEL: "The Social Club," New York: National Association for Mental Health, 1966.

POLAK, P. R., and KIRBY, M. W.: "A Model to Replace Psychiatric Hospitals," *Journal of Nervous and Mental Disease*, 162:13–22, 1976.

RACHLIN, STEPHEN, GROSSMAN, SAUL, and FRANKEL, JAY: "Patients Without Communities: Whose Responsibility?" *Hospital and Community Psychiatry*, 30:1:37–40, January 1979.

ROSEN, JOHN: *Direct Analysis*. New York: Grune & Stratton, Inc., 1953.

SCHWING, GERTRUD: *A Way to the Soul of the Mentally Ill*. New York: International Universities Press, 1954.

SECHEHAYE, MARGUERITE: *Autobiography of a Schizophrenic Girl*. New York: Grune & Stratton, Inc., 1951.

———: *Symbolic Realization*. New York: International Universities Press, 1951.

SILVERSTEIN, MAX: *Psychiatric Aftercare*. Philadelphia: University of Pennsylvania Press, 1968.

STANTON, A. H., and SCHWARTZ, M. S.: "Observations on Dissociation as Social Participation," *Psychiatry*. 12:339–54, 1949.

SULLIVAN, H. S.: *The Interpersonal Theory of Psychiatry*. New York: W. W. Norton & Co., Inc., 1953.

TAUBE, CARL A., and REDICK, RICHARD: *Utilization of Mental Health Resources by persons Diagnosed with Schizophrenia*. Washington, D.C.: U.S. Government Printing Office, 1973, Department of Health, Education, and Welfare Publication No. (HSM) 73–9110.

TEST, MARY ANN, and STEIN, LEONARD: "Community Treatment of the Chronic Patient: Research Overview," *Schizophrenia Bulletin*, 4:3:350–364, 1978.

TUDOR, GWEN E.: "A Sociopsychiatric Nursing Approach to Intervention in a Problem of Mutual Withdrawal on a Mental Hospital Ward," *Psychiatry*, 15:193–217, May 1952.

WARD, ANITA H.: "My Silent Patient," *Perspectives in Psychiatric Care*, 7:2:87–91, 1969.

WEBSTER, JANICE: "Nursing Families," in Barnes, Elizabeth, ed.: *Psychosocial Nursing*. London: Tavistock Publications, 1968, p. 176.

WILLIAMS, HAROLD L., Morris, Garyo., and Lubin, Archie: "Illusions, Hallucinations and

Sleep Loss," in West, Louis Jolyn, ed., *Hallucinations.* New York: Grune & Stratton, June, 1962.

WILMER, HARRY: *Social Psychiatry in Action.* Springfield, Ill.: Charles C. Thomas, 1958.

Suggested Readings

AHMED, M. B., and YOUNG, ESTELLE L.: "The Process of Establishing a Collaborative Program Between a Mental Health Center and a Public Nursing Division: A Case Study," *American Journal of Public Health,* 64:9:880–85, September 1974.

ALLEN, PRISCILLA: "A Consumer's View of California's Mental Health Care System," *The Psychiatric Quarterly,* 48:1:1–14, 1974.

ARIETI, SILVANO: "An Overview of Schizophrenia from a Predominantly Psychological Approach," *American Journal of Psychiatry,* 131:3:241–49, March 1974.

ARNOLD, H. M.: "Working with Schizophrenic Patients—Four A's: A Guide to One-to-One Relationships," *American Journal of Nursing,* 76:6:941–943, 1976.

BARTON, GAIL M., and KRONE, CAROLYN H.: "Creation of an Aftercare Program," *American Journal of Nursing,* 78:5:864–867, May 1978.

BAYER, MARY: "Easing Mental Patients' Return to Their Communities," *American Journal of Nursing,* 76:3:406–408, March 1978.

BELLAK, LEOPOLD: "A Drug Free Week After Admission," *Schizophrenia Bulletin,* 3:3:342–344, 1977.

BECK, JAMES C.: "Social Influences on the Prognosis of Schizophrenia," *Schizophrenia Bulletin,* 4:1:86–101, 1978.

BLATT, SIDNEY J., and WILD, CYNTHIA M.: *Schizophrenia: A Developmental Analysis.* New York: Academic Press, 1976.

BUDSON, R. D.: *The Psychiatric Halfway House: A Handbook of Theory and Practice.* Pittsburgh: University of Pittsburgh Press, 1978.

BURNHAM, DONALD, GLADSTONE, ARTHUR I., and GIBSON, ROBERT W.: *Schizophrenia and the Need-Fear Dilemma.* New York: International Universities Press, 1969.

CARPENTER, MARY D.: "Residential Placement for the Chronic Psychiatric Patient: A Review and Evaluation of the Literature," *Schizophrenia Bulletin,* 4:3:384–398, 1978.

CATTELL, JAMES P., and CATTELL, JANE SCHMAHL: "Depersonalization: Psychological and Social Perspectives," in *American Handbook of Psychiatry,* Vol. III. New York: Basic Books, Inc., 1974, pp. 766–99.

DENNEHY, ANNE: "Nursing Intervention in the Hallucinatory Process," American Nurses'

Association, Regional Clinical Conferences, 1965, pp. 22–25.

DUBIN, WILLIAM R., and CIAVARELLI, BEATRICE: "A Positive Look at Boarding Homes," *Hospital and Community Psychiatry,* 29:9:593–595, September 1978.

FROMM-REICHMANN, FRIEDA: "Some Aspects of Psychotherapy with Schizophrenics," in Brody, E. B., and Redlich, F. C., eds.: *Psychotherapy with Schizophrenics.* New York: International Universities Press, 1952, pp. 89–111.

GOLDSTEIN, WILLIAM N.: "Toward an Integrated Theory of Schizophrenia," *Schizophrenia Bulletin,* 4:3:426–435, 1978.

GRUBER, LOUIS N., BROWN, ADA, and MAZOROL, CAROL: "Ex-patient Visitors to the Hospital Psychiatric Unit," *Hospital and Community Psychiatry,* 29:11:731–734, November 1978.

HAMMER, MURIEL, MAKIESKY-FARROW, SUSAN, and GUTWIRTH, LINDA: "Social Networks and Schizophrenia," *Schizophrenia Bulletin,* 4:4:522–545, 1978.

Harvard Law Review: "Developments in the Law: Civil Commitment of the Mentally Ill," 87:1190:1191–1403, April 1974.

JEFFREY, W. D., KLEBAN, C. H., and PAPERNIK, D. S.: "Schizophrenia: Treatment in Therapeutic Community," *New York State Journal of Medicine,* 76:3:384–390, 1976.

JONES, MAXWELL: "Community Care for Chronic Mental Patients: The Need for a Reassessment." *Hospital and Community Psychiatry,* 26:2:94–98, 1975.

JONES, SUSAN L.: "The Double Bind as a 'Tested' Theoretical Formulation," *Perspectives in Psychiatric Care,* XV:4:162–169, 1977.

KINCHELOE, MARSHA, and HAGAR, LORRAINE: *Out the Back Wards' Door,* 1974. Available from Marsha Kincheloe, 130 East 4th South, #11, New York City, N.Y. 10003.

KLERMAN, GERALD L.: "Better but not Well: Social and Ethical Issues in the Deinstitutionalization of the Mentally Ill," *Schizophrenia Bulletin,* 3:4:617–631, 1977.

LEONARD, A. R., and KING, E. S.: "Involving Public Health Nurses in Mental Health Work with Patients and Families Before and After Discharge," *Hospital and Community Psychiatry,* 19:321–24, 1968.

LIDZ, THEODORE: *The Origin and Treatment of Schizophrenic Disorders.* New York: Basic Books, Inc., 1973.

LUDWIG, E. G., and COLLETTE, JOHN: "Dependency, Social Isolation and Mental Health in a Disabled Population," *Social Psychiatry,* 5:2:92–95, April 1970.

LYON, GLEE GAMBLE, and HITCHENS, EMILY A.: "Ways of Intervening with the Psychotic Individual in the Community," *American Jour-*

nal of Nursing, 79:3:491–493, March 1979.

MEINHARDT, KENNETH: "Nonhospital Alternatives for Acute Psychiatric Care in California." *Hospital and Community Psychiatry,* 29:4:437–442, July 1978.

MELEHOV, D. E., GROSSMAN, A. V., and PETRUNEK, A.: "Industrial Rehabilitation of Psychiatric Patients in Open Industry and in Special Workshops," *Social Psychiatry,* 5:1:12–15, January 1970.

MELLOW, JUNE: "The Experimental Order of Nursing Therapy in Acute Schizophrenia," *Perspectives in Psychiatric Care,* 6:249–55, November–December 1968.

MUELLER, P. S., and ORFANIDIS, M. M.: "A Method of Co-therapy for Schizophrenia Families," *Family Process,* 15:2:179–191, 1976.

NUSSBAUM, KURT: "Psychiatric Disability Determination Under Social Security in the U.S.," *Psychiatric Quarterly,* 48:1:63–72, 1974.

OPLER, MARVIN: "Schizophrenia and Culture," *Scientific American,* 197:2:103–10, August 1957.

———: *Culture and Social Psychiatry.* New York: Atherton Press, 1967.

———: *Culture and Mental Health.* New York: Macmillan Publishing Co., Inc., 1959.

OSTENDORF, M.: "Dan is Schizophrenic: Possible Causes, Probable Course," *American Journal of Nursing,* 76:6:944–947, 1976.

PASAMANICK, BENJAMIN, SCARPITTI, FRANK R., and DINITZ, SIMON: *Schizophrenics in the Community: An Experimental Study in the Prevention of Hospitalization.* New York: Appleton-Century-Crofts, 1967.

PEPLAU, HILDEGARD: *Interpersonal Relations in Nursing.* New York: G. P. Putnam's Sons, 1952.

ROGERS, JOANNA, and GRUB, PEARL: "The VA Psychiatric Patient: Resocialization and Com-munity Living," *Perspectives in Psychiatric Care,* XVII:2:72–76, March–April 1979.

RUBIN, THEODORE ISAAC: *Jordi; Lisa and David.* New York: Ballantine Books.

SARTORIUS, N., and JABLENSKY, A.: "Transcultural Studies of Schizophrenia," *WHO Chronicle,* 30:12:481–485, December 1976.

SCHRODER, PATRICIA J.: "Nursing Intervention with Patients with Thought Disorders," *Perspectives in Psychiatric Care,* XVII:1:32–39, Jan.–Feb., 1979.

SHERSHOW, JOHN C., ed.: *Schizophrenia: Science and Practice.* Cambridge: Harvard University Press, 1978.

SOKOLOVSKY, JAY, COHEN, CARL, BERGER, DIRK, and GEIGER, JOSEPHINE: "Personal Networks of Ex-mental Patients in a Manhattan SRO Hotel," *Human Organization,* 37:1:5–15, 1978.

SPIVAK, MARK: "A Conceptual Framework for Structuring the Housing of Psychiatric Patients in the Community," *Community Mental Health Journal,* 10:3:345–50, Fall 1974.

STRAUSS, JOHN S., and CARPENTER, WILLIAM: "Prediction of Outcome in Schizophrenia. II. Five-year Outcome and its Predictors: Follow-up Data on the U.S. IPSS Patients." *Archives of General Psychiatry,* 34:159–163, February 1977.

TEST, MARY ANN, and STEIN, LEONARD: "Training in Community Living: A Follow-up Look at a Gold Award Program." *Hospital and Community Psychiatry,* 27:193–194, 1976.

TEST, MARY ANN, and STEIN, LEONARD, eds.: *Alternatives to Mental Hospital Treatment.* New York: Plenum Press, 1978.

WYNNE, L. D., CROMWELL, R. L., and MATTHYSSE, S. eds.: *The Nature of Schizophrenia: New Approaches to Research and Treatment.* New York: John Wiley and Sons, 1978.

10

The Psychotic Child

LEARNING OBJECTIVES / Persons studying this chapter should be able to:

1. Describe infantile autism
2. Describe the phases and subphases of the separation—individuation process according to Mahler
3. Discuss theories of the determinants of etiology of infantile autism according to Bettelheim, Mahler, and Rimland
4. Discuss differences and similarities between early infantile autism and childhood schizophrenia
5. List ten guidelines important for the nurse in relating to psychotic children

The right to affection, love, and understanding. The right to adequate nutrition and medical care. The right to free education. The right to full opportunity for play and recreation. The right to a name and nationality. The right to special care, if handicapped. The right to be among the first to receive relief in times of disaster. The right to learn to be a useful member of society and to develop individual abilities. The right to be brought up in a spirit of peace and universal brotherhood. The right to enjoy these rights, regardless of race, color, sex, religion, national, or social origin.[1]

The Skin Horse had lived longer in the nursery than any of the others. He was so old that his brown coat was bald in patches and showed seams underneath, and most of the hairs in his tail had been pulled out to string bead necklaces. He was wise, for he had seen a long succession of mechanical toys arrive to boast and swagger, and by-and-by break their mainsprings and pass away, and he knew that they were only toys, and would never turn into anything else. For nursery magic is very strange and wonderful, and only those playthings that are old and wise and experienced like the Skin Horse understand all about it. "What is REAL?" asked the Rabbit one day, when they were lying side by side near the nursery fender, before Nana came to tidy the room "Does it mean having things that buzz inside you and a stick-out handle?" "Real isn't how you are made," said the Skin Horse. "It's a thing that happens to you. When a child loves you for a long, long time, not just to play with, but REALLY loves you, then you become REAL." "Does it hurt?" asked the Rabbit. "Sometimes," said the Skin Horse, for he was always truthful. "When you are REAL you don't mind being hurt." "Does it happen all at once, like being wound up," he asked, "or bit by bit?" "It doesn't happen all at once," said the Skin Horse. "You become. It takes a long time. That's why it doesn't happen to people who break easily, or have sharp edges, or who have to be carefully kept. Generally, by the time you are REAL, most of your hair has been loved off, and your eyes drop out and you get loose in the joints and very shabby. But these things don't matter at all, because once you are REAL you can't be ugly, except to people who don't understand!"[2]

[1] UN Declaration of the Rights of the Child, International Year of the Child, 1979.

[2] Williams, Margery: *The Velveteen Rabbit or How Toys Become Real.* Garden City, N.Y.: Doubleday & Company, Inc , 1958, pp. 16–17.

As nurses most of you will have contact with many children throughout your life. Therefore, it is most important that you learn to recognize aspects of autism and schizophrenia so as to be of assistance in early diagnosis and treatment of the children and to be of help to their families. Autism is a syndrome wherein the child is self-absorbed, inaccessible, and unable to relate to others. The child often appears to be retarded. Autism refers to that condition in which the child has never participated; therefore, it is different from withdrawal. An autistic child is remote from people but active with the inanimate world. He clings to things, manipulates them, and likes to spin objects adeptly. Autistic children like sameness and have a fantastic memory for the placement of objects around them, even remembering which colors are up or down in a playroom of scattered blocks and toys.

Early Infantile Autism

Early infantile autism was first described by Kanner (1946). At about the same time, Bradley (1942–43), working independently, described childhood schizophrenia. Infantile autism begins before the age of thirty months (Rutter, 1975). Autistic children may appear healthy during the first four months of life but some may have a feeding problem, some may appear apathetic, and others may cry a lot. The first awareness of parents that something is wrong may be that the baby does not assume an anticipatory posture before being picked up. Head banging may then occur, and by the fourteenth to eighteenth month the child clearly occupies himself with rocking and head banging and is apathetic and disinterested.

The autistic child can sit motionless for hours staring, appearing deep in thought, very preoccupied, He gives no sign of recognition of people and may flash a pensive smile, which has been described in conjunction with his intelligent appearance as silent wisdom. Kanner (1973, p. 139) considers autistic aloneness as one of the two major diagnostic signs of autism. He also believes that the aloneness from the beginning of

life makes it difficult to view autism as due to faulty parent–child relationships.

About two years of age and thereafter the child presents additional problems. The child insists upon the preservation of sameness, which is the second of the major diagnostic signs. His behavior is very repetitive and he is preoccupied with mechanical objects. Feeding problems may get worse and the parents begin to look for help. The child is often misdiagnosed as mentally retarded, at this stage, although these children are agile, graceful, do not appear retarded, and have excellent memories for spatial arrangements, objects in the physical environment, and music. However, 50 percent of these children do not speak. If they do speak, it may be in a monotone, high-pitched and echolalic. Bettelheim (1967) points out that autistic children avoid using "I" at all and this indicates a confusion between the "me" and the "not me." The word "you" is used for the word "I" and is termed by others the pronominal reversal (Kanner, 1946). They also avoid the use of "yes" as much as "I" and Bettelheim ascribes this to negativism.

ETIOLOGICAL DETERMINANTS

Although there is controversy over the issue, Kanner (1973) describes the parents of autistic children as cold, formal, detached intellectual types. He referred to them as "refrigerator-type" parents who seldom divorce, although at no time did he cite this as a direct cause–effect relationship. Some parents and researchers have challenged this notion. Kanner also states that, so far, research has not produced any evidence "of any consistent neurologic, metabolic, or chromosomal pathology which can be connected with the etiology of autism" (Kanner, 1973, p. 139). Proponents of the genetic theory readily admit that they do not know the phenotypical expression of the genotypical defect. Nature versus nurture hypotheses are still being studied,

Bettelheim (1967) has long been a strong proponent of the theory that it is the child's fear of destruction that leads him to autism. He considers the autism as a defensive denial against destruction and that the syndrome results from pathological child–parent relationships with emphasis upon the mother–child relationship.

Margaret Mahler (1971) in her work as pediatrician and adult and child psychoanalyst provides us with concepts of child development pertinent to childhood psychoses. Her emphasis is on emergence and development of the ego and phases of development involving separation–individuation. The *first phase, autism,* covers the first few weeks of life, in which the infant does not distinguish between himself and the external environment. Gradually the infant learns to differentiate between pleasure and pain. The *second phase* is termed *symbiotic* and occurs at about the age of one month. It refers to the closeness with the mother in which the infant does not differentiate between himself and the nonself. Some characteristics of symbiosis are evident in many instances of childhood psychosis. An early realization of separateness, according to Mahler, is also a danger signal for normal development. It is also thought that a very early awareness of being separate coupled with defensive maneuvers is a very visible part of many cases of childhood psychoses. On the other hand, a delay in differentiation where the symbiosis was not satisfactory may allow time for the ego to develop. Children who remain in the symbiotic phase exhibit very little curiosity and/or exploratory behavior.

According to Mahler's theory, in the normal child, the *third phase,* that of the *separation–individuation process,* begins at four or five weeks of age. Examination of the mother's face and locomotion helps this "hatching" process.

The separation–individuation phase includes not only separation from the mother but individuation itself. It has four subphases. The subphases, as identified by Mahler, are as follows: (1) The subphase of *differentiation* begins at five to ten months and emerges with locomotion, creeping, climbing, scanning, coordination of hand and mouth, pleasure in the motions of the body, interest in objects, and games where the child plays in a territory close to the mother. The game peek-a-boo is played often as the child examines his mother's face; he is delighted when the mother's face appears again and again. (2) The subphase of *practicing* occurs at ten to fifteen months wherein the child is curious and exploratory. He also seems oblivious to knocks and falls. He practices his motor skills and has a great interest in his own functions. Although the child stays by his mother, strange adults are accepted quite readily. (3) The subphase of *rapprochement* occurs at fourteen to twenty-two months. Separation begins to be actively resisted and individuation has rapid growth. The toddler vocalizes and knows "me" and "mine" and "no." The child now realizes the power of locomotion in that he can move away from mother and becomes constantly concerned about where she is. Mahler believes that a sudden deprivation of the power of moving away from mother and the ability to return for "refueling" may be an etiological factor in the development of depression in later life. (4) The subphase of *object constancy* occurs at eighteen to thirty-six months when the child develops intrapsychic representations of the mother and father (or substitutes). Verbal communication develops rapidly, resistance to the demands of adults appears, a sense of time develops, and the child engages in make-believe.

Mahler (1965) believes that autism is secondary to symbiosis and that both result from disturbances in the symbiotic relationship. In her theory she suggests that the autistic child is constitutionally unable to use the maternal ego to develop his own ego.

A study was made by Massie (1977) of patterns of mother–child behavior during the infancy of children who later on were diagnosed as suffering early childhood psychosis. He analyzed home movies to determine the attachment behavior of the infant and the reciprocal behavior of the mother. In the case study, the infant exhibited normal attachment behavior but the mother did not reciprocate. Currently the importance of maternal–infant bonding is receiving more attention (Klaus & Kennell, 1976).

Rimland (1964) hypothesizes that the child with early infantile autism has a maldevelopment of the reticular formation and that it may be therefore a sensory deprivation psychosis. He makes a connection between early infantile autism and the behavior of people with sensory deprivation. In essence, he describes autism as a condition where the brain takes in and sends out but does not analyze or sort. The neural structure does not permit stimuli to register. The child apprehends stimuli but does not comprehend. Rimland (1964, p. 86) refers to this as the closed-loop phenomenon. Recently, autism has been associated with meningitis, maternal rubella, encephalitis, and epilepsy (Wing, 1978).

Rutter and Schopler (1978) in a review of advances and development of autism conclude there is no definitive evidence that psychogenic stress is consistently associated with autism and that development of autism occurs where there is a biological deficit *and* psychogenic stress.

A definitive treatment for autism is not known at this time. Each child is different and an individualized approach to helping is essential. The increasing use of psychotropic drugs in the treatment of children within this decade calls for a more scientific approach to its use. Behavioral treatment of autism is cited as an approach that can have a significant effect on problems associated with this disorder (LaVigna, 1978). Ethical questions concerning the use of physical punishment, especially electric shock, in the treatment of autistic children are raised by Webster (1977). Helpers of parents of psychotic children should focus on their strengths as well as their problems.

The prognosis of autism is influenced by whether or not mental retardation is also present. Almost all autistic children who are also severely mentally retarded remain dependent and in need of supervision. About half of autistic children of normal nonverbal intelligence eventually work during their adult life (World Health Organization, 1977, p. 17). The emotional and developmental needs of autistic people need more research in order to find ways to help them have a better quality of life.

Difference Between Early Infantile Autism and Childhood Schizophrenia

Differences between the child with early infantile autism and the schizophrenic child have been described in that early infantile autism is present from the beginning of life, there are no hallucinations, and the parents seldom divorce, whereas the child with schizophrenia has hallucinations, both visual and auditory, may have delusions, may be disoriented, is poorly coordinated, and is likely to come from a broken home.

Szurek (1971) and associates report from their clinical work of twenty to thirty years that the psychotic child incorporates and identifies with the disorders of both parents and that the schizophrenic attempts, from the oral phase, both to be like and to rebel against parental solutions of their own conflicts. The problems of parents of psychotic children, on first review, are not as evident to some interviewers as they may be to an *experienced clinician.*

Children who are diagnosed as schizophrenic may exhibit *movements* of self-spinning, jumping, flapping, toe walking, and other marked mannerisms. With regard to *speech,* it may not be used, pronouns may be reversed, echolalia present, or phrases used repetitively. These children, in the auditory area, may cover their ears, be distressed at noise, or behave as if deaf. In the area of repetitive-ritualistic behavior, they may have elaborate food fads, live with patterns and objects, spin objects, be involved in carrying, banging, or twirling objects, and be highly involved in other elaborate ritualistic play. They insist on the sameness of objects and on the sameness of events.

Psychotic children use the receptors of touch, taste, and smell; they tend to avoid the use of the distant receptors such as hearing and vision (Hingtgen, 1972). Often they do not respond to questions and will not establish eye contact. When physically close to a person, the child may stare straight at the individual but fix his gaze above the head, avoiding eye contact. One child moved about as though he were a puppet on a string. These children engage in repetitive stereotyped behavior such as watching records go around all day. These rituals may be a safety measure to strengthen the ego for the battle with the drives.

Whether or not the psychotic child is basically autistic or schizophrenic is yet to be clearly established. Also yet to be determined is the etiology of childhood psychosis. The direction now seems to be that of careful studies of the organic–somatic, ethological, and psychosocial factors in addition to the intrapsychic point of view.

Relating to Psychotic Children

The student who works with psychotic children is most certainly in line for a more thorough understanding of self. Since changes in the children may be slow to emerge and small, this realization helps students be more objective about what can be accomplished with patients in general and with psychotic children in particular. Some students who are easily discouraged and want fast, vast changes and rapid progress in patients may only be frustrated by working with children, especially with those who give no verbal communication of their thoughts, needs, and so forth. Commonly, students also feel they will undo whatever else another therapist has built up with the child. Children are sensitive to anxiety in others and thus there is a testing-out phase of the developing relationship. Uncertainty and apprehension of the student may be reflected in the child. When the student begins to see the child as being a child in addition to being a child with problems, the child then is accepted, feels accepted, and work can begin. Students are fearful of even the tiniest children because they do not know what to expect of them in this phase of the relationship. Nonverbal children who do not exhibit eye contact or verbal awareness of the student usually pose an entirely different situation for the student to deal with than previous experiences have provided. Students who are themselves in Erikson's (1963) stage of intimacy versus isolation may especially have some difficulty where they are physically enveloped by a nonverbal child; i.e., the child hugs and kisses, sits on his/her lap, and in other ways is involved in the intimate territory of the student. Touch and contact comfort may become central in the care of the patient in the form of cuddling, holding, and rocking him.

The life-space interview is based upon the actual day-to-day living experiences of the child (Redl, 1959). The principle of the life space also applies to other age groups. Issues that have been identified as central to treatment become the focus of the interviewer, who is someone with a clear role and power in the life experience of the child and who shares his life space. Helping the psychotic child in all the big and small events of the day and night becomes the treatment focus (Bettelheim, 1974, pp. 426–27). In the use of the life-space interview, students who work with psychotic children develop trusting relationships and afford interpersonal contacts by playing games, drawing pictures, and planning costumes for parties. Playing on slides, swings, singing, playing tag, dancing, cooking, bathing, going to the bathroom, and going to the store are other activities.

ASSESSMENT OF NEEDS

Assessment of needs emerges from where the child is developmentally in terms of physical, psychological, sociocultural, and educational factors. An additional category that rounds out these factors is that of self-care activities. From this assessment by an interdisciplinary team, a treatment plan is developed for the child. It does not get made in one week, but is incremental. One student's part in the treatment plan of a child with whom she worked for one semester started with the baseline that the staff were more occupied with the other children on the unit than with Cissie. Consequently, the student chose to work with this child who was receiving less attention than the others. The decision was made in consultation with the nursing team and was aimed toward the overall goal of increasing the affectional response of the child.

Cissie, now ten years old, does not speak. However, she vocalizes and communicates nonverbally by tugging and pulling. She can count to eight, print, match words with pictures, and keep some attention on stories and lessons through music and records. She dresses herself, bathes, and helps set the table and clean up after meals. She can swim, use the playground, and cook. She likes to go for walks. At times, when she is thwarted, she bites, scratches, kicks, and pulls hair.

The student identified her aims as follows: (1) to establish rapport, (2) to focus on recognition and organization of her own feelings and actions, (3) to note activities of mutual enjoyment between student and child in order to determine emotional expression, (4) to continue to participate in the games of mutual enjoyment to increase the child's affectional response or expression of joy, and (5) to prepare for termination.

In working with the psychotic child, verbalizations assume a great importance. For example, say to the child, "I hope it is O.K. with you for me to be your nursing student. I'll be here at . . . (days) and from . . . (time) and sometimes we can be together, just the two of us, and at other times we will be with the others in group activities." During the times on the unit, let the child know where you are and how long you will be there, for example, when you leave for your own meals, when you will be in the playroom, and so forth.

HELPING ESTABLISH EGO BOUNDARIES

Through the processes of feeding, bathing, and going to the toilet, there are many opportunities for helping the psychotic child know who he is and where he is. Our own attitudes toward the child influence him. If we are hopeless about his condition, then he will feel it and it will further increase his psychotic condition. Feelings of hopelessness should be talked out with your nursing team. Often it becomes a process of taking a more realistic view of what actually is possible to accomplish for the psychotic child. It is generally accepted that the earlier the psychotic process occurs in life, the more severe the handicap, for later years.

Setting limits helps establish ego boundaries in that it communicates to the child that you care enough to see what he does. Giving a child time to complete an activity is essential and then toward the end of that

time giving a five-minute warning. Being present when the child is going through something difficult such as going to the store and buying something for the first time uses the concept of proximity touch control. Going with the child to his space, offering a new person with whom to relate, provides an experience for the psychotic child to differentiate himself and to feel an affectional response for another person.

The following summary portrays some aspects of a relationship with one child:

I have seen Johnny, age ten, in one-hour sessions for a period of 16 weeks. In addition, I have made one home visit. My chief impression in the home visit centered around the coldness, overprotectiveness, and need for control presented by the mother and the fact that the father, although present, said very little. With Johnny, my primary objective has been to help him relate to me. Relating to another person, I felt, would be the first step in helping him to face reality and to be stimulated toward more appropriate communication. Specifically, my contacts emphasized ego support, through helping him to identify himself and to perform self-care. Part of this was accomplished through play; during our first sessions, he spoke very little but expressed much of his feeling in drawing. Although his drawings were primitive, he worked methodically and described a specific meaning for each part. Invariably, his drawings were of men surrounded by a box. Frequently, they expressed Johnny's misconduct or unhappiness. One drawing, which he interpreted as showing a "bad boy," consisted of a figure with an upside-down heart and buried legs. Johnny can do simple arithmetic and can spell second-grade words. Although much of the time he sits twirling a string or wishes to have his back rubbed, this is becoming less frequent. Recently, he has pointed out things in the environment such as airplanes and cows. His speech is still difficult for me to understand but he is beginning to speak more in sentences from which one can deduce the general meaning. At times, he speaks clearly. Unless encouraged, he uses few words. Lately he has expressed a fear of dying because he feels cold, and due to this he can often be found sitting on the ward heater. Many of his thoughts are verbalized as going "far, far, away." He says that he can do this by flying or disappearing in the ground. He cannot elaborate on this but the verbal expression follows some frustrating event. Although withdrawn and passive most of the time, he does express his displeasure by screaming, followed by hitting his head with one hand and running or by kneeling and rocking. Once, when we stopped for me to speak with someone else, he lay down in front of an oncoming car and had to be picked up bodily and carried out of the way.

When I first began seeing him, the activity he enjoyed most was eating candy. This has declined to the point where he simply stores the candy in his pocket. His range of activities has reached the point where he will swing and throw a ball. Although his progress is slow, he is responding to individual attention. His ward job has helped to develop some interest. Johnny's mother has been considering home care supplemented by a nearby day school.

SELF-UNDERSTANDING

When you work with psychotic children it must be understood that how you felt during your own childhood may be reactivated—how you felt about yourself, your relationships to your parents and to your siblings. There are times when the behavior of children may exceed your defensive capabilities. The psychotic child who kicks, spits, and bites may arouse your own aggressive impulses and you may feel guilty because of them.

Your own rage may surface if you have unresolved sibling rivalry and if you see one child preferring another nurse to yourself. It is very helpful to discuss your feelings fully with your instructor or preceptor.

Summary

This chapter presents some aspects of work with psychotic children. Early infantile autism and childhood schizophrenia are described. Some theories about the etiology of childhood psychoses are presented and some aspects of relating to psychotic children are discussed.

References

BETTELHEIM, BRUNO: *Love is Not Enough.* Glencoe, Ill.: Free Press, 1950.

————: "Joey—a Mechanical Boy," *Scientific American*, 200:3:116ff., March 1959.

————: *The Empty Fortress: Infantile Autism and the Birth of the Self.* New York: Free Press, 1967, pp. 426–27.

————: *A Home for the Heart.* New York: Alfred A. Knopf, 1974.

BRADLEY, C.: "Biography of a Schizophrenic Child," *Nervous Child*, 1:141–71, 1942–43.

ERIKSON, ERIK H.: *Childhood and Society.* New York: W. W. Norton and Company, Inc., 1963.

HINGTGEN, J. N., and BRYSON, C. O.: "Recent Development in the Study of Early Childhood Psychosis: Infantile Autism, Childhood Schizophrenia and Related Disorders," *Schizophrenia Bulletin*, 5:8–62, 1972.

KANNER, LEO: "Early Infantile Autism," *American Journal of Psychiatry*, 103:242–46, 1946.

————: "Child Psychosis: A Personal Overview," *Journal of Autism and Childhood Schizophrenia*, 1:1:1479, 1971.

————: *Child Psychiatry*, 4th ed., Springfield, Ill.: Charles C Thomas, 1972.

————: *Childhood Psychosis: Initial Studies and New Insights.* New York: John Wiley & Sons, 1973, p. 139.

KLAUS, MARSHALL and KENNELL, JOHN H.: *Maternal-infant Bonding.* Saint Louis: C. V. Mosby Company, 1976.

LaVIGNA, GARY W.: "The Behavioral Treatment of Autism," *Psychiatric Clinics of North America*, 1:2:247–161, 1978.

MAHLER, MARGARET S., and GOSLINER, BERTRAM J.: "On Symbiotic Child Psychosis: Genetic, Dynamic and Restitutive Aspects," in Eissler, Ruth, ed.: *The Psychoanalytic Study of the Child*, Vol. X. New York: International Universities Press, Inc., 1955, pp. 195–212.

———— and FURER, MANUEL: "Certain Aspects of the Separation–Individuation Phase," *The Psychoanalytic Quarterly*, 32:1:1–14, 1963.

————: "On Early Infantile Psychosis: The Symbiotic and Autistic Syndromes," *Journal of the American Academy of Child Psychiatry*, 4:554–68, 1965.

————: "A Study of the Separation–Individuation Process and Its Possible Application to the Borderline Phenomena in the Psychoanalytic Situation," in Eissler, Ruth S. et al., eds.: *The Psychoanalytic Study of the Child*, Vol. XXVI. New York: Quadrangle Books, 1971, pp. 403–24.

MASSIE, HENRY N.: "Patterns of Mother–Infant Behavior and Subsequent Childhood Psychosis: A Research and Case Report," *Child Psychiatry and Human Development*, 7:4:211–230, 1977.

REDL, FRITZ: "A Strategy and Technique of the Life-Space Interview," *American Journal of Orthopsychiatry,* **29**:1–17, January 1959.

RIMLAND, BERNARD: *Infantile Autism: The Syndrome and Its Implications for a Neural Theory of Behavior.* New York: Appleton-Century-Crofts, 1964, p. 86.

RUTTER, MICHAEL; SHAFFER, DAVID; and SHEPHERD, MICHAEL: *A Multi-Axial Classification of Child Psychiatric Disorders.* Geneva: World Health Organization, 1975.

RUTTER, MICHAEL, and SCHOPLER, ERIC: *Autism: A Reappraisal of Concepts and Treatment.* New York: Plenum Press, 1978.

SZUREK, STANISLAUS A.: "Psychiatric Problems in Children," reprint from *California Medicine,* 5 & 6:3–15, May–June 1950.

———— and BERLIN, I. N.: "Elements of Psychotherapeutics with the Schizophrenic Child and His Parents," reprint from *Psychiatry: Journal for the Study of Interpersonal Processes,* **19**:1:1–9, February 1956.

————: "A Child Psychiatrist's Comments on Therapy of Schizophrenia," in Szurek, S. A., et al., eds.: *Inpatient Care for the Psychotic Child,* Vol. 5. Palo Alto, Calif.: Science & Behavior Books, Inc., 1971, p. 32.

———— et al., eds.: *Inpatient Care for the Psychotic Child.* Palo Alto, Calif.: Science & Behavior Books, Inc., 1971.

WEBSTER, C. D.: "A Negative Reaction to the Use of Electric Shock with Autistic Children," *Journal of Autism and Childhood Schizophrenia,* 7:2:199–202, 1977.

WILLIAMS, MARGERY: *The Velveteen Rabbit or How Toys Become Real.* New York: Doubleday & Co., Inc., 1958.

WING, LORNA: "The Aetiology and Pathogenesis of Early Infantile Autism," *Trends in Neurosciences,* 1:1:7–8, 1978.

WORLD HEALTH ORGANIZATION: *Child Mental Health and Psychosocial Development.* Geneva: World Health Organizaition, 1977.

Suggested Readings

ANTHONY, E.. JAMES: "Child Therapy Techniques," in Arieti, S., ed.: *American Handbook of Psychiatry,* Vol. II. New York: Basic Books, Inc., 1974, pp. 147–63.

ARNOLD, EUGENE: *Helping Parents Help Their Children.* New York: Brunner/Mazel, 1978.

BARUCH, DOROTHY: *One Little Boy.* New York: Julian Press, 1952.

BISHOP, BARBARA R.: "The Psychiatric Nurse as Therapist—Not Baby-Sitter!" *Perspectives in Psychiatric Care,* 10:1:41–43, 1972.

————: "A New Look for the Psychiatric Nurse: The Child-Care Specialist," *Perspectives in Psychiatric Care,* 11:1:16–19, 1973.

BOATMAN, MALETA J., PAYNTER, JANE, MEJIA, BERTA, and MILNES, ESTER: "The Integration of Activities on a Children's Ward," in Szurek, S. A., et al., eds.: *Inpatient Care for the Psychotic Child.* Palo Alto, Calif.: Science & Behavior Books, 1971.

BRONFENBRENNER, URIE: *Two Worlds of Childhood.* New York: Russell Sage, 1970.

CASOLY, ROSE MARIE: "Affective Development in a Psychotic Boy," *Perspectives in Psychiatric Care,* 9:1:34–37, 1971.

CLARK, DEBORAH A., and LONG, KATHLEEN ANN: "Nurses as Health Educators with Emotionally Disturbed Children." *Perspectives in Psychiatric Care,* **XVIII**:4:167–175, July–August 1979.

CRITCHLEY, DEANE L.: "Nursing Intervention with the Disturbed Latency-Age Child," in Fagin, Claire M., ed.: *Nursing in Child Psychiatry.* St. Louis: C. V. Mosby, 1972, pp. 28–45.

DESLAURIERS, A. M., and CARLSON, C. F.: *Your Child Is Asleep: Early Infantile Autism.* Homewood, Ill.: The Dorsey Press, 1969.

FAGIN, CLAIRE M., ed.: *Nursing in Child Psychiatry.* St. Louis: C. V. Mosby, 1972.

GAMER, ENID, GALLANT, DAVID, GRUNEBAUM, HENRY U., and COHLER, BERTRAM J.: "Children of Psychotic Mothers: Performance of 3-year-old Children on Tests of Attention," *Archives of General Psychiatry,* 34:5:592–597, 1977.

GARDNER, LYETT I.: "Deprivation Dwarfism," *Scientific American,* 227:1:76–83, July 19, 1972.

GARMEZY, NORMAN: "Children at Risk: The Search for the Antecedents of Schizophrenia. Part I. Conceptual Models and Research Methods," *Schizophrenia Bulletin,* 8:14–90, Spring 1974.

————: "Children at Risk: The Search for the Antecedents of Schizophrenia. Part II. Ongoing Research Programs, Issues and Intervention," *Schizophrenia Bulletin,* 9:55–125, Summer 1974.

GINOTT, HAIM G.: *Group Psychotherapy with Children.* New York: McGraw-Hill Book Co., Inc., 1961.

GREENFIELD, JOSH: *A Child Called Noah.* New York: Warner, 1973.

————: *A Place for Noah.* New York: Holt, Rinehart and Winston, 1978.

HARRIS, FAYE G.: "Failure at Four," in *American Nurses' Association, ANA Clinical Conferences.* New York: Appleton-Century-Crofts, 1969, pp. 259–65.

HARRIS, MERRIL: "Understanding the Autistic

Child," *American Journal of Nursing* **78**:10: 1682–1685, 1978.

HYDE, NAIDA D.: "Play Therapy: The Troubled Child's Self Encounter," *American Journal of Nursing,* **71**:1:1366–70, July 1971.

Joint Commission on Mental Health of Children: *Crisis in Child Mental Health: Challenge for the 1970's.* New York: Harper & Row, 1970.

KAHAN, V. L.: *Mental Illness in Childhood.* New York: J. B. Lippincott Co., 1971.

KRAMER, E.: *Art as Therapy with Children.* New York: Shocken Books, 1971.

MAHLER, MARGARET S.: *On Human Symbiosis and the Vicissitudes of Individuation. Vol. I. Infantile Psychosis.* New York: International Universities Press, Inc., 1968.

MCDEVITT, JOHN B., and SETTLAGE, CALVIN F., eds.: *Separation–Individuation: Essays in Honor of Margaret S. Mahler.* New York: International Universities Press, Inc., 1971.

MIDDLETON, AGNES B., and POTHIER, PATRICIA C.: "The Nurse in Child Psychiatry," *Nursing Outlook,* **18**:5:52–57, May 1970.

MINSKI, LOUIS: *Non-communicating Children.* New York: Appleton-Century-Crofts, 1970.

NEUBAUER, PETER B.: "Disorders of Early Childhood," in Arieti, S., ed.: *American Handbook of Psychiatry,* Vol. II. New York: Basic Books, Inc., 1974, pp. 51–67.

NORDOFF, PAUL: *Therapy in Music for Handicapped Children.* New York: St. Martin's Press, 1972.

O'GORMAN, GERALD: *The Nature of Childhood Autism.* London: Butterworth's, 1967.

OREMLAND, EVELYN K., and OREMLAND, JEROME D., eds.: *The Effects of Hospitalization on Children.* Springfield, Ill.: Charles C Thomas, 1973.

PAPPENFORT, DONNELL M., KILPATRICK, DEE MORGAN, and ROBERTS, ROBERT W., eds.: *Child Caring: Social Policy and the Institution.* Chicago: Aldine Publishing Co., 1973.

PARK, CLARA CLAIBORNE: *The Siege.* New York: Harcourt, Brace & World, 1967.

PINDERHUGHES, CHARLES A.: "Differential Bonding: Toward a Psychophysiological Theory of Stereotyping," *American Journal of Psychiatry,* **136**:1:33–37, 1979.

REXFORD, EVEOLEEN N., SANDER, LOUIS W., and SHAPIRO, THEODORE, eds.: *Infant Psychiatry: A New Synthesis.* New Haven: Yale University Press, 1976.

RIBBLE, MARGARET A.: *The Rights of Infants.* New York: Columbia University Press, 1965.

ROLLINS, NANCY: *Child Psychiatry in the Soviet Union.* Cambridge, Mass.: Harvard University Press, 1972.

RUBIN, THEODORE ISAAC: *Jordi; Lisa and David.* New York: Ballantine Books, 1960.

RUTTER, MICHAEL: "Childhood Schizophrenia Reconsidered," *Journal of Autism and Childhood Schizophrenia,* **2**:315–37, 1972.

SCHOPLER, ERIC: "The Development of Body Image and Symbol Formation Through Body Contact with an Autistic Child" *Journal Child Psychology,* **3**:191–202, July–Dec. 1962.

———: "Early Infantile Autism and Receptor Processes," *Archives of General Psychiatry,* **13**: 327–35, October 1965.

———: "Discussion of Two Definitions of Autism," *Journal of Autism and Childhood Schizophrenia,* **8**:2:167–169, 1978.

SOLOW, ROBERT A.: "The Use of Phenothiazines in Children," *Western Journal of Medicine,* **129**:6:489, 1978.

SPITZ, RENE A.: *No and Yes: On the Genesis of Human Communication.* New York: International Universities Press, Inc., 1957.

———: *The First Year of Life: A Psychoanalytic Study of Normal and Deviant Development of Object Relations.* New York: International Universities Press, Inc. 1965.

STEWART, MARK A., and GATH, ANN: *Psychological Disorders of Children: A Handbook for Primary Care Physicians.* Baltimore: Williams and Wilkins, 1978.

SZUREK, STAINISLAUS ANDREW: *Clinical Studies in Childhood Psychoses: 25 Years in Collaborative Treatment and Research.* The Langley Porter Children's Service. New York: Brunner/Mazel, 1973.

WEISS, SANDRA J.: "The Language of Touch." *Nursing Research,* **28**:2:76–80, March–April 1979.

WILSON, L.: *This Stranger, My Son.* New York: G. P. Putnam's Sons, 1968.

WING, J. K.: *Early Childhood Autism: Clinical, Educational, and Social Aspects.* London: Pergamon Press, Inc., 1966.

WINNICOTT, D. W.: "The Development of the Capacity for Concern," *Bulletin of the Menninger Clinic,* **27**:167–76, 1963.

WOLMAN, BENJAMIN B.: *Children Without Childhood: A Study of Childhood Schizophrenia.* New York: Grune & Stratton, Inc., 1970.

World Health Organization: *Mental Disorders: Glossary and Guide to their Classification in Accordance with the Ninth Revision of the International Classification of Diseases.* Geneva: World Health Organization, 1978.

11

Acting Out Behavior

LEARNING OBJECTIVES / Persons studying this chapter should be able to:

1. Compare and contrast admissions of patients under eighteen to mental-health services for 1971 and 1975
2. Define: acting out, antisocial personality disorder, conduct disorder
3. Discuss the genesis of acting out according to Szurek, Rexford, and Bowlby.
4. Describe the behavior of the person who develops an antisocial personality disorder
5. Discuss treatment approaches of the acting-out individual
6. List ten guidelines important in the nursing care of the acting-out patient

Problems of young people have increased rapidly during the past few years. Between 1971 and 1975, there has been an increase of admissions under eighteen years of age of approximately 50 percent to inpatient and outpatient mental-health services. Most of the under-eighteen age group were treated in community mental-health centers in 1975, maintaining the trend of 1971. From 1971 to 1975 numbers of admissions under eighteen to state and county mental hospitals and general-hospital psychiatric inpatient services decreased but increased in private psychiatric hospitals, community mental-health centers, and outpatient psychiatric services (see Table 3, p. 18). For admissions under age eighteeen, males outnumbered females for both 1971 and 1975. For the under-eighteen age group, admission rates per one hundred thousand population increased between 1971 and 1975 from 638 to 989. Approximately 55 percent were diagnosed as having transient situational disturbances and behavior disorders of childhood and adolescence; the next most frequent diagnosis was schizophrenia (18 percent) followed by personality disorders (10 percent). Services of residential treatment centers for emotionally disturbed children are excluded from these tabulations.

The main emphasis in this chapter is on understanding some aspects of acting-out behavior in youth.

Definition

Acting out refers to the impulsive expression of feelings through body language instead of words. It was first recognized by Freud as a defiant attitude of the patient toward the psychoanalyst, which in fact was a reproduction of past attitudes of the patient toward his parents. He considered acting out to be a representation of the past through action instead of memory, the action serving to discharge inner impulses.

Now, acting-out behavior is widely accepted to be the tendency of some persons to express unconscious conflicts, or feelings of hostility or love, by actions, rather than words without conscious awareness of this fact. It may be harmful or it may be beneficial in situations, for example, such as play therapy (American Psychiatric Association, 1980). Acting out may therefore occur during psychoanalysis, during psychotherapy, in all the developmental phases of life, in psychoses, and at other times. Acting out may be episodic or a life pattern. The term "acting out" is often used in an indiscriminate manner for any aggressive or antisocial action. In this latter context, it is imprecise.

Genesis of Acting Out

Freud thought that criminal acts performed by children were attempts to establish a realistic basis for unconscious guilt feelings, which he thought originated from the oedipal period. He also acknowledged that there are adult criminals who commit crime without any sense of guilt, who have developed no moral inhibitions, and/or who are in conflict with society and feel justified in their behavior (Freud, 1949). Alexander and Stauf (1931), elaborating on Freud's theory, delineated acting-out behavior to be an expression of the unconscious need for punishment.

The concept of superego lacunae in the genesis of acting out is a contribution of Johnson and Szurek (1969). The defects in the superego, in this theory, are usually limited to lack of control over impulses such as lying and stealing. According to Szurek (1969), the antisocial child can feel guilt, regret, and anxiety, but usually *after* committing the deed. Intellectually, he differentiates between right and wrong but cannot learn from experience; that is, despite frequent transgressions, he continues to seek immediate gratification of impulses; he continues to have a low frustration tolerance and cannot postpone action. The parents are found to achieve vicarious gratification of their own impulses in the acting-out behavior of the child; therefore, the act-

ing out is *unconsciously fostered and sanctioned by a parent, who, through the child's behavior, receives vicarious gratification of his own antisocial impulses.* The defects in the superego of the child correspond to those of parents, which, in turn, are derived from their parents, and thus the intergenerational pattern is perpetuated.

In the study of families and family interaction of acting-out children by Rexford (1966), the fathers were found to be passive–aggressive men with many dependency needs and confused sexual identification, whereas the mothers were unable to view the needs of their children as separate from their own. In addition, the mothers were unable to provide the children with warmth and appropriate limit setting at the various developmental phases. The principal concern of the parents was to control the behavior of the child; they did not look favorably upon the idea of and the opportunity to understand the feelings of the children. The families were also found to be ambivalent and inconsistent in dealing with the conflicts and anxieties of the children, and encouragement of direct instinctual expression was prevalent. With this kind of family interaction, the child becomes deficient in a moral sense. The more important parent, usually the mother, encourages the antisocial behavior of the child.

Lidz (1966) found that mothers of acting-out children have more serious superego defects than simply lacunae and that the fathers are weak men with poor impulse control. The acting-out child is of unique significance to the parents or parent and is unconsciously selected from several children. With this child, the parents alternately infantilize and expect perfection and therefore give an uncertain permissiveness.

Therefore, acting out is in direct response to another person; the acter outer unconsciously aims to influence another person primarily through nonverbal communication. He cannot internalize conflicts due to his developmental defects and is very sensitive to the id impulses of others.

The genesis of acting out has also been cited as due to the lack of opportunity for forming an attachment to a mother figure during the first three years of life, deprivation of a mother figure for three to six months during the first three years, changes from one mother figure to another during the same period, and masked deprivation in which the mother is unable to view the child as separate from herself (Bowlby, 1969, 1973).

Another aspect of acting out has been portrayed by Blos (1966, p. 136) who describes acting out as a phase-specific mechanism of adolescence and relates four characteristics of adolescence to it: (1) the alternation between progression and regression, (2) disengagement from internalized, earlier love objects, (3) fear of ego impoverishment and a seeking for compensation in external events, and (4) attempts to achieve ego synthesis.

Perhaps in no other phase of life is there so much physical, hormonal, and intellectual growth as in adolescence. Urges to taste the experiences of life are hindered by authority figures and fears of loss of security of childhood.

Because of the phase-specific acting out of adolescence it is difficult to distinguish between normal and psychopathological behavior during this phase of life.

The genesis of acting out is very complex and is considered by Chwast (1977) to derive from socioeconomic and political factors as well as from individual factors.

Antisocial Personality Disorder

Antisocial personality disorder was previously called antisocial reaction (sociopathic personality disturbance) and before that was referred to as "psychopathic personality" or "constitutional psychopathic state." The term "moral insanity" was used more than one hundred years ago to refer to this disorder.

When the antisocial pattern occurs in a child or adolescent under the age of eighteen it is diagnosed as a "conduct disorder" (*Diagnostic and Statistical Manual of Mental Disorders*. III, 1980).

Patients with severe acting-out problems who are diagnosed as antisocial personalities and conduct disorders are seen in juvenile guidance centers, group homes, special schools, facilities of youth authorities, outpatient clinics, psychiatric inpatient units, home visits, residential treatment centers, and prisons.

CLINICAL PROFILE

Although the development of antisocial personality has been associated with low socioeconomic status, it occurs in every social stratum. Antisocial personality disorder occurs more in males than females. They seem incapable of forming meaningful relationships with others and rarely feel sorry for what they do. Although the mental status may be normal for the most part they may complain of boredom, tension, and depression. Their mood can change rapidly from superficial charm to aggressive acts.

In childhood, stealing, lying, fighting, and truancy are some of the signs of this disorder. When school authorities and others confront the parents, they often deny the facts, downplay the behavior, or defy the authorities themselves. One mother asked, "If the school can't handle him how do you expect me to?" Thus, the child is in a situation where parental discipline is either inconsistent or absent and he doesn't learn what is prohibited and what is socially acceptable. The following describes a child whose discipline was inconsistent:

Harry, an eight-year old child, got into a fight most every day on his way to school. He often burned his lunch, set fire to dry grass in vacant lots, and was truant. In addition he threw stones at the neighbors' houses, defaced one house with eggs, vandalized a lily pool, killed all the goldfish, and destroyed the plants in a greenhouse. When parents were confronted, the mother denied he did it and the father beat him.

The child may run away, have tantrums, seek the company of older "bad" companions, quarrel with everybody, be obstinate, and rebel against everything. The child is restless in school, constantly challenges the teacher, rarely remembers to bring pencil and paper, disrupts the class, cuts class, breaks windows, goes off the school grounds at lunch, and refuses to admit he is doing anything wrong.

At age fifteen, Bill is in the ninth grade at a junior high school. He is the youngest of three boys; one brother is seventeen and the other is twenty. Four years ago his parents divorced and since that time the children move back and forth between them. Each time Bill was in trouble at school (suspension or student–teacher–parent conference) he moved to the home of the other parent. Minor disruptions occurred while Bill was in the sixth, seventh, and eighth grades and his grades began to slip. He began the ninth grade at a private boy's school but was thrown out after one semester of "F's" in all courses.

Within three months at a public, junior high school he was suspended three times; once for disrupting and cutting classes and the second time because he was found with the keys to the school display cases. Eight display cases had been broken into and materials stolen from them. The third time he was suspended for being late for typing—twelve times out of twenty-one—for disrupting the metals class, and for swearing at the teacher.

A nursing student worked with Bill for seven weeks during the latter half of the spring semester as a counselor. In her assessment she felt he was immature for his age, had an undeveloped superego, attempted to handle authority by anger and belligerence, and was concerned mostly with the "here and now." Moving from school to school had not helped him develop relationships with peers (most students in the school had known each other for two years). In addition his support system had been shattered since the divorce of his parents.

In this situation, the student was careful to set realistic goals of establishing trust, taking one day at a time and helping Bill work on that day's expectations and problems and give praise for appropriate behavior. If he made it through one day being on time and attending classes, he was praised and encouraged. Long-term goals were to help him take responsibility for his own actions (he denied everything) and to help him prepare for the next year (the parents had decided to send him to a boarding school in another city).

In the counseling sessions, the student listened to what Bill had to say about what had transpired and tried to be nonjudgmental. Then she would read the teacher's version, discuss the discrepancies, and make a plan for the next day. For example, how to arrive on time, how tardiness affected himself and others, why he didn't like the class, and what he was going to do about it. The counseling sessions also included praise for projects he completed. Bill often came by at the end of the day to report that he had made it through the day without getting kicked out of class.

As adolescents, drinking alcohol, use of illicit drugs, and early sexual behavior are added to the earlier behavior. In adulthood, these patterns of behavior continue. As a result of this disorder, the individual may spend many years of his life in an institution.

The following patient was admitted to the psychiatric unit after slashing his wrists.

Michael, now fourteen years old, has been living with his father, an iron worker, in a nearby city. The parents have been divorced for six years. The father remarried and has three children by the second wife.

Michael's brother lives with his mother in another state. Two years ago, Michael was up for grand larceny, was made a ward of the court, and was put on probation. One year ago he was up for auto theft and sent to live with his mother, where he stole a gun and threatened two girls with it. He also violated the curfew and was picked up driving a stolen car. Returning to his father's house to live, he has now stolen another car and is under the care of the youth authority. He states that he is depressed although no depression is evident. He also relates that he sees himself in a house surrounded by fire and that he has confusing dreams. Michael has completed the seventh grade; he likes baseball and swimming and wants to be a psychologist or a chemist.

Another patient, Johnny, now eleven years old, is admitted to the psychiatric unit from the youth authority because of a suicide attempt.

Johnny's parents separated when he was five, at which time he stayed with his father, who remarried. The stepmother was described as strict; therefore, Johnny managed to stay mostly with his own mother. He has an urge to set fires; he has burned one hotel and set fires in several residences by putting rags inside rooms. In school, he set a girl's coat on fire; he has burned one house completely.

In school, he is average in courses, is good in sports, and was noted by teachers to be "an enjoyable and normal boy in most aspects." He states that he tried to hang himself at juvenile hall "for no reason, just to do it."

Cindy, a twelve-year-old girl, was admitted to the children's unit of a state mental hospital. The treatment team thought the acting out was due to depression.

Cindy came from a broken home and has a long history of acting-out delinquent behaviors in school. These behaviors led to her referral to the community mental-health center in her catchment area and to her admission. On the ward, a main problem was stealing. Every day she was found to have taken something from another patient's belongings—a radio, blouse, hairbrush, and the like—and to have given it to another patient.

When the nursing student was able to get her to talk about her feelings of depression, the stealing diminished.

The escapades of delinquents in state mental institutions are well known to those who have worked with this age group. In addition to techniques for helping patients develop internal controls, the treatment group must be prepared for riots, fire setting, stealing, and escapes. The following is an example of a rather common event and how it was handled by the nursing staff.

One day at the noon meal on a locked male psychiatric unit it was noted that the transistor radio for the ward dining room was gone. At community meeting, no one admitted knowing where it was. The nursing staff, knowing the patients, thought the culprit could be only one person. Since some of the other patients had already suffered things stolen from them by this patient, his reputation was known to the group. In a nursing conference it was decided that no one would have a pass outside the ward until the radio was found. This restriction mobilized the group of patients to put pressure on this patient, who finally came around to the head nurse (with whom he had a positive relationship) and pointed out the radio hidden behind a stack of sheets in the linen room.

The following case is an example of the complexities in treatment of a voluntary patient.

Margaret, a native American, now twenty-two years old, is admitted to the psychiatric unit for dependency on heroin. She has been on drugs since the age of fourteen. Twice married, she has a daughter, age five, who is developmentally disabled and who lives with the grandmother of the patient. The patient's mother keeps the household together by working in a beauty shop

and pays for the daughter's drugs in an attempt to keep her away from prostitution. The present husband (it is a mixed marriage) is very much in love with the patient and is trying to get her to stay away from drugs.

On the unit she glibly speaks of her first husband being a hit man for a revolutionary group. In most every contact with her, she has a different, elaborate, embroidered story to relate about herself. One time it was about being the daughter of a famous Indian chief and the next time it was a fantastic story about life among the revolutionaries and being kidnapped and sold into white slavery.[1]

In telephone conversations with her mother she speaks in loud, angry tones and often shouts and cries, but refuses to see her. The patient, despite being married only two weeks, takes up with a young blond male patient on the unit and they are found almost in bed together by the night nurse.

The patient's treatment program includes psychotherapy with a psychiatrist of which she never fails to remind the nurses and the other patients. On the unit, she consistently refuses to attend community meetings, occupational therapy, and group therapy. She often refuses to get up for breakfast but talked another patient into bringing her breakfast in bed.

She was put on a detoxification schedule, detoxified, and referred to vocational rehabilitation. She delayed going for vocational rehabilitation; instead, she made very unrealistic plans to follow in the footsteps of the young male patient who was being discharged to a live-in drug-treatment program in another city. The patient refused home visits to members of her family. Upon discharge, she was thought to be free of drugs but flew across the country the next day ostensibly to visit her first husand. Further follow-up was complicated by the fact that she did not show up for outpatient treatment.

Criteria for diagnosis of antisocial personality are set forth in the *Diagnostic and Statistical Manual of Mental Disorder.* III, 1980. In general, the individual (1) must be eighteen years of age with a history of chronic antisocial behavior, (2) must have had the onset before the age of fifteen with two or more incidents of a long list of behaviors, some examples of which are: truancy, thefts,

[1] This characteristic is similar to the fantasies of childhood. It is a fantastic storytelling called *pseudologia phantastica.*

vandalism, and so on, (3) must have had at least three incidences *since* the age of fifteen of another list of behaviors some examples of which are poor job or school performance, illegal occupation, and repeated thefts, (4) and no period of five years or more free from antisocial behavior between the ages of fifteen and the beginning of the adult antisocial behavior.

In many cases, individuals with severe acting-out problems will not come to treatment unless they are institutionalized or it is made a condition of their probation parole. There is general agreement that they need specialized treatment facilities. Some prison systems have developed active treatment services for these individuals.

TREATMENT APPROACHES

Aichorn (1935) was one of the first to report results from milieu treatment of delinquent boys. It has been said that he helped the young patients verbally plan their escapes with the expectation that it was only a plan and not to be acted upon. The process of verbal planning gratified the impulses, and what the sanctions and consequences would have been had they carried out the action were fully discussed.

Aichorn provided a corrective emotional experience with others as the treatment modality, and the transference relationship was considered to be the basis for change. In addition to milieu treatment, he made use of individual, group, and family treatment as well.

The work of Bettelheim (1955), Redl (1951), and Slavson (1965), with delinquent youth, reflects the influences of Aichorn's treatment methods.

Maxwell Jones (1953) at Belmont Hospital, England, reported successes with the use of the therapeutic-community concept in the treatment of unemployed, underprivileged, antisocial adults.

The group work of Anton Semyonovich Makarenko (1957) in the Soviet Union is noteworthy. He organized rehabilitation colonies for wandering children and youth, orphaned and displaced by the revolution and World War I. Principles of group work formulated by Makarenko are in use today;

for example, at the Moscow Institute of Psychiatry, Professor E. E. Lukomsky[2] used them in the treatment of patients with alcoholism.

Szurek (1969) recommends treatment that includes filling the superego lacunae and an analysis of conflicts. Like identification with the parent, identification is more with the behavior of the therapist than with what the therapist says; it is also with what he does, and these two things have to be congruent for the patient to begin to develop a sound superego. On the other hand, Cleckley (1964) states that one of the prohibitive influences in treatment is the inability of the patient to form a transference.

Gianascol (1969) reports that in his experience, some acting-out behavior by a delinquent represents a plea for external control as the patient himself recognizes that he has poor control of his impulses. Therefore, the treatment group must take seriously any threats the patient makes.

Brief psychotherapy for acting-out problems is described by Small (1979).

A community-based program based on sociopsychological principles and emphasizing containment of the acting out is described by Grant (1977). In this program resolution of internal conflicts and achieving effective inner controls are the goals.

Acting out has to be considered in relation to its origins in order to establish a rational therapeutic approach.

It is important to understand that acting-out behavior occurs very fast; it is impulsive and done without thinking about either the behavior or its consequences. Often the behavior scapegoats others and gets them fighting.

In order for the patient to be helped, he must experience a warm, trusting environment and develop a trusting relationship with someone of the treatment team or with a group and learn socially acceptable behavior since he has not developed a socialized superego and ego ideals. A warm, authoritative parental figure, one with whom the patient can identify, may be the most effective. The antisocial individual does not have long-lasting goals and aims in his life. He

---

[2] Personal communication, October 20, 1970, Moscow.

needs to learn the problem-solving process and to use it. One-to-one relationships and/or problem-solving groups may help the antisocial person move toward this goal.

Each acting-out event needs to be thoroughly discussed with the patient in terms of its consequences and social reality.

Realistic goals need to be set for the acting-out patient. The therapist needs to be flexible, to avoid being manipulated, and to help the patient learn to tolerate anxiety. Manipulation[3] is common and should be anticipated, although this should not be confused with acting out, which is unconscious.

With the antisocial patient, one should be aware of one's own involvement in acting out. Finding one's self in provocative behavior, setting up new limitations and rules, being very angry, and being very pleased by the behavior of the patient are warning points.

Countertransference acting out can occur and professionals need to be constantly aware of this possibility (Berry, 1977). The antisocial person is a master as a "con artist" and appears self-confident, having lived by his wits. Some people get talked into doing most anything by their winning ways and superficial charm. The nurse needs to be constantly alert to behavior and its meaning; protection of other patients is often necessary. Suicide gestures may be made to get attention, such as asking for something for pain, or to get admitted to a psychiatric unit instead of going to the youth authority or to prison. Although these patients do not intend to kill themselves, the pseudosuicide plan may fail and become a reality.

The nurse should be ready to set limits and to stand by these limits, despite vitriolic verbal abuse. Setting limits on behavior carries with it two parts: One part states what one cannot do, and the second part states clearly what one can do, thereby setting up consistent behavioral expectations and counteracting the uncertainty experienced by the patient in his family relationships. The nurse must be fair in the use of authority and avoid being punitive. Overidentification with the patient can be a problem in the treatment team where one member

sides with the patient or takes on the mode of dress and behavior of the patient.

A tendency for patients to separate team members, especially the psychiatrist and the nursing staff, and play one against the other occurs. Usually the good behavior is shown to the psychiatrist and the aggressive behavior to the nursing staff. Having team members participate in patient–staff meetings greatly reduces incidents of patients' acting out (Ploye, 1977).

The confrontational approach should be used in helping the patient to verbalize feelings instead of acting out. The nurse can teach this by modeling. In addition, when acting-out behavior occurs on a psychiatric ward, an emergency community meeting can be called to confront the patient and to encourage verbalization of feelings of everyone concerned.

Group treatment is likely to be the milieu in which the patient identifies with the group and learns socially acceptable behavior.

Some drug-treatment programs organized to use the therapeutic potential of the group center around the idea of teaching responsibility to the patient. Accepting the idea that the patient is not sick but irresponsible, the group through the use of discipline and small-group interaction teaches behavioral control. After behavioral control is managed, other aspects such as motivation to change and responsibility, i.e., work and awareness of the consequences of one's action, are approached.

All members of the treatment group therefore have to know what is going on between the patient and themselves. This is the basis for the rule in therapeutic communities that there can be no *privileged communication.* Full discussion at team meetings, reports, community meeting, and in charting is essential for treatment; otherwise, the treatment team may repeat the unresolved conflicts of the patient.

Everyone who exhibits acting-out behavior in childhood and adolescence does not develop an antisocial personality. Persons in the helping professions are now more in tune with helping children and adolescents with their feelings and problems of living, for example, when parents divorce, and with their problems in school. How-

---

[3] Manipulation is coercion of another person to do something to meet some need of one's own.

ever, the incidence of problems of youth continues to increase. New types of guidance need to be found to assist children and youth during the complex passage from childhood to adult in modern societies. Specialized health-care services need to be developed to assist in these transitional situations and linked with educational and social services, if youth is to move toward valued social roles. The World Health Organization (1977) has brought attention to these worldwide needs.

Summary

This chapter presents some aspects of acting-out behavior in youth. Various theoretical points of view are presented. A general clinical profile of the person with a conduct disorder and an antisocial personality is included, some patients are described, and treatment approaches are discussed; guidelines for nursing care are given.

References

AICHORN, AUGUST: *Wayward Youth.* New York: Viking Press, 1955.

ALEXANDER, FRANZ, and STAUF, H.: *The Criminal, the Judge, and the Public.* Translated by Gregory Zilborg. New York: The Macmillan Co., 1931.

American Psychiatric Association: *A Psychiatric Glossary.* Washington, D.C.: American Psychiatric Association, 1980.

———: *Diagnostic and Statistical Manual of Mental Disorders.* III. Washington, D.C.: American Psychiatric Association, 1980.

BERRY, THOMASIN J.: "Countertransference with the Borderline Patient," *Smith College Studies in Social Work,* 48:1:44, 1977.

BETTELHEIM, BRUNO: *Truants from Life: The Rehabilitation of Emotionally Disturbed Children.* New York: The Free Press, 1955.

BLOS, PETER: "The Concept of Acting Out in Relation to the Adolescent Process," in Rexford, Eveoleen N., ed.: *A Developmental Approach to Acting Out.* New York: International Universities Press, Inc., 1966, p. 136.

BOWLBY, JOHN: *Attachment and Loss: Attachment,* Vol. I. New York: Basic Books, Inc., 1969.

———: *Attachment and Loss: Separation, Anxiety and Anger,* Vol. II. New York: Basic Books, Inc., 1973.

CHWAST, JACOB: "Psychotherapy of Disadvantaged Acting-Out Adolescents," *American Journal of Psychotherapy,* 31:2:216–26, 1977.

CLECKLEY, HERVEY: *The Mask of Sanity.* St. Louis: C. V. Mosby Co., 1964, pp. 362–63.

FREUD, SIGMUND: "Criminality from a Sense of Guilt," in *Collected Papers,* Vol. IV. London: Hogarth Press, 1949, p. 343.

GIANASCOL, A. J.: "Psychiatry and the Juvenile Court: Patterns of Collaboration and the Use of Compulsive Psychotherapy," in Szurek, Stanislaus A. *et al.,* eds.: *The Antisocial Child: His Family and His Community.* Palo Alto, Calif.: Science and Behavior Books, 1969, pp. 149–59.

GRANT, DENNIS H.: "A Community Based Program for Acting Out Adolescents," *Military Medicine,* 142:12:932–34, 1977.

JOHNSON, ADELAIDE M., and SZUREK, STANISLAUS A.: "The Genesis of Antisocial Acting Out in Children and Adults," in Szurek, S. A., *et al.,* eds: *The Antisocial Child: His Family and His Community.* Palo Alto, Calif.: Science and Behavior Books, 1969, pp. 13–28.

JONES, MAXWELL, et al.: *The Therapeutic Community.* New York: Basic Books, Inc., 1953.

LIDZ, THEODORE, in Rexford, Eveoleen N., ed.: *A Developmental Approach to Problems of Acting Out.* New York: International Universities Press, Inc., 1966, pp. 6–17.

LUKOMSKY, E. E.: Personal communication, October 20, 1970.

MAKARENKO, ANTON SEMYONOVICH: *Pedagogical Poem.* Kiev: Ministry of Culture, 1957.

PLOYE, P. M.: "On Some Difficulties of Inpatient Individual Psychoanalytically Oriented Psychotherapy," *Psychiatry,* 40:2:133–145, 1977.

REDL, FRITZ: *Children Who Hate.* New York: The Free Press, 1951.

———: *Controls from Within: Techniques for the Treatment of the Aggressive Child.* Glencoe, Ill.: The Free Press, 1952.

———: "A Strategy and Technique of the Life Space Interview," *American Journal of Orthopsychiatry,* 29:1–17, January 1959.

REXFORD, EVEOLEEN N.: "A Developmental Concept of the Problems of Acting Out," in *A Developmental Approach to Problems of Acting Out.* New York: International Universities Press, Inc., 1966, pp. 6–17.

SLAVSON, S. R.: *Reclaiming the Delinquent.* New York: The Free Press, 1965.

SMALL, LEONARD: *The Briefer Psychotherapies.* New York: Brunner/Mazel, 1979.

SZUREK, STANISLAUS A.: "Childhood Origins of Psychopathic Personality Trends," in *The Antisocial Child: His Family and His Community.*

Palo Alto, Calif.: Science and Behavior Books, 1969, pp. 2–12.

U.S. DEPARTMENT OF HEALTH, EDUCATION, AND WELFARE: *Statistical Note 90.* 1973.

————: *Memorandum #37.* April 7, 1978.

WORLD HEALTH ORGANIZATION: *Health Needs of Adolescents. Report of a WHO Expert Committee.* Geneva: World Health Organization, 1977.

Suggested Readings

BERNFELD, SIEGFRIED: *Sisyphus or the Limits of Education.* Berkeley: University of Calif. Press, 1973 (originally published 1925).

BIRD, BRIAN: "A Specific Peculiarity of Acting Out," *Journal of the American Psychoanalytic Association,* 5:4:630–47, October 1957.

BRONFENBRENNER, URIE: "The Origins of Alienation," *Scientific American,* 232:2:53–61, August 1974.

BURGESS, ANTHONY: *A Clockwork Orange.* New York: W. W. Norton Co., 1963.

FEINSTEIN, SHERMAN C., and GIOVACCHINI, PETER L.: *Adolescent Psychiatry: Developmental and Clinical Studies.* Vol. 6. Chicago: University of Chicago Press, 1978.

FREUD, ANNA: "Adolescence," *Psychoanalytic Study of the Child,* Vol. 13. New York: International Universities Press, Inc., 1938, pp. 255–78.

FROSCH, JOHN: "The Relation Between Acting Out and Disorders of Impulse Control," *Psychiatry: Journal for the Study of Interpersonal Processes,* 40:4:295–314, 1977.

GROUP FOR THE ADVANCEMENT OF PSYCHIATRY: *Power and Authority in Adolescence: The Origins and Resolutions of Intergenerational Conflict.* New York: Group for the Advancement of Psychiatry, 1978.

HARRIS, FAYE, and FREGLY, MARILYN S.: "An Adolescent Struggle for Independence," in Fagin, Claire M.: *Nursing in Child Psychiatry.* St. Louis: C. V. Mosby Co., 1972, pp. 82–104.

HENDERSON, JOHN M.: "The Doing Character," *Adolescence,* 7:26:308–26, 1972.

HENDIN, HERBERT: *The Age of Sensation.* New York: W. W. Norton, 1975.

HERSCHMAN, PETER L.: "Team Transference and Resistance in the Treatment of Patients Who Act Out," *The Psychiatric Quarterly,* 46:2:220–34, 1972.

KENISTON, KENNETH: *All Our Children: The American Family Under Pressure.* New York: Harcourt, Brace, Jovanovich, 1977.

KOLB, LAWRENCE C.: *Modern Clinical Psychiatry.* Philadelphia: W. B. Saunders Co., 1977, pp. 609–618.

OFFER, DANIEL: "Rebellion and Antisocial Behavior," *American Journal of Psychoanalysis,* 31:1:13–19, 1971.

RAJOKOVICH, MARILYN J.: "High Schools Need Nurse Counselors, Too," in Fagin, Claire M., ed.: *Readings in Child and Adolescent Psychiatric Nuring.* St. Louis: C. V. Mosby Co., 1974.

RAPPEPORT, JONAS R.: "Antisocial Behavior," in Arieti, Silvano, ed.: *American Handbook of Psychiatry,* Vol. III. New York: Basic Books, Inc., 1974, pp. 255–69.

SCHIMEL, JOHN L.: "Problems of Delinquency and Their Treatment," in Arieti, Silvano, ed.: *American Handbook of Psychiatry,* Vol. II. New York: Basic Books, Inc., 1974, pp. 264–74.

SOROSKY, ARTHUR D.: "The Psychological Effects of Divorce on Adolescents." *Adolescence,* 12:45:123–36, 1977.

U.S. DEPARTMENT OF HEALTH, EDUCATION, AND WELFARE: *Depression in Childhood: Diagnosis, Treatment, and Conceptual Models.* Washington, D.C.: U.S. Government Printing Office, 1977.

12

Drug Abuse and Drug Dependence (Refer to Appendix D)

The main thesis of this chapter is that drug abuse can apply to any drug. However, the main interest is in drugs that produce changes in mood and behavior since these have the greatest potential for abuse. We live in a society in which drugs are advertised on the mass media as being the answer to many problems. In many cases, the abuse of drugs simply brings on more problems.

The effect of drugs has been known since antiquity. The drunkenness of Noah is mentioned in the Bible and displayed in sculpture by a fifteenth-century artist on a corner of the Doge's Palace in Venice. The Sumerians in Mesopotamia knew about opium, the dried juice of the opium poppy, in 300 B.C. *Cannabis* and coca leaves seem to have been known since recorded history. Other drugs have appeared on the scene more recently. Almost all drugs have some beneficial use and it is only in drug abuse that something needs to be done. Drug abuse refers to taking drugs to the extent that they result in damage to the individual or to the community by upsetting and disturbing its way of life (World Health Organization, 1967). Tranquilizers, antidepressants, sleeping pills, coffee, alcohol, and tobacco have widespread use in our society. The use of hallucinogenic drugs assumed epidemic proportions in the sixties, followed by heroin and other drugs. These are three terms that are frequently confused in discussions of drug abuse:

Addiction. Dependence on a chemical substance to the extent that physiologic dependence is established. The latter manifests itself as withdrawal symptoms (the abstinence syndrome) when the drug is withdrawn.[1]

Habituation. A condition, resulting from the repeated consumption of a drug, which involves little or no evidence of tolerance, some psychological dependence, no physical dependence, and a desire (not a compulsion) to continue taking the drug for the feeling of well-being that it produces.[2]

Drug dependence. Habituation to, abuse of, and/or addiction to a chemical substance. Largely because of psychologic craving, the life of the drug-dependent person revolves about the need for the specific effect of one or more chemical agents on mood or state of consciousness. The term thus includes not only addiction (which emphasizes physiologic dependence), but also drug abuse (where the pathologic craving for drugs seems unrelated to physical dependence). Alcoholism is a special type of drug dependence. Other examples are dependence on opiates, synthetic analgesics with morphine-like effects, barbiturates; other hypnotics, sedatives, some antianxiety agents, cocaine, marijuana; psychostimulants; and psychotomimetic drugs.[3]

The World Health Organization has recommended that the term "drug dependence" be used instead of "addiction" and "habituation."

Alcoholism

Alcoholic individuals may be defined as "excessive drinkers, irrespective of the cause, so dependent on alcohol as to be disturbed in physical or mental health or in social activities. The assessment of consumption can only be made in relation to accepted local and national drinking habits."[4] Because of the increase in medical and nonmedical use of drugs, greater attention needs to be given to the dangers of the interaction of drugs with alcohol. The use of alcohol with other drugs results in 20 percent of the total accidental and suicidal drug related deaths per year (Surgeon General, 1979). Some descriptions of drug interactions are given as follows:

Tolerance. More and larger doses of a drug are required to achieve the equivalent effect. The person who is dependent on heroin may tolerate very large doses that would result in death in a nontolerant person. Heroin users who are detoxified may die if they resume their heroin use at the same high dose as prior to detoxification.

Potentiate. A drug that makes the effect of another drug greater.

Cross-tolerance. Occurs where a larger amount of another drug has to be given because of the presence of an original drug. For example, patients with alcohol have to have larger amounts of anesthesia to produce sleep. However, after the first phase of anesthesia, alcohol can result in a supra-additive interaction where a deep, lethal narcosis occurs (*FDA Drug Bulletin,* 1979).

Antagonist. A drug that counteracts the action of another drug. In this situation, the effect of the two drugs taken together is less than if they were taken separately.

Additive. Two drugs taken together induce an effect equal to the effect if taken separately.

Synergistic. When two drugs are taken together the effect is greater than the two drugs taken separately. For example, with alcohol, the lethal dose of barbiturates is much lower.

More than one half of the one hundred most frequently prescribed drugs contain at least one thing that is known to react adversely to alcohol and many of the interactions are related to dosage, particularly those that are metabolized by the liver and

---

[1] American Psychiatric Association: *A Psychiatric Glossary.* Washington, D.C.: 1980.

[2] Department of Defense: *Drug Abuse: Game Without Winners.* Washington, D.C.: Superintendent of Documents, 1968.

[3] American Psychiatric Association: *A Psychiatric Glossary.* Washington, D.C.: 1980.

[4] World Health Organization: "WHO and Mental Health, 1949–1961," *WHO Chronicle,* 16:5:177, May 1962.

those that affect the central nervous system (*FDA Drug Bulletin,* 1979). An interaction between alcohol and another drug is any change in the pharmacologic effects of one due to the other. There are many effects of a drug and viewing a drug as having *one* effect is not acceptable (Nowlis, 1978). The anticoagulant properties of warfarin-type drugs can be dangerously increased by alcohol. Various oral antidiabetic medications and alcohol may produce disulfiram-like reactions (U.S. Dept. of Health, Education, and Welfare, 1978c). Alcohol is also one cause of cancer.

Alcohol may increase the lowering of blood pressure in conjunction with antihypertensives. The combination of alcohol and barbiturates can be lethal. Alcohol and phenothiazines can result in respiratory depression—severe and possibly fatal—and toxicity due to impaired liver function. Repeated use of alcohol appears to increase sensitivity to morphine and vice versa (*FDA Drug Bulletin,* 1979).

ETIOLOGY

There is no general agreement about the etiology, psychodynamics, and treatment of alcoholism. The theories advanced about the etiology of alcoholism are numerous but no single theory explains it sufficiently. Four principal theories of etiology are: (1) *genetic,* (2) *pathophysiological,* (3) *psychological,* and (4) *sociocultural.*

Since alcoholism tends to run in families, it is thought by some workers that the alcoholic has inherited a susceptibility to it. At this time, this theory has not been proven but is still being studied. The theory that the alcholic has an abnormal craving for the drug due to an inherited enzyme system different from that of nonalcoholics is an additional unproved biological theory.

The pathophysiologic point of view purports that there is a dysfunction of the endocrine system, the hypophysis, adrenal, or other metabolic functions. The prevailing point of view, however, is that the endocrine dysfunction is the result of the alcoholism, not the origin of it.

Psychological theories include the *personality trait theory* in which it is hypothesized that the alcoholic is dependent, feels inferior, is fearful, and has a low frustration tolerance. There is some evidence that the alcoholic individual does have a high psychopathic deviate score (which is connected with the antisocial personality) on the Minnesota Multiphasic Personality Inventory test (U.S. Department of Health, Education, and Welfare, 1972, p. 66). *Learning theory* attempts to show us that drinking is a reflex response to a stimulus and that the drinking behavior relieves the individual of tensions or unpleasantness. However, the alcoholic, by the very fact of his ingestion of the drug, experiences discomfort and pain, and this in itself seems to disclaim the learning theory point of view. However, therapists are using aversive conditioning in the treatment of patients with alcoholism. *Psychoanalytic theory* postulates that the alcoholic is fixated at the oral phase of development, that self-destruction is high, and that unconscious homosexuality is a factor. The alcoholic is passive, dependent, and fixated at narcissistic levels.

Wurmser (1977) describes affect regression and breakdown of affect defense as occurring in people dependent on drugs. For the alcoholic the feelings denied are guilt, loneliness, shame, shyness, and social isolation. Gratification lies in the expression of repressed or suppressed anger. Under the influence of alcohol, the person experiences camaraderie and acceptance in a regressed state.

The *sociocultural theory* by Bales describes four cultural attitudes toward drinking: abstinence, ritualistic, convival, and utilitarian. These four attitudes toward drinking influence the rates of alcoholism in a society.

It is thought, for example, that the low incidence of alcoholism among Italians and Jews is due to the fact that wine is part of the culture (ritualistic), used at ceremonials, and is taken for granted. It is a part of family life and nothing much is made of it. In other cultures many young people reaching the legal birthday enter a bar to celebrate the event, people try to outdrink each other, in all age groups much attention is given to how well one holds one's liquor, and strong liquor is the accepted drink.

Convivial drinking is widespread in our culture as exemplified in the cocktail hour.

Utilitarian drinking, for example, as used in business transactions, is also widespread.

Bales relates social organization and cultural practice to the incidence of alcoholism and describes the bases for the relationship as being the attitudes toward drinking produced by the culture, the degree that the culture produces inner tensions, and the degree that the culture provides substitute means of satisfactions. The deviant behavior theory postulates that there is a strain between the perceived goals and the means for achieving them and that the mode of adaptation is alcoholism. This theory describes the interaction of the individual with sociocultural factors that are omitted by the learning theorists.

The life histories of alcoholics encompass almost all of the neuroses, the functional psychoses, and the personality disorders. In addition, the physical problems that result as a consequence of alcoholism are many.

The alcoholic is involved in the following circular process: excessive drinking—disapproval—self-recrimination—guilt—rationalization and other defense mechanisms, such as denial and projection—excessive drinking.

The difference between the social drinker and the pathological drinker therefore refers to excessiveness, interference with work and social adjustment, and production of a pathological emotional reaction. The one characteristic common to all alcoholics is that they drink too much. The idea of an alcoholic personality is no longer acceptable. The search for causes for drinking too much has obscured the search for understanding of the mechanism of alcoholism. There are always reasons why people behave the way they do. It is thought that people drink excessively as a defense against anxiety. But there is no clarification as to why alcohol is chosen as a defense against anxiety.

Synonyms for alcohol are ethanol, ethyl alcohol, grain alcohol, and spirit of wine (Thomas, 1973). It is readily absorbed from the gastrointestinal tract. Being a central nervous system depressant, it exerts its first action upon the reticular activating system. Alcohol depresses this system and the cortex is released from its integrating control (Goodman and Gilman, 1970, p. 135).

Thus, the higher centers of judgment, self-criticism, learning, and memory are affected by alcohol. Excitement comes from the resultant lowering of inhibitions. The superego of the individual has been said to be part of the person that is most soluble in alcohol. Oxidation of alcohol is slow and occurs as follows: alcohol: acetaldehyde: acetic acid: $CO_2 + H_2O$. It is thrown off from the body through the breath and the urine.

The hangover results from excessive use of alcohol and is characterized by gastritis, nausea, vomiting, dizziness, headache, malaise, dehydration, and excessive thirst. Himwich (1956, p. 348) cites accumulation of acetaldehyde, retention of potassium, and lactacidemia as possible causes of the hangover. No two hangovers are alike in their emotional pain. It is difficult to adequately describe their affects of despair. Although many "remedies" are suggested for a hangover, the best treatment is probably aspirin, rest, and ingestion of food.

Alcohol has seven calories per milliliter and is therefore classified by some as a food; others consider it a drug. Ethyl alcohol is made (1) by fermentation of carbohydrates and (2) by the addition of water to ethylene, using sulfuric acid as a catalyst (Grillot, 1964).

Ethyl alcohol has been known since early antiquity. In the human body, alcohol is readily absorbed from the stomach and the small intestine. The rapidity of absorption depends on the speed of ingestion, concentration of alcohol, volume of alcohol, and the presence and character of other food within the stomach; however, within approximately five minutes after alcohol intake, some of it is in the bloodstream. It is almost completely oxidized; in the process, energy is released and carbon dioxide and water are given off.

Although the initial feeling after intake of alcohol is one of expansiveness and euphoria, it is a depressant, not a stimulant. The feeling of well-being is caused by the lowering of inhibitions, and the effect of the drug leads the drinker to feel that his performance is improved when, in actuality, it has been impaired. Alcohol taken in moderation stimulates the flow of the digestive juices and thereby aids digestion. Dilation

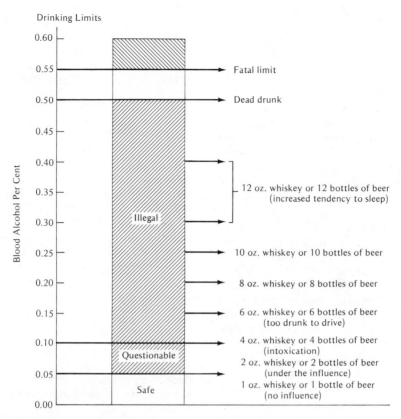

Drinking Limits

FIGURE 11. Alcohol Intake Based on Responses of a 150-Pound Person.

of the blood vessels results in perspiration and heat loss; therefore, use of alcohol to keep warm in a cold climate can have disastrous results. Hot toddies for colds and for sleep probably encourage relaxation more than anything else.

Intoxication depends upon the amount of alcohol in the bloodstream. A concentration of 0.10 to 0.20 percent in the blood indicates intoxication, whereas 0.50 to 0.90 is in the fatal range. Four bottles of beer or four highballs or cocktails will take a 150-pound person up to 0.10 percent level (Fig. 11).[5]

Acute alcoholic intoxication is characterized by euphoria, increased motor activity, clumsiness, incoordination, diplopia, staggering gait, nausea, vomiting, poor control of urination, and finally, loss of conscious-

ness, stupor, and profound coma. Associated with chronic alcoholism are alterations in personality, *delirium tremens,* acute alcoholic hallucinosis, Korsakoff's syndrome, Wernicke's syndrome, cirrhosis of the liver, pellagra, alcoholic polyneuritis, tuberculosis, cardiovascular disease, gastric ulcers, malnutrition, and the various resultant social conditions.

The National Council on Alcoholism identifies the following factors as placing persons at higher risk of alcoholism: (1) family history of alcoholism, (2) teetotalism in the family, (3) teetotalism in the spouse or in the family of the spouse, (4) a broken home or home with severe parental discord, (5) a child in the latter half of a large family or the last child of a large family, (6) heavy drinking is often associated with heavy smoking, (7) having women relatives of more than one generation who have had recurrent depressions, and (8) some cultural groups (the Irish and Scandinavians) have

[5] The alcohol in a highball or cocktail is based on the use of one ounce of 100-proof whiskey or gin (Department of Public Health, San Francisco, 1979).

been described as having more alcoholism than others; however, alcoholism can occur in any cultural group.

EPIDEMIOLOGY

Alcohol is one of the most dangerous drugs and the drug most frequently abused in the United States. The number of alcoholics in the United States is unknown; however, it is now estimated that there are 10 million adults and 3.3 million youths between 14 and 17 years of age with an additional 40 million being affected by it. Alcoholism is America's third most serious health problem (U.S. Department of Health, Education, and Welfare, 1978c). The problem of alcohol and its consequences has been given highest priority by the Center for Disease Control, the watchdog of public health in the United States. It is also estimated that there are two male alcoholics for each female alcoholic. Alcoholism seems more prevalent within the middle-age group. Analysis of the demography of a particular county or metropolitan area yields valuable information as to how many alcoholics there actually may be within the area. The incidence of cirrhosis of the liver was formerly used as an indicator. Cirrhosis of the liver is certainly associated with alcoholism, but there are other causes of it. An annual expense of $100 million for handling drunkenness arrests is an estimate of cost for the nation.

The magnitude of the problem of alcoholism is shown in that during 1975 it was the second-ranked primary diagnosis for admissions to state and county mental hospitals (U.S. Department of Health, Education, and Welfare, 1978a). The percentage of admissions reached almost 50 percent in the forty-five to fifty-four age group. The median group for admissions with a primary diagnosis of alcohol disorders was forty-four years (U.S. Department of Health, Education, and Welfare, 1977a). In 1972 the National Council on Alcoholism noted that the youngest alcoholics dropped from the age of fourteen years to twelve. Alcohol has a part in half of all fatal car crashes; in 1976 this comprised forty-seven thousand deaths. It has a part in a fourth to a third of all

serious accidents: 1.8 million (U.S. Department of Health, Education, and Welfare, 1977b). The economic cost to the nation was $43 billion in 1975 (U.S. Department of Health, Education, and Welfare, 1978c).

USERS OF ALCOHOL

Alcohol is available worldwide, although there are areas in which its use is prohibited, for example, in the Moslem countries, India, and "dry" counties in the United States. Its use is associated with tension release and social interaction such as cocktail party, conventions, picnics, business luncheons, and adolescent get-togethers.

WHO IS THE ALCOHOLIC?

Although the people on Skid Row[6] have formerly been thought of as comprising the alcoholic population, these individuals are not all alcoholic and make up only 5 percent of alcoholics. The incidence of alcoholism has increased among women or at least is more visible and therefore counted among the statistics. At present the male-to-female ratio is considered to be 2:1.

FETAL ALCOHOL SYNDROME

Heavy use of alcohol during pregnancy may result in fetal abnormalities, for example, craniofacial anomalies, mental retardation, brain, cardiac, liver, and other anomalies. Safe drinking levels during pregnancy are not known but risk is established above six drinks per day (Noble, 1978). Pregnant women and those likely to be pregnant should therefore abstain from the use of alcohol. Fetal alcohol syndrome is the third leading cause of birth defects with associated mental retardation.

---

[6] The term "Skid Row" probably originated in Seattle in the late nineteenth century. Yessler Street was greased to skid logs down the slope into the water. Taverns, hotels, and other places for the loggers lined the street (Pittman, 1967).

TREATMENT OF THE ALCOHOLIC PATIENT AND HIS FAMILY

In his message to the Congress on health, former President Lyndon B. Johnson called for a new program in the treatment of alcoholism (1966). He said:[7]

"The alcoholic suffers from a disease which will yield eventually to scientific research and adequate treatment. Even with the present limited state of our knowledge, much can be done to reduce the untold suffering and uncounted waste caused by this affliction. I have instructed the Secretary of Health, Education, and Welfare to appoint an Advisory Committee on Alcoholism; establish in the Public Health Service, a center for research on the cause, prevention, control, and treatment of alcoholism; develop an education program in which to foster public understanding based on scientific fact; and work with public and private agencies on the state and local level to include this disease in comprehensive health programs."

Authorizations under the Alcoholic and Narcotic Addict Rehabilitation Amendments of 1968 and 1970 provided for development and expansion of services for the treatment and prevention of alcoholism.

During 1970, the Comprehensive Alcohol Abuse and Alcoholism Prevention, Treatment, and Rehabilitation Act. (S. 3835, Senator Bayh) was passed by the Senate in August. It became Public Law 91–616 on December 31, 1970, and called for the establishment of the National Institute on Alcohol Abuse and Alcoholism, within the National Institute of Mental Health, with the responsibility for formulation of national policies and goals regarding prevention, research, training, control, treatment, and rehabilitation of alcohol abuse and alcoholism, and for developing and conducting programs and activities aimed at these goals. It also called for the establishment of a National Advisory Council on Alcohol Abuse and Alcoholism to make recommendations to the Secretary of the Department of Health, Education, and Welfare. The Act required that comprehensive state health plans include services for pre-

vention and treatment of alcoholism and forbade discrimination against admitting alcoholic individuals to hospitals receiving grants under the Act. This Act was a declaration of national policy that alcohol is not a crime but an *illness*. The National Institute of Drug Abuse is now organized under Alcohol, Drug Abuse and Mental Health Administration (ADAMA). Community mental-health services provided by Public Law 88–164 also aid the alcoholic patient.

DETOXIFICATION CENTERS

In contrast with the punitive approach, the illness approach requires immediate attention to the alcoholic. Detoxification centers now provide the facilities for drying out, thereby replacing jails. This system is used successfully in Czechoslovakia. Some *communities have established detoxification units as part of comprehensive treatment programs.* In the detoxification center, attention is given to a thorough health examination, including a urine test for sugar and acetone. No glucose is given to the acute alcoholic until it is determined whether or not he is diabetic. High-protein meals with vitamin and mineral supplements are provided. Twenty-four-hour bed rest and tranquilizers and antacids for gastritis are used. Close observation and caring for the alcoholic are often necessary to prevent suicide.

Clothing, a bath, laundry facilities, and some recreational activities are provided. Patients are counseled by the staff members; regular lectures, group therapy, films, work projects, vocational rehabilitation, and Alcoholics Anonymous meetings are part of the program. After drying out, the patient may be referred for further treatment.

DISULFIRAM (ANTABUSE) THERAPY

Tetraethylthiuram disulfide, first used in Copenhagen in 1948, can be effective in the treatment of alcoholism (Larsen, 1948). A patient may be given a trial reaction in the hospital in which the drug is administered and he is then given his favorite drink. The oxidation of the alcohol is delayed at

[7] Johnson, Lyndon B.: Health Message to Congress, 1966.

the acetaldehyde stage and an unpleasant reaction ensues; therefore, the patient avoids drinking alcohol to avoid the unpleasant consequences. The reaction of disulfiram with alcohol occurs rapidly (within minutes). The face, at first, becomes flushed and red and the vasodilation becomes generalized. A severe headache ensues with nausea, vomiting, chest pain, respiratory difficulties, hypertension, syncope, anxiety, weakness, vertigo, blurred vision, and marked pallor. The blood pressure may dip very low. The success of this treatment depends upon whether the patient takes the medication. Compulsive individuals may be more successful in taking the medication every day than others. Patients are instructed to take their daily dose in the early morning. They should carry identification stating they are on the drug and be instructed to avoid medications and food containing alcohol. Because of the slow elimination of the drug from the body, sensitization to alcohol lasts six to twelve days after ingestion. Another drug, calcium carbimide (Temposil), has a similar action to Antabuse. Antabuse implants are being used in Poland[8] and more recently in Canada.

OTHER THERAPIES

Conditioning and conditioned aversion therapies are being revived once more with some success. The impact of modern learning theory in the behavioral sciences gives impetus to these therapies. An excellent and scholarly review of these treatment approaches from the thirties is that of Franks (1966). The new annual review of behavior therapy includes recent noteworthy articles (Franks et al., 1978). Modeled upon conditioning principles, electro-conditioning therapy of alcoholics sets the sequence (drinking—painful stimulation—no reward) in treatment (Hsu, 1965). Other therapies, individual psychotherapy, family therapy, group psychotherapy, and milieu therapy are also used for the treatment of the alcoholic patient and his family.

SELF-HELP GROUPS

Alcoholics Anonymous is a fellowship group established in 1935 in Akron, Ohio, to help people stop drinking and stay sober. It is conducted by former alcoholics and organized to provide help to alcoholics on a twenty-four-hour basis all over the nation. Every night in the week there is an AA meeting somewhere in every metropolitan area. Every sizable town has its local chapter. It is organized around a religious–social theme and uses many principles of group psychotherapy. A call from an alcoholic at any time of day or night is answered by one of the members. Group loyalty is high and, in the group, catharsis is experienced and the alcoholic is accepted as he is *except for his drinking behavior.* Anonymity is guarded in AA groups.

Professionals and AA groups now cooperate in their efforts to aid the alcoholic to stop drinking. Alcoholics are helped in the rehabilitation process through the houses run by the AA and in other ways as well.

Al-Anon Family Groups are rather new, incorporating in the midfifties. All are self-supporting. *Al-Anon* is a fellowship of men, women, and children whose lives have been affected by the alcoholic. It is organized for the purpose of helping families and friends of alcoholics. This purpose is reached by:

- Offering comfort, hope, and friendship to the families and friends of compulsive drinkers
- Providing the opportunity to learn to grow spiritually through living by the Twelve Steps adopted from Alcoholics Anonymous
- Sharing experience in coping with the disease of alcoholism and how the program helps in giving understanding and encouragement to the alcoholic.[9]

Alateen groups are organized for teenagers who have a parent who cannot stop drinking. These groups were started in California in 1957 by a boy whose father was

[8] Department of Health, Poznan, Poland, personal communication as a World Health Organization fellow, 1970.

[9] Al-Anon Family Group Headquarters, Inc., 1974 (P.O. Box 182, Madison Square Station, New York, N.Y. 10010).

an alcoholic in AA. His mother was a member of an Al-Anon Family Group. Alateen is patterned along the lines of Al-Anon (Al-Anon, 1979). Alateen now has over two thousand groups that meet to help each other.

THE ROLE OF THE NURSE

One of the first hurdles for the nurse is self-awareness with regard to one's own attitude toward the alcoholic. If the nurse has a moralistic attitude, the patient will feel it and will probably further lower his self-esteem. At the other end of the scale, the nurse may think instant reform is possible. An objective attitude is called for in working with the alcoholic patient. When diabetic patients go off their diets and have to be regulated, the nurse is not likely to moralize. Is not the chronic alcoholic patient in a similar situation? If the nurse derogates the returning alcoholic patient with the greeting, "What! You again?" his self-esteem is further lowered.

Alcoholic patients are frequently admitted to general hospitals for surgery and for other treatments. While undergoing these procedures, treatment for the alcoholism may be ignored and daily doses of *spiritus frumenti* ordered by the attending physician. Such situations need to be changed. A health team that heals a surgical wound and ignores the alcohol problem sentences the patient to continued psychic pain. Caring enough about the patient to discuss the alcoholic problem with him may be the catalyst for progress. Admission of alcoholic patients to general hospitals under other diagnoses still occurs and supports continuation of stigma.

Accidents and alcoholism are connected and, unless the accident victim is intoxicated or a very thorough history is taken, the hospitalized patient may not be diagnosed as alcoholic and may go into *delirium tremens* and die unless preventive measures are instituted. Preventive action could include, for example, a soft high-vitamin, high-caloric diet with adequate fluid intake and between-meal feedings; a box of hard candy by the bedside will assist in the carbohydrate intake. Chlordiazepoxide is usually given. Anticonvulsants and vitamin therapy may also be ordered by the physician.

Visual hallucinations may be the first sign of impending *delirium tremens,* as well as nausea and vomiting. Because *delirium tremens* is a medical emergency, it must be treated at once. The syndrome is also characterized by auditory hallucinations, illusions, disorientation, tremors, fear, restlessness, and insomnia. Recognition of the early signs of *delirium tremens* will aid in early treatment and recovery of the patient.

The patient with *delirium tremens* needs someone at his bedside continuously to allay apprehension and to prevent injury in response to the hallucinations. A light should be left on in the room to aid orientation, and shadows from its parabola avoided, if possible. The hallucinations are usually very frightening to the patient. They may sometimes *be* pink elephants marching along at the end of the bed. *Restraints should not be used because they tend to further agitate the patient.*

In the treatment of *delirium tremens* all alcohol and alcohol-like medication are usually stopped. Cough medicines that are made with alcohol should not be given to the patient. Paraldehyde, which is synergistic with alcohol, was once generously used in treatment but is now largely replaced by other hypnotics and by tranquilizers. When phenothiazines are used, it must be remembered that they potentiate alcohol and that another side effect is orthostatic hypotension. In acute *delirium tremens,* the first tranquilizer should be given intramuscularly. If the patient cannot tolerate oral liquids, they should be given intravenously. Orange juice with ½ ounce of dextro-maltose to a 10-ounce glass is given at frequent intervals to replenish glycogen stored in the liver, for vitamin C, sodium chloride, and potassium content. The patient should receive multivitamins, and appropriate electrolytes. A nonbarbiturate sedative should be given for insomnia. Withdrawal is treated by various medications; there is no single protocol for treatment.

Patients withdrawing from alcohol need constant observation, monitoring of vital signs, and level of consciousness. Patients may die in *delirium tremens;* therefore, early recognition and treatment are of utmost importance. With adequate treatment, the syndrome of *delirium tremens* is reversible.

Community nurses who are in the homes of families have an important part to play in the treatment of the alcoholic. They also see people in clinics, schools, industries, and community activities. The community nurse is in a position where high visibility of alcoholism aids identification of cases early in onset. Warning signs of alcoholism should alert the nurse in early recognition of this mental disorder. Some are as follows:

Drinking alone
A feeling of having to have a drink
Missing a day's work due to a hangover
Drinking in the morning
Missing a social engagement due to drinking
Drinking instead of eating
Excessive drinking at mealtime

Constructive suggestions to the alcoholic and his family may aid them in seeking help with their problem. For the helping person, knowing one's own limitations in the treatment of the alcoholic person and motivating the alcoholic to accept help are important. Knowing where to get help for the patient is a must whether it be a day treatment center, a rehabilitation center, a community mental-health center, a clinic, a psychologist, a physician, psychiatrist, AA, Al-Anon, or Alateen Group. Of equal importance to the nurse is knowing the agencies to approach for consultation and advice such as the local community mental-health services.

Specialist community mental-health nurses may provide treatment themselves in terms of family therapy, group psychotherapy, and individual psychotherapy. In milieu therapy, the nurse also acts as a role model for the alcoholic patient.

Where the nurse has contact with people in schools, universities, industry, and community activities, an educational program about the use and abuse of alcohol can aid in prevention. In schools, the nurse may set up an educational program for the teachers so that they can better help their students with the question of drinking alcohol.

In one's own life, preventive techniques may be applied, for example, entertaining without the use or overuse of alcohol. I have gone to cocktail parties where the guests were met at the door with a tray of drinks. Pushing drinks onto guests at some parties seems to be taken as generosity of the host, when, in actuality, it may be doing the guests a disservice. If alcohol is served, a wide array of nonalcoholic drinks can also be made available and offered to the guests.

If people must drink, impress upon them the importance of eating. There does seem to be some evidence that early contact with alcohol within the family, at meals and at ceremonials, teaches moderation, the difference between safe and unsafe drinking, and avoidance of a later alcoholic problem. Helping others to understand abstinence with complete social acceptance of those who choose to abstain or drink very little is another preventive angle.

Since the greatest impact on alcoholism in the future may come from research rather than from services, nurses have an important role also in this area.

Other Drugs

Drug abuse arises from a complex interaction of psychosocial forces, the individual who uses it, the social and cultural content, the availability of the drug, the opportunity to take the first dose, and the continuance of its use. Kolb (1977) describes individuals who depend on drugs as mostly antisocial personalities but also includes neurotic and psychotic individuals because of their emotional problems. Kolb (1977, p. 602) cites the largest group of individuals who depend on drugs as being those with personality disorders who become dependent on drugs through other addicts. There are many ideas about the causes of drug abuse; the pervasive alienation in our society is one thesis. Certain aspects of our society are relevant to understanding drug dependence: the drug-saturated society itself, the glorification of drugs by the mass media, the role modeling done by the older generation on drug taking, peer-group pressure, overavailability, the interrelatedness of tobacco smoking and cannabis smoking, and anxiety (Fort, 1969a, 1969b). Wurmser (1977, p. 48) describes the basic affects and moods of persons dependent on drugs as: "disappointment, disillusionment, rage, shame, loneliness and a panicky mixture of terror and despair." The highest incidence is among those of low income, poor education, and broken homes, although this picture is rapidly changing. On the other hand, use of hallucinogens is widespread in middle-class youth, with an upswing in heroin dependence, cocaine and polydrug dependence.

Drug abusers are from every social class, occupation, and walk of life. Young people seem to be the most involved in drug abuse. Children at grade-school age are now part of the drug-abuse scene. Drug ingestion by children in the home has been a leading problem for years.

Because drugs that affect mood and behavior are most likely the ones that will be abused, some of these are discussed below. They are categorized as *depressants, volatile chemicals, narcotics, stimulants, hallucinogens,* and *cannabis.* Alcohol is the most abused depressant and, because of its epidemiology, has been discussed in the first part of this chapter.

DEPRESSANTS

The depressant effect of a drug is on the central nervous system; it is related to the concentration in the blood. The higher the concentration in the blood, the greater the depressant effect. Tolerance in most cases develops with repeated doses.

BARBITURATES

Barbital, the first barbituric acid derivative, was introduced to medicine in the early 1900s; although more than twenty-five hundred barbiturates have been synthesized since that time, about thirty are now in widespread use. Barbiturates are useful drugs for relief of anxiety and insomnia. They are the most commonly used of the various hypnotics. They have widespread use as sleeping pills, in suicide attempts (overdose is the leading cause of death by poisoning), and are used now in epidemiological proportions by children. Illicit traffic in the barbiturates profits many individuals who make trips to Mexico to pick up large supplies, distributed there by the drug companies, return to this country, and resell them (Rice, 1969). Other places where large quantities of barbiturates are obtained illicitly are the supply depots of the armed services. Excess barbiturates are also widely obtained through prescriptions.

The abuser administers barbiturates orally, rectally, or intravenously. They are water-soluble and can therefore be reduced to liquid. When injected, they cause what is described as an immediate flash that releases tension and spreads throughout the body. The sensation is described as similar to being drunk. The pleasure is the flash and is called the high. There is loss of coordination and emotional control.

The danger of abuse of barbiturates is the development of tolerance and psychological and physiological dependence. When a person is physiologically dependent, abrupt withdrawal is dangerous and requires medical supervision. After ten to twelve hours without drugs, there are signs of increasing anxiety, muscle twitching, tremors, weakness, insomnia, nausea, and orthostatic hypotension; changes in the electroencephalogram occur with convulsions. Convulsions may occur within sixteen hours or as late as the eighth day in the barbiturate withdrawal syndrome (Department of Defense, 1968). Confusion, agitation, delirium, and hallucinations may also occur.

In addition to the barbiturates, other central nervous system depressants that may cause dependence are: chloral hydrate, methaqualone, glutethimide (Doriden), ethchlorvynol (Placidyl), methyprylon (Noludar), and ethinamate (Valmid).

ANTIANXIETY DRUGS

The antianxiety drugs meprobamate (Equanil, Miltown), chlordiazepoxide (Librium), oxazepam (Serax), chlorazepate potassium (Tranxene), and diazepam (Valium) are drugs of abuse.

VOLATILE CHEMICALS

Inhaling fumes from glue, gasoline, kerosene, paint thinner, or lighter fluid produces an effect similar to that of a general anesthetic such as ether (Schieser and Cohen, 1968). Glue is squeezed into a rag or bag, which is placed over the nose and mouth. Kerosene, gasoline, and paint-thinner fumes may be inhaled directly from the container. The effect of inhalation of these volatile chemicals is excitement and exhilaration, hallucinations, blurring of vision, and slurred speech; ringing in the ears and staggering also occur. Further inhalation may lead to unconsciousness of about one hour's duration.

Repeated use suggests the development of psychological dependence; other effects are damage to the kidneys, liver, heart, blood, and nervous system. A danger is death by suffocation and the development of psychotic behavior. Sudden death (after deep inhalations) may occur especially when inhaling in a physically stressful situation such as running.

Aerosols are liquids, solid, or gaseous products discharged by a propellant force of compressed gas from a container. Over three hundred different types are now on the market. The large majority who inhale the foregoing volatile chemicals are between the ages of ten and fifteen years.

The anesthetics have restricted availability; nitrous oxide is the most widely used.

MORPHINELIKE NARCOTICS[10]
(OPIATES)

Narcotics are the most powerful analgesics known. Some are used for coughs and diarrhea. Narcotics tend to cause lethargy, apathy, drowsiness, constipation, pinpoint pupils, and decreased vision. Large doses depress respirations. Coma, slow, shallow respirations, cold, clammy skin, limp body, and convulsions may ensue. Narcotics produce tolerance and dependence, both psychological and physical.

---

[10] The medical meaning of the term *narcotic* refers to a drug that depresses the central nervous system for the relief of intense pain and produces stupor or sleep.

On the street they may be taken orally, by sniffing, smoking, subcutaneously, intramuscular and intravenously. Persons dependent on narcotics become preoccupied with getting and taking drugs and tend to neglect themselves. Contaminated equipment results in septicemia, hepatitis, abscesses, and endocarditis. The sticky resin from the capsule of the poppy *Papaver somniferum* is opium. It may be eaten, drunk, or smoked in the crude form. Opium and its derivatives exert a depressant effect upon the central nervous system. They relieve pain and anxiety and comprise one of the most powerful narcotics. Alkaloids of opium, morphine and codeine, are widely used in medicine today. All other pain-relieving drugs are compared with morphine in estimation of their effectiveness.

Heroin, a derivative of morphine, is sold as diluted powder in packets called decks or bags or in capsules. It is prepared and administered intravenously or sniffed. On the average, the abuser of heroin takes about 3 mg (one bag) per day. Being a central nervous system depressant, it diminishes hunger, thirst, sexual urges, fear, and pain and relieves anxiety. It produces a sense of well-being and reduces sensitivity to psychological and physical stimuli. Under the influence of the drug, the user is lethargic and indifferent to his personal situation. Heroin produces tolerance and physiological and psychological dependence. Psychological dependence is the more serious because it continues after the drug is discontinued. The pregnant user will continue the drug with full knowledge that the baby will also be addicted and will die after birth unless treated. As the need for the drug increases, the activities of the user are concentrated on how to get a "fix."

Without drugs, withdrawal symptoms develop within twelve to sixteen hours, and without treatment, the withdrawal syndrome is called cold turkey due to the resemblance of the "gooseflesh" of a plucked turkey. The withdrawal syndrome occurs as follows: the first signs of the withdrawal syndrome are yawning, lacrimation, rhinorrhea, sneezing, and perspiration. This is followed by dilated pupils, "gooseflesh," tremors, and anorexia. Within thirty-six hours, cramps of the back, abdomen, and legs appear, with uncontrollable muscle twitching and hot and cold flashes. These aspects are followed by vomiting, diarrhea, restlessness, insomnia, increased blood pressure, pulse, temperature, and respiration. Depression and an obsession to get a "fix" follow.

This syndrome reaches its height forty-eight hours after the last drug use and continues for seventy-two hours, then subsides during the following five to ten days. In contrast with alcoholic and barbiturate withdrawal, this one does not include convulsions. Users know the routine of the different treatment centers and will sometimes turn themselves in to the ones that give the best withdrawal treatment. Detoxification may be done by administration of morphine in diminishing doses or by the use of methadone in diminishing doses or a combination of both drugs. Methadone maintenance programs modeled after Nyswander et al. (1958) are now developed on an outpatient basis. In these programs, after withdrawal from other addicting drugs, methadone is administered to patients on a long-term basis. They are then able to go about their usual activities such as work and school without spending all their time searching for other drugs. Methadone can be given orally.

Other opium derivates may be abused, for example, codeine, Dilaudid, and metopon. Demerol, although not chemically related to the opiates, is addicting. One of the dangers of all these drugs is death from overdosage.

STIMULANTS

Coffee, tea, and colas are stimulants and are widely used in our culture.

TOBACCO DEPENDENCE

The psychological and physiological dependence of millions of people in this country and elsewhere on tobacco is now widely accepted as drug dependence. Despite the relationship between heart disease, cancer, and cigarette smoking, the dependence continues.

When information about the harm of tobacco cigarette smoking became widespread in the 1960s the percentage of adolescent boys taking up smoking stopped but the percentage of adolescent girls beginning to smoke increased. Now the rates are about the same. Smoking has decreased in adult men and women but the increase in smoking by younger women has resulted in the rise of tobacco smoking (Horn, 1977).

Throughout the world tobacco smoking is correlated with socioeconomic status and level of education. Blue-collar workers and those without secondary education smoke most (World Health Organization, 1979b).

Biofeedback techniques have been used successfully to demonstrate the hazards of smoking to high-school students. Withdrawal clinics emphasize the group-therapy approach with group discussion, support, health information, and general advice on how to stop smoking. Drug films and lectures may also be used as well as individual psychotherapy. The tension, hunger, and craving of withdrawal can be treated by tranquilizers. Some use an amphetamine-barbiturate mixture. Lobeline, which is an alkaloid from *Lobelia inflata,* an Indian tobacco plant, has been used to substitute for nicotine. Buffered nicotine chewing gum is now being used. Aversion therapy, satiation, sensory deprivation, and psychoanalysis have been used in treatment. At this time there is no evidence of effectiveness for specific therapeutic modalities; however, support and guidance is better than no treatment (Raw, 1978).

Treatment methods have been described as relatively unimportant compared with the determination and motivation of smokers to stop smoking (World Health Organization, 1979b).

COCAINE

Cocaine is a strong stimulant; legally, it is a narcotic. Cocaine is an active ingredient of the South American coca plant. In the Andes, leaves are chewed for refreshment. The leaves of the coca plant (decocainized) are used in the United States for flavoring cola drinks. Medical use is now limited to ear, nose, and throat surgery.

Cocaine is available on the street as a

white crystalline powder. It is called "Bernies, Big C, C, Coke, Dream, Flake, Nose Candy, Snow," and other names. Cocaine is administered by sniffing, orally or intravenously.

The stimulant effect is excitement, overtalkativeness, intense euphoria, and a sense of increased physical strength. It dilates the pupils, there is an increase in blood pressure, pulse, and temperature. Users may have delusions of persecution and agitation and experience frightening hallucinations after the initial feelings of pleasure. Delusions of jealousy are very common and violence may result. As the effects of the drug wear off, depression ensues and the patient becomes restless and irritable. Tremors, palpitation, gastrointestinal disturbances, and specks in front of the eyes may occur. One of the characteristic effects of cocainism is the feeling that there are insects beneath the skin. Because of its pleasurable effects a strong psychological dependence can occur. Withdrawal is not accompanied by the tendency to collapse as seen in opium derivatives (Kolb, 1977).

A patient, Mr. M. A., in his midthirties was admitted to the inpatient psychiatric unit by a friend. He had hit six objects in one block while driving away from his home. He had also bought a carbine, threatened a man who double-parked with it, and said he was going to kill his punk brother. He was dirty, dishevelled in appearance, in constant motion, and continuously eating. He was also irritable, loud, provocative, tremulous, scared, jumpy, with a labile mood, but wanted to be withdrawn from the drug. He stated that he was taking 1 gm of cocaine (at four hundred dollars) per day and thought he was going to die. He had threatened arson, shot holes in the wall of his home, and torn the place apart.

Medications given were diazepam and chloral hydrate. Other treatments were milieu in a locked psychiatric unit and psychotherapy.

AMPHETAMINES

Amphetamines have been in medical use since the 1930s. In medicine today they are used for depressive patients as psychostimulants and also as anorectics for obese patients. They are also used to counteract drowsiness caused by the sedative drugs.

Amphetamines produce an initial increase in blood pressure, palpitations, pallor, dilated pupils, dry mouth, headache, and diarrhea; they also increase alertness and produce euphoria.

Athletes have taken amphetamines to improve performance; they have been given to race horses for the same reason. Truck drivers take them to stay awake and students use them as stimulants to stay up and study. They are called bennies and highs (amphetamine), Christmas tree (dextroamphetamine and Amytal), Dexies (dextroamphetamine), and "crystal" and "speed" (methamphetamine). Amphetamines are taken orally and intravenously. Methamphetamine is now one of the most commonly abused drugs of this group.

The user of these drugs takes large doses over a period of four or five days, without eating or sleeping. The episode can lead to severe weight loss, malnutrition, and psychosis requiring hospitalization. The individual frequently becomes extremely suspicious and this may merge into a paranoid psychosis. The person is at a high energy level; his behavior unpredictable and may be violent.

Amphetamine withdrawal is characterized by insomnia, apathy, and an increase in rapid eye movement (REM) sleep. Suicides have also occurred during the withdrawal phase.

Tolerance and psychological dependence occur. Most authorities agree that amphetamines do not produce physiological dependence or withdrawal syndrome, although fatigue, exhaustion, and severe depression are experienced after withdrawal.

HALLUCINOGENS

Dream images, distortions of perceptions, and hallucinations are characteristic of hallucinogen use. These drugs are also referred to as psychotomimetic[11] or psychedelic. They have no widespread medicinal use, although LSD has been used experimentally with alcoholics and patients with terminal cancer (Pahnke et al. 1969).

[11] Psychotomimetic refers to mimicking the psychoses, which the hallucinogens were at first thought to do.

LSD

Lysergic acid diethylamide, or LSD, has been known since 1938. This acid is present in ergot, a rye fungus. It is now derived from the chemical laboratory in large quantities for illicit use on a wide scale.

LSD may be obtained as a small white pill, as a powder in capsules, or as a tasteless, colorless, odorless liquid in ampules. It is referred to as acid. It primarily affects the central nervous system. The user of acid may have dilated pupils, tremors, increased temperature and blood pressure, and hyperactive reflexes. The LSD trip involves changes in sight, hearing, touch, body image, and time; sensitivity to sound increases; synesthesia[12] occurs, disorientation and cognitive changes appear. The environment is perceived in an entirely new way. Nausea and vomiting may also occur. The "bad trip" refers to perceptual alterations that result in panic where the individual loses control of himself and reacts self-destructively. Trivial events take on great significance and any mood may ensue. LSD may create tolerance and psychological dependence may develop, but it is seldom intense; physiological dependence does not occur. Recurrent hallucinations may occur even some months after LSD has been taken.

Other hallucinogens include mescaline from the Mexican cactus (peyote); psilocybin from certain mushrooms found in Mexico; D.M.T. (dimethyltryptamine), now prepared synthetically but a natural constituent of the seeds of certain plants in the West Indies and South America; S.T.P.—Serenity, Tranquility, and Peace—(dimethoxymethylamphetamine) and M.D.A.—Mellow Drug of America—(methylenedioxyamphetamine). Some morning glory seeds are also known for their hallucinogenic effect.

PHENCYCLIDINE (PCP)

PCP is a veterinary anesthetic that can be taken orally, sniffed, injected, or smoked. It is a white crystalline powder readily soluble in water and ethanol.

Phencyclidine was tested as an anesthetic

[12] The translation of one sensory phenomenon into another; for example, sounds become visualized.

for humans in the 1950s but clinical use was discontinued because it caused delirium in some individuals. During 1967 it was introduced as a veterinary anesthetic (Sernylan).

PCP is available illicitly in powder, tablet, in capsules, in a leaf mixture, and as crystal forms. It is known on the street as "crystal," "angel dust," "PCP," "PC Pill," "Hog" and "DOA."

PCP has the potential for inducing bizarre and violent behavior in the user as well as severe anxiety and depression and thinking disorders.

Acute PCP intoxication may appear as (1) an acute confused state or (2) stupor or coma. In the acute confused state the patient appears awake but verbally uncommunicative and may respond with nodding or moving his eyes. He may be disoriented, confused, fearful, and amnesic. The patient's eyes are open and staring, nystagmus is present (it may be horizontal, rotary, or vertical), and the corneal reflex may be absent. The patient is ataxic, restless, has facial grimaces and rigid muscle tone, and the deep tendon reflexes are increased. The patient may be anxious, agitated, and excited; depersonalization may occur. As stupor and coma emerge, the patient's blood pressure may be variable, arrhythmias appear, urinary output and respirations decrease (apnea can occur), and convulsions are possible. No antagonist is known for counteracting the toxic effects of phencyclidine (Burns and Lerner, 1976).

Many deaths are associated with PCP intoxication. Because of confusion and incoordination, drowning is common.

To assist a PCP user, the patient should be put in a quiet, dark place and physical touch should be avoided. Patients who are agitated must be cared for in a controlled environment and vital signs monitored as unobtrusively as possible. Patients who take high doses need gastric lavage, toxicological examination of urine and blood, monitoring of vital signs, neurological status, fluid intake, and urinary output. Cranberry juice and ascorbic acid are given to the alert patient for urine acidification that aids excretion of the drug (Vourakis et al., 1979). The phencyclidine delirium may be followed by a psychosis resembling schizophrenia. Careful studies need to be made of individuals who use this drug.

Recently the human and veterinary anesthetic Ketamine[13] is growing in abuse. Common street names are "green," "1980 Supergrass" (when used with marijuana), "K," "Super Acid," "Purple," and "Mauve."

Complications of its use are delusional states, confusion, and hallucinations. Surgical patients (about 12 per cent) experience these complications. Recurrences of hallucinations can occur without additional drug and repeated use can result in psychosis *(FDA Drug Bulletin, 1979).*

CANNABIS SATIVA

Cannabis is the generic name of Indian hemp *(Cannabis sativa). Cannabis sativa* may be divided into two groups: (1) *Cannabis sativa indica,* which is grown in India, and (2) *Cannabis nonindica,* grown elsewhere. The active ingredients are tetrahydrocannabinols, which affect the mind and body in various ways. Marijuana, the popular name for the plant, is also the dried leaves and flowering tops of the plant. Hashish is the resin from the flowers of *cannabis.* It is much richer in cannabinols than the leaves and tops. Hashish oil is a concentrate of *cannabis.* It is an extract, a dark viscous liquid. A drop or two is equal in effect to a marijuana cigarette. For high potency of the plant, a high temperature and low humidity are necessary (Advisory Committee on Drug Dependence, 1968). Marijuana was once used extensively in medicine. Although there is controversy over the abuse of *Cannabis sativa,* the World Health Organization Expert Committee on Dependence Producing Drugs states:[14]

There is agreement that Cannabis produces hilarity, talkativeness, and increased sociability. A sufficiently strong dose will distort perception, particularly of time and space, and impair both judgment and memory. There is also a warping

of emotional reactions that may take the form of irritability or confusion. For some people, the drug acts as an hallucinogen and lowers the sensory threshold, making paintings seem more vivid and the experience of listening to music more intense. Anxiety and aggressiveness may result from intellectual and sensory confusion. There is no development of physical dependence, nor unequivocal proof that lasting mental disturbances have been produced by Cannabis, although predisposed people may have temporary psychoses.

Treatment of Patients with Drug Dependence

Nyswander and associates (1958) have shown that outpatient treatment of persons dependent on drugs has some success. In these programs, methadone is administered to the patient who must come to the clinic for his dose. Methadone blocks the action of heroin and relieves the craving for drugs. The patient is therefore relieved of the need to look for a "fix."

Psychotherapy, both group and individual, and family therapy are used in the treatment of the person who depends on drugs. Although difficult to establish, it should be begun during the withdrawal phase, if possible.

SELF-HELP GROUPS

Narcotics Anonymous is modeled after Alcoholics Anonymous. There are various other self-help groups such as NARCO (Narcotic Addiction Research and Community Opportunities, New Haven, Connecticut). Daytop Village has branches over the country. Reality therapy is emphasized and professionals work in this organization. Delancey Street Foundation emphasizes rehabilitation independent of government assistance.

Teen Challenge centers its therapy on God; it was founded by David Wilkerson, an evangelist, in 1959. Teen Challenge has headquarters in Brooklyn, New York, and has activities in San Francisco, Boston, Philadelphia, Chicago, Dallas, and Toronto, Canada.

---

[13] An arylcyclohexylamine marketed as Ketalar, Ketaject, and Ketavet. It was first marketed as an anesthetic in the 1970s. It is chemically related to phencyclidine (PCP).

[14] World Health Organization: "Drugs, What They Are," *World Health,* p. 8, July 1967.

THE ROLE OF THE NURSE

A main focus for all helping professionals is to take the myth out of the use of drugs. Young people want to know the facts and telling them only about the bad effects of drugs omits the fact of the initial pleasure. Many youngsters take drugs without knowing what they are and what the results may be. If the group culture is to experiment with drugs, then, in order to be accepted in the group, there will be strong pressure to also experiment. School nurses and other community nurses in public health and community mental-health programs are especially in a position to use preventive measures. Students may need assistance in asserting their own independence of social pressure to conform and take drugs and to find other ways of relating to peers. Role playing and discussion are of value in these endeavors. Parents can also be assisted in meeting with each other and setting limits on drug-taking behavior. Teachers need to know about the dangers of drugs and what to do about them.

With regard to the use of barbiturates, the nurse has an important role in teaching moderation of use. Barbiturates are commonly prescribed as sleeping medication in hospitals and given matter-of-factly by the nurse. Sometimes more simple measures to help sleep are superior: a back rub, hot milk, a quiet environment, or a bedtime chat. The same measures can be repeated, if the patient awakens in the middle of the night. These measures should especially be provided for patients who are hospitalized for long periods of time, due to the adaptation and adjustment problems that they have. Although the nurse singlehandedly cannot reroute our drug-oriented society, in home visits families can be taught the fallacy of taking a drug for everything. Helping the parents look at their own modeling to their children and changing it if necessary is another approach. If the nurse is dependent on drugs, nicotine, for example, the patient being taught to quit smoking perceives the hypocrisy and whatever is taught will probably be ignored. Helping people to "turn on" to things other than drugs is another track.

Drug abuse is common in the professions. Among occupational groups, physicians, pharmacists, and nurses have a high rate. Early detection of drug abuse and help at that point or referral may be the deterrent to chronic use. Setting in motion the procedures for dealing with social and emotional problems requires knowing the specific resources of a community.

A nonjudgmental attitude is required in working with people who depend on drugs. Help the individual who has been occupied with the drug culture to communicate about something else; often that is the only thing that he has been able to talk about. The individual may need help with the basic necessities of life and these have to be provided for in some way.

In withdrawal, the nurse has a central role in the success of the effort. Patients who are being withdrawn will wheedle, cajole, develop myriad symptoms, threaten suicide, and even attempt suicide to try to get their dose of the drug. It takes consistent limit setting to achieve the withdrawal. Even a ten-minute leeway on the time that the next dose is due is pleaded for most strongly. Addicts know how to run up the mercury on a thermometer, put blood in their stools, and various other devices to fake physical illness and therefore be in line for more medication. If the withdrawal is to be successful, the environment has to be controlled so that the patient gets only his prescribed dose.

The nurse's observation and reporting of signs and symptoms are an essential part of the treatment process.

Patients who depend on drugs are still admitted to general hospitals without this fact being recorded on their admitting diagnosis. Nursing care can sometimes be very difficult when such facts about the patient are not shared with them. Some orthopedic patients who are immobilized for long periods are subject to drug dependence.

Narcotic orders are written by licensed physicians, and no nurse should continue giving narcotics for very long without requesting reassessment by the physician. Some hospitals have a policy that narcotics orders automatically expire within forty-eight hours. Others require consultation with the supervising nurse before dispensing. The order "q 4 h prn" requires judgment from the nurse as to its administration. Judicious use of narcotics by nurses can prevent dependence. On the other hand, I have seen nurses verbalize fear that their patients would become addicted when, in fact, they were on the brink of death and regular use of the narcotics that were ordered would give relief to suffering.

Summary

In this chapter, drug abuse and drug dependence have been discussed, with particular emphasis on the epidemiology of alcoholism and other drugs most commonly abused. Therapeutic modalities are outlined and the role of the nurse discussed.

References

AL-ANON: *Youth and the Alcoholic Parent.* New York: Al-Anon, 1979.

AMERICAN PYSCHIATRIC ASSOCIATION: *A Psychiatric Glossary.* Washington, D.C.: American Psychiatric Association, 1980.

BALES, ROBERT F.: "Cultural Differences in Rates of Alcoholism," *Quarterly Journal of Studies on Alcohol,* 6:480, 1946.

BURNS, R. STANLEY, and LERNER, STEVEN E.: "Perspectives: Acute Phencyclidine Intoxication," *Clinical Toxicology,* 9:4:477–501, 1976.

DEPARTMENT OF DEFENSE: *Drug Abuse.* Washington, D.C.: U.S. Government Printing Office, 1968.

DEPARTMENT OF HEALTH, POZNAN, POLAND: Personal communication as a World Health Organization Fellow, 1970.

FDA Drug Bulletin, 9:2:10–12, June 1979.

FORT, JOEL: Notes taken from lecture on "Sex, Drugs, and Society," San Francisco, August 1969a.

————: *The Pleasure Seekers: The Drug Crisis, Youth and Society.* New York: The Bobbs-Merrill Co., 1969b.

FRANKS, CYRIL M.: "Conditioning and Conditioned Aversion Therapies in the Treatment of the Alcoholic," *The International Journal of the Addictions,* 1:2:61–98, June 1966.

FRANKS, CYRIL M., and WILSON, TERENCE, eds.: *Annual Review of Behavior Therapy.* Vol. 6. New York: Brunner/Mazel, 1978.

GOODMAN, LOUIS S., and GILMAN, ALFRED: *The Pharmacological Basis of Therapeutics.* New York: Macmillan Publishing Co., Inc., 1970, 4th ed.

GRILLOT, GERALD F.: *A Chemical Background to*

Nursing. New York: Harper & Row, Publishers, 1964.

HIMWICH, HAROLD E.: "Alcohol and Brain Physiology," in Thompson, George N.: *Alcoholism.* Springfield, Ill.: Charles C Thomas, 1956, pp. 291–408.

HORN, D.: "Smoking and Disease—What must be Done," *WHO Chronicle,* 31:355–361, September 1977.

HSU, JOHN J.: "Electroconditioning Therapy of Alcoholics," *Quarterly Journal of Studies on Alcohol,* 26:3:499–59, September 1965.

JOHNSON, PRESIDENT LYNDON B.: "Health Message to Congress," 1966.

KOLB, LAWRENCE C.: *Modern Clinical Psychiatry.* Philadelphia: W. B. Saunders Co., 1977.

LARSEN, VALDEMAR: "The Effect on Experimental Animals of Antabuse (Tetraethylthiuramdisulfide) in Combination with Alcohol," *Acta Pharmacologia,* 4:321–22, 1948.

MARTIN, E. W.: *Hazards of Medication.* Philadelphia: J. B. Lippincott Company, 1971, p. 435.

NATIONAL COUNCIL ON ALCOHOLISM, INC., 1979.

NOBLE, ERNEST P.: "Statement: Fetal Alcohol Syndrome," in U.S. Department of Health, Education, and Welfare: *The Community Health Nurse and Alcohol Related Problems.* Washington, D.C.: U.S. Government Printing Office, 1978, p. 283.

NOWLIS, HELEN: *Drugs Demystified.* Paris: United Nations Educational, Scientific and Cultural Organization, 1978.

NYSWANDER, MARIE, et al.: "The Treatment of Drug Addicts as Voluntary Outpatients," *American Journal of Orthopsychiatry,* 28:714–27, 1958.

PAHNKE, WALTER H., KURLAND, ALBERT A., GOODMAN, LOUIS E., and RICHARDS, WILLIAM A.: "LSD-Assisted Psychotherapy with Terminal Cancer Patients," in Hicks, Richard E., and Fink, Paul Jay: *Psychedelic Drugs.* New York: Grune & Stratton, Inc., 1969, pp. 32–42.

PITTMAN, DAVID J.: "Public Intoxication and the Alcoholic Offender in American Society," in the President's Commission on Law Enforcement and Administration of Justice: *Task Force Report: Drunkenness.* Washington, D.C.: U.S. Government Printing Office, 1967.

RAW, MARTIN: "The Treatment of Cigarette Dependence," in Israel, Yedy, et al.: *Research Advances in Alcohol and Drug Problems.* Vol 4. New York: Plenum Press, 1978, pp. 441–485.

RICE, DONALD: Testimony to the U.S. House of Representatives, Select Committee on Crime, San Francisco, October 23, 1969.

SCHIESER, DAVID W., and COHEN, SEYMOUR:

"Drugs and Their Effects," *California's Health,* 25:8:2 ff., February 1968.

SMITH, DAVID: "Fetal Alcohol Syndrome: A Tragic and Preventable Disorder," in Estes, Nada J., and Heineman, M. Edith: *Alcoholism: Development, Consequences, and Interventions.* Saint Louis: C. V. Mosby Company, 1977, pp. 144–152.

SURGEON GENERAL OF THE U.S. PUBLIC HEALTH SERVICE, 1979.

THOMAS, CLAYTON L., ed.: *Taber's Cyclopedic Medical Dictionary.* Philadelphia: R. A. Davis, 1973.

U.S. DEPARTMENT OF HEALTH, EDUCATION, AND WELFARE: *First Special Report to the U.S. Congress on Alcohol and Health.* Washington, D.C.: U.S. Government Printing Office, 1972, p. 66.

————: *Statistical Note 138.* Washington, D.C.: U.S. Government Printing Office, 1977a.

————: *Drugs and Driving.* Washington, D.C.: U.S. Government Printing Office, DHEW Publication N. (ADM) 432, 1977b.

————: *NIAA Information and Feature Service,* January 24, 1977c.

————: *Statistical Note No. 148.* Washington, D.C.: U.S. Government Printing Office, 1978a.

————: *The Community Health Nurse and Alcohol Related Problems.* Washington, D.C.: U.S. Government Printing Office, 1978b.

————: *Third Special Report to the U.S. Congress on Alcohol and Health.* Washington, D.C.: U.S. Government Printing Office, 1978c.

U.S. DEPARTMENT OF JUSTICE: *Drugs of Abuse.* Washington, D.C.: U.S. Department of Justice, 1976.

————: *Drugs of Abuse.* Washington, D.C.: U.S. Government Printing Office, 1979.

VOURAKIS, CHRISTINE, and BENNETT, GERALD: "Angel Dust: Not Heaven Sent," *American Journal of Nursing,* 79:4:649–653, April 1979.

WORLD HEALTH ORGANIZATION: "Drugs, What They Are," *World Health,* July 1967.

————: *WHO Expert Committee on Drug Dependence.* Technical Report Series, No. 437 and No. 460, Geneva, 1970.

————: "Tobacco Smoking in the World," *WHO Chronicle,* 33:94–97, March 1979a.

————: "Treatment of Cigarette Dependence," *WHO Chronicle,* 33:98–100, March 1979b.

WURMSER, LEON: "Mr. Pecksniff's Horse? Psychodynamics in Compulsive Drug Use," in U.S. Department of Health, Education and Welfare: *Psychodynamics of Drug Dependence.* Washington, D.C.: U.S. Government Printing Office, 1977, pp. 36–72.

Suggested Reading

BURKHALTER, P.: *Nursing Care of the Alcoholic and Drug Abuser.* New York: McGraw-Hill Book Company, 1975.

CHAFETZ, MORRIS E., HERTZMAN, MARC, and BERENSON, DAVID: "Alcoholism: A Positive View," in Arieti, Silvano, ed.: *American Handbook of Psychiatry.* Vol. 3. New York: Basic Books, Inc., 1974, pp. 367–392.

DE BARD, MARK L: "Diazepam Withdrawal Syndrome: A Case of Psychosis, Seizure, and Coma," *American Journal of Psychiatry,* 136:1:104–105, 1979.

DERICCO, DENICE A., BRIGHAM, THOMAS A., and GARLINGTON, WARREN K.: "Development and Evaluation of Treatment Paradigms for the Suppression of Smoking Behavior," *Journal of Applied Behavior Analysis,* 10:2:173–181, Summer 1977.

ESTES, NADA J. and HEINEMANN, M. EDITH, eds.: *Alcoholism: Development, Consequences, and Interventions.* St. Louis: The C. V. Mosby Company, 1977.

LEVINE, DAVID G.: "A Historical Approach to Understanding Drug Abuse Among Nurses," *American Journal of Psychiatry.* 131:9:1036–37, September 1974.

MAYKOSKI, KATHLEEN A., RUBIN, MARILYN B., and DAY, SR. AGNITA CLAIRE: "Effect of Cigarette Smoking on Postural Muscle Tremor," *Nursing Research,* 25:1:39–43, January–February 1976.

SCHMID, NANCY J., and SCHMID, DONALD T.: "Nursing Students' Attitudes Toward Alcoholics," *Nursing Research,* 22:3:246–48, May–June 1973.

STACEY, B., and DAVIES, J.: "Drinking Behavior in Childhood and Adolescence: An Evaluative Review," *British Journal of Addictions,* 65:203–212, 1970.

STEINGLASS, P.: "Family Therapy in Alcoholism," in Kissin, B., and Begleiter, H., eds.: *The Biology of Alcoholism. Volume 5. Treatment and Rehabilitation of the Chronic Alcoholic.* New York: Plenum Press, 1977, pp. 259–99.

U.S. DEPARTMENT OF HEALTH, EDUCATION, AND WELFARE: *Phencyclidine (PCP) Abuse: An Appraisal.* Washington, D.C.: U.S. Government Printing Office, NIDA Research Monograph, 1978.

WORLD HEALTH ORGANIZATION: "Alcohol Control Policies: A Public Health Issue," *WHO Chronicle,* 30:243–246, June 1976.

————: "Safe Use of Psychotropic and Narcotic Substances," *WHO Chronicle,* 33:12–15, January 1979.

13

Psychogeriatrics

LEARNING OBJECTIVES / Persons studying this chapter should be able to:

1. Define psychogeriatrics
2. List the ten questions for psychiatric assessment of organic brain syndrome in older persons
3. List five aspects of persons with organic mental disorder
4. Describe characteristics of the acute confusional state
5. Describe characteristics of senile dementia
6. Describe characteristics of multi-infarct dementia (cerebral arteriosclerosis)
7. Define reality orientation; list nine nursing actions in nursing care that aid reality orientation

Psychogeriatrics refers to mental disorders of old age, their epidemiology, prevention, etiology, and treatment. It is especially concerned with those disorders that first appear after sixty-five years of age (World Health Organization, 1972).

Until the advent of Medicare and Medicaid, large numbers of older persons with mental disorders were sent by the counties to state mental hospitals where the state paid for their care. Now, with federal financing, alternatives to state mental hospitals are available. Although nationally, both the total number and rate of additions of persons sixty-five and over at state and county mental hospitals decreased between 1971–1975, thirteen states reported increases. These states are: Alaska, Colorado, District of Columbia, Florida, Louisiana, Missouri, Nebraska, North Carolina, North Dakota, Oklahoma, South Dakota, Texas, and Wisconsin. (U.S. Department of Health, Education, and Welfare, 1978.)

The kinds of facilities in which older persons are cared for vary within the different states. Health professionals of all disciplines now have more older persons in their practices. Professionals untrained or uninterested in problems of aging may misdiagnose older persons as being senile when, in fact, they may have a treatable organic mental disorder or depression.

Common problems encountered in older persons in psychiatric practice are: (1) depression, (2) paranoid trends, and (3) organic mental disorder. Because depression and paranoid trends are not exclusively problems of aging, the reader is referred to Chapters 6 and 7 for a full discussion of these problems. Although organic mental disorders can occur at any age, they are prevalent among older persons and the most prevalent are presented here.

Psychiatric Assessment

Nurses have a highly important role in clinical assessment and the ensuing treatment and nursing care. In nursing practice, there is a tendency in some areas to expect that older people will be confused upon hospitalization and no attempts made to definitely assess the confusion or to help clear it up. There is a tendency, for example, to record "Patient confused" and let it go at that.

Assessment of the older person involves the same components as that for a younger person and the reader is referred to Chapter 4 for the mental-status examination. However, additional tools of more specific aspects are useful for a definitive clinical assessment of the older person. For the mental-status examination of the older person, the ten questions should be used to assist in the evaluation of impairment (see Table 6).

Goldfarb has found these ten questions the best indicators to use as a test for assessment of the presence and extent of brain syndrome in older persons (personal communication). If the individual gives one incorrect answer, he has mild or no brain syndrome; if he gives three to eight incorrect answers, he has moderate to severe brain syndrome and nine to ten incorrect answers suggest severe brain syndrome. The examiner may, of course, ask additional questions helpful in assessment, for example, "What time is it now?" (orientation to time), "What is the name of this place?" (orientation to place), and 'What did you eat for breakfast?" (recent memory), "Where were you born?" (remote memory), and "What is my job?" (orientation to person). For a complete assessment of the older person Butler (1977) uses a twenty-two-page data sheet.

Organic Mental Disorders

Persons with organic mental disorders have conditions caused by or associated with impairment of brain tissue function. Five aspects of these disorders are: (1) memory loss, (2) disorientation, (3) impairment of intellectual function, (4) impaired judgment, and (5) labile affect (Butler, 1973).

Table 6.   Ten Questions*

Question	Measures Orientation for
1. Where are we now?	Place
2. Where is this place (located)?	Place
3. What is today's date—day of month?	Time
4. What month is it?	Time
5. What year is it?	Time
6. How old are you?	Memory—recent or remote
7. What is your birthday?	Memory—recent or remote
8. What year were you born?	Memory—remote
9. Who is the President of the U.S.?	General information—memory
10. Who was the President before him?	General information—memory

* From Goldfarb, Alvin I.: "Psychiatry in Geriatrics," *Medical Clinics of North America.* 51:6:1521, November 1967. By permission.

The following conditions are some of the causes of organic mental disorders: brain tumors, head trauma, infections, dehydration, electrolyte imbalance, anemia, malnutrition, avitaminosis, cardiac and circulatory disorders, genito-urinary problems, postoperative complications, fever, fecal impaction, and intoxication from drugs (including alcohol) and poisons. The syndrome may appear suddenly in the older person as a result of stress or some specific physiological problems.

Although symptoms vary, organic brain syndrome may begin with mild intellectual changes, the older person recognizes it, and resolves the problem:

Mrs. Jones, now in her seventies, lives in a small apartment downtown. She takes several prescribed medications, cooks her own meals, and belongs to a downtown senior center. She recognizes her failing memory so as she takes her medications, she places each bottle on another table labeled TAKEN. One afternoon while out shopping she forgot which direction she lived so now she carries her apartment key, name, and address around her neck. She makes lists of things to do each day on her calendar and checks them off as they are accomplished.

Older persons with advancing organic brain syndrome may be socially adequate but have difficulty in thinking clearly and focusing attention. They may repeat themselves over and over without realizing it. Although they try very hard, there are certain things they cannot remember. Nightime is difficult because the sensory cues for orientation are diminished.

Another patient, B. P., now in her seventies, very depressed and on the verge of chronic organic brain syndrome, adjusted quickly to the set routine of the psychiatric hospital. The manager of her hotel had been instrumental in her admission because of her failing memory. The hotel was located in a nice part of the city and meals were served in a lovely dining room. Fiercely independent for many years as an employee of the local internal revenue office, she was now in painful conflict about what to do about her living arrangements. She greeted the nurse, pleadingly, with the following: "I want Jesus to just fold me up in his arms and take me. Now that I've ended up in a place like this, well, just let me die, I just want to die. I've never done anything to anyone in my life and

I don't know why I should be punished like this." The few times she seemed delighted and smiled were when she wore red and when she was asked about her airplane rides with Charles A. Lindbergh in her youth.

Nursing care involved helping B. P. with her personal hygiene. She made no effort to bathe, change her clothes, or otherwise groom herself unless someone suggested it. Confusion and confabulation were present at times but she stood her ground when another younger manic patient criticized her. Otherwise, as her mood improved, most of the time she covered up her memory gaps by telling jokes and smiling. At times, she sat thoughtfully and would say, "I don't know whatever will become of me." She had no relatives or close friends with the exception of one younger man who lived in an adjacent county who used to work with her. After her depression lifted, she insisted on returning to her hotel, which she did, but follow-up visits by nursing students found her again staying in her hotel room without even going to the dining room for meals. She seemed to have lost track of time; soon she was readmitted, placed in a board and care home for a short period, and soon afterward was admitted to a convalescent hospital where she died within a few months.

As the brain syndrome advances, impaired attention, memory, retention, and recall occur; judgment and orientation are impaired. Disturbances of perception, i.e., misinterpretations may be present, and the person becomes confused. In addition, decreased or increased psychomotor activity may be present.

The patient, M. V., aged eighty-one, an Italian-American, was admitted to the psychiatric hospital when the neighbors reported her strange behavior to the geriatric screening unit of the community mental-health services. In the home visit to assess the situation, M. V. was found putting away the Christmas tree, although it was now April. There were candles and flashlights but no heat, water, light, or gas in the house. A tier of newspapers about fourteen feet long lined the hall. The neighbor stated that no one had visited the patient for ten years. When asked about her family, the patient stated, "My son is not dead but was buried fourteen years ago in a large hole." Pointing to the manhole in front of the house, she said, "My son, son-in-law, my sister are all in that hole. They're not dead. They would not give me welfare." The patient was admitted to the psychiatric hospital to evaluate organic deficits, to provide basic needs until the staff could locate and contact the family, to secure a possible conservatorship and placement. Milieu therapy and Haldol, 1 mg. b.i.d. were ordered. A temporary *conservatorship*[1] was secured so the locksmith could open up the house. Her bankbook of the last month showed five dollars in savings but the bank knew nothing of her family. An address led to a local real-estate man who said that she owned her house and lot and had formerly rented out a flat. He also indicated that she had some family still alive. Checking the welfare central index yielded the startling fact that three years previously she brought in her welfare checks and said she did not want them anymore. Her history stated that in 1957 her son had cancer and had asked her to come out west from the East Coast. He soon died and the children were made wards of the court. Another son was deceased but the patient had two daughters living on the East Coast and a niece was listed as living in a small town about fifty miles away. M. V. was also known to the Italian Welfare Agency. The daughters were contacted and one made plans to come out for two weeks.

M. V. continued to show some confusion and confabulation but maintained good spirits. She claimed a picture of Prince Charles and the Queen of England as part of her family. She also had the delusion that Vittorio Emmanuele, late King of Italy, was her relative. She was able to perform self-care in the hospital and displayed anger when the daughter did not come and visit her every evening. She was liked by the staff and other patients and expressed some hostility about no one caring for her for years and "now everybody wants to visit me and take me away." Although she had lucid moments, it was determined that she needed a more sheltered environment than afforded by her own home; therefore, she was presented with a choice of residential care homes and chose to live in one near her old neighborhood.

[1] *Conservatorship:* This is a legal process that allows another individual or agency to act on the person's behalf and to protect his interest when he is unable to care for himself. When a professional person in an agency providing comprehensive evaluation or a facility providing intensive treatment determines that a person in his care is gravely disabled as a result of mental disorder or impairment by chronic alcoholism and is unwilling to accept, or incapable of accepting, treatment voluntarily he may recommend conservatorship to the officer providing conservatorship investigation of the county of residence of the person prior to his admission as a patient in such a facility. (State of California—Health and Welfare Agency: *California Mental Health Services Act.* Sacramento: California Office of State Printing, 1979, p. 44.)

ACUTE CONFUSIONAL STATE (DELIRIUM)

Characteristics of the confusional state are exemplified by delirium: alterations of level of consciousness, i.e., clouding, fluctuations and rapid variations, disorientation, illusions, hallucinations, fear, bewilderment, and paranoid trends. Also, delusions may appear as well as generally disorganized behavior and ego functions become progressively impaired. Sleep disturbances are present.

Mr. A. R., age sixty-six, was admitted to the psychiatric unit in an acute confusional state. A janitor in a local hospital, he had suddenly become agitated and combative when his supervisor enquired why he forgot one work assignment that day. Very little was known about him. He carried no identification; no home address was known. The supervisor could give little information except that he lived alone and that his work had been excellent. Mr. R. could give no information about himself. He wore a puzzled, bewildered expression and walked around the unit as though trying to figure out what was happening to him. He needed assistance in finding his way about the unit and readily accepted assistance. A nursing student approached him with friendliness, stayed with him and explained what had happened, the purposes of the tests ordered by the psychiatrist, and developed trust. He seemed to want to answer questions asked of him but could not remember. No one on the psychiatric team had been able to find out where Mr. R. lived. The nursing student and Mr. R. paged through current magazines and newspapers together to help his memory. She thought he was not psychotic and presented this information to the psychiatric team. She also got the idea to get a street map and ask him to point out the section of the city where he lived. Although he could not remember the street, his face lit up when he recognized his neighborhood on the map (near San Francisco's Chinatown). So the student and a psychiatric technician took him for a visit to the area and he went right to his hotel. Glad to find him, the manager greeted him happily. Mr. R.'s confusion cleared up gradually over a two-week period. The diagnosticians called his condition "organic brain syndrome of unknown cause."

Early treatment of the acute confusional state is of utmost importance. With proper treatment, the acute confusional state may clear up completely. Nurses are often in a position to do early assessment of older persons in these acute confusional states. Too many times the symptoms of delirium have been considered chronic and people have been sent on to long-term institutions instead of receiving treatment. These disorders may also accompany chronic diseases such as diseases of the heart or diabetes. Older persons who are depressed show signs that simulate organic brain syndrome, therefore, careful assessment is of utmost importance. Because depression and organic brain syndrome may co-exist, a trial regimen of antidepressant drugs may be the only way to differentiate. If the patient has an affective disorder, it is important to know this because it is responsive to treatment.

SENILE DEMENTIA

Here, the older person experiences an insidious decrease of intellectual functioning. Major memory deficits occur, judgment is severely impaired, major personality changes occur, and the person may experience loss of impulse control. Loss of memory for recent events is the cardinal symptom. Deficits in memory are both anterograde and retrograde. Memory of early childhood events may be recalled vividly but the older person may not be able to recall what he had for breakfast. Forgetting to extinguish cigarettes and turn off the gas are extremely hazardous. Wandering away and getting lost are constant worries of those supervising their care. This wandering may occur at night and create added problems for family members. Some older persons are constantly on the go collecting and moving objects from one place to another. Inhibitions may be decreased and sexual indiscretions occur. The older person's affect may be labile, changing quickly from being calm and cheerful to crying. Ability to think abstractly is lost. Ability to dress, button clothes, and tie shoes is decreased. The older person may withdraw, be argumentative, and physically resist anyone who tries to help.

Mr. A. O., a former author, is now in his upper seventies. He readily verbalizes and carries on necessary activities of daily living under the constant supervision of his wife, who is in her late sixties and who has a pacemaker. The content of his language is confined to events that occurred thirty years previously. A tall, muscular man, he physically resists getting dressed and undressed and cannot be reasoned with in this regard. All other aspects of daily living he follows amiably. Mrs. O. rarely leaves him for anything, fearful that he will die and she will not be present.

In the most advanced stages of senility, the older person becomes helpless, incontinent, and apathetic. There is a steady decline and the average survival is five years (Butler, 1977). The cause of senility is unknown.

MULTI-INFARCT DEMENTIA (CEREBRAL ARTERIOSCLEROSIS)

The core feature of this disorder is a gradual decrease of intellectual functioning, the result of which interferes with the older person's occupational or social activities. Memory deficits tend to fluctuate, the older person forgets one minute and remembers the next. The first symptoms are headaches, dizziness, and lassitude. Some attacks occur suddenly; others come on gradually and there is a tendency for the course of the disorder to occur stepwise, that is, to remit and fluctuate. Mental status rapidly changes with clearly defined attacks of confusion. Some cognitive functions are impaired whereas others are intact. The older person may have insight and judgment, but may become delirious and hallucinate. Focal neurological signs and symptoms are present. Because of the multiple infarcts, the physical condition of the older person is worse than in senile dementia. Death may come rapidly or the condition may be prolonged. Special medical and nursing care are required because of the physical involvement. When the person is in remission, other treatments can be beneficial: psychotherapy, physical therapy, occupational therapy, for example. Depression often accompanies this disorder, and suicide is a danger. There are no specific treatments for senile dementia and cerebral arteriosclerosis but much can be done in terms of providing an environment at home or in an institution in which the older person does as much self-care as possible where the milieu is familiar, simplified, and the older person's daily schedule made rather constant. Clear communication, a balance of stimulation and quiet, occupational therapy, and recreation are helpful.

Facilities that encourage patients to produce useful objects are for the most part absent in institutions for older persons in the United States. Convalescent Home #20 for two hundred older people in Moscow provides a contrast. In this home, older people garden, take care of the house plants, and make useful objects in a well-stocked sewing room. A library is available with daily newspapers, *Krokodil* (the Russian humor magazine), and books in Russian and German. A social hall enables residents to get together for lectures, plays, and informational meetings.[1] Patients' rooms hold personal objects, no patient was in bed, and everything was spotlessly clean.

A comparative study of institutionalized older people in Scotland and the United States by Kayser-Jones (1979) cites the importance of institutionalized older persons having something to exchange with the caretakers in order to participate in social relationships. Drastic changes need to be made in our institutions for older people to make them humanistic. Butler (1977) often advises psychotherapy for the older person and his family. Medications may be prescribed for agitation, but many older persons receive much too much antipsychotic drugs. Nurses have a responsibility to prevent this occurrence. In the nursing-care plan, perhaps nothing is as important as reality orientation and resocialization.

Nursing Care: Reality Orientation and Resocialization

Reality orientation refers to knowing your name, the place where you are, who the people are around you, and the time (month, year, date, and day of the week). It is a part of rehabilitation for the confused

[1] Site visit by the author, August 1978.

or disoriented person. A formal program of reality orientation has been developed and used at the Veterans Administration Hospital, Tuscaloosa, Alabama (Folsom, 1968). Reality orientation aims to aid the older person with organic mental disorder move toward awareness of himself and his environment.

Hogstel (1979) evaluated reality orientation with older, confused patients in a nursing home. No *significant* differences were found in the degree of confusion of the older persons after a three-week orientation program. However, many patients were reported less confused after the program.

In the care of older persons requiring reality orientation, assess individual needs and make the nursing-care plan. Set realistic expectations, be sincere, firm, and consistent. Nursing actions are discussed as follows:

1. All communication should be stated clearly and not necessarily loudly. Learn how hearing aids work and check to see if the patient's is working; if it is not, see that it gets repaired. If patients are rambling in their speech, tell them about it. Avoid saying that you understand something when you actually did not. This kind of communication only adds to the confusion.

2. Call the patient by name and do this consistently, beginning with awakening the patient. Put the name of the patient on the door of his room and on his closets. These names may easily be made by the patient in occupational therapy. Some system for marking clothes and safekeeping of possessions is necessary; otherwise, confused patients collect clothes and possessions of other patients and add to the unreality. Placecards at dining help orientation. Wear your own nametag as a memory aid.

3. In order to aid orientation, remind patients of the time and the date over and over. A schedule of daily events on the unit itself posted in a prominent place aids failing memories.

4. A calm, simplified, bright, and cherry environment with a set routine helps the confused older person to help himself. One therapist sprays cologne around the room before group psychotherapy for sensory stimulation (Oberleder, 1969). Easy access to bathing facilities, clothes, toilet, occupational therapy, and the like, is necessary; if required, guide patients to and from their destination.

The use of a multipurpose room for various activities helps disoriented and confused patients as opposed to directing them to various rooms for different activities. For example, the dayroom can be used for serving meals; it can also be set up for occupational-therapy projects, films, and exercise groups. As the preparations are under way, patients can be involved in them and see for themselves what is going on around them. Dayrooms located where patients can watch staff and visitors come and go may assist in orientation. Walks in the neighborhood and in the garden and gardening itself help the confused elderly person to think about where he is.

5. *Encourage visits by family and friends;* they assist in maintaining reality contacts.

6. *Encourage self-help* in activities of daily living. It is important to help older people maintain what physical capabilities they still possess. Simple exercises such as standing, sitting down, and walking aid in this process. Older people need assistance with bathing, toileting, brushing their teeth, cleaning their spectacles, keeping their clothes clean and mended, clipping their fingernails and toenails, and other grooming activities. It does not help the patient for you to do these things for him when he is able to do them for himself. A daily exercise group meeting is helpful in maintaining active body processes. Excellent exercises can be performed while sitting.

7. *Encourage patients to help each other* by request and example. One patient with organic brain syndrome had been admitted from her own home because of inability to care for herself. In the psychiatric unit, another patient became interested in her, assisted her at mealtimes and with her personal hygiene. The relationship seemed mutually beneficial.

8. Above all, avoid *infantilizing* the older person by using first names, putting their hair in pigtails and ribbons, and doing things for them that they are capable of doing for themselves. Your expectations influence behavior. Set your expectations at a level toward which the patient can move.

9. Recognize the unique cultural aspects of the older person of diverse cultures as well as the longitudinal changes within a particular culture.

Depression and the Older Person

Perhaps in no other age group is depression more common than in the older person. Because depression frequently accompanies organic mental disorders, it is briefly mentioned here. (Refer to Chap. 6 for a full discussion of depression.) For the older person who is mildly depressed, self-renewal may be all that is needed. Taking up a new hobby and useful roles where one is welcomed and loved may be the effective treatment. Suicide is a danger in the depressed older person and lethality must always be assessed. Hospitalization, psychotherapy, antidepressants, and/or electroconvulsive therapy may be used.

The condition of the following patient represents an example of the presence of both depression and organic mental disorder.

The patient was admitted to the psychiatric unit after a nurse on an outreach team made a home visit.

Mrs. M. G., seventy-four years old, was brought to the psychiatric inpatient unit for seventy-two-hour observation by the outreach team of the community mental-health center. A neighbor, not having seen the patient and her husband go in and out of the house for days, telephoned the police. On arrival, they found the corpse of the husband on the couch in the living room and the patient sitting with the body. He had been dead four days. She was anxious, agitated, and unable to answer questions. The outreach team was brought in. Mrs. G. denied that her husband was dead, stating that "voices say ugly things to me." The patient was feeble, depressed, and would not give any information. She spoke out to say, "Leave me alone, don't bother me" and "That man in my house was not my husband," moaning quietly but continuously. The neighbors stated that it was customary for the old couple to go out to dinner every evening. They had known them for twenty-five years and reported that the patient had been well dressed until the last two years. Addresses of two physicians were found in her telephone book—they were contacted; one had been her physician until seven years ago and stated that she had been depressed for many years. The husband had been under his care but had missed his appointments during the past few months. The husband had reported to him that his wife had taken to wandering away from home and he had once found her in the back of a truck down the street. Milieu therapy and amitryptyline (Elavil), 25 mg t.i.d., were prescribed at the hospital. Being severely depressed and unwilling or unable to participate in making plans for herself or burial of her husband, she was recommended for a conservatorship. The patient, in group therapy, said that she did not want to share her business but did give the name of her sister. From the sister, it was learned that she had seen the patient two years previously and found her doing all right then. In the hospital, Mrs. G. continued to be depressed and frightened and said that she heard voices saying, "You are not Martha G." The sister took a temporary court guardianship so she could bury her brother-in-law. Three plans for care were proposed: (1) residential care home, (2) intermediate care facility, and (3) home care with home visits and participation in a day-treatment program. The patient's depression lifted somewhat. It was later determined that she also had chronic organic brain syndrome. Although she had gotten along at home as long as her husband was alive, she now could not manage alone; therefore, she was placed in an intermediate care facility.

Common topics in group therapy with the aged in psychiatric units are depression, drinking, suicide, and death. The affects of depression and anger are present and expressed. It is not uncommon for the therapist to be greeted with "Dearie, I am ready for death."

One patient, Mr. B. G., now seventy-six, Italian, and formerly a longshoreman, was admitted to the psychiatric hospital from a general hospital where he had a prostatectomy and in convalescence had slit his wrists and also struck out at a nurse. He was still markedly depressed and spoke of contemplating suicide every day and was thinking that he would carry it out but he did not want to get blood all over everything and make a mess. This patient was living in a residential care home where he had his own little apartment. Divorced for many years, the patient had only one relative, a son who visited him periodically from his ranch in the nearby grape-growing areas. The patient expressed much anger toward his son whom he had helped as a child and who now would not let him live with him, because the patient and the daughter-in-law did not get along. This patient assumed some leadership in the therapy group and assisted other patients to speak of their feelings of being lonely and alone. He gradually seemed to accept his situation and made plans to live in a downtown hotel, after discharge.

Often the aged person in the psychiatric unit denies the death of spouse or idealizes the dead person.

One patient, Mr. D. N., in his seventies, with unresolved grief and mourning and who was severely depressed, spoke constantly of his dead wife in group therapy in a sad, slow, stentorian voice. Although married late in life to each other they had been together every day for thirty years and it had never occurred to him that she would die first. Both had been very active in the theater on the East Coast and now her death had left him completely alone.

This patient recovered from his acute depression, was assisted to find a residential care home with some other men of his intellectual level, and was maintained by antidepressant medication and group psychotherapy on an outpatient basis.

Mrs. F. P., now in her eighties, was admitted to the psychiatric hospital for depression. A beauty queen at age eighteen in the Midwest with two marriages that ended in divorce, she now spent most of her time in the local bar. On admission she was markedly depressed and had all the signs and symptoms of the late stages of alcoholism plus a large decubitus ulcer infected with staphylococci. "No one wants to listen to me. I'm too sick to do anything. I'm too old to bother with. Why do you want me to do anything when you know I'm old and weak? Just let me lie here and die," she verbalized over and over. Milieu therapy, group psychotherapy, individual psychotherapy, an antidepressant drug, and one-to-one nurse–patient relationships helped this patient toward recovery. Nursing care involved helping the patient ventilate feelings with regard to her increasing helplessness, ego-building actions such as insistence on grooming, bathing, changing clothes, participation in activities, and complimenting the patient. Cigarettes were limited; otherwise she chain-smoked. This patient was also encouraged to renew her contacts with her sister in the Midwest, who, in fact, flew out with her husband to visit. Deciding not to return to the Midwest to live with her sister, she was discharged back to her apartment, refusing referral to a local senior center and Alcoholics Anonymous.

Summary

In this chapter, psychogeriatrics as a fairly new field of practice is defined. Selected common organic mental disorders of older persons are described and reality orientation outlined. Some case vignettes of depressed older persons are presented.

References

AMERICAN PSYCHIATRIC ASSOCIATION: *Diagnostic and Statistical Manual of Mental Disorders III,* Washington, D.C.: American Psychiatric Association, 1980.

BUTLER, ROBERT N., and LEWIS, MYRNA, I.: *Aging and Mental Health: Positive Psychosocial Approaches.* St. Louis: C. V. Mosby, 1973, p. 69.
_____: Aging and Mental Health: *Positive Psychosocial Approaches.* St. Louis: C. V. Mosby Co., 1977.

CALIFORNIA, STATE OF: *California Mental Health Services Act.* Sacramento: California Office of State Printing, 1974, p. 23.

FOLSOM, JAMES C.: "Reality Orientation for the Elderly Mental Patient," *Journal of Geriatric Psychiatry,* I:2:291–307, Spring, 1968.

GOLDFARB, ALVIN J.: "Psychiatry in Geriatrics," *Medical Clinics of North America,* 51:6:1515–27, November 1967.

GROUP FOR THE ADVANCEMENT OF PSYCHIATRY: *The Aged and Community Mental Health: A Guide to Program Development.* Vol. VIII, Report No. 81. New York: Group for the Advancement of Psychiatry, 1971.

HOGSTEL, MILDRED O.: "Use of Reality Orientation with Aging Confused Patients," *Nursing Research,* 28:3:161–165, May/June 1979.

KAYSER-JONES, JEANIE: "Care of the Institutionalized Aged in Scotland and the United States: A Comparative Study," *Western Journal of Nursing Research,* 1:3:190–200, Summer 1979.

NURSING SERVICE, VETERANS' ADMINISTRATION HOSPITAL: "Guide for Reality Orientation," Tuscaloosa, Alabama, 1970.

OBERLEDER, MURIEL: "Emotional Breakdowns in Elderly People," *Hospital and Community Psychiatry,* 20:7:191–196, July 1969.

U. S. DEPARTMENT OF HEALTH, EDUCATION, AND WELFARE: *Statistical Note No. 149.* Washington D.C.: U.S. Government Printing Office, 1978.

WORLD HEALTH ORGANIZATION: *Psychogeriatrics,* Geneva: World Health Organization, 1972, p. 11.

Suggested Readings

BEREZIN, MARTIN A. and CATH, STANLEY H., eds.: *Geriatric Psychiatry: Grief, Loss and Emotional Disorders in the Aging Process.* New York: International Universities Press, Inc., 1965.

BROCK, ANNA M., and MADISON, ANN S.: "The Challenge of Gerontological Nursing," *Nursing Forum,* XVI:1:95–105, 1977.

BURNSIDE, IRENE MORTENSON, ed.: *Nursing and the Aged.* New York: McGraw-Hill Book Company, 1976.

GLASSCOTE, RAYMOND, et al.: *Old Folks at Homes: A Field Study of Nursing and Board-and-Care Homes.* Washington, D.C.: American Psychiatric Association, 1976.

GRESHAM, MARY L.: "The Infantilization of the Elderly," *Nursing Forum.* XV:2:195–210, 1976.

HENKER, III, FRED O.: "Organic Brain Syndrome: A Psychosomatic Approach," *Psychosomatics.* 19:5:270–272, May 1978.

METZ, ELEANOR L.: "Assessing the Older Psychiatric Patient," in Dunlap, Lois Craft, ed.: *Mental Health Concepts Applied to Nursing.* New York: John Wiley and Sons, 1978, pp. 204–209.

RYPINS, RUSSEL F., and CLARK, MARY LOU: "A Screening Project for the Geriatric Mentally Ill," *California Medicine,* 109:273–78, October 1968.

TEETER, RUTH B., GARETZ, FLOYD K., MILLER, WINSTON R., and HEILAND, WILLIAM F.: "Psychiatric Disturbances of Aged Patients in Skilled Nursing Homes," *American Journal of Psychiatry,* 133:12:1430–1434, December 1976.

VLADECK, BRUCE C.: *Unloving Care: The Nursing Home Tragedy.* New York: Basic Books, Inc., 1980.

14

Psychotherapy

L E A R N I N G   O B J E C T I V E S / Persons studying this chapter should be able to:

1. Define psychotherapy
2. Name and describe three types of psychotherapy

3. Name six stages of the process of crisis intervention and describe the components of each stage

Psychotherapy is a treatment for patients with emotional problems by psychological means. In psychotherapy, a formal, contractual, structured relationship is established between a trained person and the patient for the objective of alleviating emotional distress, changing disturbed behavior, and fostering personality growth and development. Psychotherapy includes established and respected methods of individual therapy, group therapy, and family therapy (American Nurses Association, 1976). The reader is referred to Chapter 4 for a discussion of the one-to-one nurse–patient relationship.

The American Nurses' Association designates psychotherapy within the scope of psychiatric and mental-health nursing practice. To be a psychiatric mental-health nursing specialist ". . . demands expertise in the psychotherapeutic methodologies" (American Nurses' Association, 1976, p. 11).

The American Psychiatric Association describes psychotherapy as a contractual interaction with a psychotherapist in which a person desires to relieve symptoms, resolve problems of living or is seeking personal growth (American Psychiatric Association, 1980).

Types of Psychotherapy

Wolberg (1967) distinguishes three types of psychotherapy:

1. *Supportive,* in which the objects are to alleviate symptoms, strengthen defenses, and restore equilibrium. Supportive therapy is recommended for individuals who have sound egos but are temporarily disrupted, for those who need ego strengthening, and for those who need assistance in equilibrium maintenance. Counseling and educational guidance fall in this category. Crisis intervention, now widely used as short-term psychotherapy (Ewing, 1978), falls under this heading. In supportive psychotherapy, the therapist must have a warm, caring, helpful attitude toward the patient but at the same time be objective in order to be helpful. If the therapist does not like the patient or cannot empathize deeply with the patient, therapy will probably not take place. Supportive psychotherapy does not focus on past events unless the patient connects present with past. The therapist facilitates verbalization, and catharsis, listens, communicates, encourages, reassures, uses suggestion, persuasion, and guidance.

2. *Re-educative.* Here the objectives are to gain insight into conscious conflicts, reach one's highest potentialities, and to modify behavior. In order to attain the objectives, the ways that the patient relates are scrutinized and techniques for changing behavior are carried out. Re-educative therapy is recommended for persons who are expected to be able to examine their own behavior and attempt new behaviors. Relationship therapy, behavior therapy, and psychodrama are examples of re-educative therapy.

In re-educative psychotherapy, the therapist may use a variety of techniques to modify the behavior of the patient or, together with the patient, examine interpersonal relationships with the aims of modification of behavior and personal growth. Where the relationship with the therapist is the central factor, the therapist needs to be skilled in management of transference, countertransference, and resistance.

3. *Reconstructive.* Here the objectives are for the patient to gain insight into unconscious conflicts, their origins, and to change the personality. The process of therapy is based upon the genetic–dynamic theory of personality and the relationship to the present. Included under reconstructive therapy are Freudian psychoanalysis, neo-Freudian psychoanalysis, egoanalysis, and psychoanalytically oriented psychotherapy. Patients undergoing psychoanalysis must be prepared with time, money, and strength to undergo major challenges to defenses and reintegration through intensive sessions four to five times a week over a period of two to five years (Wolberg, 1967).

Although concern for psychological aspects of people is evident throughout history, we are indebted to Freud for a scientific psychological approach to the inner person called psychoanalysis. Psychoanalysis is a theory of psychology of human development, a form of psychotherapy, and a method of research. Fundamental to Freud's theory is the principle that mental activity results from what has preceded it. The second fundamental principle is the existence of the unconscious. Psychoanalysis is a method of indirect study of the unconscious life of the individual. Through free association, interpretation of dreams and resistance, and transference, the patient's unconscious thoughts, feelings, and motivation are uncovered and inferences can be made about them. During psychoanalysis, the patient lies on a couch without facing the analyst.

Psychoanalytically oriented psychotherapy is derived from psychoanalysis; however, free association is not promoted and the transference is not so intense. The therapist listens via the face-to-face posture, empathizes, provides the development of trust, and the patient has a feeling of being helped. Painful feelings of anxiety, guilt, fear, and shame are cleared up through catharsis and early processes are modified.

Crisis Intervention

Crisis intervention developed as a technique for primary prevention (see Chap. 1). It is also known as psychiatric first aid (Evans, 1968) and psychological first aid (Klinman, 1978). Crisis intervention has assumed an important position in community mental-health services. The development of crisis theory, community mental-health centers, the acceptance of people in crisis of reaching out for assistance to these centers, and the focus on prevention have contributed to the widespread use of crisis intervention. The acceptance by professionals in the field of psychiatry of the concept of outreach services to the home has also been an important factor in the development of crisis intervention. For many years, the field of psychiatry held to the expectation that unless the patient came to the professional, therapy could not begin.

At times of crises, family and friends and others may be of assistance to the person experiencing the crisis. Crisis intervention is therefore not performed only by professionals. Volunteers such as those in disasters, suicide-prevention centers, and other areas intervene in crises as well as family members, neighbors, and friends.

Life's crises are currently being accepted by persons experiencing them as events where help from community mental-health services are appropriate (Carter, 1977). For example, young couples getting a divorce are now more likely than in the past to seek assistance for helping the children understand the process.

CRISIS INTERVENTION AS SHORT-TERM PSYCHOTHERAPY

Crisis intervention as short-term psychotherapy is now widely used in many clinical practice areas, for example, for persons who are sexual trauma victims, families where sudden infant death has occurred, as well as other special groups (Ewing, 1978).

Individuals with initial mental disorder are now treated on a short-term basis in community mental-health centers where a full range of services can help avoid long-term institutionalization, thus providing secondary prevention. Twenty-four-hour emergency services, with a multidisciplinary staff, provide crisis intervention by telephone, walk-in, and by appointment. Staff sometimes spend two to three hours or more upon first contact with a patient encouraging catharsis, listening, and helping problem-solve. At these crisis points, medications may also be prescribed by the physician. For those who need more help, alternatives to hospitalization are now developed in some communities for short stays in a structured environment. For example, one catchment area of San Francisco houses its crisis unit in an open Victorian house with twenty-four-hour supervision by mental-health workers. This kind of facility provides a small number of beds to enable patients who do not need inpatient treatment to stay a few days up to two weeks until they are once more in equilibrium. Other patients may only require an overnight stay in the inpatient service.

Large numbers of persons with chronic mental disorder now live in their communities and frequently are in need of crisis intervention. With these persons, intervention is tertiary prevention. The full range of treatment facilities must include not only walk-in services, but outreach, home visiting, inpatient beds available at all times, transitional facilities with a variety of levels of structure and supervision of patients. Outpatient departments, halfway houses,

acute day-treatment centers, supervised residential (twenty-four-hour) programs, and extended day-treatment programs organized to meet the needs of the patients are necessary for crisis intervention with this population. Many problems exist in providing these persons with the help that they need. To ensure that the person in crisis gets appropriate assistance, linkage to other agencies via person-to-person contacts must be developed by the multidisciplinary team in crisis-intervention programs.

PROCESS OF CRISIS INTERVENTION

If crisis intervention is to be effective, action must be taken right away to aid the person experiencing the crisis to regain his former equilibrium. Caplan describes six weeks as the crisis period. The crisis can be a growth experience in that new problem-solving techniques can develop as a result of the crisis. If not resolved appropriately, the crisis can result in further disorganized behavior.

Crisis intervention requires careful consideration of the individual's situation, if the therapist is to be of assistance. The following process may be helpful to follow: (1) rapport, (2) assessment, (3) planning, (4) intervening, (5) planning for the future and termination, and (6) follow-up.

Rapport. The therapist's attitude of caring, interest, willingness to help, and warmth, both verbal and nonverbal, assist in the establishment of rapport. Unless rapport is established, therapy may not occur.

Assessment. During the first interview, data must be gathered for delineating the problem. Levels of anxiety, ego functioning, and affect should be assessed. Reduction of anxiety also begins as support is given and as the data are being obtained.

In order to identify the problem, the therapist facilitates the relating of the problem by the patient. "What happened?" "What brings you here today?" demonstrate the kinds of questions that may be asked about the precipitating event. The therapist needs to know what precipitated the crisis, the events leading up to it, how the patient functioned before the crisis, and available sources of support. The patient may elaborate a great deal on many problems but be unable to pinpoint the specific problem that brought him in. The therapist listens for a theme, in order to begin making a plan (Enelow, 1977). Some patients are highly anxious, very verbal, and excited. Others are fearful, vague, or silent. In *data gathering,* the family members, and/or significant others may also be of assistance, if they are available. A short review of the patient's recent life situation may elicit the life crisis (i.e., work, school, family, and social activities). The data gathering and *evaluation* of the situation occur simultaneously. A crisis center may require a form to be filled out before the interview with the therapist. Identifying data of age, occupation, home address, education, Medicaid number, if any, position in family, and so on, may therefore have already been obtained by someone else in the facility. Previous and current treatment history should also be obtained. The therapist facilitates expression of feelings, listens, gathers data, and evaluates the situation of the patient as an ongoing process. At some point the therapist, using clinical judgment, makes a decision whether the patient can be helped in the crisis center or needs to be referred somewhere else, for example, to a psychiatrist. If the patient cannot be evaluated in the crisis center, then he needs to be referred to where he can be evaluated. This may be the inpatient psychiatric service or a detoxification unit, for example. Motivation of the patient to work on his problem is assessed.

In urban areas, many persons with mental disorder are estranged from their families and live alone in downtown hotels, apartments, and residential care homes in the poorer sections of the city. Crisis workers may engage the assistance of hotel managers, and residential care home operators as sources of support. If the patient needs a different level of support than that available in the crisis center to re-establish equilibrium, a wide range of services is helpful for appropriate choices to be made and the crisis intervention should then be continued in the appropriate program.

Crisis intervention with persons with mental disorder requires careful assessment.

While a full mental-status examination may not be done in a crisis center, some aspects of it are of vital importance. *Affect* must be assessed. Is the patient depressed? If so, suicidal risk must be evaluated. The therapist has the responsibility for determining if the patient is of danger to himself or others. Direct questions may elicit suicidal thoughts, for example, "Have you thought of hurting yourself?" A lethality rating should be done (see Chap. 8). Although there is no foolproof method for predicting violence, a history of assault, homicidal threats and current threats, possession of weapons, and plans for homicide need to be assessed, and some clinical judgment made on these points. Hoff (1978) advises that this type of assessment be done by anyone who assumes the helping role in crisis intervention. If in doubt, it is better to be on the safe side and get a protected environment for the patient if he is dangerous to himself or others.

Planning. When the problem has been delineated and agreed upon, and the therapist thinks that the patient will benefit from crisis intervention, a plan is made. If possible, a contract is made with the patient. The contract structures time, place, and emphasizes the time-limited focus of treatment. The contract may be verbal or written. If it is written, it is signed by both the therapist and the patient. The contract should include time and number of sessions, the specific problem to be worked on, and the responsibilities of both the therapist and the patient.

Intervening. The purpose of the intervention is to restore equilibrium. Intervention really begins on initial contact with the patient. Intervention depends upon the circumstances of the patient, the skills of the therapist, and the availability of resources in the community. Intervention can be accomplished in many ways, some of which are as follows:

- *Facilitating catharsis* by listening and helping the patient recognize his feelings and the relationship between his feelings and the precipitating event. The therapist listens for a theme.
- *Confrontation.* The therapist may need to

point out self-defeating behavior, and when the patient cannot verbalize strong feelings.

- *Explore alternative coping mechanisms.* The patient is encouraged to consider coping mechanisms that have been successful in the past and to consider alternatives to those that have not worked for him.
- *Giving emotional support.* A place to go for resolution of crises, and a therapist who is accepting, empathetic, nonjudgmental, and willing to hear the patient's view of things may be all that is needed. The importance of spontaneous human reactions expressed to the person in crisis by the therapist are very important. The refusal of the therapist to express feeling may appear as unfeeling to the patient and add to his feelings of isolation. Some patients depend on the helping institution and feel better once they have made the decision to go there and seek help.

Encouraging the patient to ask significant others to help, giving information, advocacy, and using community resources may also be helpful in crisis intervention (Ewing, 1978). One to five sessions may be required to restore the equilibrium.

Planning for the Future and Termination. It is in this phase that the therapist and patient review the contract and summarize the accomplishments. In all cases, the therapist assists the patient to discuss his feelings about ending treatment and to make realistic plans for the future.

Follow-up Evaluation. More research needs to be done on the effectiveness of crisis intervention. A follow-up telephone call or appointment may be made to determine the condition of the patient and to evaluate the effectiveness of the intervention.

Summary

In this chapter a brief overview of psychotherapy is presented. Crisis intervention as short-term psychotherapy is described and the process outlined.

References

AMERICAN NURSES' ASSOCIATION: *Statement on Psychiatric and Mental Health Nursing Practice.* Kansas City, Mo.: American Nurses' Association, 1976.

AMERICAN PSYCHIATRIC ASSOCIATION: *A Psychiatric Glossary.* Washington, D.C.: American Psychiatric Association, 1980.

CARTER, FRANCES MONET: "Presentation to President's Commission on Mental Health," Unpublished manuscript, 19 June 1977.

ENELOW, ALLEN J.: *Elements of Psychotherapy.* New York: Oxford University Press, 1977.

EVANS, FRANCES MONET CARTER: *The Role of the Nurse in Community Mental Health.* New York: The Macmillan Company, 1968.

EWING, CHARLES P.: *Crisis Intervention as Psychotherapy.* New York: Oxford University Press, 1978.

HOFF, LEE ANN: *People in Crisis: Understanding and Helping.* Menlo Park, Calif.: Addison-Wesley Publishing Company, 1978.

KING, JOAN: "The Initial Interview: Basis for Assessment in Crisis Intervention," *Perspectives in Psychiatric Care,* **IX**:5:247–256, 1971.

KLINMAN, ANN S.: *Crisis/Psychological First Aid for Recovery and Growth.* New York: Holt, Rinehart, and Winston, 1978.

WOLBERG, LEWIS R.: *The Technique of Psychotherapy.* Vol. I. New York: Grune and Stratton, 1967.

Suggested Readings

CLARK, TERRI PATRICE: "Counseling Victims of Rape," *American Journal of Nursing,* 76:12:1965–1966, December 1976.

DECKER, BARRY, and STUBBLEBINE, J. M.: "Crisis Intervention and Prevention of Psychiatric Disability: A Follow-up Study," *American Journal of Psychiatry,* 129:6:725–729, June 1972.

NAKUSHIAN, JANET MICHEL: "Restoring Parents' Equilibrium After Sudden Infant Death," *American Journal of Nursing,* 76:10:1600–1601, October 1976.

NELSON, ZANE P., and MOWRY, DWIGHT D.: "Contracting in Crisis Intervention," *Community Mental Health Journal,* 12:1:37–44, Spring 1977.

ORNE, MARTIN T.: "Psychotherapy in Contemporary America: Its Development and Context," in Arieti, Silvano, ed.: *American Handbook of Psychiatry,* Vol. 5. New York: Basic Books, Inc., pp. 3–33. 1975.

PARAD, HOWARD J., ed.: *Crisis Intervention: Selected Readings.* New York: Family Service Association, 1965.

PISARCK, GAIL, ZIGMUND, DIANE, SUMMER-

FIELD, RITA, MIAN, PATRICIA, JOHANSEN, PAMELA, and DEVERAUX, PAULINE: "Psychiatric Nurses in the Emergency Room," *American Journal of Nursing,* 79:7:1264–1267, July 1979.

ROSENBAUM, C. P., and BEEBE, J. E.: *Psychiatric Treatment: Crisis , Clinic and Consultation.* New York: McGraw-Hill, 1975.

SMITH, W. G.: "Critical Life-Events and Prevention Strategies in Mental Health," *Archives General Psychiatry,* 25:103–109, August 1971.

WILLIAMS, REG ARTHUR: "Crisis Intervention," in Longo, Dianne C., and Williams, Reg Arthur: *Clinical Practice in Psychosocial Nursing.* New York: Appleton-Century Crofts, 1978, pp. 191–209.

15

Group Psychotherapy

LEARNING OBJECTIVES / Persons studying this chapter should be able to:

1. Define T-Groups and group psychotherapy and differentiate between the two
2. Describe factors for change that occur in group psychotherapy
3. Specify the responsibilities of the therapist in determining the composition of a group for group psychotherapy
4. Describe the phases of group psychother-

apy and the role of the therapist in each
5. Discuss common problems encountered in group psychotherapy
6. Describe psychodrama, play therapy, occupational therapy, and activity therapy
7. Specify the responsibilities of the nurse in preparation for activity groups, and outings from inpatient psychiatric units

This chapter presents some of the more traditional group therapies currently in use for persons with mental disorder (see Chap. 2 for family therapy and Chap. 3 for milieu therapy).

Although T-groups, sensitivity groups, and encounter groups are not treatment modalities, they are mentioned here because of their widespread influence in our society and because of the need to differentiate between them and group psychotherapy.

T-groups[1]

The T-group differs from the therapy group in that it is concerned with conscious or preconscious behavior rather than unconscious motivation. T-group participants are presumed to be well rather than ill (Bradford et al., 1964). In T-groups a participant learns human relations, communication, and leadership skills. He learns about behavior of himself and the other group members by being in the group under the guidance of a trainer. The T-group is not designed or practiced as therapy.

T-groups originated at the National Training Laboratory (NTL) at Bethel, Maine, in 1947; the focus was on using this method in human-relations training. Subsequently, regional laboratories were established, and the initial summer laboratory of 1947 expanded into a year-around program. Other countries have established laboratories, and participants come to NTL[2] from all continents.

Broad objectives of training are self-insight; better understanding of other persons, and awareness of one's impact upon them; better understanding of group processes and increased skill in achievement

---

[1] T-groups are *training* groups.

[2] NTL is now the NTL Institute for Applied Behavioral Sciences.

of group effectiveness; increased recognition of the characteristics of larger social systems; and greater awareness of the dynamics of change. At NTL, other laboratories are held in areas such as community-leadership training, school administration, and higher education. Some of the early work on the integration of the school system in St. Louis was done by a group of teachers in consultation with the late Hilda Taba, and NTL alumna.

The T-group is composed of twelve to fifteen individuals who work together on an intensive schedule perhaps six hours a day for two weeks. To meet personal goals of improvement in sensitivity and skills, the following conditions should be met: (1) *presentation of self*—the individual shares his thoughts and feelings; (2) *feedback*—a continuously operating system that reflects relevancy of behavior; (3) *climate*—a group atmosphere of trust is necessary for persons to be able to reveal their thoughts and feelings; (4) *cognition*—knowledge from theory and research aids the individual to understand his own experience; and (5) *experimentation*—an opportunity to try new behavior is necessary for it to become part of a person. A chance to practice new approaches also aids in helping the individual accept being different. Unless these new learnings can be applied at home, they will probably not last very long.

The process of learning from this presentation–feedback–experimentation process has to be learned and is one of the most valuable aspects of the experience. Peculiar to the T-group is its process of inquiry, exploration, and experimentation relative to its own activities. As the trainer creates a vacuum by abandoning the usual leadership role, other members of the group enter into the act.

A model to assist in thinking about interpersonal relations called the Johari window is an example of a cognitive aid used in the early T-groups (see Fig. 12). Block one is the public self (known to self and known to others); block two is the blind area (unknown to self but known to others); block three represents a hidden area (known to self but unknown to others); and block four represents the area unknown to self and unknown to others. In the T-group, by presen-

1. Known to self and known to others	2. Unknown to self but known to others
3. Known to self but unknown to others	4. Unknown to self and unknown to others

FIGURE 12. The Johari Window. (Adapted from Luft, Joseph: *Group Processes: An Introduction to Group Dynamics.* Palo Alto, Calif.: National Press, 1963.

tation of self and feedback, block one is expected to increase, and blocks two and three to diminish in size. Although block four is recognized as being very influential, it is not expected to change by experience in T-groups.

Nursing students can benefit from T-group experience or modifications of it. Some nursing schools offer T-groups to all students as part of the curriculum. They are an aid in the identification of feelings and in the fostering of the conscious, therapeutic use of self. This kind of group also assists students to become aware of the universality of feelings. The following comments from students about what they got out of such groups speak for themselves:

From the group, I learned to look for the patient's feelings rather than concerning myself with what the patient thought of me.

Last Friday, I conducted a patient-centered conference; so I had an excellent opportunity to find out the facets of a group. It isn't easy when there is opposition in a group. I used all I had learned to bring out the ideas of the opposition without antagonism within myself. It worked!

In such groups, feelings of confusion, worry about grades, fear, pressure, anger, inferiority, and identification with the problems that patients have can all be aired. Awareness and sharing of such feelings develop an ability to respond to peers and the needs of patients. Students demonstrate to each other ways of helping people surmount stress and of caring for their patients.

Since the advent of T-groups, a variety

of groups have emerged usually emphasizing some particular technique and with very vague purposes. The T-group first emphasized teaching in human relations, and as the focus shifted from education to change in the person, T-groups became known as sensitivity groups, and later as encounter groups. Now, under the heading of encounter group, there are so many types of groups they defy description. Whereas the T-group was designed for normal, healthy leaders in society, to assist them to develop greater effectiveness in the leadership role, encounter groups may now claim that they are offering therapy for normal people.

ENCOUNTER GROUPS

The popularity of encounter groups in the United States is probably due to alienation resulting from the disappearance of the extended family and the small community where people felt they belonged and where much emotional support was available. The disorganization of the nuclear family adds its effect to widespread alienation. The affluence of society provides some people with the time and money to participate and mass conformity to the tastemakers also exerts its influence. A society in which fads receive wide attention and following undoubtedly influences the variety of groups that have arisen.

Role Playing

Role playing is a technique useful in solving human-relations problems. The steps in role playing are as follows:

"Warming up" the group
Selecting the participants
Preparing others to observe
Role playing
Discussion and evaluation
Replaying the revised roles
Sharing the experiences and generalizing

1. *The warm-up—for awareness and identification.* In the warm-up a member of the group describes a particular situation in which he has experienced a human-relations problem. The warm-up serves several very important functions. It acquaints the participating group with the problems at hand and arouses awareness of their need to learn ways of dealing with the problem. It involves the group emotionally in a specific situation and thereby helps each to identify with the situation.
2. *Selection of participants for role playing.* After a short discussion, the leader asks the group to describe briefly the characters in the situation and to tell how they felt. Then, volunteers are requested to play these characters' parts in acting out an ending to the story.
3. *Preparing others to observe and role play.* Before the role playing starts, the leader prepares the listening group for participant observation.
4. *The role playing.* The role players then perform their enactment. The actual performance may be brief or quite extended; length is not necessarily important. The actors may end the role playing with a question-and-answer session; or they may work out a solution.
5. *Discussion and evaluation.* The next step is discussing and evaluating how the actors portrayed the roles they assumed and how the problem of human relations was solved.
6. *The replay.* Replay is the next step in role playing. It is not always necessary, and some leaders omit it. So often in life one wishes for a second chance to solve a dilemma. In role playing, there is a second chance to try out new approaches to problems.
7. *Sharing experience and generalizing.* This is the last step and usually ends with a short summary by the leader.

Sociograms

For the person who is beginning the study of groups, a method of visualization of the quantity and quality of communication within the group structure can be helpful. An example of the communication within a psychotherapy group is shown in Figure

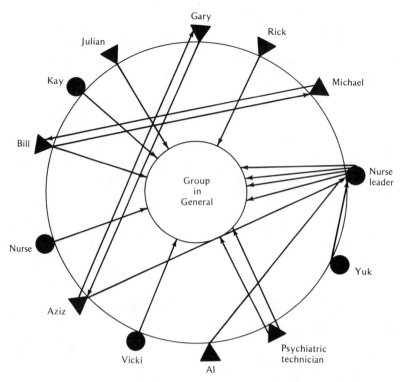

FIGURE 13.   Communication within a Psychotherapy Group.

13. The observation in this instance only recorded the quantity of remarks. Qualities of communication could also be visualized through the use of various configurations or colors.

Written notes of the verbal and nonverbal interactions of a group are also aids to studying groups. Audiotapes, videotapes, and/or a one-way mirror afford useful opportunities for the study of groups. An observer who does not verbally or nonverbally participate in the group can offer valuable contributions.

Group Psychotherapy

Group psychotherapy was introduced in this country by Joseph Pratt in 1905 at a Boston dispensary. He worked in internal medicine with groups of patients with tuberculosis, diabetes, and hypertension in a program designed to assist them with prob-

lems of morale (Bowman, 1958). Although group techniques were used by various physicians thereafter, the push in group psychotherapy came about during World War II, due in part to the great shortage of psychiatrists. The involvement of nurses in this therapeutic work was accelerated by the federal funds available for education of nurses through the National Mental Health Act of 1946 and establishment of the National Institute of Mental Health. An important contribution to group psychotherapy in nursing practice has been made by Armstrong and Rouslin (1963). Marram's (1978) work focuses on the group approach not only in psychiatric mental-health nursing but in general practice as well.

Group psychotherapy is the application of psychotherapeutic techniques to a group, including use of the group interaction of its members.

Forces that affect the behavior of individuals within a group are many and dynamic. We know that members of a group interact and influence each other; how others view us is a part of the self-concept. Because the study of group dynamics has permeated educational and work situations and the mass media, the idea of psychotherapeutic groups is widespread.

TYPES OF GROUP THERAPY

Some types of groups used in psychiatry are given below.

ANALYTIC

In this type of intensive, insight-oriented group therapy, changes in the intrapsychic structure of the person are expected. The classical techniques of psychoanalysis are used: free association, reality testing, catharsis, interpretation, dream analysis, and analysis of resistance. Resolution of the transference is central to this treatment.

NONDIRECTIVE

In this type of group therapy, gaining of insight into the more conscious aspects and mobilizing the strengths of the individual are expected. The focus is upon the here-and-now interpersonal problems of the patient. These groups are also referred to as interactional groups or process-oriented groups. Encouragement of free expression on any topic related to the problems of the patient is the main focus of this group. Rogers (1952, 1969) has made the major contribution to nondirective techniques. The therapist, who listens and tries to empathize deeply with the group members, gives feedback about what he perceives from others and about his own feelings toward them. The group members gain trust and therefore can be more open and gain a more objective view of self.

PROBLEM-SOLVING GROUP THERAPY

These groups are centered toward guidance. Through sharing with others, ego strength is increased and the patient is better able to cope with the problem at hand. In this group a specific problem is identified by the group for discussion, for example,

the effect of ECT, discharge, or a job interview.

DIDACTIC

The aim of the didactic group is to motivate the patient toward recovery. It may also assist in health maintenance and survival. This is a group in which content is introduced by a leader; the material might consist of a lecture about the relationship of emotions to bodily changes, a book, or a movie that will subsequently be discussed. This was the type of group used effectively during World War II for patients with neuroses; it is now used for various patients, especially in resocialization programs. It may be especially helpful to those patients who need an authority figure. Remotivation groups fall under this heading; lectures on nature with nature walks are an example.

SUPPORTIVE

In this type of group therapy, the goal is to restore emotional equilibrium. Supportive group therapy may be used as a principal therapeutic modality or as an adjunct. Occupational therapy, therapeutic social clubs, and milieu therapy, for example, fall under this heading. In one sense all types of group therapy are supportive.

ACTIVITY

Emphasis in this group is upon verbal and nonverbal expression with the use of art materials, body movement, or other types of activity. Socialization is a goal of activity groups.

REPRESSIVE–INSPIRATIONAL

Although this type of group does not make use of a professional leader, it is used successfully in many cases, for example, by Alcoholics Anonymous. Coercion, persuasion, and other techniques are used to assist the patient in giving up a symptom or a way of life for other things. Inspiration is used to aid the patient to repress his problems.

Generic nursing students are probably most often involved in supportive-didactic-activity type groups. The American Nurses' Association Division on Psychiatric and Mental Health Nursing sets forth the expectation that nurses who practice group psychotherapy have preparation in this treatment method, including graduate study of theory and supervised clinical experience (American Nurses' Association, 1976). Psychiatric mental-health nurses are now prepared as clinical specialists and have been prepared for their roles in group psychotherapy. Analytic group psychotherapy must be conducted by someone well trained in psychoanalytic technique.

FACTORS FOR CHANGE

Important factors that occur in group process that can be conducive to change and growth in the individual are:

- *Catharsis.* Self-disclosure and talking-out of thoughts and feelings gives the person an opportunity to learn what others think and feel about his situation.
- *Tolerance and courage.* Experiencing and sharing a wide variety of feelings as expressed in the group without being overwhelmed can give courage for continued work on one's problem.
- *Hope*—the desire that problems will eventually be solved.
- *Identification.* The group offers many opportunities for learning what others do and imitating their behavior.
- *Sharing of information.* The exchange of information among group members can aid in better self-understanding as well as understanding of each other.
- *Universalism*—the comfort of knowing that "all are in the same boat," that one is not so different from others.
- *Altruism*—the unselfish desire to help others.
- *Socialization*—a give and take of interaction of the individual and the group. Perceptions about how others view the group member can aid in the development of new social skills.

Group psychotherapy offers a broader area for *transferences* to occur than individual psychotherapy. Transferences with other group members are possible in addition to transference to the therapist. An older female member among a group of varied ages may become the mother figure. The youngest patient may be viewed as the baby of the group, create sibling rivalry and infantile behavior from other members. Transference relationships that occur in the group can be more intimate than the original one (Foulkes and Anthony, 1957). Strong transferences occur in group therapy; working through these feelings are important milestones to the patient. *Countertransference* can be a problem for the group therapist. Supervision and consultation can assist the group therapist, if this occurs. More *resistance* will probably occur in members who have not chosen group psychotherapy for themselves. When the distress of the patient leads him to enter group psychotherapy, it may be only halfheartedly.

In psychotherapeutic groups, there are always two major aspects for the therapist to observe: manifest and latent, conscious and unconscious, overt and covert activities. Emphasis is upon:

- Communication, both verbal and nonverbal
- Group interaction among members, position within the group and subgroups
- The present state
- Group themes

Group members may find support from other members, get criticism of feelings and ideas that may be helpful for adjustment and growth. Group psychotherapy offers practice in relating to others, development of communication skills, identification with others, and a situation for self-expression with a minimum of anxiety and fear. The dynamic processes that occur in individual psychotherapy also occur in group psychotherapy (Slavson, 1957).

Techniques of group psychotherapy vary according to the theoretical orientation, experience, and background of the therapist and treatment goals for the individual members. In practice, most group psychotherapists are probably eclectic unless they are leaders of a particular technique they have founded, for example, the nondirective mode of Carl Rogers.

GROUP CLIMATE

A group climate of acceptance is essential for members to be able to face and solve difficulties arising within it. Defensiveness and feelings of rejection can thereby be minimal. The leader can affect the group climate by being permissive, accepting, and thereby role-modeling to the other group members. Meeting in a well-lighted, attractive, and ventilated room with chairs arranged in a circle can set the climate for ease of communication.

Feelings of universalism, sympathy, love, trust, affinity, attraction, and interest operate in groups as well as anger, fear, hatred, rivalry, and mistrust. As a group is formed, interaction occurs, communication takes place, and members begin to understand themselves and others better. As conflicts are verbalized and understood, therapy is in process. Every psychotherapeutic group develops characteristics of its own. Because people in psychotherapeutic groups are usually experiencing conflict and suffering, deeply hidden facts of life emerge and interaction with others occur. Just talking about problems in a group can be helpful for some persons. Some persons can more readily speak about their problems in a group than in an individual interview situation.

COMPOSITION OF GROUPS

Therapy groups may be comprised of families, couples, patients with the same diagnosis, relatives of patients, or a number of other combinations. The ideal number of people in a therapeutic group is six to eight. If the group is much larger or smaller, interaction is impeded. Traditional therapy groups meet periodically in a time frame mutually agreed upon with the therapist, usually one hour and fifteen minutes to one hour and forty-five minutes. Group psychotherapy offers the person an opportunity to work out earlier disturbing experiences through the medium of the group. There are no formulas to determine if a patient will benefit from group psychotherapy; it is not a substitute for individual therapy. Some persons find the intensive one-to-one relationship of individual psychotherapy much too threatening for a variety of reasons but are benefited by treatment in a group.

Choosing patients for a therapy group is one of the most important actions of the therapist. Here again, there are no set rules. Most any patient who is excluded from a group by one therapist may be included by another. In the screening process, patients are usually interviewed and experienced clinicians may seek heterogeneity of conflict and coping and homogeneity of ability to withstand anxiety as criteria for composition (Yalom, 1975). Age, sex, diagnosis, and intelligence are also criteria that are used by some clinicians. The work of the leader in preparation of the group is to: (1) decide on record keeping and consultation; (2) select the members usually by a screening interview; (3) agree on a contract and set a time and frequency for meeting (some groups meet five times per week or once a week); (4) find a suitable place for meeting that is comfortable and private; (5) notify all the members of time and place; and (6) inform members of the purpose of the group. At the first meeting of the group, introduce all members and restate the purpose of the group. Expectations are restated: attendance, punctuality, expected number of sessions, no physical violence, confidentiality, verbalization, acceptance, and the like, and the stage is set for the group culture to develop. The leader tries to develop a facilitating atmosphere for the group. In addition, a method of communication in case of emergency is determined.

PHASES

What a therapist does in group therapy is determined by the therapeutic goals, theoretical orientation, and composition of the group. After the selection of the group members, group therapy has three phases: (1) group cohesion, (2) working through, and (3) group termination.

GROUP COHESION

The goal of the group is to provide an experience in which change can occur. Members question how the group will help and size up the other members. Members direct their comments and questions to the leader and look politely for similarities among each other. Advice is sought by members and guidance given. Then rebellion and hostility begin to occur with much criticism of each other and the leader. Members take sides; some support the leader while others criticize. Then, morale increases, ventilation increases, and there is an atmosphere of trust and support. In this phase, the therapist notes who speaks, the verbal and nonverbal communication, reflects, clarifies, draws members out, promotes group interaction, listens for group themes, and asks the group members for their reactions. When cohesion occurs, then the group goes into its working phase.

WORKING THROUGH

In this phase the factors contributing to change occur. The therapist tries to foster the factors for change. Anxiety, conflict, projection, hostility, rivalry, and scapegoating may occur and the therapist helps explore their origins. Transference, countertransference, and resistance can play their part in this phase. The skills of the therapist in therapeutic use of self comes into play, especially in this phase. Confrontation characterizes this phase. Members no longer address themselves to the therapist but address the group. The group becomes a place to take risks and test out expressions of anger, for instance. The group helps by giving perceptions of these negative feelings, both verbally and nonverbally. Thus, the group works toward the goal of change for the individuals within it.

TERMINATION

Groups are terminated for a variety of reasons but ideally when the therapeutic goals have been reached. Separation anxiety, loss, and pain have to be dealt with as members realize the group will never meet again. If the group denies concern about termination, the therapist must confront the group. Group members themselves may decide how they wish to end it. The foremost task of the therapist is to facilitate the members to express their thoughts and feelings about termination; however, it is expected that the thoughts and feelings of the therapist will also be verbalized.

COMMON PROBLEMS ENCOUNTERED IN GROUP THERAPY

If *dropouts* occur below five members, new members are usually sought for the effectiveness of the group. Although cancellation of the group may be discussed by its members, experienced clinicians will not cancel without first doing everything to keep the group intact. *Lateness* and *absences* often occur with various reasons given for it. A mechanism for follow-up should be established in case an emergency has occurred. If the lateness and absences are assessed as resistances, the feelings should be explored. Exploring resistances make up a large part of group sessions.

The formation of *subgroups* may be a disruptive influence. Some therapists discourage social relationships outside the group. Others feel the subgrouping itself may not be so deleterious as the silence about it in the group (Yalom, 1975).

Hostility is expected to be expressed in group therapy. When it is expressed toward other members or the therapist, it is important to help the patient identify the feeling and the origin of it. When hostility is expressed, there is a tendency for group members to take sides; usually there is also support in every group.

If a member *monopolizes,* the group can be asked for responses and efforts made to help the patient see how he appears in the group and the response of the other members. The therapist does not want to silence the patient; however, if the patient *cannot* stop monopolizing (as in the case of some manic patients), he may be requested to leave temporarily until he can control himself.

Pairing frequently occurs in group therapy where two people carry on their own conversation about the group interaction. They can be asked directly to share their observations with the group.

Leaving the group session before it is over

occurs frequently on inpatient units. The therapist should restate the expectation that the patient should remain and if the patient cannot comply, ask that he return.

Patients in group therapy often ask *direct personal questions* of the group therapist. Clinicians may deflect this type of question by commenting, "I am wondering why you ask that."

The *silent* patient may present the greatest challenge to the therapist and to the group. All efforts should be made to recognize the silence, learn the reasons for it, and draw the patient out. Comments on nonverbal behavior and process checks (Yalom, 1975) such as "How did it feel when he just said that?" should be made periodically. Patients do learn vicariously. One patient in a therapy group that I conducted did not say anything in the group for two months of hourly meetings twice a week. However, she participated nonverbally, her appearance changed markedly for the better and after the two months she opened up. Therapists should not give up on a person who is silent.

PSYCHODRAMA

Psychodrama is a technique of group therapy in which individual problems or group-centered problems are dramatized. Psychodrama was introduced by Moreno (1946). The therapist–director may select a conflicting episode in the life of the patient or the patient or group may choose the situation to be dramatized. Others may act as auxiliary egos representing the inner life of the patient. Significant others in the life of the patient enter into the drama and the patient can relive a problem situation. A chair may become a prop and represent a place where an imaginary person sits. In psychodrama, very intense emotions may be aroused and catharsis experienced. The director–therapist directs and interprets the action.

PLAY THERAPY

In this therapy, child's play is the modality for expression and communication between the therapist and the child. It may be con-

ducted with one child in a session (Baruch, 1964) or with a group of children. If with a group, the focus of treatment is always the individual child (Ginott, 1961). Play therapy is usually conducted in a playroom prepared with child's toys selected with a rationale in mind. Careful consideration is given to grouping children together in play therapy.

OCCUPATIONAL THERAPY

In occupational therapy, patients are offered opportunities for expression of feelings through the medium of arts and crafts. Through creative work, the patient can develop skills and increase self-esteem. Currently, occupational therapy may be prescribed by the psychiatrist or, more often, suggested to the patient by the occupational therapist. It may be offered in a separate department or room, or the therapist may bring materials to where the patient is, if, for example, the patient is not permitted to leave a locked psychiatric unit. In my community, patients in day-treatment centers may make objects and sell them at periodic bazaars or as street merchants, putting part of the sales back into a "kitty" to purchase more supplies. Thus, occupational therapy can teach a vocation as well. Currently, art therapy is very popular. In art therapy, patients can express themselves nonverbally. A variation is where the therapist brings simple materials, patients draw or paint an individual picture, and then each patient describes it. Or, a group mural may be made where a mutually agreed upon theme is carried out such as "love," "childhood," and so on. One nursing student skilled in art therapy held regular therapy sessions with very regressed patients on a psychiatric ward of a local prison. Following the theme of "home," one patient drew an outline of the prison itself. Publication of a newsletter affords a means of occupation, an expressive medium for drawings, poetry, prose, and the like, and requires taking on responsibility for its publication including editorializing, production, and circulation. It can also serve as a means to educate the public.

ACTIVITY THERAPY

Slavson (1943) originated activity group therapy from his work with children with behavior disorders. One of the purposes of an activity group is to provide an informal focus for an individual to react with others and thereby aid the socialization process. Other purposes of activity groups refer to ego building through restoration of self-confidence, learning new skills, and developing old ones, to experience joy and thereby increase the affectional response. The activity group may meet around art materials, music, body movement, or many other types of activity.

Physical exercise is an important part of health maintenance. Patients of various age groups need different kinds of exercise. Nursing staff can implement regular morning exercises with patients. Walks, volley ball, swimming, and bowling are popular group activities for exercise. The current interest in exercising gives impetus to this as an activity group.

Music, group singing, and *dancing* are widely used activity therapies. For older people, familiar songs from their youth bring forth a mosaic of feelings. Folk circle dances can be fun to accompany the music and anyone can join in. Current disco dancing is popular with all age groups. Specialists in music and dance therapy are employed by some psychiatric facilities for this treatment.

Various techniques of muscle *relaxation* and tension release are currently popular. Patients have often learned these techniques elsewhere and their expertise can be shared with the relaxation group. Activity groups form an integral part of psychiatric mental-health nursing.

The presence of large numbers of formerly institutionalized patients in community mental-health services present an almost overwhelming need for these groups. In addition, short-term hospitalization has increased the need for activity groups in day-treatment programs.

Nursing staff may plan and carry out activity groups. If activity group specialists are available, nursing staff can help actualize the activities.

Outings are for fun and meet the human need for recreation and new experiences. They are planned by staff and patients together. In my community, a trip to the conservatory in Golden Gate Park, picnics combined with outdoor swimming in the adjacent counties with warm climates, ferryboat rides, a ride on the motorized cablecar, and trips to the zoo are popular. For patients in day-treatment programs, longer trips may be planned such as weekend camping. One board and care home caretaker organizes a yearly group trip to Hawaii (the residents have to save a long time for this) where they all stay with relatives of the caretaker. If the patient is on a locked inpatient unit, a physician's written order for a pass must be secured for activities off the unit. In preparation for an activity group it is essential to:

- Assess the needs of the group individual members. This includes their abilities and weaknesses.
- Hold a group meeting so that the patients can participate in decision making about the activity.
- Collaborate with team members.
- Secure and prepare necessary materials.
- Make an alternate plan in case of unanticipated events such as inclement weather.
- Plan ahead so that hours of activities do not conflict with other plans of the patient, for example, appointments with therapists.

Through the activity group, antisocial behavior can be directed into socially acceptable behavior. The interpersonal contact may reduce social isolation of the patient by encouraging him to take the risk of developing a significant interpersonal relationship. Activity groups can also provide outlets for hostility, aggression, and other emotions. It is essential that the group leader know all the names of patients, how to spell them, and how to pronounce them correctly. Patients should be addressed often by their correct name in conversation and all involved should show an attitude of care and concern.

The importance of the dependability and reliability of the therapist cannot be overes-

timated. Patients who have been institutionalized for many years have been disappointed many times; they do not need
additional disappointments.

The use of holiday themes in activity
groups aids reality testing. For example, a
popular activity is a trip to the country at
Halloween to pick pumpkins for later carv-
ing into jack-o'-lanterns. Others, related to
health, are dental-hygiene classes where patients use disclosing tablets and dental floss
in front of a large mirror and first-aid classes
in which all steps of what to do in case of
an accident are rehearsed.

In preparation for an outing from an inpatient unit, the nurse is responsible for:

• The final determination of who can go
  (conditions of patients can change since
  pass orders were written).
• Determination of staff needed to accompany the group.
• Safety of the patient.
• Administering medications at the designated times.
• Making a list of those going and leaving
  a copy at the desk with the destination
  and expected time of return.
• Seeing that the patients are appropriately
  dressed.
• Knowing where to go and how to get
  there.

In situations where patients have no
money, knowledge of free activities is helpful in planning outings.

Community survival groups are groups
where resources and materials available in
the community for financial assistance, housing, food, transportation, clothing, recreation, socialization, health care, and the like
are shared, discussed, and feelings expressed. Field trips to these designated areas
may be part of the group activity. Trips to
teach patients where the facilities are located, for example, parks, churches, stores,
and museums, and how to use the public
transportation are useful. *Know your neighborhood and community* is the theme. Patients
with very little money to spend may also
need to be introduced to the next-to-new
shops in order to replenish clothing. Pa-

tients often need help with finding good
places to buy new clothes.

Summary

In this chapter a discussion of T-groups
was presented and the distinction made between T-groups and group psychotherapy.
The process of role-playing was described,
the use of sociograms in the study of groups
was presented. Various types of group therapy were outlined with emphasis upon the
nondirective and activity groups.

References

AMERICAN NURSES' ASSOCIATION: *Statement on Psychiatric and Mental Health Nursing Practice.* Kansas City, Mo.: American Nurses' Associa-tion, 1976.

ARMSTRONG, SHIRLEY W., and ROUSLIN, SHEILA: *Group Psychotherapy in Nursing Practice.* New York: The Macmillan Co., 1963.

BARUCH, DOROTHY: *One Little Boy.* New York: Dell, 1964.

BOWMAN, KARL: "Group Psychotherapy—His-torical Perspectives," in *Proceedings of the Second Annual Western Regional Meeting,* American Group Psychotherapy Association, 1958, p. 42.

BRADFORD, LELAND, GIBB, JACK R., and BENNE, KENNETH D.: *T-Group Theory and Laboratory Methods.* New York: John Wiley and Sons, Inc., 1964.

FOULKES, S. H., and ANTHONY, E. J.: *Group Psychotherapy: The Psycho-analytic Approach.* Bal-timore: Penguin, 1957.

GINOTT, HAIM G.: *Group Psychotherapy with Children.* New York: McGraw-Hill Book Co., 1961.

LUFT, JOSEPH: *Group Processes: An Introduction to Group Dynamics.* Palo Alto, Calif.: National Press, 1963.

MARRAM, GWEN D.: *The Group Approach in Nursing Practice.* St. Louis: The C. V. Mosby Company, 1978.

MORENO, J. L.: *Psychodrama.* New York: Beacon House, 1946.

ROGERS, CARL: *Client-Centered Therapy.* Boston: Houghton-Mifflin Co., 1951.

_____: "The Group Comes of Age," *Psychology Today,* 3:3–27, December 1969.

SLAVSON, S. R.: *An Introduction to Group Therapy.* New York: The Commonwealth Fund, 1943.

————: "Are There 'Group Dynamics' in Therapy Groups?" *International Journal of Group Psychotherapy.* 7:2:131–154, April 1957.

YALOM, IRVIN D.: *The Theory and Practice of Group Psychotherapy.* New York: Basic Books, Inc., 1975.

Suggested Reading

ENELOW, ALLEN J.: *Elements of Psychotherapy.* New York: Oxford University Press, 1977, pp. 125–144.

McLAUGHLIN, FRANK E., DAVIS, MARY L., and REED, JOHN L.: "Effects of Three Types of Group Leadership Structure on the Self-Perceptions of Undergraduate Nursing Students," *Nursing Research,* 21:3:244–257, May–June 1972.

NAKAGAWA, HELEN: "Group Theory in Nursing Practice," in Huey, Florence L., compiler: *Psychiatric Nursing 1946–1974: A Report on the State of the Art.* New York: The American Journal of Nursing Company, 1975.

SAMPSON, EDWARD E., and MARTHAS, MARYA SAMPSON: *Group Process for the Health Professions.* New York: John Wiley and Sons, 1977.

SWANSON, MARY G.: "A Check List for Group Leaders," *Perspectives in Psychiatric Care,* Vii:3:120–126, 1969.

THOMPSON, VAIDA D., LAKIN, MARTIN, and JOHNSON, BETTY SUE: "Sensitivity Training and Nursing Education: A Process Study," *Nursing Research,* 14:2:132–137, Spring 1965.

16

Somatic Approaches to Treatment

LEARNING OBJECTIVES / Persons studying this chapter should be able to:

1. Identify four major groups of drugs discussed in this section that are used in the treatment of patients with mental disorder
2. Describe the biogenic amine hypothesis as it relates to antipsychotic and antidepressant drugs
3. Name the five classes of antipsychotic drugs
4. With chlorpromazine (thorazine) as the prototype phenothiazine derivative antipsychotic drug, describe the therapeutic aim, toxic and side effects, precautions, and nursing actions associated with its use
5. Name three classes of antiparkinsonian drugs commonly used for treatment of the extrapyramidal syndrome
6. With trihexyphenidyl (Artane) as the prototype anticholinergic drug, describe the therapeutic aim, toxic and side effects, precautions, and nursing actions associated with its use
7. Name the two major classes of antidepressant drugs
8. Describe the therapeutic aim, toxic and side effects, precautions, and nursing actions associated with the use of the tricyclic antidepressants
9. Describe the therapeutic aim, toxic and side effects, precautions, and nursing actions associated with the use of the MAO inhibitors
10. Describe the therapeutic aim, toxic and side effects, precautions, and nursing actions associated with the use of lithium
11. Describe the therapeutic aim, toxic and side effects, precautions, and nursing actions associated with the use of the antianxiety agents: benzodiazepines and propanediols
12. Outline the nursing care of a patient receiving ECT

Pharmacotherapy

INTRODUCTION

Rauwolfia serpentina (India snake root) was used in the 1930s and 1940s as a treatment for mania. It was synthesized in 1952 but was soon found to cause depression and fell out of favor. Chlorpromazine was synthesized at the Rhône Poulenc Laboratories in France by Charpentier in 1950 and offered for treatment of schizophrenic patients in 1952.

The treatment and care of persons with mental disorder has radically changed since 1952 due to many factors, one of which is the advent of the phenothiazine drugs. These drugs have relieved symptoms and made other symptoms more bearable for many persons. As a result of the discovery of the phenothiazines, renewed interest in the biochemical aspects of mental disorder, especially schizophrenia, depression, and mania, has occurred and many research projects have been funded by the National Institute of Mental Health (and others) for biochemical investigations.

Drugs used in the treatment of mental disorder have powerful effects and require close monitoring by knowledgeable people. Drug dosages are tailored to the individual patient; dosages therefore vary widely. The higher the dose, the greater is the chance for adverse reactions. Knowledge of the action of these drugs, their interactions with each other, with other medications and foods is very important for the clinician. These drugs have greatly relieved the suffering of many persons and have assisted them to return to living in the community. However, they do not take the place of caring human relationships necessary for psychosocial needs. Because of their widespread use in psychiatry, major groups of drugs prescribed for patients with mental disorder discussed here are antipsychotics, antidepressants, antimanic, and antiparkinsonian.

The amine hypothesis is presented as it relates to the phenothiazines, monoamine oxidase inhibitors, and the tricyclics. These drugs have similar chemical structures and side effects but differ in their physiological action.

BIOGENIC AMINE HYPOTHESIS

One of the current hypotheses relating to variability of affect centers around the nerve ending, the synapse, and the receptor site, norepinephrine, a biogenic amine, is thought to be the neurotransmitter[1] of the nerve impulse from nerve endings in the brain to receptor sites. Norepinephrine, dopamine, and serotonin are three biogenic amines thought to act as neurotransmitters. As can be viewed in Figure 14, there is

a dynamic equilibrium between the synthesis, metabolism, storage, release, and recapture of the neurotransmitters in the nerve ending. Norepinephrine is shown here as one of the biogenic amines.

Norepinephrine is stored in the nerve ending; released within the cell, it is inactivated by the enzyme monoamine oxidase. When discharged at the synapse, it is inactivated by the extracellular enzyme catecholomethyltransferase. Monoamine oxidase regulates the levels of norepinephrine within the nerve cells.

The monoamine oxidase inhibitor drugs prevent metabolism of norepinephrine, whereas the tricyclic drugs block the recapture of norepinephrine after its release from the nerve endings, prohibiting less released epinephrine to return to the neuron and resulting in both cases in *increased levels of amines.* These two groups of drugs therefore have a similar effect through a different mechanism.

When more transmitter is present to be received by the effector cells, mental depression is relieved, whereas when the transmitters are depleted, depression is produced, for example, by reserpine. From these actions, the amine hypothesis of depression was formulated: *a decrease of brain amines is associated with causing depression, and an increase of brain amines relieves depression.* Drugs that increase or potentiate norepinephrine have antidepressant effects.

Phenothiazines and the tricyclic imipramine deplete permeability of the cells. Phenothiazines block the central adrenergic transmission by making the receptor sites less permeable so that the effect of norepinephrine, the transmitter, is reduced. The reduction of the effect of norephinephrine on the receptor site, brought about by the phenothiazines, causes sedation. The therapeutic result for the patient is psychomotor slowing, calm, and an affective indifference. This is referred to as the *neuroleptic syndrome* (Goodman and Gilman, 1970, p. 156).

All antipsychotic drugs block the dopamine receptors and increase the rate of dopamine turnover (Goodman and Gilman, 1975). This action is associated with relief of symptoms in schizophrenia. The antipsychotic drugs affect the function of three ma-

---

[1] A neurotransmitter is a chemical that is discharged from a nerve fiber ending (Axelrod, 1974).

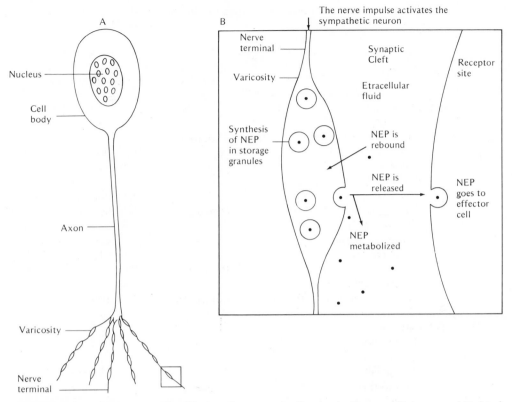

FIGURE 14. The Dynamic Equilibrium Between the Synthesis, Storage, Release, and Rebinding of the Neurotransmitters at the Nerve Ending. (Adapted from Axelrod, Julius: "Neurotransmitters," *Scientific American,* **230**:6,60, June 1974.)

jor systems of the brain: the reticular activating system, the hypothalamus (pituitary endocrine–autonomic), and the limbic systems. In addition they also affect the globus pallidus and corpus striatum with the extrapyramidal syndromes occurring as side effects.

ANTIPSYCHOTIC DRUGS

At present, there are five major classes of antipsychotic drugs used in this country: phenothiazines, butyrophenones, thioxanthenes, dihydroindolones and dibenzoxazepines (refer to Table 7). These drugs are also known as major tranquilizers, neuroleptics, and ataractics. A major purpose of the antipsychotic drugs is to modify the signs and symptoms of schizophrenia. For a patient with a high degree of agitation and who is combative, an antipsychotic such as chlorpromazine or thioridazine may be prescribed by the physician. For a patient with a thought disorder who is withdrawn, a more potent antipsychotic drug such as fluphenazine, thiothixene, or haloperidol may be prescribed. The major actions of the antipsychotic drugs are similar.

PHENOTHIAZINES

Because the phenothiazines are the most widely used of the antipsychotic drugs they are discussed here. They are divided into three subgroups based upon the differences in the side chain (refer to Table 7). The aliphatic and piperidine subgroups are more sedative than the piperazine subgroup. Parkinsonian effects are more likely to occur in the piperazine subgroup than in the other two subgroups (Kolb, 1977).

Table 7. Selected Antipsychotic Drugs Commonly Used

Names		Antipsychotic
Generic	*Representative Brand*	*Range Daily Dose*
1. *Phenothiazines*		
Aliphatic Subgroup		
Chlorpromazine HCL U.S.P.	Thorazine	300–1200 mg
Promazine HCL N.F.	Sparine	500–1000 mg
Triflupromazine	Vesprin	100– 300 mg
Piperidine Subgroup		
Mepazine	Pacatal	50– 400 mg
Thioridazine	Mellaril	100– 500 mg
Piperazine Subgroup		
Acetophenazine	Tindal	30– 120 mg
Fluphenazine	Permitil	2– 10 mg
	Prolixin	
Perphenazine	Trilafon	16– 32 mg
Prochlorperazine N.F.	Compazine	75– 100 mg
Trifluoperazine	Stelazine	3– 15 mg
2. *Butyrophenones*		
Haloperidol	Haldol	2– 15 mg
3. *Thioxanthenes*		
Thiothixene	Navane	6– 30 mg
Chlorprothixene	Taractan	30– 200 mg
4. *Dihydroindolines*		
Molindone	Moban	20– 225 mg
5. *Dibenzoxazepines*		
Loxapine	Loxitane	20– 250 mg

Of the phenothiazines, chlorpromazine is presented here as the prototype drug. There are perhaps two dozen or more phenothiazines on the market now; all have a similar chemical formula. They differ somewhat in side effects, potency, and intensity of side effects.

Therapeutic Aim. Patients who receive phenothiazines are relieved of agitation, feel drowsy, lethargic, unconcerned, somnolent, affective indifference, and a state of being unaware, but the person can be aroused from this state. Loss of ego control can be one of the most frightening experiences to a person. Patients in acute psychotic states who are out of control can now quickly regain control by taking phenothiazines. Patients who are in high states of excitement and who need rapid tranquilization may receive chlorpromazine 100 to 150 mg IM, repeated every hour until calm. For more moderate states of psychosis, chloropromazine 100 mg qid is the usual starting drug and the dose may be adjusted as required. Patients are calmed without being put to sleep. Delusions, hallucinations, agitation, and aggression are decreased. The drug can decrease the fears of psychotic patients, who will state that the fears are still there but that they are not bothered by them. Thus, an affective indifference to these fears may be maintained, and the patient becomes more communicative. The liquid form of the drug may be used when patients refuse the pills or hoard them.

The selection of the specific drug for the individual patient depends upon: age, diagnosis, mental and physical status, goals of treatment, response of the individual to medication, the compliance with the therapeutic regime, availability of medication, and the patient's previous response to the drug.

Toxic and Side Effects. Deaths from overdose of antipsychotic drugs are rare and most deaths from these drugs have occurred in children. Overdose results in drowsiness leading to coma. Hypotension, convulsions, hypothermia, extrapyramidal syndromes, and cardiac arrhythmias may occur with overdose.

AUTONOMIC EFFECTS. The patient may appear pale, feel weak, cold, dizzy, and faint, indicating orthostatic (postural) hypotension. The patient should be instructed to get up gradually and lie down if he feels faint. It may be prevented by instructing the patient to lie down for thirty minutes after the dosage.

Anticholinergic effects are blurred vision, xerostomia (dry mouth), tachycardia, constipation, and urinary retention. Patients may also complain of nasal congestion.

CENTRAL NERVOUS SYSTEM EFFECTS. Oversedation may occur with these drugs. If the patient is sleeping all the time, the dose may be reduced or given as a single dose in the evening so that a peak blood level occurs while the patient is asleep.

The extrapyramidal syndrome is common to all classes of antipsychotic drugs. There are four types of the extrapyramidal syndrome: (1) *pseudoparkinsonism*—a masked facies, slow movements, shuffling gait, "pill rolling" movements of the fingers that stop, for instance, when the patient picks up a cup, rigidity and tremors of the extremities at rest occur in this syndrome. Dosage and type of drug being received by the patient require reassessment when this syndrome occurs. Antiparkinsonian drugs may be prescribed for this syndrome. (2) *Akathisia.* This is restlessness that cannot be controlled by the patient. It must be differentiated from agitation. It may be alleviated by reduction of dosage, or administration of an antiparkinsonian drug. (3) *Acute dystonia.* This syndrome has a sudden onset and is seen more

often in young people. It involves the muscles of the shoulders, neck, and face, and sometimes the spine and extremities. Grimacing, tortocollis, trismus, sialorrhea, opisthotonous, oculogyric crisis, dysphagia, and agitation may occur suddenly. Medication to counteract this syndrome should be administered as soon as possible. Diphenhydramine (Benadryl), Benztropine (Cogentin), or Trihexyphenidyl (Artane) counteract the syndrome; parenteral preparations should be readily available. The patient should be informed of what is happening to him and reassured that it can be counteracted. This syndrome is sometimes mistaken for hysteria by the uninitiated professional. (4) *Tardive dyskinesia.* This syndrome is characterized by involuntary movements of the tongue, lips, and jaw and puffing and blowing movements of the cheeks. Sucking and smacking movements of the lips occur, the tongue makes darting movements, the jaws move from side to side, and the patient may also have choreic movements of the extremities. It appears late in the use of antipsychotic drugs, even after six years on the medications. There is no known treatment for this syndrome. The darting movement of the tongue is the first sign and the drug should be discontinued at once. To prevent tardive dyskinesia, patients should have drug holidays.

CARDIAC EFFECTS. Arrhythmias may occur when patients are on these drugs. Cardiac changes are associated with thioridazine (Hollister, 1977).

ALLERGIC REACTIONS. Agranulocytosis, a potentially fatal toxic effect on the bone marrow, if it occurs, usually appears early in treatment (six weeks). It is manifest by sore throat and fever. The drug must be discontinued at once and measures instituted to protect the patient from infection, i.e., reverse isolation, antibiotics, and supportive measures.

Skin reactions may occur with these drugs. Photosensitivity is common and dermatitis, both general and contact, may occur. Rashes tend to clear when the drug is discontinued and may not reappear when the drug is restarted. Photosensitivity may be prevented by keeping the patient covered with long sleeves, hats, and by the use of sun screens. Pigmentation, a gray-blue skin color where the patient has been exposed to the sun, may occur with long-term use of phenothiazines in high doses, most often chlorpromazine.

Cholestatic jaundice sometimes occurs but is declining. The syndrome occurs soon after initiation of the drug and is manifest by fever, eosinophilia, rashes, bile in the urine, pale stools, anorexia, and yellow sclera. If jaundice appears, the drug should be discontinued and treatment instituted (Kolb, 1977).

METABOLIC AND ENDOCRINE EFFECT. Weight gain is very common and difficult to manage. Menstrual irregularities and amenorrhea may occur. Gynecomastia, galactorrhea, and decreased libido sometimes occur; ejaculation may be inhibited and impotence can be a problem. Where the patient lives in a hot climate hyperpyrexia is a danger and must be treated immediately by placing the patient in a cool environment and sponging with alcohol, i.e. (Hollister, 1977, p. 143).

MISCELLANEOUS EFFECTS. The antipsychotic drugs may lower the convulsive threshold. Pigmentary retinopathy may occur with irreversible loss of vision with large doses of thioridazine, i.e., above 800 mg, per day. Opacities in the cornea and lens may occur without loss of vision.

Precautions

1. Potentiation with other drugs, for example, with alcohol, barbiturates, analgesics, sedatives, hypnotics, and narcotics.
2. Antipsychotic drugs should be discontinued before surgery (usually two to four days). Check for the use of these drugs on all unconscious patients, if possible. The interaction of phenothiazines with anesthetics may dangerously lower the blood pressure; therefore, the anesthesiologist must be aware of this fact.
3. Toxic reactions may occur where patients also receive anticholinergic, antiparkinsonian, and tricyclic drugs.
4. Because these drugs may interfere with the temperature-regulating mechanism, e.g., hypothermia, infection may be masked.

5. Because of their antiemetic effect (except thioridazine [Mellaril]) these drugs may mask nausea and vomiting.
6. After prolonged use, sudden withdrawal of chlorpromazine may result in restlessness, tremors, insomnia, and perspiration.

For administration of these medications, the oral route is preferred. Some medications are in tablets, capsules, suppositories, syrup, elixir, concentrate; others are in vials, ampules, or syringes. They vary widely in potency. The liquid form of the drugs may be used when the patient refuses the tablets or hoards them. Rates of absorption vary according to the form of the medication and the route of administration, parenteral being the most rapid.

After the individual is over the acute phase, drugs should be gradually reduced. On long-term pharmacotherapy, patients should also have drug holidays. Most everyone who depends on some medication wants to find out now and then if he can get along without it. Many patients, especially those with schizophrenia who are on long-term drug therapy, may have exacerbations if their medications are discontinued.

Because of the effect of the human relationship in the administration of any drug, development of rapport with the patient is essential. In this section, however, nursing actions are primarily directed toward the drugs themselves.

Nursing Action

1. Inform the patient, family member or significant other of the medication by name, dose, the reason for taking it, and the side effects.
2. Observe for therapeutic effect of the drug, toxicity, and side effects.
3. Take the blood pressure, both before and several times after administration of the drug.
4. If orthostatic hypotension occurs, instruct the patient to lie down for thirty minutes after taking the drug. Instruct the patient to rise slowly after sitting on the side of the bed for a few minutes.
5. Monitor vital signs carefully until the

therapeutic dose is determined and periodically thereafter.

6. Monitor safety needs of the patient who may be slowed down by the medication, for example, when going on walks, crossing the street, and so on. Patients who are on high doses of antipsychotics should not drive a car or any other moving vehicle or work in high places.

7. Acute dystonic reactions require quick action. The patient should be assisted to a quiet room to decrease stimulation, informed of what is happening to him, and not left alone. Notify the physician and have the medications ready for counteracting the syndrome.

8. Daily exercise is important to help overcome weight gain. Reducing diets may be necessary to avoid weight gain.

9. Diet, liquids, and exercise may help prevent constipation; however, patients may need a daily stool softener. It is important to monitor bowel movements because fecal impaction can occur. I have seen a patient who was thought to be six months pregnant by the psychiatric staff but was found by the gynecologist to have a fecal impaction!

10. Monitor urinary output because of the possibility of urinary retention. A simple urine test may also be done for the detection of bile.

11. Xerostomia is very uncomfortable for patients (paradoxically, sialorrhea may occur). Fluids, rinsing the mouth with a sugar-free breath freshener or sugar-free chewing gum help. (Sugar provides a culture for oral monilia.)

12. Blurred vision may increase the anxiety of the patient who wears glasses or otherwise uses his eyes a great deal. The patient should be instructed to delay buying glasses or getting them changed until the drug is regulated.

13. Teach the patients to monitor their own symptoms; for example, they should be taught to report sore throat or fever, pale stools, and yellow sclera right away.

14. To prevent contact dermatitis, avoid direct contact with the drug.

15. Patients should be warned of the interactive effects of antipsychotic drugs with alcohol, barbiturates, narcotics, and the like. Combinations of antipsychotic drugs and narcotics can dangerously lower the blood pressure.

16. Mix concentrates with fruit juice to minimize irritation.

17. Report signs and symptoms of toxicity to the physician immediately, i.e., sore throat, fever, jaundice, acute dystonic reactions, low blood pressure, brownish vision, or decrease in visual adaptation to darkness.

18. Keep appropriate emergency drugs on hand.

19. If the patient lives in a hot climate, special care must be taken to avoid overheating.

20. Patients should be instructed to stay out of the sun or wear hats, long sleeves, and use a sunscreen.

A patient on long-term drug therapy should be advised to continue use of the drug although he feels well. He needs to be aware of potentiation with alcohol. Where there is a family physician and other professionals involved in the care of the patient, they should also be informed and some definite arrangement made for a supply of medications and follow-up on same. Many chronic schizophrenic patients formerly in large state mental institutions who now live in their own communities in residential care homes are especially in need of follow-up care. Professionals and others involved in their care need to be especially knowledgeable about drugs used in the treatment of patients with mental disorder, the dosages, side effects, and general management. Since phenothiazines potentiate with narcotics, patients should be aware of this in our society where narcotics are sold on the streets. Fluphenazine hydrochloride (Permitil, Prolixin) is the most potent phenothiazine available. It is now commonly used intramuscularly for patients on an outpatient basis; it retains physiological activity longer than any other phenothiazine. A dose of 25 mg every two weeks of fluphenazine enanthate or fluphenazine decanoate is helpful to many patients.

After prolonged use, sudden withdrawal of chlorpromazine may result in restlessness, tremors, insomnia, and perspiration.

BUTYROPHENONES

Haloperiodol (Haldol) has been used in the United States since 1967. The action of this drug has been hypothesized to be similar to that of the phenothiazines. Therapeutic use of the butyrophenones for psychiatric patients is the same as for the phenothiazines.

It is considered by some to have a more rapid therapeutic effect for patients with acute schizophrenia. The butyrophenones have less anticholinergic effects and produce less orthostatic hypotension than do the phenothiazines. This drug lowers temperature, pulse, respiration, and blood pressure and extrapyramidal syndromes occur. Leukopenia, agranulocytosis, and liver changes are toxic effects. Butyrophenones also potentiate analgesics, barbiturates, and anesthetics.

THIOXANTHENES

The actions of this group are similar to the phenothiazines in the piperazine group.

ANTIPARKINSONIAN DRUGS

These drugs are used for the extrapyramidal syndromes induced by the use of antipsychotic drugs (see Table 8). These drugs can mask the development of tardive dyskinesia, which is irreversible. They should not be prescribed prophylactically (Goodman and Gilman, 1975).

THERAPEUTIC AIM

The purpose of their use with psychiatric patients is to decrease the extrapyramidal effect of the antipsychotic drugs.

The action of the anticholinergics is thought to (1) block the re-uptake of dopamine by the nerve terminals in the striatum, and (2) partially block cholinergic receptors in the striatum (Goodman and Gilman, 1975).

The antihistamine diphenhydramine (Benadryl) is sometimes used; it has fewer side effects than the anticholinergics but is not so effective in amelioration of the extrapyramidal syndrome. Amantadine, an antiviral agent, is now being used for the extrapyramidal syndrome.

TOXIC AND SIDE EFFECTS

Trihexyphenidyl (Artane) is discussed here as the prototype anticholinergic drug used to decrease the extrapyramidal syndrome. Side effects of this drug are xerostomia, blurred vision, urinary retention, and constipation. In large doses, atropinelike intoxication may occur characterized by confusion, delirium, hallucinations, ataxia, and somnolence.

PRECAUTIONS

Additive effects occur with the antipsychotic, MAO inhibitors, and anticholinergic drugs. The anticholinergics are contraindicated for patients with glaucoma and with urinary problems due to disorders of the prostate. For acute dystonias, these drugs should be available for parenteral administration.

Nursing Action

1. Observe for therapeutic and side effects.
2. Observe for toxicity. If the patient's hallucinations and confusion increase, reevaluation of the drug is necessary.
3. Monitor vital signs.
4. Monitor stool and urine output.
5. Encourage fluids, mouth rinse with a sugar-free breath freshener or sugar-free chewing gum for xerostomia.
6. Instruct the patient if sleepy not to drive a car or any other moving vehicle or work in high places.
7. Instruct the patient, a family member, or significant other the reason for taking the drug, dosage, action, and its interactions with other drugs.
8. Exercise, fluids, and roughage in the diet assist with the problem of constipation.

Table 8. Selected Antiparkinsonian Drugs Commonly Used for the Extrapyramidal Syndrome

Names		*Usual Daily Dosage*
Generic	*Representative Brand*	
1. *Anticholinergics*		
Trihexyphenidyl	Artane	1– 15 mg
Benztropine Mesylate	Cogentin	1– 4 mg
Procyclidine	Kemadrin	6– 20 mg
2. *Antihistamines*		
Diphenhydramine	Benadryl	25–100 mg
3. *Antiviral*		
Amantadine	Symmetrel	200–300 mg

ANTIDEPRESSANT DRUGS (REFER TO TABLE 9)

TRICYCLICS

These drugs are antidepressants; on the other hand, they tend to tranquilize the normal person. Imipramine (Tofranil) has been in use since 1957. Imipramine as the prototype drug in this group blocks the re-uptake of cerebral neurotransmitters (norepinephrine and serotonin) at the nerve ending, thus increasing their availability. Drugs that ameliorate depression affect the metabolism of norepinephrine; however, the definitive relationship between these biochemical changes and depression are unknown.

Therapeutic Aim. The purpose of the antidepressant drugs is to relieve the suffering of depression. If the tricyclics are taken over a period of time by a depressed person, the mood becomes elevated. It takes two weeks for them to begin to take effect and three to four weeks to achieve the maximum therapeutic effect.

Toxic and Side Effects

AUTONOMIC EFFECTS. The tricyclics are potent anticholinergics; therefore, xerostomia, blurred vision, constipation, urinary hesitancy, and urinary retention are side effects. Paralytic ileus may occur. The

severe anticholinergic effects are more common in the older person.

CARDIOVASCULAR EFFECTS. Palpitations, tachycardia, orthostatic hypotension, arrhythmias, and cardiac conduction disturbances may occur with these drugs.

CENTRAL NERVOUS SYSTEM EFFECTS. Oversedation may occur with the use of these drugs. The parkinsonian-like syndrome does not occur but the patient may have a fine tremor. Insomnia, agitation and restlessness, and seizures sometimes occur.

MISCELLANEOUS EFFECTS. Mild cholestatic jaundice and skin allergies may occur. Hyperhidrosis (excessive perspiration) about the head and neck may occur with the use of the tricyclics. Patients may also complain of headache, weakness, and fatigue. Transition from depression to hypomania may occur. Overdosage may result in agitation, seizures, paralytic ileus, mydriasis, hypertension, high fever, and coma. Overdosage can result in very serious poisoning. Nausea and vomiting occur when the drug is withdrawn.

Precautions

1. Severe reactions have occurred when these drugs were given concurrently with the MAO inhibitors.

Table 9. Selected Antidepressant Drugs Commonly Used

Names		Usual Daily Dosage
Generic	Representative Brand	
1. *Tricyclics*		
Amitriptyline	Elavil	25–150 mg
Desipramine	Norpramine	25–150 mg
Imipramine	Tofranil	50–200 mg
Nortriptyline	Aventyl	20– 50 mg
Protriptyline	Vivactil	15– 40 mg
Doxepin	Sinequan	50–100 mg
2. *Monoamine Oxidase Inhibitors*		
Tranylcypromine	Parnate	10– 30 mg
Phenelzine Sulfate	Nardil	30– 45 mg
Nialamide	Niamid	75–200 mg
Isocarboxazid	Marplan	10– 30 mg

2. Tricyclics have an additive effect to other anticholinergic drugs, for example, antipsychotics, antiparkinsonian, antihistamines, Donnatal, and the like.
3. Additive effects occur between the tricyclics and other central nervous system depressants, alcohol, for example.
4. Tricyclics can prevent the antihypertensive effect of quanethidine (Ismelin).
5. Great caution should be exerted if these drugs are given to patients with cardiovascular disease, narrow-angle glaucoma, prostate problems, or a history of urinary retention.
6. Older people are subject to depression and it is this age group in which severe toxic reactions occur, for example, toxic psychosis, and anticholinergic reactions.
7. Because of the danger of suicide, lethality must be carefully assessed before sending the patient home with these drugs.
8. Tricyclics may precipitate hypomania.

Nursing Action
1. Because of the danger of suicide, careful attention must be given (as with any drug) that the patient does not hoard the medication.
2. Inform the patient, a family member, or a significant other, of the drug, the reason for its use, dosage, action, and interaction

with other drugs. Point out that the medication takes effect in about two weeks.
3. Observe and assess the therapeutic effect. As the depression lifts, the patient sleeps better, has an increased appetite, gains weight, and is less self-depreciating.
4. Monitor vital signs. If orthostatic hypotension occurs, instruct the patient to arise gradually by first sitting on the side of the bed for a few minutes.
5. Monitor urine and stool output. If constipation occurs, encourage fluids, exercise, and roughage in the diet. The patient may require a laxative or a stool softener. If paralytic ileus and severe retention occur, the drug has to be discontinued.
6. For xerostomia, encourage fluids, rinsing of the mouth with a sugar-free breath freshener or sugar-free chewing gum.
7. Patients with severe anticholinergic toxicity may be given physostigmine while on cardiac monitor (Tinklenberg and Berger, 1977).

MONOAMINE OXIDASE INHIBITORS

In 1951, isoniazid and iproniazid were developed as treatments for tuberculosis. They were soon found to have mood-elevating effects. In 1957, they were introduced to psychiatry, but have not found great favor in the United States due to their toxicity. Some of the MAO inhibitors have been removed from the market because of their toxicity. Some clinicians avoid the use of the MAO inhibitors entirely; others use them with great caution.

The use of these drugs for the depressed person relates to the hypothesis that the biogenic amines in the brain are decreased in depression. Monoamine oxidase is one of the regulators of the cerebral neurotransmitters: norepinephrine, epinephrine, dopamine, and serotonin (Goodman and Gilman, 1975). When monoamine oxidase is inhibited, the brain biogenic amines increase and this increase is associated with the relief of depression. With the use of these drugs, there is an inactivation of the brain enzyme monoamine oxidase; when this enzyme is inhibited, regeneration of it takes weeks. It must be understood that the MAO inhibitors inhibit not only the monoamine oxidase enzyme, but other enzymes as well. Therefore, there are additional side effects due not only to the inhibition of the monoamine oxidase but to the additional inhibiting action. Tranylcypromine (Parnate) is discussed here as the prototype drug in this group.

THERAPEUTIC AIM

These drugs are mood elevators that produce stimulation of euphoria and an increase in mental alertness and activity. They are used to relieve depression. Like the tricyclics the MAO inhibitors may require two to three weeks to affect the depression; however, toxicity may appear within a few hours. Overdosage may result in agitation, hallucinations, high fever, and convulsions.

TOXIC AND SIDE EFFECTS

The most serious side effect is the hypertensive crisis associated with the ingestion of certain foods; the crisis may occur from two to twenty hours after ingestion. The hypertensive crisis is manifested by: severe headache, usually occipital, hyperpyrexia, chest pain, muscle twitching, elevated blood pressure, apprehension, pallor, nausea, vomiting, excessive perspiration, and rest-

lessness. Intracranial bleeding can occur and this crisis can be fatal.

Tyramine, a pressor amine is normally oxidized by monoamine oxidase. Because of the MAO inhibitors, tyramine is not deaminated and the result is their high concentration and the hypertensive crisis (Goodman and Gilman, 1975). Foods containing tyramine are: cheeses, wine, chicken livers, yeast, beer, pickled herring, coffee, bean pods, and canned figs. All foods containing tyramine must be avoided by persons taking the MAO inhibitors.

The MAO inhibitors may prolong and potentiate the effects of many drugs including the tricyclics, barbiturates, alcohol, amphetamines, ephedrine, epinephrine, and methylphenidate. Patients, family physicians, their families, or significant others must fully understand the foods to be avoided and that no medication whatsoever should be taken without prior approval, including over-the-counter drugs.

Autonomic Effects. Both hypotension and hypertension have occurred. Xerostomia, blurred vision, constipation, hesitancy in urination and bowel function, dizziness, vertigo, fainting, and orthostatic hypotension have also occurred.

Central Nervous System Effects. Because of their central stimulating effect, insomnia, restlessness, tremors, convulsions, agitation, and irritability can occur.

Hepatic Effects. Liver toxicity may occur in a syndrome similar to viral hepatitis; it is serious and the medication should then be discontinued.

Miscellaneous Effects. Inhibition of ejaculation, impotence, skin rashes, and red-green color blindness have occurred. Patients often complain of weakness and fatigue.

PRECAUTIONS

1. There are so many adverse interactions of these drugs with other drugs that no other drug should be given unless its interaction with these drugs is known.
2. Because of the danger of suicide, lethal-

ity should be carefully assessed and the risk evaluated because of the potentially fatal effect of the interactions of these drugs with tyramine-containing foods.

NURSING ACTION

In addition to nursing actions already discussed for the anticholinergic syndrome, the following are recommended:

1. Assess lethality. Patients who are suicidal may attempt suicide by overdosage, taking additional incompatible drugs, and/ or eating the tyramine-containing foods.
2. Instruct the patient, a family member, or significant other of the drug and its action and interaction with other drugs. The patient must be warned not to take any medication prescribed or over-the-counter drugs without prior approval.
3. Monitor vital signs.
4. Observe for therapeutic, toxic, and side-effects.
5. The onset of headache requires immediate withdrawal of the drug.
6. Make a list of forbidden foods and instruct the patient, the dietitian, the family and/or significant other, and the family physician that these foods must be avoided.

ANTIMANIC DRUG

Although other drugs have the ability of calming the manic patient, lithium is currently the drug of choice and is discussed in this section.

LITHIUM

In 1949, John F. J. Cade of Australia introduced lithium as an antimanic drug; however, it was not generally used in the United States until 1969. In mania, it is thought that the cerebral neurotransmitters should be decreased. Although the specific action of lithium in the relief of manic disorders is not known, it has been suggested that it acts to decrease norepinephrine at the synaptic cleft in the central nervous system and thereby reduces euphoria. Recently, lithium is also being used for the treatment of depression.

Therapeutic Aim. The purpose of the use of lithium in the treatment of individuals with manic disorders is to decrease the spiraling mood, the psychomotor activity, and to help them get some rest. The therapeutic serum lithium level is between 0.6 and 1.5 mEq. per liter. The toxic level, 2.0 mEq. per liter, is very close to the therapeutic level. Some manic patients take lithium as a preventive measure. With lithium there is a delayed onset of action; it takes from three to ten days for it to reach the antimanic effect.

Toxic and Side Effects. Patients receiving lithium may have mild adverse reactions after the first two or three doses: nausea, vomiting, diarrhea, muscular weakness, fatigue, and abdominal pain. Other adverse reactions are polyuria, polydipsia, leukocytosis, slowing of the EEG, pretibial and hand edema, weight gain, fine tremors of the lips and hand, slurred speech, and ataxia. These initial reactions disappear after one or two weeks; however, toxicity is demonstrated by a reoccurrence of the initial symptoms: increased lip and hand tremors, weakness, drowsiness, ataxia, slurred speech, nausea, and vomiting. Severe toxicity is characterized by severe tremors, incontinence, blurred vision, arrhythmias, disorientation, confusion, restlessness, muscular hyperirritability, convulsions, stupor, coma, and death.

Lithium is distributed throughout the body water; it is not metabolized and is excreted primarily by the kidneys. Excretion of lithium is often decreased in the older person. Coma and severe electrolyte imbalance may ensue where there is a low sodium level in the body; lithium excretion is inhibited, and toxicity is increased. When lithium was formerly used as a salt substitute for cardiac patients on low-salt diets, lithium poisoning was the result. Dosages of lithium are tied to the serum lithium level. An initial dose of 900–1200 mg per day in divided doses is used by many clinicians. Patients who receive lithium describe their feelings as being "internally curbed" and state they are "now able to face issues."

Precautions

1. The safety of this drug in pregnancy has not been established. Various lithium registries are now collecting data on the effect of lithium on pregnant women and all cases should be reported to them.
2. When sodium intake is lowered, lithium excretion is slowed down; therefore, lithium should not be given to patients on a salt-free diet. Diarrhea and excessive perspiration also deplete sodium and may result in toxicity.
3. Lithium is contraindicated for patients with thyroid, renal, cardiac, or central nervous system dysfunctions.
4. Antipsychotics, because of their antiemetic effect, if given in conjunction with lithium, may mask nausea, which can be an indication of lithium toxicity.
5. Lithium levels must be measured and monitored because the therapeutic and toxic levels are very close. The serum lithium level should not be allowed to rise above 2 mEq. per liter. Lithium levels should be taken at the same time of the day eight to ten hours after the last dose. The lithium level should be taken every two or three days until the therapeutic level is maintained and once weekly thereafter; if the patient is on maintenance therapy, once monthly is recommended. If a single nighttime dose is given, a morning blood level will be significantly higher than that from divided doses.
6. Patients should not be given diuretics while on lithium because of the danger of sodium depletion.

Nursing Action. Manic patients are sometimes in seclusion until the drug takes effect; antipsychotics may be prescribed for the interim period.

1. Instruct the patient, a family member, or significant other about the drug, reasons for taking it, dosage, and side effects.
2. Observe for therapeutic effect, toxicity, and side effects.
3. Because the drug causes polyuria and polydipsia, provide frequent fluids and opportunities to empty the bladder throughout the twenty-four hours.

4. It is important that the patient eats and takes in a normal amount of sodium chloride to prevent toxicity that accompanies sodium depletion and the use of lithium.
5. Sodium depletion brought on by diaphoresis from hot weather or activity should be avoided while on lithium therapy.
6. Manic patients, with their racing ideas and short attention span, may not dwell on their physical ailments; therefore, pay particular attention to complaints.
7. Give lithium with meals or snacks to avoid nausea.
8. Nursing mothers on lithium should not breast feed; the lithium may cause toxicity in the nursing infant.
9. Monitor urine and stools. If the kidneys decrease in function, toxicity can increase. Older persons are particularly susceptible to decreased excretion of lithium.
10. If maintenance drug therapy is indicated, instruct the patient to take the medication exactly as prescribed. Adherence to the prescribed regimen is necessary for maintenance of a therapeutic blood level. Patients learn to manage their own therapeutic level; for example, after a hard game of golf on a hot day, the patient may decide to skip a dose.
11. Instruct the patient of the dangers of going on crash diets while on this drug.
12. Instruct the patient of the dangers of giving the medication to anyone else.

Antianxiety Drugs

Antianxiety drugs are widely used in our society for the relief of anxiety and tension associated with functional and psychosomatic disorders (see Table 10).

They are also used in the management of acute drug withdrawal syndromes (alcohol, barbiturates, and narcotics). Antianxiety drugs are readily available from both legitimate and illegitimate sources. Currently, diazepam (Valium) is the most frequently prescribed drug in the United

Table 10. Selected Antianxiety Agents

Names		Antianxiety Range Daily Dose
Generic	Representative Brand	
1. *Benzodiazepines*		
Chlordiazepoxide	Librium	20–60 mg
Diazepam	Valium	5–20 mg
Oxazepam	Serax	30–90 mg
Chlorazepate	Tranxene	15–60 mg
2. *Propanediols*		
Meprobamate	Equanil Miltown	400–1200 mg
Tybamate	Solacin Tybatran	500–1500 mg
3. *Sedative/Antihistaminics*		
Hydroxyzine	Atarax Vistaril	25–150 mg
Diphenhydramine	Benadryl	75–300 mg
4. *Sedative/Antidepressants*		
Doxepin	Sinequan	75–200 mg

States. Treatment with antianxiety drugs is based upon the behavior of the individual and is advocated for use where a specific function of the person is impaired.

Some clinicians recommend their use only in conjunction with psychotherapy and for short periods.

BENZODIAZEPINES

Many physicians prefer these drugs because the margin between the therapeutic dose and the lethal dose is very wide. The effect of these drugs upon the brain is not well known (Goodman and Gilman, 1975). Overdose is frequent but not likely to be lethal, duration of action is long, and drug interactions are few except for an additive effect with central nervous system depressants (Goodman and Gilman, 1975, p. 191). These drugs increase the seizure threshold and can be used as hypnotics. They potentiate the anticholinergic effects of antipsychotic and antidepressant drugs.

Toxic and Side Effects

Drowsiness and ataxia may appear. Skin rash, nausea, headache, dizziness, vertigo, impaired sexual function, agranulocytosis, menstrual irregularities, and failure to ovulate may occur. Paradoxical excitement in the form of increased hostility (except with the use of oxazepam), and increased anxiety may occur.

Precautions

On high doses, patients may have suicidal impulses or become psychotic. Tolerance and dependence occur with the use of these drugs. Tobacco cigarette smoking may decrease their effectiveness. Withdrawal after high doses may result in seizures.

Nursing Action

1. Because the placebo effect cannot be separated out from the physiological effect of these drugs, a positive attitude by the nurse is important in the success of their use.
2. Inform the patient, family member, or significant other of the medication by name, dose, the reason for taking it, and the side effects.
3. Observe for therapeutic effect of the drug, toxicity, and side effects.
4. Caution the patient of the potentiation of the sedative effects of these drugs with central depressants such as alcohol. Over-

the-counter drugs should not be taken unless they are checked out beforehand with the clinician.

5. Instruct the patient not to drive a car, other moving vehicles, work in high places, or other activity requiring alertness.

6. Caution patients to not stop taking these drugs unless under supervision.

7. Because some side effects of these drugs are very similar to anxiety itself, careful continuous assessment of their effect is required.

8. Watch your own attitude toward patients who are dependent on these drugs; nurses can be overly moralistic toward patients who depend, for instance, on Valium.

PROPANEDIOLS

Meprobamate and tybamate are the two drugs in this group with meprobamate being the most frequently used of the two. The margin between the therapeutic dose and lethal dose is narrow and deaths do occur (Tinklenberg, 1977). Meprobamate sedates and relaxes the patient but the mode of action is not known.

Toxic and Side Effects

Drowsiness, ataxia, headache, dizziness, hypotension, slurred speech, palpitations, nausea, vomiting, and rashes may occur. Blood dyscrasias and porphyria have been reported. With the use of meprobamate, tolerance and dependence occur, but not with tybamate (Goodman and Gilman, 1975, p. 189).

Precautions

Interactions with other drugs can occur with the use of meprobamate because it can induce microsomal enzyme systems in the liver (Goodman and Gilman, 1975). Safety in pregnancy has not been established. Suicide attempts with these drugs may be lethal. Delirium and seizures may ensue within thirty-six to forty-eight hours upon withdrawal from large doses of these drugs.

Nursing Action

1. Inform the patient, family member, or significant other of the medication by name, dose, the reason for taking it, and the side effects.

2. Observe for therapeutic effect of the drug, toxicity, and side effects.

3. Caution the patient not to stop these drugs unless under supervision.

4. Give careful attention that the patient does not hoard or give away these potentially lethal drugs.

5. Because the safety of use in pregnancy has not been established, instruct the pregnant patient not to take these drugs.

OTHER

Antihistamines are sometimes used as antianxiety agents. Side effects are drowsiness, dry mouth, blurred vision, and paradoxical excitement. Tolerance to these drugs can occur. A sedative antidepressant, Doxepin, is sometimes recommended, especially for patients with anxiety and depression.

The beta-adrenergic blocking agent propranolol (Inderal) is being used to reduce anxiety although it has not been approved by the Food and Drug Administration for treatment of anxiety alone (Dennis, 1979).

Barbiturates are also used by some physicians for anxiety and a wide array of other conditions. Many physicians prefer the use of other drugs as antianxiety agents. Nevertheless, patients can easily get barbiturates in large quantities from legitimate and illegitimate sources. One action of the barbiturates is depression of respiration. Drowsiness, ataxia, lethargy, "hangover," headache, rashes, depression, nausea, hypotension, and impairment of judgment and fine motor skills can occur as side effects. Barbiturates interact with other central nervous system depressants. Withdrawal is severe. They also cross the placental barrier and the fetus may exhibit withdrawal symptoms. These drugs are commonly used to commit suicide and for suicidal attempts. Tolerance and dependence easily develop with their use and they interfere with the metabolism of anticoagulants (Coumadin). Doses large enough to affect anxiety often sedate the patient to the point where he cannot be alert.

Sleep therapy induced by barbiturates was once frequently used for excited psychiatric inpatients and is still widely used in the USSR.

Convulsive Therapy

Convulsive therapy used as a primary treatment to alleviate the depressive affect is discussed as follows:

ELECTROCONVULSIVE THERAPY

Electroconvulsive therapy was introduced to psychiatry by Ugo Cerletti and Lucio Bini in 1938. Although many theories, both psychological and physiological, have been advanced as to why it is effective, at this time the action is unknown. One theory is that the shock serves an unconscious need for punishment in the depressed patient. Another is that the treatment provides an experience of death and a feeling of rebirth. Recently, it is thought by some theorists that ECT has an effect on the cerebral neurotransmitters and that this effect alleviates the depression. However, certain aspects of the process of ECT are known: (1) The changes in the patient result from the cerebral seizures. (2) Improvement of the patient is independent of the mode of induction of the seizure. (3) The number of treatments required varies with the symptoms and age of the patient. (4) Changes in appetite, menses, libido, and other physiology also occur. (5) Effects of seizures are affected by medications, and the effects of seizures are reversible in time (American Psychiatric Association, 1978).

In the early days of the use of ECT, before muscle relaxants were discovered to be useful in conjunction with it, compression fractures of the vertebrae occurred. During the 1940s and 1950s, small doses of curare were given to offset the danger of fractures. During those times, patients were not anesthetized before treatment.

ECT consists of administering an electrical stimulus via electrodes placed on the temples from a machine constructed for treatment purposes. A grand mal convulsion is the desired reaction. The treatment is given for the most part to patients with severe depressions; however, it is also given to patients with certain schizophrenic disorders and acute mania.

Preceding this treatment, the patient receives a thorough physical examination, which may include an x-ray of the chest and x-rays of the spine. An ECG and EEG may also be done. The treatment is explained to the patient and the consent form for electroconvulsive therapy is then signed according to the laws within the state and the policies within the specific hospital.

Once the consent form is signed, the nurse and the psychiatrist schedule the patient for treatment. Most patients fear ECT but others may welcome it, fully expecting death. The treatment is usually given in a special treatment room removed from the unit or set apart from the psychiatric ward in some manner. Techniques vary with treatment teams. All personnel on the treatment team should be well trained in the treatment technique and be known by the patients receiving it.

NURSING CARE OF THE PATIENT RECEIVING ECT

The nurse is responsible for setting up the treatment room and for the safety of the patient. Supplies of medications and equipment to be used during the treatment need to be on hand. The electrodes are soaked in a solution of 25 percent sodium bicarbonate in water to aid conduction. Resuscitation equipment, oxygen, drugs, and other equipment should be on hand.

The following drugs and equipment are recommended by the American Psychiatric Association.[1]

1. *Drugs*
   - atropine sulfate = 0.4 mg/ml
   - calcium chloride—10% solution—10 ml vial (emergency syringe)
   - dexamethasone (Decadron)—4 mg/ml and/or 24 mg/ml

[1] American Psychiatric Association: *Electroconvulsive Therapy.* Washington, D.C.: American Psychiatric Association, 1978, pp. 11–12. By permission.

- dextrose—5% in water—250 ml units
- diazepam 5 mg ml—2 and 19 ml vials
- epinephrine—1:10,000 solution—10 ml (emergency syringe)
- lidocaine (Xylocaine): Special preparation for use in cardiac dysrhythmias—2% solution = 5 ml = 100 mg in emergency syringe
- metaraminol (Aramine)—1% solution—10 ml vial sodium bicarbonate—7.5% solution = 44.6 mEq.—50 ml (emergency syringe)
- L-norepinephrine (Levophed)—2 mg/ml—4 ml ampuls.

2. *Equipment*
   - Suction tested for proper function
   - Needles
   - Infusion sets
   - Electrocardiograph
   - Defibrillator
   - Emergency Crash Cart or similarly equipped unit.

The nurse prepares the medications and places the patient's chart and treatment record in the room. Any changes in the patient's condition such as high anxiety level, and the like, should also be verbally reported to the psychiatrist.

Nursing care of the patient receiving ECT occurs in three phases: (1) Pre-ECT, (2) during ECT, and (3) post-ECT.

Pre-ECT. Establish a trusting nurse–patient relationship. The procedure should be explained to the patient as he will experience it, and the patient encouraged to ask questions and to express thoughts and feelings. Likewise, the family and/or significant other should be informed about the procedure and the temporary confusion and memory loss following ECT.

Because the treatments are usually given during the morning hours, the patient's breakfast is withheld. All lab reports must be on the patient's chart. Vital signs are checked upon awakening the patient; if there are abnormalities, the treatment may be cancelled. Atropine may be ordered to be given twenty minutes prior to treatment to decrease secretions in the respiratory tract. All metallic objects are removed from the patient such as hairpins, watches, and rings. Valuables of patients are placed in safekeeping; dentures are removed before

treatment but partial plates are sometimes left in to avoid breaking the remaining teeth during the tonic phase of the convulsion. The patient wears a hospital gown, robe, and slippers. The patient should void before the treatment to prevent possible rupture of the bladder or incontinence. Because patients ambulate to the treatment room, glasses or contact lens should be removed after they arrive there.

During ECT. The patient is accompanied to the treatment room, removes robe and slippers, and places himself on the treatment table in a dorsal recumbent position. A short-acting anesthetic such as methohexital (Sodium Brevital) is given followed by intravenous succinylcholine chloride (Anectine) to block the transmission of the motor nerve impulse to the skeletal muscles, reducing the severity of the convulsion and preventing fractures. The most frequent fracture is a compression fracture of the vertebrae. Because succinylcholine chloride also temporarily relaxes the respiratory muscles, careful attention must be given to respiration. A mouth gag is placed between the teeth to avoid injury to the tongue and teeth, and one operator holds the jaw firmly upward to prevent injury. Electrode paste is rubbed onto the designated area on the head, and the electrodes are firmly applied to these areas. The button is pushed by the psychiatrist and the patient is unconscious immediately after the current is applied. The patient goes into the tonic phase of the convulsion, which lasts about ten seconds. Following the tonic phase of the convulsion is the clonic phase, which lasts longer.

Following the clonic phase is a period of apnea. An airway may be inserted and artificial respiration instituted, followed by administration of oxygen by positive pressure. The electrode paste is cleansed from the skin of the patient. The abdomen of the patient is exposed to ascertain respirations. Once breathing is restored, the patient is positioned on his side to prevent inhalation of any secretions and removed to a recovery room by stretcher.

Post-ECT. The nurse checks for cyanosis and adequate respiration. The patient remains unconscious for five to ten minutes and then slowly regains consciousness. The nurse checks vital signs at regular intervals and orients the patient. A period of confusion follows the treatment, and the patient needs side rails up on the bed and should be observed closely for twenty minutes to one hour. He may then be given a light breakfast and get dressed.

If the patient remains sleepy, he may need to rest longer in his own bed. He may also require being oriented repeatedly. Afterward, patients should be encouraged to engage in the usual activities of the hospital unit. Patients receiving this treatment may have headaches. Most physicians leave standing orders for aspirin, 0.65 gm p.r.n. Patients may also complain of soreness in their jaws and limbs. Patients also complain of memory loss caused by the treatment; they need to be reassured that their memory will be regained; the loss is temporary. Nurses may set up group meetings for patients on electroconvulsive therapy so that they can better understand what is happening to them and can receive help and reassurance from others.

If the patient is being given ECT on an outpatient basis, he should be oriented before he leaves the hospital, instructed not to drive a car, and accompanied home by a responsible person.

There is no set number of treatments required. The number and frequency of treatments depend upon the severity of the patient's mental disorder. He may have two to three per week, two per day for two to three successive days, a total of six treatments, or as many as twenty-five or thirty. Some patients with frequent psychotic episodes may have had fifty to one hundred treatments.

Many patients who received ECT in the early days of its use are often very afraid of it because they may have received it without the benefit of *any* premedication. The observations of the nursing staff are important to note the degree of confusion of the patient while on a course of treatment. Patients with many successive treatments may become aphasic or confused. Since this severely confused state is not the desired effect, treatments may be discontinued immediately or tapered off. It usually takes longer for older patients and for patients who are already confused from other treatments to regain consciousness immediately after a treatment.

During the convalescent period (one to three weeks) patients should not resume their usual work, drive a car or other hazardous vehicle; they should be supervised during this period by a responsible person until the temporary memory loss is abated.

TEAM WORK

Usually a treatment team gives the electroconvulsive therapy. One person is responsible for preparation of the medications, the mouth gag, holding the jaw; another lightly restrains the patient during the tonic phase lest this cause a fracture in itself. Another person is responsible for the patient in the recovery room and still another is responsible for serving breakfast. If more than one patient receives ECT, another staff member should stay with the patient before ECT for reassurance. The physician administers the anesthetic, muscle relaxant, sets the machine, holds the electrodes, and pushes the button. A careful recording of each treatment is made on a special treatment sheet as well as on the nurses' notes.

INHALATION CONVULSIVE THERAPY

Hexofluorodiethyl ether (Indoklon) produces convulsions. Introduced by Karliner and Padula (1959) in the treatment of psychiatric patients, it is usually applied as an inhalant. A mild and brief convulsion is produced. Previous to the application of the ether, the patient receives a short-acting anesthetic such as methohexital (Sodium Brevital) and succinylcholine chloride (Anectine) intravenously. After anesthesia and relaxation are produced, the ether is given by the use of a mask and a vaporizer; respiration is assisted by the use of oxygen. Patients are often less fearful of this treatment than they are of electroconvulsive therapy (Kiening, 1974).

Hydrotherapy

To aid in calming the patient, hydrotherapy in the form of continuous tubs and wet sheet packs as well as other modalities were used in the treatment of psychiatric patients before antipsychotic drugs were discovered. Nurses who administered hydrotherapy formed many one-to-one relationships with patients receiving this treatment although the emphasis during those times was upon the procedure. New hydrotherapy units in mental hospitals in the United States were still being built and widely used in the 1950s; however, they have now been converted to other uses. Hydrotherapy is still a major treatment for patients with mental disorder in other countries, for example, the USSR.

Summary

In this chapter some current established somatic therapies are described. Major drugs used in the treatment of persons with mental disorder are discussed and nursing actions outlined. Nursing care of the patient receiving electroconvulsive therapy is presented.

References

AMERICAN PSYCHIATRIC ASSOCIATION: *Electroconvulsive Therapy*. Washington, D.C.: American Psychiatric Association, 1978.

AXELROD, JULIUS: "Neurotransmitters," *Scientific American*, 230:6:59–71, June 1974.

BARCHAS, JACK D., BERGER, PHILIP A., CIARANELLO, ROLAND D., and ELLIOTT, GLEN R., eds.: *Psychopharmacology: From Theory to Practice*. New York: Oxford University Press, 1977.

BARCHAS, JACK D., AKIL, HUDA, ELLIOTT, GLEN P., HOLMAN, R. BRUCE, and WATSON, STANLEY J.: "Behavioral Neurochemistry: Neuroregulators and Behavioral States," *American Association for the Advancement of Science*, 200:26:964–973, 26 May 1978.

DENNIS, GARY: "Anxiety," Lecture, San Francisco, Calif., 23 June 1979.

GOODMAN, LOUIS S., and GILMAN, ALFRED: *The Pharmacological Basis of Therapeutics*. 4th ed. New York: MacMillan Publishing Co., Inc., 1970.

———. eds.: *The Pharmacological Basis of Therapeutics*. 5th ed. New York: MacMillan Publishing Co., Inc., 1975.

HOLLISTER, LEO E.: *Clinical Use of Psychotherapeutic Drugs*. Springfield, Ill.: Charles C Thomas, 1973.

———: "Antipsychotic Medications and the Treatment of Schizophrenia," in Barchas, Jack D., et al: *Psychopharmacology: From Theory to Practice*. New York: Oxford University Press, 1977, pp. 121–150.

KARLINER, W., and PADULA, L. J.: "Improved Technique for Indoklon Convulsive Therapy," *American Journal of Psychiatry*, 116:358, 1959.

KIENING, SISTER MARY MARTHA: Personal Communication, June 1974.

KOLB, LAWRENCE C.: *Modern Clinical Psychiatry*. Philadelphia: W. B. Saunders Company, 1977.

TINKLENBERG, JARED R.: "Antianxiety Medications and the Treatment of Anxiety," in Barchas, Jack D., et al, eds.: *Psychopharmacology: From Theory to Practice*. New York: Oxford University Press, 1977, pp. 226–242.

TINKLENBERG, JARED R., and BERGER, PHILIP A.: "Treatment of Abusers of Nonaddictive Drugs," in Barchas, Jack D., et al: *Psychopharmacology: From Theory to Practice*. New York: Oxford University Press, 1977, pp. 386–403.

Suggested Readings

CARLSSON, ARVID: "Antipsychotic Drugs, Neurotransmitters, and Schizophrenia," *American Journal of Psychiatry*, 135:2:164–174, February 1978.

DAVIS, JOHN M.: "Overview: Maintenance Therapy in Psychiatry: I. Schizophrenia," *American Journal of Psychiatry*, 132:12:1237–1245, December 1975.

———: "Overview: Maintenance Therapy in Psychiatry: II. Affective Disorders," *American Journal of Psychiatry*, 133:1:1–13, January 1976.

KLINE, NATHAN S.: "Psychotropic Drugs," *American Journal of Nursing*, 73:1:54–62, January 1973.

MANN, STEPHAN C., and BOGER, WILLIAM P.: "Psychotropic Drugs, Summer Heat and Humidity, and Hyperpyrexia: A Danger Restated," *American Journal of Psychiatry*, 135:9:1097–1100, September 1978.

MCAFEE, HEIDI ANN: "Tardive Dyskinesia,"

American Journal of Nursing, 78:3:395–397, March 1978.

SPRING, GOTTFRIED K.: "The Current Role of Lithium in the Treatment of Affective Disorders," *Psychosomatics,* 17:3:151–156, September 1976.

WORLD HEALTH ORGANIZATION: "Psycho-tropic Drugs and Mental Illness," *WHO Chronicle,* 30:10:420–424, October 1976.

_____: "Drugs for Treating Mental Illness and Epilepsy in Developing Countries," *WHO Chronicle,* 31:2:53–55, February 1977.

_____: "Controlling Psychotropic Substances," *WHO Chronicle,* 32:1:3–8, January 1978.

17

History of Psychiatric Nursing

LEARNING OBJECTIVES / The reader of this chapter should be able to:

1. Describe common practices in the care and treatment of mental patients in England preceding the humanitarian movement
2. Name three principal individuals who headed the humanitarian movement in France and England
3. Describe the treatment methods and nursing care at the York Retreat, England
4. Describe common practices in the treatment and care of mentally disordered persons in America: (1) early America, (2) moral treatment, (3) cult of curability, (4) custodial era, (5) reform and education
5. Identify contributions of Phillippe Pinel, Jean Baptiste Pussin, William Tuke, Dorothea Lynde Dix, Linda Richards,

Clifford Whittingham Beers, Harriet Bailey, Esther Garrison, Marion Kalkman, Hildegard Peplau
6. Describe the rise of institutions, the middle class, and the professions and the emergence of psychiatric mental health nursing practice from its beginnings to World War II
7. Identify major factors influencing psychiatric mental-health nursing since World War II
8. Consider and discuss the role of knowledge of history in planning and decision making in relation to psychiatric mental-health nursing
9. Name the two types of certification for psychiatric mental-health nursing and the requirements for each

History of Psychiatric Nursing

We fear also, it must be admitted, that brute force is the means by which in one form or another, a large majority of mankind seek to accomplish their purposes in their intercourse with the weak; and it cannot be conceded, that the exclusion of straps and strait waistcoats necessarily banishes every form in which that vulgar power can be exercised.[1]

[1] *York Retreat Reports*, 1846, p. 28.

In the year 1247 the Bethlem Hospital was founded by the Brothers of Bethlehem. The monastery of St. Mary's of Bethlehem was one of the first asylums where the Church opened its doors to the persecuted. It was common during that time for the monasteries to hide people or take them in without too many questions. The hospital later became known as "Bedlam" and is referred to in Shakespeare. Bethlem was seized in 1375 during the reign of Edward

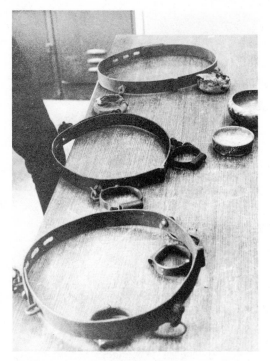

FIGURE 15. Restraints Used on Mental Patients, England (Courtesy, Guildhall Museum, London). Photograph by the author.

III. This is the first time that we learn that mental patients were kept there. A Report of the Royal Commission showed "six men lunatics there." These individuals were outcasts and treated worse than lower animals. They were shackled and chained and slept with only straw as a bed, no toilet facilities, and little food. One can still see the iron shackles and chains used during this period at the Guildhall Museum, London (see Figs. 15 and 16).

King Henry IV had Bethlem investigated in 1403 but changes in care were not made. The Reformation in England resulted in the closing of many small ecclesiastical institutions that had provided asylum for the sick and poor of all stations of life. When King Henry VIII, during his reign (1509–1547), handed over certain dissolved religious houses to the City of London, he included Bethlem. Later, the Elizabethan Poor Laws (1601) made the local communities responsible for the care of mental patients, the government began to provide care, and so did private patrons. During this time, the mildly mentally ill wandered about or were in almshouses, and the violent were locked up at home under their keepers, beaten, or put in jail.

Common Practices Preceding the Humanitarian Movement: England

At Bethlem, the practice was to chain all the patients by arm and leg as they lay on filthy straw covered with a rug. In another hospital, patients were chained to bedstocks at night regardless of their state of mind. The York Lunatic Asylum (now Naburn) was founded in 1772 and opened in September, 1777.

George III was mechanically restrained by his doctor's orders (Dr. Willis, a clericomedical doctor) but was brutally knocked down by his keeper. In April, 1789, he went to St. Paul's to give thanks for his recovery; he remained lucid until 1801 (Tuke, 1892).

Iron handcuffs that each weighed one pound five ounces and iron hobbles that weighed three pounds eight ounces were used as late as 1829 in the Lincoln Asylum.

Enlightenment

PHILIPPE PINEL, JEAN BAPTISTE PUSSIN, AND WILLIAM TUKE

The period of enlightenment began with the work of Philippe Pinel, a French physician, who struck off the chains of mental patients at Salpetriére and Bicêtre in 1793 and put these patients to work doing chores on the farm. Recently, Jean Baptiste Pussin, hospital superintendent, is cited as initiating the reform for which Pinel has received credit for almost two hundred years (Weiner, 1979). About the same time, William Tuke, a tea dealer and a Quaker in York (population sixteen thousand in 1792), became interested in the fact that a friend, Hannah Mills, had died under questionable circumstances at the York Lunatic Asylum. On April 30, 1790, an investi-

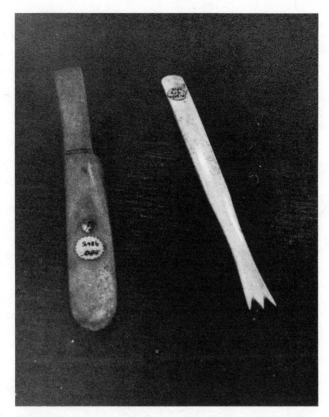

FIGURE 16. Bone Knife and Fork Used by Mental Patients (Courtesy, Guildhall Museum, London). Photograph by the author.

gation was ordered. During the investigations, one wing was burned involving the deaths of patients and the destruction of much that was believed they wished to conceal.

At a later time, William Tuke visited St. Luke's Hospital, London, and saw patients chained and lying on filthy straw. A female patient was chained to the wall.

FOUNDING OF THE RETREAT, YORK[2]

This mental hospital founded by William Tuke, a Yorkshire Quaker, opened in 1796. At the time of its founding, the two principal asylums for the insane were Bethlem, London, and the York Lunatic Asylum; St.

[2] For the material relating to the Retreat, York, I wish to thank the Quaker Library, London, and Mr. Milligan, librarian.

Luke's and Guy's Hospital also accepted lunatics. The Retreat has the distinction of being the first mental hospital in England where patients were regarded as being ill and requiring sympathy and scientific treatment. The establishment of the Retreat with its humanitarian philosophy had a deep influence on public opinion and resulted in major reform in mental hospitals.

The York Retreat was established as a distinct establishment for the mental patients of the Society of Friends. When the Retreat opened, one male patient was admitted who could not walk; later, he regained the use of his legs and called the Retreat Eden.

The Retreat was a place without the appearance of a prison. It was conceived of as a place "in which the unhappy might obtain refuge, a quiet haven in which the shattered bark might find the means of reparations of safety" (*York Retreat Reports,* 1846,

p. 11). *No iron manacles were provided at the Retreat.* However, they did use bleeding, purgatives, and emetics. They also used seclusion, leather belts to confine the arms, and also the "strait waistcoat." Attention was given to the general health of the patient and to the provision of a homelike atmosphere. The attitudes of kindness and consideration established the fundamental principles of moral treatment. No chains were used on the patient, good food was provided, and tea parties were regularly scheduled as part of the treatment. In addition, women visitors were appointed by the hospital committee to make regular visits.

The original officers of the Retreat were the *treasurer–manager, visiting physician, matron, and superintendent.* William Tuke managed it for the first twelve months and was the treasurer until 1819 at which time he was eighty-eight years old. He died in 1822 at the age of ninety-one. Dr. Fowler was the visiting physician. The founders of the Retreat did not consider the visiting physician as charged with the general and moral treatment of the patients. Dr. Fowler[3] at once saw the distinctions and developed the "expectant system," and in cases of melancholy, instead of attempting to purge the "black bile," he attempted to strengthen the patient by diet, fresh air, and exercise (*York Retreat Reports,* 1846, p. 38). The matron appointed was Katharine Allan and the superintendent was George Jepson (they married in 1806 and worked until 1822). George and Katharine Jepson[4] made the Retreat homelike. The superintendent gave medications and was the apothecary. The matron superintended the domestic arrangements, the women patients, and the servants. She also had the authority to discharge the servants. The superintendent gave the same attention to the men patients. In addition, the matron had under her care the physically sick patients of both sexes. The Grand Duke Nicholas, later czar of Russia, visited the Retreat and was much impressed with the matron Katharine Jepson (Tuke, 1892).

During 1813, due to the publication of

the facts of sixteen years of the humanitarian treatment instituted at the York Retreat, the Superintendent of the York Lunatic Asylum took offense. His views were published in the York newspapers and a controversy arose. A Yorkshire magistrate sent to the newspapers a letter detailing a case of gross ill treatment in the York Lunatic Asylum. Subsequently, investigations were ordered, and during a site visit to the York Lunatic Asylum, Godfrey Higgins, of Lancaster, asked the attendant where a certain door led to that was just off the kitchen. The attendant denied that the key could be found. Higgins found a key at the fireside, a poker. Inside the door, there were four cells; thirteen patients had slept in the filthy straw.

After the investigations, all resident officers, keepers, and nurses[5] were discharged; the steward refused to hand over the books and, instead, burned them. George and Katharine Jepson, superintendent and matron of the York Retreat, were brought in from the York Retreat to reform the internal management and supervision of the patients at the York Lunatic Asylum until new staff could be recruited. The exposure of the condition of these patients in the York Lunatic Asylum finally led to legislation for the purpose of ameliorating the cruel treatment and bad conditions.

In 1815 Mr. Haslam testified to the House of Commons that there were 122 patients at Bethlem, three male keepers, two female keepers, and ten patients in chains. In the same year, when a matron was elected to Bethlem, she found one female patient who had been chained for eight years. Samuel Tuke (1819), architect of the Wakefield Asylum, now Stanley Royd Hospital, Wakefield, Yorkshire, in his studies of asylums noted that chains were almost universally attached to the beds.

---

[3] Dr. Fowler originated Fowler's solution.
[4] George Jepson died in 1836 at the age of ninety-three; Katharine Jepson died in 1844 at the age of seventy-nine.

[5] *York Retreat Reports.* York: John L. Linney, 15, Low Ousegate, 1846, p. 51. This is the earliest reference to nurses that I found in the *New Retreat Reports.* Nurses are again mentioned in Tuke, Daniel Hack: *Chapters in the History of the Insane in the British Isles.* London: Kegan, Paul, Trench and Co., 1882. Daniel Hack Tuke became the visiting medical officer of the Retreat in 1854. That yearly report shows only four cases of mechanical restraint for the preceding five years, two of whom were surgical cases in addition to their mental condition.

Lord Ashley and Lord Shaftesbury were responsible for the Lunacy Bill of 1845–1846. By this Act, commissioners were appointed to inspect the conditions of all places where lunatics were kept except Bethlem Hospital. What had arisen as a local matter caused a fundamental change in the attitude toward mental patients in England and abroad.

SOME SIGNIFICANT EVENTS AT THE YORK RETREAT RELATING TO NURSING AND THE CARE OF PATIENTS (1839–1936)

In the earliest days of the Retreat, a patient could bring his own servant and not mix with the other patients. In 1839, a resident medical officer, Dr. Thurman, was charged with the immediate care of the patients and the direction of the attendants in order to get better observations of patients and to improve the records (York Retreat Reports, 1846, p. 38). Events significant to the development of psychiatric nursing are recorded during the subsequent years at the Retreat.

Both staff and patients took rail journeys to the seaside. "Persons of colour" gave lectures to the patients; attendants formed a mutual improvement society of which patients were members, and sometimes an extra female nurse was placed on the ward to work with a female patient.[6] The matron was expected "to cheer and sympathize with those who are under her care" (York Retreat Reports, 1874, p. 6).

As new officers of the institution came and went, changes were made. One superintendent advised adding a more educated class of attendants ". . . whose duties shall be more 'aesthetical' than 'menial' " (York Retreat Reports, 1875, p. 22). In this program for improvement he noted that "the employment of educated Nurses, except when associated with some Religious Order, has not however, on the whole, been successful in England, but in a few of the best asylums in America, it is said to have proved a success" (York Retreat Reports, 1875, p. 15).

It was during this time that Turkish baths were installed and many people came to

the York Retreat for these baths who were not mental patients.

Staff lived on the grounds of the institution, attendants lived in the wards with the patients, and the matron assumed the bulk of the responsibility for the women patients. In the evening, ladies and companions assembled for reading, music, and games in the pattern of the Philadelphia Hospital for the Insane. By the 1880s the matron had become a companion to patients, not a housekeeper. The uniform was introduced for nurses; however, on a walk or drive they were not permitted to wear them. As a result of the uniform it was noted that the "improvement in the general appearance of the nurses is very marked" (York Retreat Reports, 1883, p. 18).

A head nurse's room was set aside and a separate report on nursing was introduced when Bedford Pierce was employed (in 1892) as the chief medical officer. Gradually more than one matron appeared, a housekeeper was added, and a supervisor of nurses was mentioned (York Retreat Reports, 1887, p. 14, and 1894).

The hours of nurses were still very long. Their visits to patients were registered on a central instrument called the telltale clock. By the end of the nineteenth century nurses were admitted on a three-month probation period during which time no salary was paid. During the remainder of the two years of training the salary was small. As late as 1900 the nurses had a weekly day or weekly one-half day off duty, Sunday leave, and one hour free daily from duty.

Other changes occurred quite rapidly in the early 1900s. Nurses in charge of the wards were called "sister" as in the general hospitals. Massage, Swedish gymnastics, medical gymnastics, and invalid cooking were added to the curriculum on nursing mental and nervous diseases. A private nursing department arose and nurses working privately made two guineas per week exclusive of traveling and laundry expenses. Applications were to be made to the matron for "The Training of Mental Nurses." Applicants were to be not less than twenty-two years old. By 1902 the course was four years with three years in the institution of which two years were probationary (plus the two months on trial) and one year as

---

[6] *State of an Institution near York Called the Retreat for Persons Afflicted with Disorders of the Mind*, 1864, p. 5 (no publisher cited).

staff nurse. The fourth year was on the private nursing staff. By 1903 three sisters helped teach Swedish gymnastics and it had been clearly established ". . . that nurses specially trained for mental work are of far greater value in the nursing of mental diseases than those who have only been trained in general hospitals" (*York Retreat Reports,* 1903, p. 21).

A trained nurses' department was set up at the Retreat by 1908 because the institution itself could not employ all the nurses they trained. The curriculum in 1909 was designated as

First year: Anatomy and physiology and first aid.
Second year: Bodily diseases and sick nursing.
Third year: Mental disorders (*York Retreat Reports,* 1909, p. 11).

A male nurses department was instituted in 1912 with the same curriculum (twenty lectures per year). It was temporarily closed in 1915 during World War I when the men went into the service. As a result, women nurses were introduced into one of the men's wards. Dr. Bedford Pierce had made many changes at the York Retreat and had been instrumental in developing and maintaining the nursing curriculum. When he came to the Retreat, there was no systematic training of nurses. Dr. Pierce also gives credit to Matron Charlotte Thomasson who had been inspired by Miss Cadbury with whom she had worked at the Queen's Hospital in Birmingham. Two editions of *The Handbook for Nurses* had been prepared at the Retreat. The 1921 *York Retreat Report* was the last one prepared by Dr. Bedford Pierce.

With the advent of the General Nursing Council in England and the Nurses' Registration Act, it was the desire of the committee of the Retreat that all nurses on their staff who held senior posts should become registered nurses, and it is duly noted that the General Nursing Council gave examinations to determine who would be on the State Register of Nurses.

Arriving at the Retreat in the fog of an English winter late afternoon in 1961, I admired the Georgian entrance and asked for the matron. She appeared in the traditional blue and white uniform, stiffly starched, and with a wide, white headdress as seen in a Flemish painting. Off we went down a long, winding white-paneled hall papered a bright blue with shiny satin floral designs. Red ceiling-to-floor curtains added a dramatic color to the many windows. The matron, Miss Vera Dodge, carried an enormous ring of keys "for elderly patients to be locked in," she stated. Patients with whom I spoke had enormous, lovely rooms with expansive views of the English countryside. The living rooms had fireplaces. On each ward that we visited, the matron knew all the staff and the patients. The hospital is constructed with suntraps and verandas overlooking the fifty-eight acres. Under the Mental Health Act of 1959, which became fully operative on November 1, 1960, the Retreat was officially designated a registered nursing home and not a registered hospital for patients with mental disorder. Thus, the patient population was composed of individuals with long-term illness. On December 1, 1960, there was a total of 212 informally admitted patients and twenty-seven detained (involuntary) patients at the Retreat. During the year there were 351 admissions of which 97 percent were informally (voluntarily) admitted.

It is recognized by this writer that other institutions were involved in the era of the humanitarian movement in the care and treatment of individuals with mental disorders. The Retreat, York, has been studied due to the leadership and involvement of William Tuke, who demonstrates for history what one person can do.

Common Practices in America

EARLY AMERICA

In our own country, the development of treatment and caretaking facilities was naturally influenced by English and Western European practices. Although during 1691–1692 Americans had participated in the witchcraft delusions, by 1760 Philadelphia itself had developed as the largest American city and from it had emerged artists and scientists making themselves known here and abroad.

In early America, mental patients wandered about and often were moved from village to village. If the village had a jail or almshouse (poorhouse), they were placed there. Each almshouse had an infirmary. The poorhouses had a crazy-house, crazy-cell, crazy-dungeon, or crazy-hall. Later, these became the municipal general hospitals and continue as this in many towns and cities in the United States as of today. I have seen rooms that were cells in every sense of the word as late as 1976 in a county facility in California. Usually attached to wards of a general hospital, these were small rooms with terrazzo floors, a drain in the center of the room, and high barred windows that let the light into the room but could not be opened; these were known as seclusion rooms. A heavy wooden or metal door had a slot for passing food into the room and a thick glassed small window enabled one to view the entire room from the outside. Patients slept on a metal bed clamped to the floor or simply a mattress placed on the floor.

Benjamin Franklin drew up a petition for the establishment of the Pennsylvania Hospital during the year 1751. This was the first institution in the English colonies to care exclusively for the sick. It was a private institution and it also provided care for mental patients.

The first public mental hospital was established in 1773 at Williamsburg, Virginia (Fig. 17), after several years of discussion in the House of Burgesses.[7] This was the first state hospital for mental patients in America and remained the only one until about fifty years later when the Eastern Lunatic Asylum was established at Lexington, Kentucky, and opened in 1824.[8] Portions of the foundation were recently uncovered in Williamsburg, Virginia. The two-story building had twelve rooms on each floor, a keeper's apartment, and a manager's room. Each patient's room was 11 feet 9 inches by 10 feet 9 inches with iron grates on the inside of the windows. All windows were padlocked. The hospital was called Eastern State Hospital upon request of the House of Burgesses of Virginia "to make provision for the support and maintenance

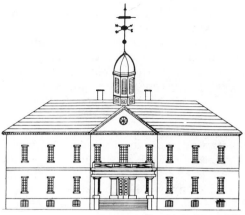

The original building of 1773

FIGURE 17. The First Public Mental Hospital for the Mentally Ill in America: the Original Building of 1773, Williamsburg, Virginia. It was first called the Hospital for Idiots and Lunatics.

of idiots, lunatics, and other persons of unsound mind." The original building was 100 feet long and 32 feet 2 inches wide.

A keeper, James Galt, was appointed and his wife was named matron. The Galt family continued in service for eighty-nine years, much like the Tuke family at the York Retreat. In 1823 there were fifty-seven patients being taken care of by the keeper, the steward, the matron, and several other white personnel and fourteen Negro slave servants (Dain, 1971, p. 43).

Much of Williamsburg has been restored in the eighteenth-century manner and plans are under way to also restore the hospital. Williamsburg was one of the earliest settlements in the country and was capital of Virginia during Colonial times. The remains of this building tell us that patients were confined; it is most likely that they were also chained.

Since the almshouses (poorhouses) had already built up a traditional attitude toward the helpless poor, the stage was set for custodial asylum for the insane.

PRIOR TO THE 1820s

Patients were chained and put on view to the public for a fee, and paupers who were both mentally ill and mentally retarded were auctioned off to work in rural

[7] Site visit, 25 July, 1974.
[8] Site visit, 22 July, 1980.

America. If the community itself did not
know what to do with one of these individuals, they were simply sent to the poorhouse,
the catchall, well into the twentieth century.
In the mental hospitals, bleeding, cupping,
leeching, and the use of purgatives and
emetics were the treatments of that time.
It must be remembered that while the issue
of the development of institutions for the
insane was being debated in the House of
Burgesses so were the beginnings of the
Revolution, and the voices of people like
Patrick Henry were being heard. The establishment of the institution at Williamsburg
set the stage for the state's responsibility
for mental patients.

Benjamin Rush[9]

Rush joined the staff of physicians at the
Pennsylvania Hospital in 1783 after the
American Revolution. He was a great humanitarian of his day despite the treatment
methods that he used and advocated in his
practice. He was a signer of the Declaration
of Independence and is known as the Father
of American Psychiatry. He was truly an
eighteenth-century man with a wide range
of interests and was involved in most of
the reform movements of his day.

Rush thought that insanity was a disease
of the arteries localized in the brain and
treated patients with venesection, cupping,
leeching, purgatives, and emetics. Hot and
cold baths were used as shock. Rush himself
designed a "tranquilizing chair" in which
the patient sat and was fixed in immobility
(see Fig. 18). The whirling gyrator was also
in use as well as the cold-water treatment
in which cold water was poured under the
sleeves of the patient's clothes so that it
might descend the body under the armpits
and down the trunk. Another treatment
used by Rush was one in which the patient
was required to stand erect for twenty-four
hours. He picked up the idea when he was
in England and saw this treatment for refrac-
tory horses (Tuke, 1885).

But it was here that patients were encouraged to record their own experiences, moral

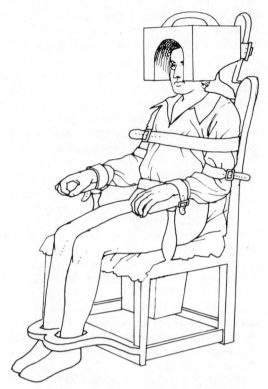

FIGURE 18.   A Tranquilizing Chair Used as
a Method of Treatment in the 1700's and Early
1800's.

suasion was begun, and the value of pleasant
companions and occupational therapy was
established.

Moral Treatment

The concept of moral treatment as set
forth by the founders of the York Retreat
emphasized an atmosphere in which kindness, cheerfulness, and contentment were
promoted, the mind and body were kept
occupied, and patients were thereby expected to recall natural and healthy trains
of thought.

Daily exercise was a part of treatment.
Patients were also employed at useful tasks
and school was held; the library included
a shell collection, stuffed animals, and
books. There were evening lectures and
the magic lantern for amusement. Moral
therapy meant the use of a kind, friendly
atmosphere in a small hospital with pleasant surroundings, amusement, games, opportunities for learning, and religious devo-

---

[9] Benjamin Rush was born in 1745 at Philadelphia
of Quaker parents. He died on April 19, 1813. Rush
was a genius of his time, and one of his radical causes
was higher education for women.

tion as replacement for brute force, confinement, and mechanical restraint. The new treatment emphasized a healthy psychological and physical environment for patients and staff. The personnel lived on the grounds and the superintendent ate with the patients.

Established in 1813 and opened in 1817 as a sectarian institution, the Friends' Asylum for the Insane at Frankford, Pennsylvania, opened to other patients in 1834. The founder of the Frankford Asylum, Thomas Scattergood, visited the York Retreat and modeled the Frankford Asylum after it, with a major emphasis upon moral treatment (Friends' Asylum for the Insane, 1813–1913). Flora B. Rowe, a graduate of the Training School for Nurses at the McLean Asylum, was employed in 1891 as "Head Nurse in charge of female attendants" (Frankford Asylum Reports, 1891).

At Frankford Asylum, patients took carriage rides, sleigh rides, and made paintings and engravings. A large circular mound of earth was reserved for excited patients to plant flowers. Patients played croquet, cricket, and football.

It must be understood that Pinel rejected the idea that insanity could occur with only physical lesions; he, therefore, paved the way for psychological treatment. Humanistic and humanitarian laymen spearheaded the concept of moral treatment both in England and in America. Despite the humanitarian movement and the improved treatment of patients, the belief that mental disorders were incurable was widespread both in America and abroad.

CULT OF CURABILITY
(1830s–1840s)

The reawakening of the humanitarian spirit through religious revival occurred in America in 1833 to 1846. Influenced by Locke that knowledge comes to the mind only through the senses, the belief arose that insanity might be due to impaired sensory organs and therefore individuals began to consider insanity as somatic in origin and therefore curable.

The optimism toward cure began with Dr. Francis Willis in his treatment of George III. In addition, when Captain Basil Hall visited the Hartford Retreat (America), glowing reports of what he observed there were widely publicized as phenomenal recoveries (Deutsch, 1937). Treatment consisted of tonic remedies such as extract of conium and carbonate of iron. Warm bathing was used and one instance cited as follows: "We put a large seton in his neck, directed opiates and some tonics" (*American Journal of Insanity,* 1844, p. 62). Quinine, nourishing food, fresh air, and exercise were prescribed. Moral treatment was used and glowing reports of phenomenal recoveries were made during this period.

As industrialization with consequent urbanization began and the population began to increase, the small therapeutic mental institution was submerged. New laws relegating the chronically ill and the dangerously insane to the mental hospitals led to the more rapid discharge of those individuals who could in fact be helped. Sometimes the number discharged was equated with cure when, in fact, they were soon to be readmitted.

A change had occurred in mental hospitals where the philosophy of treatment was determined by the physician superintendent and the ideas of dedicated laymen became less and less of an influence. Nursing religious orders were not prominent in America and trained nurses were not available. However, in the 1830s a handbook, *Directions for Attendants,* had been issued at McLean and Worcester mental hospitals. The cult of curability is cited by Deutsch as leading to the remarkable growth of mental hospitals during this period. It was at this time that the attitude of attendants began to change from that of keeper to that of nurse. The small asylums and sound buildings caring for seventy to two hundred or three hundred and fifty patients were disappearing.

CUSTODIAL ERA (1850s–1870s)

A tremendous upsurge of people moving to the cities from rural America led to an increase in the number of patients in mental hospitals and also to the transfer of the functions of the physician to the other staff who

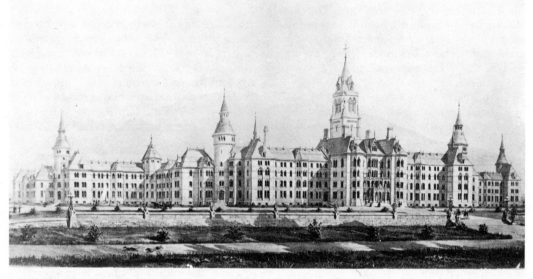

FIGURE 19. Accepted Design for Napa State Asylum for the Insane, which Opened in 1875, Imola, California.

had, for the most part, no formal training. Nurses and attendants received low salaries and had little or no experience in the care and treatment of the mentally ill, and consequently there was a high staff turnover.

Mechanical restraints and confinement once more appeared and were commonly used. Grob (1966) cites the Irish immigration as a factor in the change of attitude. Of low socioeconomic status and poor, many of these immigrants were admitted to mental hospitals. Class differences created communication problems between patients and psychiatrists and anti-Catholicism was widespread. Insanity became connected with pauperism and the thought was that the patient was insane because he was poor and poor because he came from inferior stock.

By the 1870s mental institutions had become large custodial ones for lower-class patients. Moral treatment ended and legislators related to economy instead of treatment. Very large institutions resulted and insanity was thought to be incurable. See Figures 19 and 20 for an example of an institution of those times.

Many hospital superintendents concluded that patients in the public hospitals were incurable and therefore institutions filled up with incurable cases (Dain, 1964, p. 205).

DOROTHEA LYNDE DIX[10]

Some individuals tried to change the system. Dorothea Lynde Dix, a schoolteacher who went to England to improve her health, visited Dr. Daniel Hack Tuke and the York Retreat while there. Returning to America, she succeeded in bringing the conditions of patients in mental hospitals and those who were in jails to the attention of the public. She was also appointed to the post of Superintendent of Women Nurses during the Civil War with the power to select and assign women nurses to general or permanent military hospitals (Deutsch, 1937).

Dorothea Lynde Dix made numerous visits and inspections of jails and mental institutions throughout this country. Due largely to her work, more mental hospitals were built and bad conditions within existing ones were brought to the attention of the public during her time.

Because there were no trained nurses during the Civil War, dedicated and concerned women volunteers provided the care and comfort that they knew how to give.

[10] Dorothea Lynde Dix was born on April 4, 1802, at Hampden, Maine, and died on July 17, 1887. She stayed at the New Jersey State Hospital at Trenton from 1881 until her death. She is buried at Mt. Auburn Cemetery near Boston, Massachusetts.

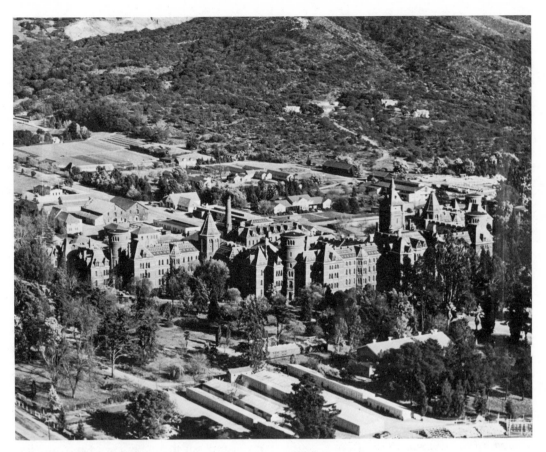

FIGURE 20. Napa State Asylum at a Later Date (1930's).

Mrs. Bickerdyke (see Fig. 21), known as Mother Bickerdyke to the soldiers, was a volunteer who carried out her labors of love and kindness to sick and wounded soldiers throughout the conflict, including Sherman's march to Atlanta (Brockett, 1866). Where there were hospitals, the practice was to employ convalescent soldiers as nurses, ward masters, and so on, but Mrs. Bickerdyke was not satisfied with their work. In defiance of military rules, she substituted "Negro women for these duties and improvement was manifest" (Brockett, 1866). Refusing to care for officers who already had their orderlies, Mrs. Bickerdyke was a mother to the private soldier. She was idolized by them for her love and kindness. In addition to washing and bandaging wounds, she garnered clothing and food for the soldiers, cooked the food herself, and refused to tolerate neglect from anyone, though they outranked her. Although a self-taught, "bornd nurse" she evidenced the comprehensive approach to patient care and the personal qualities so important to the modern psychiatric nurse in the caring and comforting roles.

REFORM AND EDUCATION
(1880s–EARLY 1900s)

It stands to reason that the mentally sick should be at least as well cared for as the physically sick. (Linda Richards, 1915, p. 108)

During the 1890s a spirit of reform again emerged in the belief that an individual can be changed by altering his environment. However, there was no scientific approach in mental hospitals.

The first permanent training school for nurses in an American institution for the insane was instituted at McLean Asylum in 1882 by Dr. Edward Cowles (Deutsch,

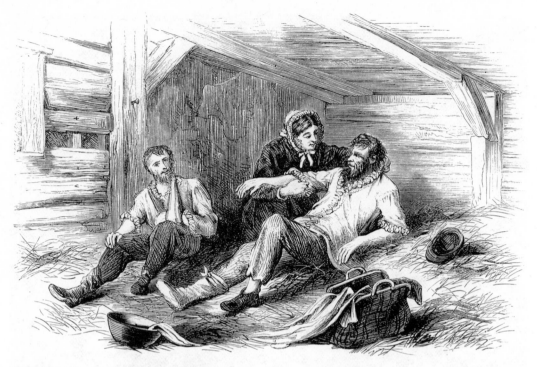

FIGURE 21. Mrs. Bickerdyke Used Her Dresses for Union Soldiers. (Author's Collection.)

1937). He also was the first to introduce women nurses to male wards.

It was during this decade that the after-care movement began in America. It was first patterned after the plans of Dr. Lind-painter, director of the Eberbach Asylum in Nassau, Germany, in 1829 (Deutsch, 1937).

Women began to take their places in public work. Freud introduced the concept that a person can be helped by psychological means and his visit to America in 1909 gave a new turn to psychiatry.

LINDA RICHARDS

Linda Richards, America's first trained nurse, graduated in 1873 from the New England Hospital for Women and Children, Boston, Massachusetts (Fig. 22). Later she visited England, met Florence Nightingale, and after returning to America organized several mental hospitals. She worked with Dr. Cowles to establish a school of nursing at Boston City Hospital and afterward at the McLean Asylum. For many years the

school at McLean Asylum was the only training school for mental nurses. Later, she led the way for establishing the first school of nursing in Japan at Kyoto.

During 1887 Nellie Bly succeeded in getting herself admitted to the New York City Lunatic Asylum, and shocked the public with her serialized articles, "Ten Days in a Mad-House," published in the *New York World.*

Due to Dr. Adolph Meyer, formal instruction began at Worcester for nurses and attendants in 1897. A training school for nurses was opened by Dr. Quinby at Worcester in 1903. When Adolph Meyer left Worcester he went to the Pathological Institute of the New York State Hospitals. He enlisted the voluntary aid of Mrs. Meyer in visiting patients and their families, thus attaining assistance in the broader social understanding of the problems of the patient, the family, and the community in relation to etiology of mental disorder (Deutsch, 1937, p. 287). He discussed his cases with Mrs. Meyer, whose opinion he highly valued (Crawford, 1974).

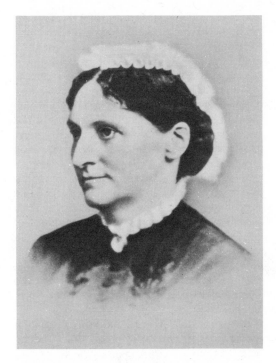

FIGURE 22. Linda Richards, America's First Trained Nurse (New England Hospital for Women and Children, October 1, 1873). (From Dolan, Josephine: *Nursing in Society.* Philadelphia, W. B. Saunders Company, 1978, p. 196.) By permission.

During this period, nurses worked seven days per week from six in the morning until eight at night and after that were on call for emergencies. Since factory workers had shorter hours and more pay, an acute shortage of labor occurred in some institutions. At Worcester, on Monday, August 26, 1902, nurses took the evening off without permission (Grob, 1966, p. 321). They did not wish to leave the patients without staff, so they drew lots to determine who would go and who would stay with the patients. Twelve of the twenty-eight left for the evening and upon return were refused entrance to their quarters. So they slept in another part of the hospital and the next day were fired. The others then resigned. The superintendent, Dr. Quinby, was then accused by these former employees of mismanagement, i.e., poor food, lack of bedding, clothing, rats and vermin, overcrowding, neglect of patients, long working hours, and staging the visits of the trustees. All the local papers

supported the Establishment except one. The nurses were very bitter because they were not permitted to testify before the examining board. Later, in 1907, an eight-hour-work-day law was passed but it did not apply to nurses and attendants. As late as 1910, nurses worked a sixty-hour week with one day off in seven. In 1916, a Central Board of Examiners of the Commission on Mental Diseases began to establish a uniform curriculum of nurses' training schools in state institutions. They set up a prescribed curriculum and uniform texts.

CLIFFORD WHITTINGHAM BEERS

Clifford Whittingham Beers, an exuberant, persuasive, and enormously energetic man, was a mental patient for three years from 1900 to 1903. Due to his experiences as a patient he saw the need for better understanding of mental disorder. He organized the Connecticut Committee on Mental Hygiene in 1908, the National Committee for Mental Hygiene in 1909, and went on to organize the First International Congress on Mental Hygiene, which was held in 1930 in Washington, D.C. His book *A Mind That Found Itself* (1908), chronicles his experiences as a mental patient.

RISE OF INSTITUTIONS, THE MIDDLE CLASS AND THE PROFESSIONS: EARLY 1900s–1920s

The development of the professions in the late nineteenth and early twentieth centuries is interwoven with the rise of institutions and the new middle class. As a profession, nursing had a late start, graduating its first trained nurse in 1873, one hundred years after the founding of the first public mental hospital in America. The development of nursing as a profession pictures the emerging role of women in the professions and the work of men who entered asylum nursing.

Treatment and care of persons with mental disorder are intertwined with the intellectual life of the era, the beliefs and actions of individuals, and with many economic and sociopolitical influences. Psychiatric mental-health nursing emerged in the context of influences that generated the rise of institutions, of the middle class, and of the professions.

INSTITUTIONALIZATION

During the last quarter of the nineteenth century, institutionalization of mentally disordered persons was in ascendance due in part to industrialization, population growth, urbanization, the belief that insanity was incurable, and the effect of the efforts of Dorothea Lynde Dix to empty the jails. Grob (1966) describes immigration as a major factor when state public asylums became large custodial places for patients of the lower classes. These asylums, often located in remote rural areas, barely sustained by meager budgets and the unpaid labor of the patients, became places where many patients spent the rest of their lives. Wards were locked, segregated by sex, and by diagnosis. Those patients able to do so worked in the laundry, bakery, kitchen, cannery, printery, dairy, poultry farm, pig stye, fields, fruit orchards, gardens, upholstery, sewing room, and so on, all run by the institution itself. Other patients, not so well, were locked inside. Staff were required to live on the grounds of the institution. Large Victorian mansions remain today that once housed superintendents, physicians, and others. Status hierarchies were evident in these authoritarian institutions where the superintendent and other physicians usually lived in the best houses whereas others, lower in the status hierarchy, were allocated more modest accommodations. Nurses' dormitories might be designated as single nurses' home and married nurses' home with the attendants quartered in the bunkhouse. Where there was an affiliation for nursing students, the superintendent of nurses might have an apartment in the nurses' dormitories.

Depressed patients were sometimes housed in small homelike cottages. Housing for the worker patients was built adjacent to the fields and patients conducted their own commercial enterprises: A small hen house could produce fresh eggs to sell to the staff and provide spending money; car washes and waxes were sources of revenue. Handmade items were sold to visitors and staff. Patients also worked as baby-sitters and maids for the staff who lived on the grounds. The staff, underpaid themselves, figured in the inexpensive housing and patient-help as fringe benefits. These jobs did assist some patients to reintegrate themselves into life outside the hospital upon discharge.

The mental institutions continued to grow larger and as they grew larger the custodial aspects became more rigid. Management of small budgets, management of patients, functional assignments in patient care, routine activities, and staff–patient interaction made up the custodial attitude. Comfortable with the status quo, once the custodial attitude occurred, it was very difficult to change.

Even in 1913 mental patients were kept in iron cages on cots with no light and no heat. As late as 1933 mentally sick inmates of a midwestern poorhouse were still being chained to trees (Deutsch, 1937, p. 452).

During the first quarter of the twentieth century, psychopathic hospitals developed. Essentially these were small psychiatric units in general hospitals, operating independently, connected with a university or connected with a mental hospital. Mental patients were admitted for diagnosis, observation, and first care. Short-term intensive treatment was provided. These units also served as clearing houses.

THE MIDDLE CLASS AND THE PROFESSIONS

Wiebe (1967) described the rise of the new middle class in the late nineteenth and early twentieth centuries as that of the professions and business in their specialized organizational clusters. These organizations provided situations where individuals from a wide variety of backgrounds and geographic areas could meet, communicate, and learn different points of view.

A spirit of reform and progressivism provided the impetus for the new organizational society. At the turn of the century, health crusades were popular causes and people organized to eradicate the "social diseases" and others as well. Mental hygiene became one of these national movements. The small community organization where everyone in a geographical unit could be a member began to be replaced by the large organization of individuals of specialized occupations (Hays, 1972). Joining an occupational group thus became a method of identification. Nursing became an organization during this era. First, the American Society of Superintendents of Training Schools for Nurses was organized in 1893; its successor was the National League of Nursing Education in 1912, which, in turn, became the National League for Nursing in 1952 (Dolan, 1978).

In 1896 the Nurses' Associated Alumnae of the United States and Canada was organized for all nurses. It was changed to the Nurses' Associated Alumnae of the United States in 1899 and became the American Nurses' Association in 1911 (Dolan, 1978). Although this was the major organization for nurses, other organizations of nurses were founded during this era. From the outset, the American Nurses Association aimed toward high standards of patient care and better welfare for nurses.

Organized under the banner of common goals, individuals with similar interest met together to achieve these goals (Israel, 1972). Thus, the idea of collective action arose. The new middle class formed according to careers necessary for the rising technological, industrial, and urban society. New occupations, identities, and careers became possible through university education in a rising scientific–industrial society (Bledstein, 1976). Professions became means of providing services to society and to better one's lot (Carter, 1978). Nursing became a means of independence, especially for women, in an era in which career choices were limited.

Organized Nursing. During the early part of this century, nursing struggled to organize good schools of nursing, both in general and mental hospitals.[11] Most schools of nursing were developed in hospitals and

---

[11] Other types of hospitals also developed schools of nursing, for example, tuberculosis sanitaria.

most nursing care around the clock was provided by the nursing students who lived on the grounds and who paid for their education by their labor.

Organized nursing studied the problems of the mental hospital training schools and began to exert leadership (Kurtz, 1912). In 1914, the National League of Nursing Education proposed that a standard curriculum in nursing include training in mental and nervous disease as part of the course in medical nursing.

Psychiatric Nursing. Psychiatric nursing arose in general hospital schools and also in asylums, both service-centered institutions. Following McLean Asylum, other asylums established schools of nursing and this type of school rapidly flourished. To complete the education of nursing students, the better asylum schools developed affiliations with general hospitals. Affiliations of general hospital schools of nursing with mental hospitals began early in this century.

Asylum schools trained nurses for work in their own institutions and also for private-duty nursing. Although desirable personal qualities and a higher education were sought in individuals for this type of nursing, standards in the asylum schools tended to be inferior to the general hospital schools. Held in low esteem, nurse graduates of asylum schools could rarely find employment in general hospitals (Goodnow, 1938).

At the Frankford Asylum, a two-year course of nurses' training was begun in 1895 taught by the medical staff. In 1896, the school also offered nurses who had already graduated special instruction in the "care of the insane." The next year seven students graduated, two men and five women. The course was described as consisting of seventy lectures with quizzes and bedside instruction. The student received ten weeks of each of the following: (1) "anatomy and physiology, (2) principles and practices of bandaging, (3) psychology and nursing in nervous diseases, and (4) materia medica, fevers, emergencies and general nursing" (Frankford Asylum Reports, 1897). An additional course of twenty lectures in massage was given by Jesse M. Ward of the Polyclinic Hospital.

In the 1897 report, Dr. Winter, a physician, was mentioned as "Directress" of the school.

It was the practice during those times for the asylums to develop their own handbooks setting forth what nurses should do.

Such instructions were contained in a handbook that designated responsibilities of the charge employee of Napa State Hospital, Imola, California (1921), and the following is one example:

All patients shall be bathed at least once a week in warm water and oftener if required. At such times underwear shall be changed. In case unusual force is required in bathing, owing to resistiveness, etc., the Matron, Supervisor, or Ward Physician shall be consulted before resorting to it. No patient shall be permitted to bathe privately except upon permission of the Ward Physician.

Professionalism. Nursing gave women an opportunity for independence and the professionalism provided purpose, dignity, and a much-needed human service.

In the interest of providing standards of comprehensive nursing care to the profession, the first curriculum guide for schools of nursing was published by the National League of Nursing Education (1917). This guide recommended that a twenty-hour course in mental and nervous disease be given in the third year (i.e., last). Lectures and clinics were to be given by a physician (neurologist or psychiatrist); nine hours by a trained nurse teacher and at least one hour by the chief of social services or a specialist in mental hygiene. Objectives of the course in mental nursing were:

1. "To teach the student nurse the relationship between the mental and physical illness and the application of general nursing principles to mental nursing
2. To teach the underlying causes of mental disease with modern methods of treatment available both in the hospital and in the community, and to endeavor to overcome the stigma attached to mental illness or mental hospital care
3. To train the nurse in observation of symptoms as expressed in early childhood and in later life through the behavior of patients, so that early signs of mental illness may be understood and appreciated, and so that nurses may give active and intelligent cooperation in movements for the prevention of illness
4. To teach the importance of directed habits of thought, desirable associations, and proper environmental conditions in early childhood and to show the relationship to mental disorders
5. To assist in developing resourcefulness, versatility, adaptability and individuality in the nurse. To emphasize qualities essential to success in mental work and the importance of special training in this branch of nursing"[12]

These objectives set the framework for a body of knowledge of psychiatric nursing essential for the definition of a profession. The objectives emphasized the importance of knowledge about the relationship between mental and physical illness and set the context of psychiatric nursing within general nursing (Objective No. 1). The objectives designated psychiatric nursing as a branch of nursing (Objective No. 5). Not only was knowledge of treatment in the hospital set forth but also in the community (Objective No. 2). The objectives clearly indicated the importance of knowledge of growth and development (Objective No. 4) and prevention (Objective No. 3). Because few general hospitals had mental departments at that time, early courses in psychiatric nursing were sometimes taken without clinical practicum with mental patients.

1915–1940s

A turning point occurred when Hideyo Noguchi and J. W. Moore (1913) identified the *Spirochaeta pallidum* as the etiological agent of general paresis. At that time 10 percent of patients in mental hospitals were admitted for this diagnosis and their life expectancy was three to five years. This was a breakthrough for psychiatry in that a definite etiology was established. Julius Wagner von Jauregg discovered fever therapy by use of the malaria *Plasmodium* for general paresis in 1917 and this treatment was introduced at St. Elizabeth's in 1922 (American Psychiatric Association, 1944). Fever therapy for general paresis remained in use until

[12] National League of Nursing Education: *Standard Curriculum for Schools of Nursing*. Baltimore: Waverly Press, 1917, pp. 109–110.

antibiotics arrived on the scene and were widely available in the 1940s. During World War II patients were still being treated with malarial therapy when penicillin was scarce and servicemen received top priority for its use. Even after penicillin was plentiful, hyperthermia induced by a machine was administered to patients with general paresis in addition to massive doses of penicillin.

Influences: World War I–World War II. Early in World War I a Division of Neurology and Psychiatry was created in the Office of the Surgeon General. It was given the responsibility for the examination of recruits, preparation of facilities for observation, treatment and care of soldiers, preparation for treatment of soldiers in the American Expeditionary Forces, and preparation for the continued treatment of those soldiers who returned home.

The development of great public interest in the war neuroses as well as their high incidence gave impetus to the mental hygiene movement after World War I.

Twenty-five years later, World War II brought to light the extreme shortages of nursing personnel. Psychiatric casualties highlighted the need for experts in the field of psychiatric nursing. Yet, some states gave no training in psychiatric nursing to their students (Fitzsimmons, 1944). A few postgraduate courses were available for the study of psychiatric nursing. The U.S. Cadet Corps (Fig. 23) gave many young women the opportunity to be nurses and therefore to choose psychiatric nursing. Of the 1,107 schools participating in the United States Cadet Corps during World War II, only 48 percent offered psychiatric nursing to all students (Favreau, 1945). At that time, there were only about three thousand psychiatrists in the United States. Many individuals, devastated by the horrors of war, required psychiatric treatment, as well as those thousands found unfit for military service due to their psychological state. Leaders in psychiatry set up treatment facilities for the Armed Forces; nurses in the service helped, and others learned from this work. After World War II, the GI Bill further assisted nurses in their educational endeavors.

During this era, the importance of psy-

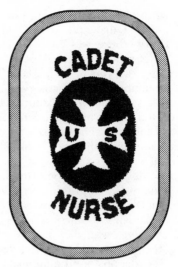

FIGURE 23. Cadet Nurse Emblem.

chogenesis of mental disorder and psychodynamics was being recognized. In private institutions, nurses acted as companions to mental patients similar to the tradition established at the York Retreat. As the practice of psychiatry widened, mental patients were often cared for at home—where families could afford to have someone else to help with the mentally disordered member; thus, private-duty home psychiatric nursing became popular. Nurses also worked in the community in mental-hygiene clinics and did psychiatric social work. Some psychiatric nurses spent many hours in the homes of psychiatric patients and took trips abroad with them (Steele, 1972). "Specialling" the patient also occurred in hospitals where patients needed additional nursing-care hours. In some instances, "specialling" was provided by the regular nursing staff who worked over and beyond their usual working hours for a fee paid by the patient or the patient's family. In one eastern, private psychiatric hospital in the 1920s and 1930s, nurses accompanied patients on walks, for dinner at restaurants, riding, on picnics, and the like, wearing knickers, riding outfits, or other clothes appropriate for the occasion. The nurse's uniform was worn only inside the hospital building (Crawford, 1974).

The Goldmark Report had warned against specialty schools of nursing (Committee for the Study of Nursing Education, 1923, p. 403). During the great Depression of the 1930s, there was an oversupply of nurses. In a report of the Committee on the Grading of Nursing Schools (1934) a recommendation was made to develop nursing schools as *educational* institutions. As a result of this study many nursing schools in general and mental hospitals were closed. Harriet Bailey published her book on *Nursing Mental and Nervous Diseases* in 1920. Katharine McLean Steele published *Psychiatric Nursing* in 1937 outlining practical procedures and other aspects of role. Later, Marion Kalkman's book, *Introduction to Psychiatric Nursing,* was the first psychiatric nursing text with psychoanalytic concepts (1950). It had a profound influence on psychiatric nursing education and practice. Theresa Muller's book, *The Nature and Direction of Psychiatric Nursing: The Dynamics of Human Relationships in Nursing,* (1950) gave impetus to the field. Hildegard E. Peplau's book, *Interpersonal Relations in Nursing,* presented a conceptual framework for psychodynamic nursing (1952).

Mellow's (1965) theory of nursing therapy evolved from its beginning in 1951 from work with the acutely ill person with schizophrenia. According to Mellow, nursing therapy is a treatment approach and a research tool. Orlando (1961), in her work on integrating mental-health principles in the basic nursing curriculum, identified function, process and principles of professional nursing practice. Bermosk and Mordan (1964) described interviewing in nursing practice. Other publications and influences were also important.

American Psychiatric Association. The American Psychiatric Association, the oldest of the medical organizations in the United States, exerted its influence in the establishment of nursing schools in asylums and on what should be taught in mental nursing. In the 1920s, the American Psychiatric Association published their accreditation requirements for mental-hospital nursing schools. Over the years, many prominent psychiatric nurse leaders were on the Committee on Psychiatric Nursing of the American Psychiatric Association; impor-

tant studies were conducted and published in the *American Journal of Psychiatry.* In 1936 there were sixty-seven schools of psychiatric nursing accredited by the American Psychiatric Association (Report of the Committee on Nursing of the American Psychiatric Association, 1936). Only in 1965 did the American Nurses' Association in a position paper on psychiatric nursing gain control of standards that had been under control of the American Psychiatric Association since 1906. It was 1968 before the American Psychiatric Association officially approved of education-centered institutions instead of hospital schools, for the education of nurses.

Treatment Approaches and Nursing Care. The idea of use of a drug to help the patient become more calm and communicative was introduced by Klaesi in 1922, and subsequently, in this country, narcosis therapy proved successful. Patients receiving this treatment were given sleeping medication periodically. It was given in dosages large enough to make the person sleepy but capable of being aroused for ambulation to the bathroom, and for eating, bathing, and so on. Patients receiving narcosis therapy required careful nursing care for positioning, safety needs, and other basic needs during the period of sedation, which usually lasted three to four days. Patients also required orientation to their surroundings and much guidance to carry out modified activities of daily living during the sleep period. This form of treatment is still widely used in the USSR. I once visited a large hospital in the Ukraine where fifteen to twenty patients were in one large room on metal cots under sleep therapy and the observation of numerous staff.

Insulin was also used during World War II and the late 1940s in some instances where patients were in acute anxiety states. In this case, subcoma therapy was used. Insulin has also been used to increase the appetite in the anorexic patient.

Metrazol shock as a convulsive agent was discovered by Ladislaus von Meduna (Hungarian) in 1935 and introduced in this country as a convulsive agent in 1937. Due to the terrifying apprehension preceding the convulsion and the introduction of electro-convulsive therapy, metrazol treatment fell into disfavor.

The use of insulin as hypoglycemic shock in the treatment of patients with mental problems was discovered by Manfred Sakel as he sought an agent to alleviate withdrawal symptoms in morphine addicts in 1933. It was introduced here by Cameron and Hoskins at Worcester State Hospital in 1936 (American Psychiatric Association, 1944). If patients were to have insulin shock treatment, a separate treatment unit was usually set up with trained staff in attendance for the duration of the treatment. Nurses were specially trained in the use of insulin therapy. In the early days of its use it was customary for a treatment team to go to Vienna and learn directly from Sakel himself. All the signs and symptoms of insulin shock and its phases had to be well known by the nurses who attended the patients in treatment. Insulin in very large doses was administered by the nurse or the physician. Patients were observed carefully by the nurses and the physician was also on hand at all times. Coma was terminated by gavage or intravenous administration of glucose and the patient was returned to his ward for lunch and the usual activities with the other patients. Careful observation of patients was required by nursing staff to prevent secondary insulin reactions. For example, a poor appetite and exercise might bring one on. Sometimes the secondary reaction occurred during sleep, so the night nurse was required to be especially vigilant. The patients themselves were usually required to be up early, have their vital signs taken, and go to the treatment unit between 6:00 and 6:30 A.M. They were also taught the signs and symptoms of insulin reaction and requested to report them at once. Patients might have anywhere from thirty to sixty comas in a course of treatment. Later, electroconvulsive treatment was combined with insulin for some patients. In these cases, the electroconvulsive treatment was given just before termination of the insulin coma. Patients might have insulin five to six days per week. Patients receiving insulin therapy received a great deal of attention from all the staff. Electroconvulsive treatment was first used in the treatment of patients with mental disorder in Italy in 1938 by Ugo Cerletti and Lucio Bini. (See Chap. 16 for discussion of ECT.)

During and after World War II, narcosynthesis was used to assist patients to relive a traumatic event. Administering an intravenous barbiturate to the patient in his own bed, the patient would be asked by the psychiatrist to recall and tell about a traumatic event. Nurses sat in on what was also termed the "Sodium Amytal interview," and monitored vital signs and the condition of the patient until the patient was free of the effects of the medication.

During this period, hydrotherapy was in wide use, for example, the continuous sedative tub with flowing water slightly under normal body temperature and the cold wet sheet pack. Steam baths, scotch douches, and salt rubs all found their therapeutic place. This era of the biological attack on mental disorder resembled the earlier "cult of curability," and some clinicians reported 90 percent of their patients to be cured by these treatments.

Occupational-therapy departments were incorporated into many psychiatric programs as the cure for mental disorder was sought. The objects that patients worked on in occupational therapy were termed "productions" and were often used in diagnosis. For example, embroidery work of the patient who could not follow a line might indicate general paresis. Definite times for occupational therapy were scheduled throughout the week and orders were written by the physician for this therapy with special reference to the occupational therapist for the kind of activity most therapeutic. Facilities in occupational-therapy departments usually included a kitchen, woodworking, metal, clay, sewing, embroidery, crocheting, finger painting, and the like. Social events such as teas were held in the occupational-therapy department for both patients and staff. Bibliotherapy and recreational therapy were also used during these times.

A General Hospital Psychiatric Unit. During this period patients in "psycho" wards in general hospitals were supervised closely; units were locked, for the most part, and all sharp items were removed from patients upon admission. Belongings of the patient were thoroughly searched and the patient was given a bath and a shampoo. If the patients were dependent upon drugs, in addition to the bath and shampoo, all body apertures were examined. Silverware and other objects useful on a ward living unit were considered sharp items and counted at the end of every shift along with the narcotics. Keys to these units were carefully controlled and all possessions of the patients were kept locked securely while the patients were dressed in hospital clothes. Objects considered harmful to patients were put on the "sharps" list to be counted and accounted for. Even bobby pins, sanitary belts, and shoestrings were listed in one psychiatric unit where I worked for a short time in 1950.

Life on the unit was organized for the patients with early rising, morning care, breakfast, medications, tests, and treatments, for example, ECT, IV vitamin therapy, or psychotherapy.

Complete neurological studies, including a spinal tap, were done on all patients as well as physical examinations, with the routine work-up of tests. Since tuberculosis was prevalent at that time, this kind of diagnostic work was important in case finding. One or two beds were available in the psychiatric unit for isolating patients with communicable disease. Patients sent in for observation and diagnosis were often found to have brain tumors. Pneumoencephalograms and EEG's were ordered for patients. Psychological testing was also available. Alcoholics in delirium tremens often had broken bones in casts.

Patients did play cards with each other and listened to the radio in the dayroom, which also served as a dining room at mealtime. Seclusion rooms were used for patients whose behavior could not be tolerated by the group and also for safety reasons since all other beds were the traditional high hospital beds. Leather restraints on wrists and ankles were used to keep patients in bed. All windows were covered with metal bars and the bathrooms and toilets were kept locked. Even the toothbrush cabinets were locked and used under supervision.

Patients were not allowed to use razors, they were shaved by the orderlies. In good weather those who were well enough might be permitted to go for a game or walk on the roof, which was caged in completely with heavy wire. In one such unit, the poor and the rich were in it together and the professors of psychiatry at the local university held rounds on the unit for the medical students and residents. Nursing students and the psychiatric nursing supervisor also attended these sessions. Principles of psychotherapy were emphasized. There was no one-to-one assignment of nursing care; all was done on a functional basis. However, certain patients were "specialled"; for example, patients receiving malarial treatment, narcosis therapy, insulin, and those who were in seclusion received more attention in terms of time. Careful recording was done on all patients and any new treatment was carefully scrutinized.

Although they were not officially recognized as such, one-to-one nurse patient relationships were developed with patients who were recovering and who might be helping the nurse with various tasks, for example, folding the sheets for the cold wet sheet packs (Paynter, 1974).

A State Hospital. One state hospital in the mid-1940s with a population of fifteen hundred patients had at most a nursing staff of six, few physicians, and one occupational therapist. Most patient-care was done by attendants. Situated on the outskirts of a town, the hospital grew its own food and patients who were trusted not to elope could volunteer to work in the fields supervised by attendants. The superintendent insisted on the patients attending the annual county fair, a big outdoor event in which selected patients and staff went together in buses chartered for the event. In the hospital itself, patients were segregated by sex and degree of disturbance. Fire drill was held routinely on all wards but was of special importance in one two-story building. In this building, from the women's disturbed ward, the fire escape was a large metal winding and sloping tube down which patients and staff slid to a locked courtyard. Assaultive and combative patients were released from their strait jackets to go down the tube.

Catatonic patients had literally to be pushed down. Bed patients were also kept on this disturbed, locked unit and nursing staff were concentrated there. A stretcher crew was supposed to come for them in case of fire. The very high ceilings of the old building with tall windows that were covered on the inside with locked steel mesh shutters guaranteed plenty of daylight but suicidal patients had to be watched closely lest they hang themselves on the gratings with their long cotton stockings. Patients who refused to eat were tube fed by the nurses. As a student, I was alone on the evening shift in this ward, when a medically ill patient died. After notification of the proper individuals and preparation of the body, I requested the stretcher crew. Because I was the only one on duty, I requested an oriented and better integrated patient to watch the other patients and use the telephone in case of emergency. (Because it was wartime, some wards *had no staff* and one patient might be designated by the supervisor to watch the patients and to use the telephone.)

In order to get the stretcher crew, I had to go a long distance across the hospital to the men's catatonic ward for the four, nonverbal, catatonic, sleepy men patients with their hand-carried stretcher. Because women were not allowed on that ward, seeing the ward from the doorway, was an event itself. When patients on that ward were in the dayroom they were required by the attendant to sit in a designated chair. I was given a large ring of enormous keys for the morgue and assured by the attendant that the patients knew exactly what to do and what keys fit particular doors. Returning to the women's ward for the body, the men patients created quite a stir because they were the only men allowed on the ward except the physician. The morgue was reached by going down stairs and through what seemed like endless miles of a dark underground tunnel lighted only by the beam of a flashlight. True enough, without saying a word, the patients knew exactly what to do.

At this hospital, women nursing personnel were not permitted on the men's wards nor were men nursing personnel permitted on the women's wards except in selected instances where the ward charge attendant agreed. On one such ward, a manic patient, a muscular, tall lumberjack was so excited that it took four attendants with the use of the firehose to get him under control. After a few days of sedation, he was working in the hospital kitchen. On this same ward, one attendant and one student often took as many as forty patients on a hike on the hospital acreage. It was difficult to keep track of forty people; the head attendant was philosophical and said, "If someone elopes, there is no place to go except home and *they'll* bring him back!"

Electroconvulsive treatment (referred to as shock) was administered in a separate building and treatment room. As many as twenty to thirty patients would be crowded in the waiting room and taken in for the treatment one by one. The superintendent psychiatrist and the superintendent of nurses administered the treatment and afterward patients were placed on mattresses on the floor in the same room for safety because there was no other staff to watch them. Patients who awakened after the treatment might observe the treatment of his fellow patients. The thinking was that it was better for the patient to know what happened during the treatment. One student was assigned to sit with the women patients in the waiting room, play cards or checkers with them in attempts to be reassuring, and one would observe in the treatment room itself.

Occupational therapy was well equipped in this hospital, and patients made items used in the hospital itself. Students rotated through designated wards, one at a time and also were assigned to occupational therapy to learn the handcrafts.

During these times all nursing care was performed on a functional basis. Patients lined up for meals and bathed on a designated day. Getting clothes, haircuts, oral care, medications, mental-status examinations, and so on, all were done by lining up. All ward cleaning was done by the patients and nursing personnel. Patients slept in large dormitories that were locked during the day; subsequently, patients were crowded into small dayrooms furnished with indestructible heavy oak benches. Patients wore clothes made and furnished to them by the hospital. Each ward had its small, locked clothes room for personal clothing of the patient. Strict accounting for all items owned by the patient was kept by the nursing staff on a clothes list placed on the patient's chart. The patients who were permitted to have visitors on Sunday were dressed in their own clothes and taken to a visitor's room off the ward and supervised.

During the era of biological attack on mental disorder it must be said that the influence of psychoanalysis became widespread and the movement was a factor in linking up psychiatry and general medicine, and psychosomatic medicine appeared. Psychotherapy became fully established as a psychiatric treatment. Although psychiatry was divided into the biological approach to treatment and the psychological approach, the two approaches were often combined.

Other Influences.   Paving the way for requirement of psychiatric nursing in the basic nursing program as essential for accreditation, accreditation of nursing schools by the profession itself began in 1939 (Dolan, 1978).

In California, the first registered nurse to be named to the post of superintendent of nurses in a state hospital was Corinne Parsons, of the Langley Porter Clinic, in 1942. This clinic was a small, one-hundred-bed psychiatric hospital located adjacent to a large university hospital and medical center and was organized primarily for the purposes of research and teaching.

In the mid-forties, the Bolton Act provided financial assistance for nurses to study advanced psychiatric nursing and courses of study were offered in a few universities as postgraduate courses for registered nurses.

The new mental-health crusade began in the minds of the framers of the National Mental Health Act of 1946 (see Fig. 24). This Act provided grants for state and private institutions for construction and for research. Through this Act, the National Institute of Mental Health (NIMH) was established in 1949. The purpose of NIMH was

To develop forward looking, useful programs that provide real specialists in the field—clinically competent people—to take care of the men-

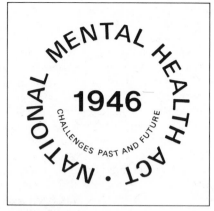

FIGURE 24.   National Mental Health Act.

tally ill, to do research in the field, to get at causes of mental illness and to deliver services.[13]

NIMH provided assistance in the development of state and community mental-health services, training of personnel, and research. Under the leadership of Esther Garrison, these grants gave impetus to the preparation and upgrading of psychiatric nursing, including master's programs.[14]

At the same time, conditions in the state hospitals had deteriorated to a new low and were well documented by Albert Deutsch (1948), who was responsible for exposing many of the very bad conditions over the nation. Thirteen state hospitals did not have a single registered nurse (Anderson, 1950). Conscientious objectors who had done their time in mental hospitals instead of in military service brought many of these conditions to light. State hospitals had become warehouses and catchalls for people not wanted in the counties.

Psychoanalysis.   Freud's discovery of infantile sexuality revolutionized child psychology. The discovery of the roots of adult

[13] Interview with Esther A. Garrison, San Francisco, 17 July 1974.

[14] For the celebration of the twenty-fifth anniversary of the enactment of the National Mental Health Act, a Special Recognition Mental Health Award was presented to Esther A. Garrison to honor distinguished achievement in the mental-health field. It cited that "since the inception of the national mental health program, she has provided innovative and vigorous leadership in the field of psychiatric nursing education."

behavior in early childhood helped us to better understand the behavior of individuals with mental disorder and gave an impetus to the psychological aspects of psychiatric treatment. Freud's structural and topographical theories of the mind gave new directions to treatment approaches. Transference, countertransference, and resistance, conceptualized by Freud as operating in psychoanalysis, have aided psychiatric mental-health nursing to move from orientation to procedures to psychotherapy. Much psychotic behavior was clarified because of the understanding of the behavior afforded by the constructs of psychoanalysis. Concepts from psychoanalysis, for example, anxiety, drives, catharsis, conflict, and mental mechanism have become so integrated into psychiatric mental-health nursing that their origin has perhaps been forgotten.

The holocaust in Europe and the annihilation of millions of Jews resulted in immigration to the English-speaking world of many psychoanalysts, including Freud himself. These individuals greatly influenced the practice of psychiatry in the United States and psychiatric nursing as well. Psychoanalytic institutes were established in large urban centers and became influential in psychiatry. Some psychiatric nurses themselves were psychoanalyzed.

IN THE 1950s

The nurse must have a thorough knowledge of psychopathology and theoretical knowledge of the various methods and technics employed in psychotherapy; specialized training as to her part in the psychotherapeutic program can then proceed. (Bennett and Carter, 1950, p. 6)

Gwen Tudor's classic study provided a perspective on the interpersonal relations of nurses with patients and personnel, the social structure of a psychiatric ward, and the interaction of these forces with regard to the problem of mutual withdrawal of patients and staff (1952).

Only in the early 1950s was psychiatric nursing required for all NLN accredited schools of nursing in the United States.

Meetings and conferences on a national level were held to stimulate growth of educational programs and better care for patients. Participants in one such meeting are shown in Figure 25.

Mental-health and psychiatric-nursing consultants at local, state, regional, and national levels met to discuss issues in order to improve the care of psychiatric patients, especially in the state hospitals (see Fig. 26). Most participants in these conferences were mental health and/or psychiatric nurses but a few were from other fields (Crawford, 1974).

Integration of Psychiatric Mental-Health Nursing. The National Institute of Mental Health funded studies for the integration of psychiatric mental-health nursing concepts in the generic nursing curricula of baccalaureate (and other) schools of nursing during the 1950s and 1960s. These projects were efforts to provide nurses with the knowledge, understandings, and skills to assist patients in all areas of nursing practice as well as the psychiatric mental-health nursing field. The National League for Nursing held many regional conferences on psychiatric-nursing education for the purpose of helping faculty to identify and integrate these concepts. Attention was called to the emotional needs of patients and of nursing students as well. Individual differences of patients were stressed, as were psychodynamics, personality development, group interaction, and the ability of the nurse to respond to the needs of patients. Individual needs of students, their strengths, weaknesses, and self-understanding received emphasis (National League for Nursing, 1958). These integration projects assisted in changing procedure-centered nursing to a person-centered comprehensive approach. They also contributed to the conceptual approach to curricular design. Because many faculty had graduated from schools of nursing that did not offer psychiatric nursing, the integration projects served as a stimulus for them to return to school and, for the first time, take classes in psychiatric nursing (Carter, 1978).

Move Toward Graduate Preparation. At a national level, a major priority in psy-

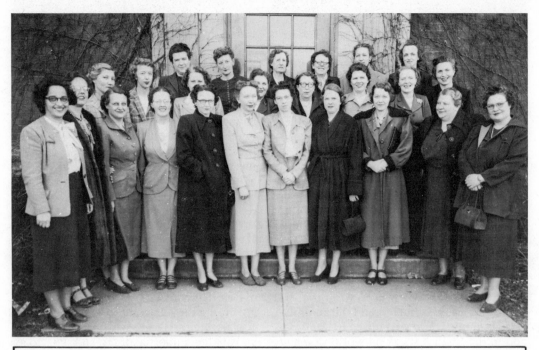

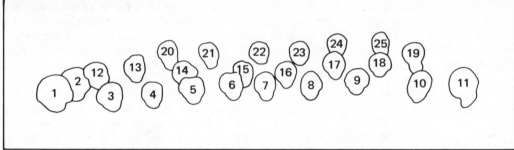

FIGURE 25. Participants in Conference on Advanced Psychiatric Nursing and Mental Hygiene Programs at the Center for Continuation Study, University of Minnesota, Minneapolis Minnesota, April 3–14, 1950. Key to schematic: 1. Ceceila Lediger, University of Minnesota; 2. Kathleen Black, Menninger Foundation; 3. Lavonne M. Frey, University of Pittsburgh; 4. Tirzah Morgan, University of Washington; 5. Esther E. Garrison, United States Public Health Service; 6. Gwen Tudor, University of Iowa; 7. Louise Moser, Duke University; 8. Mary Schmitt, National League of Nursing Education; 9. Virginia P. Crenshaw, Vanderbilt University; 10. Pearl Shalit, United States Public Health Service; 11. Martha Brown, Washington University; 12. Helen Bowditch, University of Minnesota; 13. Vivian Hansen, University of Colorado; 14. Sonia Landry, Lousiana State University; 15. Winifred Gibson, Boston University; 16. Clara M. Gilchrist, University of Cincinnati; 17. Mary M. Redmond, Catholic University; 18. Anna McQuada, Catholic University; 19. Helen Hess, Adelphi College; 20. Helen J. Weber, University of Indiana; 21. Marion Russell, Yale University; 22. Elizabeth K. Porter, Western Reserve University; 23. Ruth Von Bergen, University of Minnesota; 24. Marion E. Kalkman, University of California; 25. Hildegard E. Peplau, Teachers College. Margaret S. Taylor was present but not in the photograph.

chiatric nursing in the 1950s was toward clinically oriented, master's degree programs for nurses. The National Institute of Mental Health provided many grants to education and research. This financing made the move toward graduate preparation and clinical specialization in psychiatric nursing a reality. Discussion of a specialty board in psychiatric nursing to examine and to certify psychiatric nurses occurred at the Williams-

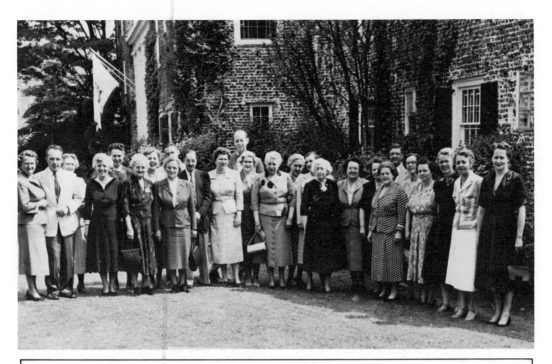

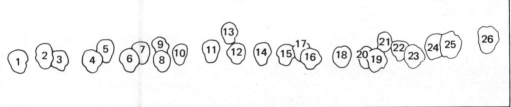

FIGURE 26. Institute for Nursing Consultants in Psychiatry, Princeton Inn, Princeton, New Jersey, May 26–29, 1954. Key to schematic: 1. Lavonne M. Frey; 2. Alphonse Sootkoos; 3. Mary Spare; 4. Lillian Salsman; 5. Margaret McConvey; 6. Laura Fitzsimmons; 7. Cecelia Abraham; 8. Florence Newell; 9. George Mason; 10. Dr. H. Beckett Lang; 11. Mary Redmond; 12. Josephine Lamb; 13. Clifford Lobel; 14. Elsie Ogilvie; 15. Theresa Muller; 16. Mary Corcoran; 17. Dorothy Hall; 18. Katharine Steele; 19. Isabel Reardon; 20. Annie Hall; 21. Daniel Blain, M.D.; 22. Kathleen Black; 23. Genevieve Noble; 24. Annine Laurie Crawford; 25. Geraldine Shoop; 26. Laura Fair.

burg conference; however, it was considered to be too soon to implement such a board (National Working Conference, 1958).

Rise of Multidimensional Approach. During this era, psychiatry became strongly influenced by the social sciences and psychiatric nurses in higher education were likely to study social sciences in their curriculum. Anthropologists and sociologists studied the organization of and interaction in mental hospitals. Psychiatric nursing concepts were considered incomplete without viewing the

patient within the context of his total environment. "Sociopsychological" needs of patients were discussed, sociopsychiatric studies conducted, and ways sought to improve the social system of the mental hospital. The effect of conflicts among the staff received wide attention.

Influenced by the public-health point of view, interest in human ecology and mental disorder arose and the effect on the individual of a peak load of stresses from the environment itself received attention in psychiatry. No longer was the intrapsychic point of view considered sufficient in evaluation of the problem of the patient. In addition to the biophysical aspects, culturological and sociological factors were added to the psychological aspects of the patient and all dimensions evaluated.

At the same time, large numbers of patients in state hospitals were still being cared for by psychiatric aides. Although state hospitals employed registered nurses for the general medical–surgical units, few were involved in other aspects of care. Despite the advances in treatment, patients were still being institutionalized for long periods, and once the patient remained in a state hospital for two or two and one-half years his hopes of ever getting out had rapidly diminished.

After the discovery of the antipsychotic drugs in the 1950s, many patients who were chronically psychotic—and others as well—were helped by them. Excited patients were calmed by these drugs and the result was an entirely different atmosphere in psychiatric units. Patients became more free of the terrifying fears, hallucinations, and delusions of the psychotic state and were able to participate in social events and to care for themselves. Now, instead of keeping excited patients in sedative baths and cold wet sheet packs, nurses took blood pressures and gave phenothiazines. Hydrotherapy departments disappeared, occupational and recreational therapy took an upswing, the concept of the therapeutic community was accepted in many institutions, locked wards were opened, patient councils were formed, staff became trained in group psychotherapy, and group nursing and one-to-one nurse–patient relationship therapy were organized and accepted.

COMMUNITY MENTAL HEALTH: 1960s AND 1970s

A new philosophy emerged in which institutionalization was clearly held to add to the problems of the mental patient instead of assisting the patient toward recovery. It held to the tenets of primary, secondary, and tertiary prevention; that is, that mental disorder could be prevented, that earlier case finding and early treatment would help reduce suffering and that rehabilitation could best occur within the home community of the patient. Thus, the ill effects of

institutionalization could be circumvented and patients would have less debilitating effects from mental disorders if treated earlier.

In 1955, an appropriation was made by the Congress to study the problem of mental disorder in the United States, to be conducted by the Joint Commission on Mental Illness and Health. The work of this group was published in 1961. The purpose of the study was to arrive at a program that would meet the needs of the mental patient. The report urged the treatment of the mental patient in his home community by a wide network of services, apportionment of funds for basic research in addition to applied research, securing the interest of young scientists in mental-health research, treatment of patients by appropriately trained individuals as opposed to quacks, wider use of parapsychiatric personnel in the treatment of mental patients, recruitment, education, and training of personnel, and providing funds at federal, state, and local levels to carry out a program for meeting the national emergency.

In order to implement the recommendations of the Joint Commission, President Kennedy sent a message to Congress asking for a bold, new approach. He said:

Under this legislation, custodial mental institutions will be replaced by therapeutic centers. It should be possible, within a decade or so, to reduce the number of patients in mental institutions by 50 percent or more. The new law provides the tools with which we can accomplish this.

Subsequently, the Mental Retardation Facilities and Community Mental Health Centers Construction Act (Public Law 88–164) and its amendments have provided financing for community mental-health centers and for staffing. As late as 1978, 647 centers were operating; another 57 funded; and an estimated 14 centers approved but unfunded.

During the past fifteen years, progress has been made toward fulfillment of the national commitment to community mental-health services. Community mental-health programs have contributed significantly to providing comprehensive services in local communities. However, in 1976, over 50 percent of the total expenditures for mental-health services were not for community mental-health programs but for services in nursing homes and public mental hospitals (President's Commission on Mental Health, Vol. I, 1978, p. 4).

Many individuals still are unserved or underserved; children, adolescents, older people, the poor, racial and ethnic minorities, and those who live in rural areas. Personnel shortages are still a problem despite the addition of thousands to the delivery system.

The *Standards of Psychiatric-Mental Health Nursing Practice* state clearly the functions of psychiatric mental-health nursing (American Nurses' Association, 1973) (see Appendix E).

In 1972, a Society of Certified Clinical Specialists in Psychiatric Nursing was founded within the New Jersey State Nurses' Association. In 1974, a Council of Advanced Practitioners in Psychiatric and Mental Health Nursing was formed within the American Nurses' Association. During 1979, the name of this group was changed to the Council of Specialists in Psychiatric-Mental Health Nursing. The First National Conference of the Council of Advanced Practitioners in Psychiatric and Mental Health Nursing was held November 11 and 12, 1974, at Atlanta, Georgia. It centered on quality development, history, and specialist certification issues. Clinical papers were presented on child psychiatric nursing, family therapy, private practice, crisis intervention, and drug and alcohol abuse. The council has taken leadership in specialist certification, third-party payment, and other issues. The American Nurses' Association now recognizes two levels of psychiatric mental-health nursing practice: (1) the psychiatric mental-health nurse generalist, and (2) the psychiatric mental-health nursing specialist (American Nurses' Association, 1976). In the interest of professional standards and accountability, both generalist and specialist credentialing in psychiatric mental-health nursing are now available within the profession itself. For the generalist, the baccalaureate degree in nursing is recommended. In addition, two years of practice in the field as a registered nurse and current practice are required. Through a formal review process by colleagues, the profession now certifies applicants who meet the standards set forth by the profession. For the psychiatric mental-health nursing specialist, the minimum level of preparation is a master's degree in psychiatric mental-health nursing. The specialist in psychiatric mental-health nursing must demonstrate a high degree of expertise in the field. Three major subspecialties are now recognized: (1) child, (2) adult, and (3) gerontological psychiatric mental-health nursing.

Graduate programs in psychiatric mental-health nursing are now well established in universities and preparation at the doctoral level is well under way. The first doctorate of nursing-science program in psychiatric nursing was developed at Boston University with the assistance of a five-year grant from the National Institute of Mental Health. It was officially approved in May, 1960. The first doctorate to be awarded in nursing came from the discipline of nursing therapy (Mellow, 1965).

The role of the psychiatric mental-health nurse is very diverse. No longer confined to mental institutions, psychiatric mental-health nurses are now involved in primary, secondary, and tertiary prevention. Psychiatric mental-health nurses do initial assessments of patients, determine the need for hospitalization or other referrals, and sign the necessary papers. They head home visiting teams and are primary therapists. They establish and maintain the therapeutic milieu in varied treatment areas, administer and monitor medications, monitor physical health, and provide appropriate nursing care for concomitant physical problems and do health teaching. Psychiatric mental-health nurses are involved in counseling and social-action work. They also coordinate and supervise the work of others. Psychiatric mental-health nurses also help develop supportive systems for patients and are involved in program planning and evaluation. Psychotherapy (individual, group, and family) is now practiced by psychiatric mental-health nurses who have advanced specialized experience. Psychiatric mental-health nurses may also be in the liaison role or the role of administrator, supervisor, educator, consultant, and researcher. A nationwide study by Jacobs (1973) showed that psychiatric mental-health nurses with higher education tended to be employed in community mental-health centers rather than hospitals. Many psychiatric mental-health nurses are now in private practice and the profession is pushing for third-party payments.

Summary

In this chapter, some aspects of practices in the care of mental patients in England and the United States during the past two hundred years have been described. An attempt has been made to present the emergence of psychiatric mental-health nursing as a profession and some major forces influencing its development.

What psychiatric nurses do, will do in the future, and have done in the past is influenced by the political and institutional social systems in which the care of mental patients is placed. The prevailing philosophy of treatment, concepts of etiology of mental disorder, and the expertise of the nurse all influence the nurse's role and derive from the culture, level of education, intellectual influences, and economic development of society.

References

AMERICAN JOURNAL OF INSANITY, edited by the Officers of the New York State Lunatic Asylum. Utica: Bennett, Backus and Haley, 1844.

AMERICAN NURSES' ASSOCATION: *Standards: Psychiatric-Mental Nursing Practice.* Kansas City, Mo.: American Nurses' Association, 1973.

————: *Statement on Psychiatric and Mental Health Nursing Practice.* Kansas City, Mo.: American Nurses' Association, 1976.

AMERICAN PSYCHIATRIC ASSOCIATION: "Report of the Committee on Nursing," *American Journal of Psychiatry,* 93:463, 1936.

————: *One Hundred Years of American Psychiatry.* New York: Columbia University Press, 1944.

ANDERSON, LELA S.: "Human Factors Involved in Providing Better Nursing Treatment and Care of Patients in Mental Hospitals," *American Journal of Psychiatry,* 106:7:786–90, January 1950.

BAILEY, HARRIET: *Nursing Mental and Nervous Diseases.* New York: The Macmillan Co., 1920.

BEERS, CLIFFORD WHITTINGHAM: *A Mind That Found Itself.* New York: Longmans, Green, 1908.

BENNETT, A. E., and CARTER, FRANCES MONET: "The Role of the Nurse in the Newer Therapies," presented at The Round Table Discussion on Psychiatric Nursing, American Psychiatric Association, Detroit, Michigan, May 2, 1950.

BERMOSK, LORETTA, and MORDAN, MARY JANE: *Interviewing in Nursing.* New York: Macmillan Publishing Co., Inc., 1964.

THE BETHLEM ROYAL HOSPITAL AND THE MAUDSLEY HOSPITAL. London: Tollit and Harvey, Ltd., 50–52 Union St., S.E.I.

BLEDSTEIN, BURTON J.: *The Culture of Professionalism: The Middle Class and the Development of Higher Education in America.* New York: W. W. Norton and Co., Inc., 1976.

BROCKETT, L. P.: *The Camp, The Battlefield, and the Hospital; or, Lights and Shadows of the Great Rebellion.* Chicago, Ill., and St. Louis, Mo.: National Publishing Co., 1866.

CARTER, FRANCES MONET: "Public Mental Health Services of San Francisco," Study made as a member of the League of Women Voters, August 1961.

————: "History of Psychiatric Nursing Since World War II," San Francisco, Calif., 1976. (Typrewritten.)

————: *Psychiatric Mental Health Nursing Curriculum in Generic, Baccalaureate Programs Accredited by the National League for Nursing in the United States.* (Ed. D. Dissertation, University of San Francisco, 1978).

COMMITTEE FOR THE STUDY OF NURSING EDUCATION: *Nursing and Nursing Education in the United States.* New York: The Macmillan Company, 1923.

COMMITTEE ON THE GRADING OF NURSING SCHOOLS: *Nursing Schools Today and Tomorrow.* New York: Committee on the Grading of Nursing Schools, 1934.

CRAWFORD, ANNIE LAURIE: Yorktown, Virginia. Interview 24 July, 1974.

DAIN, NORMAN: *Concepts of Insanity in the United States, 1789–1865.* New Brunswick, N.J.: Rutgers University Press, 1964.

————: *Disordered Minds: The First Century of Eastern State Hospital in Williamsburg, Virginia, 1766–1866.* Williamsburg, Va.: The Colonial Williamsburg Foundation, 1971.

DEUTSCH, ALBERT: *The Mentally Ill in America.* Garden City, N.Y.: Doubleday, Doran & Co., Inc., 1937.

————: *The Shame of the States.* New York: Harcourt, Brace & Co., 1948.

DOLAN, JOSEPHINE: *Nursing in Society: A Historical Perspective.* Philadelphia: W. B. Saunders Co., 1978.

EVANS, FRANCES MONET CARTER: "Nursing Education for New Roles," Paper presented at the American Psychiatric Association, Mental Hospital Institute, 1965.

————: *The Role of the Nurse in Community Mental Health.* New York: Macmillan Publishing Co., Inc., 1968.

FAVREAU, CLAIRE H.: "Existing Needs in Psychiatric Nursing," *American Journal of Nursing,* 45:9:716, September 1945.

FITZSIMMONS, LAURA: "Report of a Survey of Nursing in Mental Hospitals in the U.S. and Ontario, Canada," *American Journal of Psychiatry,* 100:9:625, March 1944.

FRANKFORD ASYLUM: *44th Annual Report on the State of the Asylum for the Relief of Persons Deprived of the Use of their Reason.* Philadelphia: William K. Bellows, 1861.

FRANKFORD ASYLUM REPORTS 1862–1886; 1887–1902.

FRIENDS ASYLUM FOR THE INSANE 1813–1913. Press of the John C. Winston Co., Philadelphia, Penn.

GARRISON, ESTHER A.: San Francisco, Calif. Interview, 17 July 1974.

GOODNOW, MINNIE: *Outline of Nursing History.* 6th ed. Philadelphia: W. B. Saunders, 1938.

GROB, GERALD N.: *The State and the Mentally Ill.* Chapel Hill, N.C.: University of North Carolina Press, 1966.

HAYS, SAMUEL P.: "Introduction—The New Organizational Society," in Israel, Jerry, ed.: *Building the Organizational Society.* New York: The Free Press, 1972, pp. 1–17.

ISRAEL, JERRY, ed.: *Building the Organizational Society.* New York: The Free Press, 1972.

JACOBS, ANGELINE MARCHESE, BROTZ, CAROL A., and GAMEL, NONA N.: *Critical Behaviors in Psychiatric-Mental Health Nursing.* Palo Alto, Calif.: American Institutes for Research, 1973.

JOINT COMMISSION ON MENTAL ILLNESS AND HEALTH: *Action for Mental Health.* New York: Basic Books, Inc., 1961, p. xvi.

KALKMAN, MARION E.: *Introduction to Psychiatric Nursing.* New York: McGraw-Hill Book Co., Inc., 1950.

KURTZ, ELLA B.: "Report of Committee on Care of Insane," *American Journal of Nursing,* XVI:198–202, December 1916.

MELLOW, JUNE: "The Evolution of Nursing Therapy and its Implications for Education," #65–9538, Boston University School of Education, Ed.D., Health Sciences, Nursing (Dissertation), 1965.

MULLER, THERESA GRACE: *The Nature and Direction of Psychiatric Nursing: The Dynamics of Human Relationships in Nursing.* Philadelphia: J. B. Lippincott, Co., 1950.

NAPA STATE HOSPITAL: *Rules and Regulations Governing the Conduct of Employees in the Care of Patients of the Napa State Hospital.* Imola, Calif.: The Imola Printery, 1921.

NATIONAL LEAGUE OF NURSING EDUCATION: *Standard Curriculum for Schools of Nursing.* Baltimore: Waverly Press, 1917.

————: *Concepts of the Behavioral Sciences in Basic Nursing Education,* Proceedings of the 1958 Regional Conferences on Psychiatric Nursing Education. New York: National League for Nursing, 1958.

NATIONAL WORKING CONFERENCE: *The Education of the Clinical Specialist in Psychiatric Nursing.* New York: National League for Nursing, 1958.

ORLANDO, IDA JEAN: *The Dynamic Nurse–Patient Relationship: Function, Process and Principles.* New York: G. P. Putnam's Sons, 1961.

PAYNTER, JANE: San Francisco, Calif. Interview. 7 July 1974.

PEPLAU, HILDEGARD E.: *Interpersonal Relations in Nursing.* New York: G. P. Putnam's Sons, 1952.

PRESIDENT'S COMMISSION ON MENTAL HEALTH: *Report to the President.* Vols. I and II. Washington, D.C.: U.S. Government Printing Office, 1978.

RICHARDS, LINDA: *Reminiscences of America's First Trained Nurse.* Boston: Whitcomb & Barrows, 1915.

SANTOS, ELVIN, and STAINBROOK, EDWARD: "A History of Psychiatric Nursing in the Nineteenth Century," *Journal of the History of Medicine and Applied Sciences,* IV:48–74, Winter 1949.

State of an Institution Near York Called the Retreat for Persons Afflicted with Disorders of the Mind, 1864 (no publisher given).

STEELE, KATHARINE MCLEAN: *Psychiatric Nursing.* Philadelphia: F. A. Davis, 1937.

————: Salem, Oregon. Interview, 10 August 1972.

TUKE, DANIEL HACK: *The Insane in the U.S. and Canada.* London: H. K. Lewis, 1885.

TUKE, D. HACK, M.D., LL.D.: *Reform in the Treatment of the Insane. Early History of the Retreat, York; Its Objects and Influence, with a Report of the Celebrations of Its Centenary.* London: J.&A. Churchill, 1892.

TUKE, SAMUEL: "A Re-Print of 'Practical Hints' by Samuel Tuke, Philanthropist and Reformer, Extracted from an Original Document Printed in 1819 Concerning the Building of Wakefield Asylum," Stanley Royd Hospital, Wakefield, Yorkshire.

WEINER, DORA, B.: "The Apprenticeship of Philippe Pinel: A New Document, 'Observations of Citizen Pussin on the Insane,' " *American Journal of Psychiatry,* **136**:9:1128–1134, September 1979.

WIEBE, ROBERT H.: *The Search for Order.* New York: Hill and Wang, 1967.

YORK RETREAT REPORTS. York: John L. Linney, 15, Low Ousegate, 1846, 1874, 1875, 1883, 1887, 1894, 1903, 1909, 1921.

Suggested Readings

AMERICAN NURSES ASSOCIATION: *Professional Development in Psychiatric amd Mental Health Nursing.* Kansas City, Mo.: American Nurses Association, 1967.

CARINI, ESTA, DOUGLAS, DOROTHY M., HECK, LOIS, D., and PEARSON, MARGUERITE: *The Mentally Ill in Connecticut: Changing Patterns of Care and the Evolution of Psychatric Nursing. 1636–1972.* State of Connecticut, Department of Mental Health, 1974.

CHURCH, OLGA M. and BUCKWALTER, KATHLEEN COEN: "Harriet Bailey—A Psychiatric Nurse Pioneer," *Perspectives in Psychiatric Care,* **28**:2:62–66, March/April 1980.

GARRISON, ESTHER A., ed.: *Doctoral Preparation for Nurses: With Emphasis on the Psychiatric Field.* School of Nursing, University of California, San Francisco, 1973.

HOLCOMBE, LEE: *Victorian Ladies at Work: Middle Class Working Women in England and Wales, 1850–1914.* Hamden, Conn.: The Shoe String Press, Inc., 1973.

HUEY, FLORENCE (compiler): *Psychiatric Nursing 1946 to 1974: A Report on the State of the Art.* New York: American Journal of Nursing Co., 1975.

HUNTER, RICHARD A.: "The Rise and Fall of Mental Nursing," *The Lancet,* **1**:98, January 14, 1956.

KALKMAN, MARION E., and DAVIS, ANNE J., eds.: *New Dimensions in Mental Health-Psychiatric Nursing.* New York: McGraw-Hill, 1974, pp. 3–30.

MCLAUGHLIN, FRANK E., and GARRISON, ESTHER A.: "Issues in Doctoral Education: Interrelationship of Research, Clinical Practicum, and Cognate Courses in Doctoral Education of Nurses," in Garrison, Esther A., ed.: *Doctoral Preparation for Nurses . . . Emphasis on the Psychiatric Field.* San Francisco: University of California, 1973.

RIDENOUR, NINA: *Mental Health in the U.S.: A Fifty-Year History.* Cambridge, Mass.: Harvard University Press, 1961.

SILLS, GRAYCE M.: "Historical Development and Issues in Psychiatric Mental Health Nursing," in Leininger, Madeleine M., ed.: *Contemporary Issues in Mental Health Nursing.* Boston: Little, Brown & Co., 1973, pp. 125–36.

SOLOMON, HARRY C.: "The American Psychiatric Association in Relation to American Psychiatry," *American Journal of Psychiatry,* **115**:1–9, July 1958.

Developmental Tasks from Infancy Through Later Maturity[1]

Infancy and Early Childhood (Birth to 6 Years)

1. Learning to walk
2. Learning to take solid foods
3. Learning to talk
4. Learning to control the elimination of body wastes
5. Learning sex differences and sexual modesty
6. Achieving physiological stability
7. Forming simple concepts of social and physical reality
8. Learning to relate oneself emotionally to parents, siblings, and other people
9. Learning to distinguish right and wrong and developing a conscience

Middle Childhood (6 to 12 Years)

1. Learning physical skills necessary for ordinary games
2. Building wholesome attitudes toward oneself as a growing organism
3. Learning to get along with age-mates
4. Learning an appropriate masculine or feminine social role
5. Developing fundamental skills in reading, writing, and calculating
6. Developing concepts necessary for everyday living
7. Developing conscience, morality, and a scale of values

[1] Havighurst, Robert J.: *Human Development and Education.* New York: Longmans, Green & Co., Inc., 1953, by permission, New York, David McKay Co., Inc. These tasks represent a maturity-expectancy score for the given periods.

8. Achieving personal independence
9. Developing attitudes toward social groups and institutions

Adolescence (12 to 18 Years)

1. Achieving new and more mature relations with age-mates of both sexes
2. Achieving a masculine or feminine social role
3. Accepting one's physique and using the body effectively
4. Achieving emotional independence of parents and other adults
5. Achieving assurance of economic independence
6. Selecting and preparing for an occupation
7. Preparing for marriage and family life
8. Developing intellectual skills and concepts necessary for civic competence
9. Desiring and achieving socially responsible behavior
10. Acquiring a set of values and an ethical system as a guide to behavior

Early Adulthood (18 to 35 Years)

1. Selecting a mate
2. Learning to live with a marriage partner
3. Starting a family
4. Rearing children
5. Managing a home
6. Getting started in an occupation
7. Taking on civic responsibility
8. Finding a congenial social group

Middle Age (35 to 60 Years)

1. Achieving adult civic and social responsibility
2. Establishing and maintaining an economic standard of living
3. Assisting teenage children to become responsible and happy adults
4. Developing adult leisure-time activities
5. Relating oneself to one's spouse as a person
6. Accepting and adjusting to the physiological changes of middle age
7. Adjusting to aging parents

Later Maturity (60 and Older)

1. Adjusting to decreasing physical strength and health
2. Adjusting to retirement and reduced income
3. Adjusting to death of spouse
4. Establishing an explicit affiliation with one's age group
5. Meeting social and civic obligation
6. Establishing satisfactory physical living arrangements

Glossary[1]

How does the ego maintain balance? Coping behavior helps people in their everyday existence. However, when individuals encounter conflicts and unhappy painful feelings, the mechanisms of defense come forward. Defense mechanisms operate unconsciously; they often occur together in an effort to protect the ego from the pain of awareness of unacceptable conflicts and unhappy, painful feelings. These mechanisms may in some way, therefore, distort reality.

Avoidance. A defense mechanism involving an active turning away from conflict-laden thoughts, objects, or experiences. In addition, *compliance* avoids issues by passive surrender and is thus similar to *avoidance.*

Compensation. A defense mechanism in which the individual attempts to make up for real or imagined deficiencies. (Compensation may also be a conscious process.)

Conversion. A defense mechanism in which intrapsychic conflicts are given symbolic external expression. The repressed conflict becomes a psychogenic paralysis; for example, a patient with an unconscious death wish toward her husband lost the use of her legs.

Denial. A defense mechanism, operating unconsciously, in which conflict and anxiety are resolved by disavowing thoughts, feelings, wishes, needs, or other reality factors that are consciously intolerable.

Displacement. An unconscious defense mechanism in which an emotion is transferred from its original object to a more acceptable substitute.

[1] Defense mechanisms mentioned in the text of this book are included here, together with additional ones for the convenience of reference. This is not a definitive list but represents common defenses.

Dissociation. A defense mechanism where emotional importance and affect are separated and detached from an idea, situation, or object. Dissociation may defer or postpone experiencing emotional impact as in selective amnesia. For example, a patient whose daughter was killed in an automobile accident where he was the driver at fault could not remember the details of the accident or her death.

Idealization. An individual overestimates an admired aspect or attribute of another person. This is commonly seen in older patients with unresolved grief and mourning who cannot say anything but praise about the deceased spouse.

Identification. A defense mechanism operating unconsciously by which an individual attempts to pattern himself after another. It is to be differentiated from imitation, which is a conscious process.

Incorporation. A defense mechanism in which the psychic representation of a person or parts of him are figuratively ingested. An example is the infantile fantasy that the mother's breast has been ingested and is part of one's self.

Introjection. A defense mechanism whereby loved or hated objects external to the individual are taken within oneself symbolically.

Isolation. A defense mechanism in which ideas are split off from the feelings usually associated with them. Fantasies of killing someone may occur without the affect of carrying it out. Therefore, the act does not take place and guilt is avoided because the thought is unacceptable to the ego. Many forms of isolation occur. In well-educated persons and individuals who have had extensive psychotherapy, intellectualizing about events reflects this defense. Obscenities and swearing can also be examples of this defense mechanism where these words are used to mask femininity.

Projection. A defense mechanism whereby that which is emotionally unacceptable in the self is rejected and ascribed to others. Projection is a very common defense mechanism and is often used in everyday life. The person becomes abrasive, irritable, critical, sarcastic, and intolerant of others. The person becomes suspicious and hostile toward other people and thereby estranged from them. Therefore, the world is perceived as hostile and a delusional system may build up as a result.

Rationalization. The individual attempts to justify motives, actions, and behavior that are unacceptable to him. A common example is the alcoholic individual who gives a myriad of reasons as to why he is drinking again.

Reaction formation. A defense mechanism in which a painful idea, action, or feelings is replaced by its opposite. For example, the patient with a colostomy who, as a consequence of the colostomy, feels that he has feces all over himself may insist on meticulous cleanliness in all aspects of his room; even the most minute speck of debris must be removed immediately.

Regression. A defense mechanism whereby the individual returns to earlier modes of adjustment. Thus, the person is at a stage where there is less conflict. If equilibrium fails at more advanced levels of adjustment, the individual returns to the earlier phases of adjustment for gratification. Thus, the person is at a stage where there is less conflict.

Repression. A defense mechanism that represents unconscious forgetting. It represents an internal flight of painful material and it is sometimes used to refer to all the defense mechanisms.

Ritualization. A defense mechanism that refers to the gratification of the need for sameness. A certain order or sameness of things or behavior is set up. Repression disguises the meaning but it is an order that has a meaning (Bibring, 1961).

Somatization. A defense that is the conversion of intraphysic conflicts into body symptoms.

Sublimation. A defense mechanism that refers to the gratification of instinctual impulse where the aim is changed from a socially unacceptable object or aim to a socially acceptable one. An example is a woman who desires to love another woman but whose superego does not permit it. As a consequence, she gets a job fitting corsets and brassieres.

Substitution. A defense mechanism whereby an unattainable or unacceptable goal, emotion, or object is replaced by one that is more attainable or acceptable. If one cannot marry Omar Sharif, one is unconsciously attracted to men with his demeanor.

Undoing. A primitive defense mechanism whereby something unacceptable and already carried out is symbolically acted out in reverse. Unacceptable behaviors are thus balanced or canceled out by the reverse process. For example, a child, angry at his brother, has a fleeting thought of seeing his brother in his coffin as he turns on the light. When he turns out the light, the act of turning the switch cancels the effect of the thought.

References

AMERICAN PSYCHIATRIC ASSOCIATION: *A Psychiatric Glossary.* Washington, D.C.: American Psychiatric Association, 1975, and 1980.

BIBRING, GRETE, DWYER, THOMAS F., HUNTINGTON, DOROTHY S., and VALENSTEIN, ARTHUR F.: "A Study of the Psychological Processes in Pregnancy and of the Earliest Mother–Child Relationship," in *The Psychoanalytic Study of the Child,* Vol. 16. New York: International Universities Press, Inc., 1961, p. 70.

FREUD, SIGMUND: "The Metapsychology of Instincts, Repression and the Unconscious," *The Standard Edition of the Complete Psychological Works of Freud.* London: The Hogarth Press, 1957, pp. 117–216.

HINSIE, LELAND E., and CAMPBELL, ROBERT JEAN: *Psychiatric Dictionary.* New York: Oxford University Press, 1960.

JOURARD, SIDNEY: *Healthy Personality: An Approach from the Viewpoint of Humanistic Psychology.* New York: Macmillan Publishing Co., Inc., 1974.

MOORE, BURNESS E., and FINE, BERNARD D., eds.: *A Glossary of Psychoanalytic Terms and Concepts.* New York: American Psychoanalytic Association, 1968.

DSM-III Classification: Axes I and II Categories and Codes[1]

All mental disorders appear in Axes I and II (refer to Chapter 3 for a description of the axes). Multiaxial diagnosis requires evaluation on all five axes.

Disorders Usually First Evident in Infancy, Childhood or Adolescence

MENTAL RETARDATION

(Code in fifth digit: 1 = with other behavioral symptoms [requiring attention or treatment and that are not part of another disorder], 0 without other behavioral symptoms.)

317.0x	Mild mental retardation, _____ [2]
318.0x	Moderate mental retardation, _____
318.1x	Severe mental retardation, _____
318.2x	Profound mental retardation, _____
319.0x	Unspecified mental retardation, _____

ATTENTION DEFICIT DISORDER

314.01	with hyperactivity
314.00	without hyperactivity
314.80	residual type

[1] From the American Psychiatric Association: *Diagnostic and Statistical Manual of Mental Disorders, III.* Washington, D.C.: American Psychiatric Association, 1980. By permission.

[2] The long dashes indicate the need for a fifth-digit subtype or other qualifying term.

CONDUCT DISORDER

312.00	undersocialized, aggressive
312.10	undersocialized, nonaggressive
312.23	socialized, aggressive
312.21	socialized, nonaggressive
312.90	atypical

ANXIETY DISORDERS OF CHILDHOOD OR ADOLESCENCE

309.21	Separation anxiety disorder
313.21	Avoidant disorder of childhood or adolescence
313.00	Overanxious disorder

OTHER DISORDERS OF INFANCY, CHILDHOOD, OR ADOLESCENCE

313.89	Reactive attachment disorder of infancy
313.22	Schizoid disorder of childhood or adolescence
313.23	Elective mutism
313.81	Oppositional disorder
313.82	Identity disorder

EATING DISORDERS

307.10	Anorexia nervosa
307.51	Bulimia
307.52	Pica
307.53	Rumination disorder of infancy
307.50	Atypical eating disorder

STEREOTYPED MOVEMENT DISORDERS

307.21   Transient tic disorder
307.22   Chronic motor tic disorder
307.23   Tourette's disorder
307.20   Atypical tic disorder
307.30   Atypical stereotyped movement disorder

OTHER DISORDERS WITH PHYSICAL MANIFESTATIONS

307.00   Stuttering
307.60   Functional enuresis
307.70   Functional encopresis
307.46   Sleepwalking disorder
307.46   Sleep terror disorder (307.49)[3]

PERVASIVE DEVELOPMENTAL DISORDERS

(Code in fifth digit: 0 = full syndrome present, 1 = residual state.)

299.0x   Infantile autism, _____
299.9x   Childhood onset pervasive developmental disorder, _____
299.8x   Atypical, _____

SPECIFIC DEVELOPMENTAL DISORDERS

(Note: These are coded on Axis II.)

315.00   Developmental reading disorder
315.10   Developmental arithmetic disorder
315.31   Developmental language disorder
315.39   Developmental articulation disorder

[3] All official DSM-III codes and terms are included in ICD-9-CM. The *International Classification of Diseases* (1977) has been modified for use in the U.S.A. and is called ICD-90-CM (clinical modification). However, in order to differentiate those DSM-III categories that use the same ICD-9-CM codes, unofficial non-ICD-9-CM codes are provided in parentheses for use when greater specificity is necessary.

315.50   Mixed specific developmental disorder
315.90   Atypical specific developmental disorder

Organic Mental Disorders

Section 1. Organic mental disorders whose etiology or pathophysiological process is listed below (taken from the mental disorders section of ICD-9-CM)

DEMENTIAS ARISING IN THE SENIUM AND PRESENIUM

PRIMARY DEGENERATIVE DEMENTIA, SENILE ONSET

290.30   with delirium
290.20   with delusions
290.21   with depression
290.00   uncomplicated

(Code in fifth digit: 1 = with delirium, 2 = with delusions, 3 = with depression, 0 = uncomplicated.)

290.1x   Primary degenerative dementia, presenile onset, _____
290.4x   Multi-infarct dementia, _____

SUBSTANCE-INDUCED

ALCOHOL

303.00   intoxication
291.40   idiosyncratic intoxication
291.80   withdrawal
291.00   withdrawal delirium
291.30   hallucinosis
291.10   amnestic disorder

(Code severity of dementia in fifth digit: 1 = mild, 2 = moderate, 3 = severe, 0 = unspecified.)

291.2x   Dementia associated with alcoholism, _____

Barbiturate or Similarly Acting Sedative or Hypnotic

305.40 intoxication (327.00)
292.00 withdrawal (327.01)
292.00 withdrawal delirium (327.02)
292.83 amnestic disorder (327.04)

Opioid

305.50 intoxication (327.10)
292.00 withdrawal (327.11)

Cocaine

305.60 intoxication (327.20)

Amphetamine or Similarly Acting Sympathomimetic

305.70 intoxication (327.30)
292.81 delirium (327.32)
292.11 delusional disorder (327.35)
292.00 withdrawal (327.31)

Phencyclidine (PCP) or Similarly Acting Arylcyclohexylamine

305.90 intoxication (327.40)
292.81 delirium (327.42)
292.90 mixed organic mental disorder (327.49)

Hallucinogen

305.30 hallucinosis (327.56)
292.11 delusional disorder (327.55)
292.84 affective disorder (327.57)

Cannabis

305.20 intoxication (327.60)
292.11 delusional disorder (327.65)

Tobacco

292.00 withdrawal (327.71)

Caffeine

305.90 intoxication (327.80)

Other or Unspecified Substance

305.90 intoxication (327.90)
292.00 withdrawal (327.91)
292.81 delirium (327.92)
292.82 dementia (327.93)
292.83 amnestic disorder (327.94)
292.11 delusional disorder (327.95)
292.12 hallucinosis (327.96)
292.84 affective disorder (327.97)
292.89 personality disorder (327.98)
292.90 atypical or mixed organic mental disorder (327.99)

Section 2. Organic brain syndromes whose etiology or pathophysiological process is either noted as an additional diagnosis from outside the mental disorders section of ICD-9-CM or is unknown.

293.00 Delirium
294.10 Dementia
294.00 Amnestic syndrome
293.81 Organic delusional syndrome
293.82 Organic hallucinosis
293.83 Organic affective syndrome
310.10 Organic personality syndrome
294.80 Atypical or mixed organic brain syndrome

Substance Use Disorders

(Code in fifth digit: 1 = continuous, 2 = episodic, 3 = in remission, 0 = unspecified.)

305.0x Alcohol abuse, _____
303.9x Alcohol dependence (Alcoholism), _____
305.4x Barbiturate or similarly acting sedative or hypnotic abuse,
304.1x Barbiturate or similarly acting sedative or hypnotic dependence, _____
305.5x Opioid abuse, _____
304.0x Opioid dependence, _____
305.6x Cocaine abuse, _____
305.7x Amphetamine or similarly acting sympathomimetic abuse, _____

304.4x   Amphetamine or similarly acting
         sympathomimetic   dependence,
         _____

305.9x   Phencyclidine (PCP) or similarly
         acting arylcyclohexylamine abuse,
         _____(388.4x)
305.3x   Hallucinogen abuse, _____
305.2x   Cannabis abuse, _____
304.3x   Cannabis   dependence,   _____
305.1x   Tobacco dependence, _____
305.9x   Other, mixed, or unspecified sub-
         stance abuse, _____
304.6x   Other specified substance depen-
         dence, _____
304.9x   Unspecified   substance   depen-
         dence, _____
304.7x   Dependence on combination of
         opioid and other non-alcoholic
         substance, _____
304.8x   Dependence on combination of
         substances, excluding opioids and
         alcohol, _____

Schizophrenic Disorders

(Code in fifth digit: 1 = subchronic, 2 =
chronic, 3 = subchronic with acute ex-
acerbation, 4 = chronic with acute exacerba-
tion, 5 = in remission, 0 = unspecified.)

SCHIZOPHRENIA

295.1x   disorganized, _____
295.2x   catatonic, _____
295.3x   paranoid, _____
295.9x   undifferentiated, _____
295.6x   residual, _____

Paranoid Disorders

297.10   Paranoia
297.30   Shared paranoid disorder
298.30   Acute paranoid disorder
297.90   Atypical paranoid disorder

Psychotic Disorders Not Elsewhere Classified

295.40   Schizophreniform disorder
298.80   Brief reactive psychosis
295.70   Schizoaffective disorder
298.90   Atypical psychosis

Neurotic Disorders

These are included in Affective, Anxiety,
Somatoform, Dissociative, and Psychosexual Disorders. In order to facilitate the identification of the categories that in DSM-II
were grouped together in the class of Neuroses, the DSM-II terms are included separately in parentheses after the corresponding categories. These DSM-II terms are
included in ICD-9-CM and therefore are
acceptable as alternatives to the recommended DSM-III terms that precede them.

Affective Disorders

MAJOR AFFECTIVE DISORDERS

(Code major depressive episode in fifth
digit: 6 = in remission, 4 = with psychotic
features (the unofficial non-ICD-9-CM fifth
digit 7 may be used instead to indicate that
the psychotic features are mood-incongruent), 3 = with melancholia, 2 = without
melancholia, 0 = unspecified.)
(Code manic episode in fifth digit: 6 =
in remission, 4 = with psychotic features
(the unofficial non-ICD-9-CM fifth digit 7
may be used instead to indicate that the psychotic features are mood-incongruent), 2 =
without psychotic features, 0 = unspecified.)

BIPOLAR DISORDER

296.6x   mixed, _____
296.4x   manic, _____
296.5x   depressed, _____

MAJOR DEPRESSION

296.2x   single episode, _____
296.3x   recurrent, _____

OTHER SPECIFIC AFFECTIVE DISORDERS

301.13   Cyclothymic disorder
300.40   Dysthymic disorder (or Depressive neurosis)

ATYPICAL AFFECTIVE DISORDERS

296.70   Atypical bipolar disorder
296.82   Atypical depression

Anxiety Disorders

PHOBIC DISORDERS (OR PHOBIC NEUROSES)

300.21   Agoraphobia with panic attacks
300.22   Agoraphobia without panic attacks
300.23   Social phobia
300.29   Simple phobia

ANXIETY STATES (OR ANXIETY NEUROSES)

300.01   Panic disorder
300.02   Generalized anxiety disorder
300.30   Obsessive compulsive disorder (or Obsessive compulsive neurosis)

POST-TRAUMATIC STRESS DISORDER

308.30   acute
309.81   chronic or delayed
300.00   Atypical anxiety disorder

Somatoform Disorders

300.81   Somatization disorder
300.11   Conversion disorder (or Hysterical neurosis, conversion type)
307.80   Psychogenic pain disorder
300.70   Hypochondriasis (or Hypochondriacal neurosis)
300.70   Atypical somatoform disorder (300.71)

Dissociative Disorders (or Hysterical Neuroses, Dissociative Type)

300.12   Psychogenic amnesia
300.13   Psychogenic fugue
300.14   Multiple personality
300.60   Depersonalization disorder (or Depersonalization neurosis)
300.15   Atypical dissociative disorder

Psychosexual Disorders

GENDER IDENTITY DISORDERS

(Indicate sexual history in the fifth digit of Transsexualism code: 1 = asexual, 2 = homosexual, 3 = heterosexual, 0 = unspecified.)

302.5x   Transsexualism, _____
302.60   Gender identity disorder of childhood
302.85   Atypical gender identity disorder

PARAPHILIAS

302.81   Fetishism
302.30   Transvestism
302.10   Zoophilia
302.20   Pedophilia
302.40   Exhibitionism
302.82   Voyeurism

302.83   Sexual masochism
302.84   Sexual sadism
302.89   Atypical paraphilia

PSYCHOSEXUAL DYSFUNCTIONS

302.71   Inhibited sexual desire
302.72   Inhibited sexual excitement
302.73   Inhibited female orgasm
302.74   Inhibited male orgasm
302.75   Premature ejaculation
302.76   Functional dyspareunia
306.51   Functional vaginismus
302.70   Atypical psychosexual dysfunction

OTHER PSYCHOSEXUAL DISORDERS

302.00   Ego-dystonic homosexuality
302.89   Psychosexual disorder not elsewhere classified

Factitious Disorders

300.16   Factitious disorder with psychological symptoms
301.51   Chronic factitious disorder with physical symptoms
300.19   Atypical factitious disorder with physical symptoms

Disorders of Impulse Control Not Elsewhere Classified

312.31   Pathological gambling
312.32   Kleptomania
312.33   Pyromania
312.34   Intermittent explosive disorder
312.35   Isolated explosive disorder
312.39   Atypical impulse control disorder

Adjustment Disorder

309.00   with depressed mood
309.24   with anxious mood
309.28   with mixed emotional features

309.30   with disturbance of conduct
309.40   with mixed disturbance of emotions and conduct
309.23   with work (or academic) inhibition
309.83   with withdrawal
309.90   with atypical features

Psychological Factors Affecting Physical Condition

SPECIFY PHYSICAL CONDITION ON AXIS III

316.00   Psychological factors affecting physical condition

Personality Disorders

(Note: These are coded on Axis II.)

301.00   Paranoid
301.20   Schizoid
301.22   Schizotypal
301.50   Histrionic
301.81   Narcissistic
301.70   Antisocial
301.83   Borderline
301.82   Avoidant
301.60   Dependent
301.40   Compulsive
301.84   Passive-Aggressive
301.89   Atypical, mixed or other personality disorder

V Codes for Conditions Not Attributable to a Mental Disorder That Are a Focus of Attention or Treatment

V65.20   Malingering
V62.89   Borderline intellectual functioning (V62.88)
V71.01   Adult antisocial behavior

V71.02　Childhood or adolescent antisocial behavior
V62.30　Academic problem
V62.20　Occupational problem
V62.82　Uncomplicated bereavement
V15.81　Noncompliance with medical treatment
V62.89　Phase of life problem or other life circumstance problem
V61.10　Marital problem
V61.20　Parent–child problem
V61.80　Other specified family circumstances
V62.81　Other interpersonal problem

Additional Codes

300.90　Unspecified mental disorder (nonpsychotic)
V71.09　No diagnosis or condition on Axis I
799.90　Diagnosis or condition deferred on Axis I

V71.09　No diagnosis on Axis II
799.92　Diagnosis deferred on Axis II

A P P E N D I X   D

Controlled Substances: Uses and Effects*

Drugs	Trade or Other Names	Medical Uses	Tolerance
Narcotics			
Opium	Dover's Powder, Paregoric, Parepectolin	Analgesic, antidiarrheal	Yes
Morphine	Morphine, Pectoral Syrup	Analgesic, antitussive	Yes
Codeine	Codeine, Empirin Compound with Codeine, Robitussin A-C	Analgesic, antitussive	Yes
Heroin	Diacetylmorphine, Horse, Smack	Under investigation	Yes
Hydromorphone	Dilaudid	Analgesic	Yes
Meperidine (Pethidine)	Demerol, Pethadol	Analgesic	Yes
Methadone	Dolophine, Methadone, Methadose	Analgesic, heroin substitute	Yes
Other narcotics	LAAM, Leritine, Levo-Dromoran, Percodan, Tussionex, Fentanyl, Darvon,† Talwin,† Lomotil	Analgesic, antidiarrheal, antitussive	Yes
Depressants			
Chloral Hydrate	Noctec, Somnos	Hypnotic	Possible
Barbiturates	Amobarbital, Phenobarbital, Butisol, Phenoxbarbital, Secobarbital, Tuinal	Anesthetic, anticonvulsant, sedative, hypnotic	Yes
Glutethimide	Doriden	Sedative, hypnotic	Yes
Methaqualone	Optimil, Parest, Quaalude, Somnofac, Sopor	Sedative, hypnotic	Yes
Benzodiazepines	Ativan, Azene, Clonopin, Dalmane, Diazepam, Librium, Serax, Tranxene, Valium, Verstran	Anti-anxiety, anticonvulsant, sedative, hypnotic	Yes
Other Depressants	Equanil, Miltown, Noludar, Placidyl, Valmid	Anti-anxiety, sedative, hypnotic	Yes

Dependence Potential		Usual Methods of Administration	Possible Effects	Effects of Overdose	Withdrawal Syndrome
Physical	Psychological				
High	High	Oral, smoked	Euphoria, drowsiness, respiratory depression, constricted pupils	Slow and shallow respirations, clammy skin, convulsions, coma, possible death	Lacrimation, rhinorrhea, yawning, anorexia, irritability, tremors, panic, perspiration, chills, cramps, nausea
High	High	Oral, injected, smoked			
Moderate	Moderate	Oral, injected			
High	High	Injected, sniffed, smoked			
High	High	Oral, injected			
High	High	Oral, injected			
High	High	Oral, injected			
High-low	High-low	Oral, injected			
Moderate	Moderate	Oral	Slurred speech, disorientation, drunken behavior without odor of alcohol	Shallow respiration, cold and clammy skin, dilated pupils, weak and rapid pulse, coma, possible death	Anxiety, insomnia, tremors, delirium, convulsions, possible death
High-Moderate	High-Moderate	Oral, injected			
High	High	Oral, injected			
High	High	Oral, injected			
Low	Low	Oral, injected			
Moderate	Moderate	Oral, injected			

	Drugs	Trade or Other Names	Medical Uses	Tolerance
Stimulants	Cocaine‡	Coke, Flake, Snow	Local anesthetic	Possible
	Amphetamines	Biphetamine, Delcobese, Desoxyn, Dexedrine, Medriatric	Hyperkinesis, narcolepsy, weight control	Yes
	Phenmetrazine	Preludin		Yes
	Methylphenidate	Ritalin		Yes
	Other stimulants	Adipex, Bacarate, Cylert, Didrex, Ionamin, Plegine, PreSate, Sanorex, Tenuate, Tepanil, Voranil		Yes
Hallucinogens	LSD	Acid, Microdot	None	Yes
	Mescaline and Peyote	Mesc, Buttons, Cactus	None	Yes
	Amphetamine Variants	2,5-DMA, PMA, STP, MDA, MMDA, TMA, DOM, DOB	None	Yes
	Phencyclidine	PCP, Angel Dust, Hog	Veterinary anesthetic	Yes
	Phencyclidine Analogs	PCE, PCPy, TCP	None	Yes
	Other Hallucinogens	Bufotenine, Ibogaine, DMT, DET, Psilocybin, Psilocyn	None	Possible
Cannabis	Marihuana	Pot, Acapulco Gold, Grass, Reefer, Sinsemilla, Thai Sticks	Under investigation	Yes
	Tetrahydrocannabinol	THC	Under investigation	Yes
	Hashish	Hash	None	Yes
	Hashish Oil	Hash Oil	None	Yes

Dependence Potential		Usual Methods of Administration	Possible Effects	Effects of Overdose	Withdrawal Syndrome
Physical	Psychological				
Possible	High	Sniffed, injected	Increased alertness, excitation, euphoria, increased pulse rate and blood pressure, insomnia, anorexia	Agitation, increase in body temperature, hallucinations, convulsions, possible death	Apathy, hypersomnia, irritability, depression, disorientation
Possible	High	Oral, injected			
Possible	High	Oral, injected			
Possible	High	Oral			
Possible	High	Oral			
None	Degree unknown	Oral	Illusions, hallucinations, poor perception of time and distance	Longer, more intense "trip" episodes, psychosis, possible death	Withdrawal syndrome not reported
None	Degree unknown	Oral, injected			
Unknown	Degree unknown	Oral, injected			
Degree unknown	High	Smoked, oral, injected			
Degree unknown	Degree unknown	Smoked, oral, injected			
None	Degree unknown	Oral, injected, smoked, sniffed			
Degree unknown	Moderate	Smoked, oral	Euphoria, relaxed inhibitions, increased appetite, disoriented behavior	Fatigue, paranoia, possible psychosis	Insomnia, hyperactivity, and decreased appetite occasionally reported
Degree unknown	Moderate	Smoked, oral			
Degree unknown	Moderate	Smoked, oral			
Degree unknown	Moderate	Smoked, oral			

* Source: United States Department of Justice: *Drugs of Abuse.* Washington, D.C.: U.S. Government Printing Office, 1979.

† Not designated a narcotic under the Controlled Substances Act.

‡ Designated a narcotic under the Controlled Substances Act.

Standards: Psychiatric–Mental Health Nursing Practice[1]

Psychiatric nursing is a specialized area of nursing practice employing theories of human behavior as its scientific aspect and purposeful use of self as its art. It is directed toward both preventive and corrective impacts upon mental illness and is concerned with the promotion of optimal mental health for society, the community, and those individuals and families who live within it. The dependent area of psychiatric nursing practice is implementation of physician's orders. The independent areas are assessment of nursing needs and development and implementation of nursing-care plans, including initiation, development, and termination of therapeutic relationships between nurses and patients. Psychiatric nursing is practiced largely in collaboration and coordination with those in a variety of other disciplines who are working concomitantly with the patient. Thus, a high degree of interdependence with colleagues from other professions is inherent.

The practice of psychiatric nursing is characterized by those aspects of clinical nursing care that involve interpersonal relationships with individuals and groups as well as a variety of other activities. These activities include: providing a therapeutic milieu, concerned largely with the sociopsychologic aspects of patients' environments; working with patients concerning the here-and-now living problems they confront; accepting and using the surrogate-parent role; teaching with specific reference to emotional health as evidenced by various behavioral patterns; assuming the role of social agent concerned with improvement and promotion of recreational, occupational, and social competence; providing leadership and clinical assistance to other nursing personnel.

Joint planning or cooperative and collaborative efforts with other professionals are an essential part of providing nursing service. Most psychiatric settings employ an interdisciplinary team approach that requires highly coordinated and frequently interdependent planning.

Direct nursing-care functions may involve individual psychotherapy, group psychotherapy, family therapy, and sociotherapy. Psychiatric nurses engaged in these therapies may employ a variety of approaches, particularly in the rapidly emerging area of sociotherapy and community mental health. With the national trend toward community mental health, psychiatric nurses are more and more involved in providing services aimed toward prevention of mental illness and reinforcement of healthy adaptations in addition to corrective and rehabilitative services.

The indirect nursing-care roles of the psychiatric nurse are those of administrator with emphasis on leadership functions; clinical supervisor with emphasis on leadership functions as well as clinical teaching; director of staff development and training in a clinical facility; consultant or resource person, and researcher. In some of these indirect care roles, nurses will also be involved in providing some direct nursing-care services to improve their own clinical skills and to serve as role models. All of these roles require coordinative and collaborative efforts with other disciplines.

The purpose of Standards of Psychiatric Nursing Practice is to fulfill the profession's obligation to provide and improve this practice. The Standards focus on practice. They provide a means for determining the quality of nursing that a client receives, regardless of whether such services are provided solely by a professional nurse or by professional nurse and nonprofessional assistants.

[1] American Nurses' Association, 1973. By permission.

The Standards are stated according to a systematic approach to nursing practice: the assessment of the client's status, the plan of nursing actions, the implementation of the plan, and the evaluation. These specific divisions are not intended to imply that practice consists of a series of discrete steps, taken in strict sequence, beginning with assessment and ending with evaluation. The processes described are used concurrently and recurrently. Assessment, for example, frequently continues during implementation; similarly, evaluation dictates reassessment and planning.

These Standards of Psychiatric Nursing Practice apply to nursing practice in any setting. Nursing practice in all settings must possess the characteristics identified by these Standards if patients are to receive a high quality of nursing care. Each Standard is followed by a rationale and assessment factors. Assessment factors are to be used in determining achievement of the Standard.

Standard I

Data are collected through pertinent clinical observations based on knowledge of the arts and sciences, with particular emphasis upon psychosocial and biophysical sciences.

RATIONALE

Clinical observation is a prerequisite to realistic assessment of a client's needs and for the formulation of appropriate intervention. Observations can be facilitated through knowledge derived from a broad general education. In addition, scholarship acquired in the study of psychosocial and biophysical sciences fosters acuity of perception and alerts the nurse to psychologic, cultural, social and other relevant clinical data.

ASSESSMENT FACTORS

1. Data-collecting activities involve observation, analysis, and interpretation of behavior patterns of clients that indicate a need for growth-promoting relationships.

2. Data-collecting activities involve identification of significant areas in which clinical data are needed.
3. Data-collecting activities involve utilization of knowledge derived from appropriate sources to gain a comprehensive grasp of the client's experience.
4. Data-collecting activities involve inferences drawn from observations that contribute to a formulation of therapeutic intervention.
5. Data-collecting activities involve inferences and treatment observations that are shared and validated with appropriate others.

Standard II

Clients are involved in the assessment, planning, implementation and evaluation of their nursing-care program to the fullest extent of their capabilities.

RATIONALE

To a very large degree, the therapeutic process is a learning process. The same principle that applies to learning also applies to therapy; that is, the learner or client must be an active participant in the process. The ability to participate in such a process will vary from person to person and, at times, even within the same person. The word "therapy" is used here in its broadest sense; that is, any behavior or planned activity that promotes growth and well-being. Thus, "nursing-care program" and "nursing therapy" are interchangeably used, although it is recognized that many other forms of therapy exist.

ASSESSMENT FACTORS

1. Client's capabilities to participate at any given time are assessed, always keeping in mind the ultimate goals mutually determined by the client and nurse.
2. Plans for achieving and re-examining the goals are developed with the client, mak-

ing whatever readjustments are necessary to progress toward them.

3. Problems are identified in collaboration with the client to determine needs and to set goals.
4. Progress of clients toward mutual goal achievement is assessed.

Standard III

The problem-solving approach is utilized in developing nursing-care plans.

RATIONALE

A nursing diagnosis is based on pertinent theories of human behavior. It is used to plan therapeutic intervention taking into consideration the characteristics and capacities of the individual and his environment in order to maximize the treatment program for the client.

ASSESSMENT FACTORS

1. The individual's reaction to the environment is observed and assessed.
2. Themes and patterns of the behavior are observed and assessed.
3. Nursing-care plans are used as a guide to nursing intervention.
4. Nursing-care plans are interpreted to professional and nonprofessional persons giving care.
5. Observations and reports of others are incorporated in the nursing-care plans.
6. Nursing-care plans are designed, implemented, and reviewed systematically by the nursing staff.

Standard IV

Individuals, families, and community groups are assisted to achieve satisfying and productive patterns of living through health teaching.

RATIONALE

Health teaching is an essential part of a nurse's role in work with those who have mental-health problems. Every interaction can be utilized as a teaching–learning situation. Formal and informal teaching methods can be used in working with individuals, families, the community and other personnel. Emphasis is on understanding mental-health problems as well as on developing ways of coping with them.

ASSESSMENT FACTORS

1. The needs of individual, family, and community groups for health teaching are identified and appropriate techniques are used in meeting these needs.
2. The principles of learning and teaching are employed.
3. The basic principles of physical and mental health and interpersonal and social skills are taught.
4. Experiential learning opportunities are made available.
5. Opportunities with community groups to further their knowledge and understanding of mental-health problems are identified.

Standard V

The activities of daily living are utilized in a goal-directed way in work with clients.

RATIONALE

A major portion of one's daily life is spent in some form of activity related to health and well-being. An individual's developmental and intellectual level, emotional state, and physical limitations may be reflected in these activities. Therefore, nursing has a unique opportunity to assess and intervene in these processes in order to encourage constructive changes in the client's behavior so that each person may realize his full potential for growth.

ASSESSMENT FACTORS

1. An appraisal is made of the client's capacities to participate in activities of daily living based on needs, strengths, and levels of functioning.
2. Clients are encouraged toward independence and self-direction by various skills such as motivating, limit setting, persuading, guiding, and comforting.
3. Each person's rights are appreciated and respected.
4. Methods of communicating are devised that assure consistency in approach.

Standard VI

Knowledge of somatic therapies and related clinical skills are utilized in working with clients.

RATIONALE

Various treatment modalities may be needed by clients during the course of illness. Pertinent clinical observations and judgments are made concerning the effect of drugs and other treatments used in the therapeutic program.

ASSESSMENT FACTORS

1. Pertinent reactions to somatic therapies are observed and interpreted in terms of the underlying principles of each therapy.
2. A patient's responses are observed and reported.
3. The effectiveness of somatic therapies is judged and subsequent recommendations for changes in the treatment plan are made.
4. The safety and emotional support of clients receiving therapies is provided.
5. Opportunities are provided for clients and families to discuss, question, and explore their feelings and concerns about past, current, or projected use of somatic therapies.

Standard VII

The environment is structured to establish and maintain a therapeutic milieu.

RATIONALE

Any environment is composed of both human and nonhuman resources that may work for or against the person's well-being. The nurse works with people in a variety of environmental settings, e.g., hospital, home, and so on. The milieu is structured and/or altered so that it serves the client's best interests as an inherent part of the overall therapeutic plan.

ASSESSMENT FACTORS

1. The effects for environmental forces on individuals are observed, analyzed, and interpreted.
2. Psychological, physiological, social, economical, and cultural concepts are understood and utilized in developing and maintaining a therapeutic milieu.
3. Communications within the environment are congruent with therapeutic goals.
4. All available resources in the environment are utilized when appropriate in the therapeutic efforts.
5. Nursing participation and its effectiveness in establishing and maintaining a therapeutic milieu are evaluated.

Standard VIII

Nursing participates with interdisciplinary teams in assessing, planning, implementing, and evaluating programs and other mental-health activities.

RATIONALE

In addition to the nurse, the number and variety of people working with clients in the mental-health field today make it imperative that efforts be coordinated to provide the best total program. Communication, planning, problem-solving, and evaluation are required of all those who work with a particular client or program.

ASSESSMENT FACTORS

1. Specific knowledge, skills, and activities are identified and articulated so these may be coordinated with the contributions of others working with a client or a program.
2. The value of nursing and team member contributions are recognized and respected.
3. Consultation with other team members is utilized as needed.
4. Nursing participates in the formulating of overall goals, plans, and decisions.
5. Skills are developed in small-group process for maximum team effectiveness.

solving, interviewing, and crisis intervention are employed in carrying through psychotherapeutic intervention.
4. Knowledge of psychopathology and its healthy adaptive counterparts are used in planning and implementing programs of care.
5. Limits are set on behavior that is destructive to self or others with the ultimate goal of assisting clients to develop their own internal controls and more constructive ways of dealing with feelings.
6. Crisis intervention is used to reduce panic of disturbed patients.
7. Long-term psychotherapeutic relationships with clients are undertaken.
8. Colleagues are utilized in evaluating the progress of the psychotherapeutic relationships and in formulating modification of intervention techniques.
9. Nursing participation in the therapeutic relationship is evaluated and modified as necessary.

Standard IX

Psychotherapeutic interventions are used to assist clients to achieve their maximum development.

RATIONALE

People with mental-health problems fashion many of their patterns of living and relating to others on a psychopathologic basis. In order to help clients achieve better adaption and improved health, a nurse assists them to identify that which is useful and that which is not useful in their modes of living and relating. Alternatives available to them are identified.

ASSESSMENT FACTORS

1. Useful patterns and themes in the client's interactions with others are re-enforced.
2. Clients are assisted to identify, test out, and evaluate more constructive alternatives to unsatisfactory patterns of living.
3. Principles of communication, problem-

Standard X

The practice of individual, group, or family psychotherapy requires appropriate preparation and recognition of accountability for the practice.

RATIONALE

Acceptance of the role of therapist entails primary responsibility for the treatment of clients and entrance into a contractual agreement. This contract includes a commitment to see a client through the problem he presents or, if this becomes impossible, to assist him in finding other appropriate assistance. It also includes an explicit definition of the relationship, the respective roles of each person in the relationship, and what can realistically be expected of each person.

ASSESSMENT FACTORS

1. The potential of the nurse to function as a primary therapist is evaluated.
2. The accountability for practicing psychotherapy is recognized and accepted.

3. Knowledge of growth and development, psychopathology, psychosocial systems, and small group and family dynamics is utilized in the therapeutic process.
4. The terms of the contract between the nurse and the client, including the structure of time, place, fees, and so on, that may be involved, are made explicitly clear.
5. Supervision or consultation is sought whenever indicated and other learning opportunities are used to further develop knowledge and skills.
6. The effectiveness of the work with an individual, family, or group is routinely assessed.

Standard XI

Nursing participates with other members of the community in planning and implementing mental-health services that include the broad continuum of promotion of mental health, prevention of mental illness, treatment, and rehabilitation.

RATIONALE

In our contemporary society, the high incidence of mental illness and mental retardation requires increased effort to devise more effective treatment and prevention programs. There is a need for nursing to participate in programs that strengthen the existing health potential of all members of society. In this effort cooperation and collaboration by all community agencies becomes imperative. Such concepts as early intervention and continuity of care are essential in planning to meet the mental-health needs of the community. The nurse uses organizational, advisory, or consultative skills to facilitate the development and implementation of mental health services.

ASSESSMENT FACTORS

1. Knowledge of community and group dynamics is used to understand the structure and function of the community system.
2. Current social issues that influence the nature of mental-health problems in the community are recognized.
3. High-risk population groups in the community are delineated and gaps in community services are identified.
4. Community members are encouraged to become active in assessing community mental-health needs and planning programs to meet these needs.
5. The strength and capacities of individuals, families, and the community are assessed in order to promote and increase the health potential of all.
6. Consultative skills are used to facilitate the development and implementation of mental-health services.
7. The needs of the community are brought to the attention of appropriate individuals and groups, including legislative bodies and regional and state planning groups.
8. The mental-health services of the agency are interpreted to others in the community. There is collaboration with the staff of other agencies to insure continuity of service for patients and families.
9. Community resources are used appropriately.
10. Nursing participates with other professional and nonprofessional members of the community in the planning, implementation, and evaluation of mental-health services.

Standard XII

Learning experiences are provided for other nursing-care personnel through leadership, supervision, and teaching.

RATIONALE

As leader of the nursing team, the nurse is responsible for the team's activities, and must be able to teach, supervise and evaluate the performance of nursing-care personnel. The focus is on the continuing development of each member of the team.

ASSESSMENT FACTORS

1. Leadership roles and responsibilities are accepted.
2. Team members are encouraged to identify strengths and abilities. A climate is provided for the continuing self-development of each member.
3. A role model in giving direct nursing care is provided for the team.
4. The supervisory role is used as a tool for improving nursing care.
5. The client's needs, as well as the abilities of each member of the nursing team, are evaluated and assignments are based on these evaluations.

Standard XIII

Responsibility is assumed for continuing educational and professional development and contributions are made to the professional growth of others.

RATIONALE

The scientific, cultural, and social changes characterizing our contemporary society require the nurse to be committed to the ongoing pursuit of knowledge that will enhance professional growth.

ASSESSMENT FACTORS

1. There is evidence of study of one's nursing practice to increase both understanding and skill.
2. There is evidence of participation in in-service meetings and educational programs either as an attendee or as a teacher.
3. There is evidence of attendance at conventions, institutes, workshops, symposia and other professionally oriented meetings, and/or other ways to increase formal education.

4. There is evidence of systematic efforts to increase understanding of psychodynamics, psychopathology, and avenues of psychotherapeutic intervention.
5. There is evidence of cognizance of developments in relevant fields and utilization of this knowledge.
6. There is evidence of assisting others to identify areas of educational needs.
7. There is evidence of sharing appropriate clinical observations and interpretations with professionals and other groups.

Standard XIV

Contributions to nursing and the mental-health field are made through innovations in theory and practice and participation in research.

RATIONALE

Each professional has responsibility for the continuing development and refinement of knowledge in the mental-health field through research and experimentation with new and creative approaches to practice.

ASSESSMENT FACTORS

1. Studies are developed, implemented, and evaluated.
2. Responsible standards of research are used in investigative endeavors.
3. Nursing practice is approached with an inquiring and open mind.
4. The pertinent and responsible research of others is supported.
5. Expert consultation and/or supervision is sought as required.
6. The ability to discriminate those findings that are pertinent to the advancement of nursing practice is demonstrated.
7. Innovations in theory, practice, and research findings are made available through presentations and/or publications.

The Code for Nurses: The Eleven Points[1]

1. The nurse provides services with respect for human dignity and the uniqueness of the client unrestricted by considerations of social or economic status, personal attributes, or the nature of health problems.
2. The nurse safeguards the client's right to privacy by judiciously protecting information of a confidential nature.
3. The nurse acts to safeguard the client and the public when health care and safety are affected by the incompetent, unethical, or illegal practice of any person.
4. The nurse assumes responsibility and accountability for individual nursing judgments and actions.
5. The nurse maintains competence in nursing.
6. The nurse exercises informed judgment and uses individual competence and qualifications as criteria in seeking consultation, accepting responsibilities, and delegating nursing activities to others.
7. The nurse participates in activities that contribute to the ongoing development of the profession's body of knowledge.
8. The nurse participates in the profession's efforts to implement and improve standards of nursing.
9. The nurse participates in the profession's efforts to establish and maintain conditions of employment conducive to high-quality nursing care.
10. The nurse participates in the profession's effort to protect the public from misinformation and misrepresentation and to maintain the integrity of nursing.
11. The nurse collaborates with members of the health professions and other citizens in promoting community and national efforts to meet the health needs of the public.

[1] American Nurses' Association, 1979. By permission.

A P P E N D I X G

A Patient's Bill of Rights[1]

The American Hospital Association presents a Patient's Bill of Rights with the expectation that observance of these rights will contribute to more effective patient care and greater satisfaction for the patient, his physician, and the hospital organization. Further, the Association presents these rights in the expectation that they will be supported by the hospital on behalf of its patients, as an integral part of the healing process. It is recognized that a personal relationship between the physician and the patient is essential for the provision of proper medical care. The traditional physician-patient relationship takes on a new dimension when care is rendered within an organizational structure. Legal precedent has established that the institution itself has a responsibility to the patient. It is in recognition of these factors that these rights are affirmed.

1. The patient has the right to considerate respectful care.

2. The patient has the right to obtain from his physician complete current information concerning his diagnosis, treatment, and prognosis in terms the patient can be reasonably expected to understand. When it is not medically advisable to give such information to the patient, the information should be made available to an appropriate person in his behalf. He has the right to know by name, the physician responsible for coordinating his care.

3. The patient has the right to receive from his physician information necessary to give informed consent prior to the start of any procedure and or treatment. Except in emergencies, such information for informed consent, should include but not necessarily be limited to the specific procedure and/or treatment, the medically significant risks involved, and the probable duration of incapacitation. Where medically signifi-

[1] The Board of Trustees of the American Hospital Association developed the Statement on a Patient's Bill of Rights that has met with considerable interest in the health-care field. This is the complete statement. Reprinted with the permission of the American Hospital Association, copyright 1975.

cant alternatives for care or treatment exist, or when the patient requests information concerning medical alternatives, the patient has the right to such information. The patient also has the right to know the name of the person responsible for the procedures and/or treatment.

4. The patient has the right to refuse treatment to the extent permitted by law, and to be informed of the medical consequences of his action.

5. The patient has the right to every consideration of his privacy concerning his own medical care program. Case discussion, consultation, examination, and treatment are confidential and should be conducted discreetly. Those not directly involved in his care must have the permission of the patient to be present.

6. The patient has the right to expect that all communications and records pertaining to his care should be treated as confidential.

7. The patient has the right to expect that within its capacity a hospital must make reasonable response to the request of a patient for services. The hospital must provide evaluation, service, and/or referral as indicated by the urgency of the case. When medically permissible a patient may be transferred to another facility only after he has received complete information and explanation concerning the needs for and alternatives to such a transfer. The institution to which the patient is to be transferred must first have accepted the patient for transfer.

8. The patient has the right to obtain information as to any relationship of his hospital to other health care and educational institutions insofar as his care is concerned. The patient has the right to obtain information as to the existence of any professional relationships among individuals, by name, who are treating him.

9. The patient has the right to be advised if the hospital proposes to engage in or perform human experimentation affecting his care or treatment. The patient has the right to refuse to participate in such research projects.

10. The patient has the right to expect reasonable continuity of care. He has the right to know in advance what appointment times and physi-

cians are available and where. The patient has the right to expect that the hospital will provide a mechanism whereby he is informed by his physician or a delegate of the physician of the patient's continuing health care requirements following discharge.

11. The patient has the right to examine and receive an explanation of his bill regardless of source of payment.

12. The patient has the right to know what hospital rules and regulations apply to his conduct as a patient.

No catalogue of rights can guarantee for the patient the kind of treatment he has a right to expect. A hospital has many functions to perform, including the prevention and treatment of disease, the education of both health professionals and patients, and the conduct of clinical research. All these activities must be conducted with an overriding concern for the patient, and, above all, the recognition of his dignity as a human being. Success in achieving this recognition assures success in the defense of the rights of the patient.

APPENDIX H

Common Objective and Subjective Descriptions of Anxiety

Alienation
Anorexia
Anxious
Amnesia
Apprehensive
Awe
Breathless
Butterflies
Cannot concentrate
Chest pains
Choking sensations
Clutched-up
Compulsions
Cramps
Diarrhea
Dizziness
Dread
Dry mouth
Easily startled
Excessive verbalization
Faintness
Fast pulse
Flushing
Giddy
Headache

Helpless
Hyperventilation
Impending doom
Inadequate
Indecisive
Insecure
Insomnia
Irritable
Jittery
Jumpy
Keyed up
Meaninglessness
Nausea
Nervous
Nothingness
Obsessions
Overconcern
Overdrinking
Overeating
Oversensitive
Pallor
Palpitations
Panic
Perspiration
Phobias

Pupils dilated
Rapid respirations
Rapid speech
Repeating speech of others
Restless
Shaky
Sighing
Syncope
Tense
Terror
Threatened
Tied-up
Tightness in chest
Tremulous
Troubled
Uneasy
Urge to Urinate and fre-
quent urination
Vertigo
Vigilant
Vomiting
Weakness
Worried
Wound up

APPENDIX I

The Florence Nightingale Pledge

I solemnly pledge myself before God and in presence of this assembly,
To pass my life in purity and to practice my profession faithfully.
I will abstain from whatever is deleterious and mischievous and will not take or knowingly administer any harmful drug.
I will do all in my power to maintain and elevate the standard of my profession, and will hold in confidence all personal matters committed to my keeping and all family affairs coming to my knowledge in the practice of my profession.
With loyalty will I endeavor to aid the physician in his work, and devote myself to the welfare of those committed to my care.

Code for Nurses: Ethical Concepts Applied to Nursing (International)[1]

The fundamental responsibility of the nurse is fourfold: to promote health, to prevent illness, to restore health and to alleviate suffering.

The need for nursing is universal. Inherent in nursing is respect for life, dignity and rights of man. It is unrestricted by considerations of nationality, race, creed, colour, age, sex, politics or social status.

Nurses render health services to the individual, the family and the community and coordinate their services with those of related groups.

Nurses and People

The nurse's primary responsibility is to those people who require nursing care.

The nurse, in providing care, promotes an environment in which the values, customs and spiritual beliefs of the individual are respected.

Nurses and Practice

The nurse carries personal responsibility for nursing practice and for maintaining competence by continual learning.

The nurse maintains the highest standards of nursing care possible within the reality of a specific situation.

The nurse uses judgment in relation to individual competence when accepting and delegating responsibilities.

[1] International Council of Nurses, 1973. By permission.

The nurse when acting in a professional capacity should at all times maintain standards of personal conduct which reflect credit upon the profession.

Nurses and Society

The nurse shares with other citizens the responsibility for initiating and supporting action to meet the health and social needs of the public.

Nurses and Co-Workers

The nurse sustains a cooperative relationship with co-workers in nursing and other fields.

The nurse takes appropriate action to safeguard the individual when his care is endangered by a co-worker or any other person.

Nurses and the Profession

The nurse plays the major role in determining and implementing desirable standards of nursing practice and nursing education.

The nurse is active in developing a core of professional knowledge.

The nurse, acting through the professional organization, participates in establishing and maintaining equitable social and economic working conditions in nursing.

A P P E N D I X   K

Format for Nurse–Patient Interaction

Date
Time
Setting
Objective(s) of Interaction
Description of Patient

What the Nursing Student Said[1]	What the Patient Said[1]	Rationale for your Actions[2]

Summary and Evaluation[3]

---

[1] Here the conversation between you and the patient is recorded as you remember it. Include any nonverbal communication in parentheses.

[2] In this section include your reasons for your actions with documentation of theoretical concepts.

[3] Describe the themes of the interaction, evaluate your actions, and include goals for the next interaction.

Index